TEXTBOOK OF
URORADIOLOGY

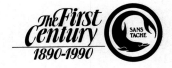

TEXTBOOK OF
URORADIOLOGY

N. Reed Dunnick, M.D.

Professor of Radiology
Director, Division of Diagnostic Imaging
Duke University Medical Center
Durham, North Carolina

Ronald W. McCallum, M.B., F.R.C.P.(C), F.A.C.R.

Professor of Radiology
University of Toronto
Radiologist-in-Chief
St. Michael's Hospital
Toronto, Ontario, Canada

Carl M. Sandler, M.D.

Professor of Radiology and Surgery (Urology)
University of Texas Medical School at Houston
Chief, Radiology Service
Lyndon B. Johnson General Hospital
Adjunct Professor of Radiology
Baylor College of Medicine
Houston, Texas

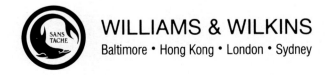

WILLIAMS & WILKINS
Baltimore • Hong Kong • London • Sydney

Editor: Timothy H. Grayson
Associate Editor: Carol Eckhart
Copy Editors: Joseph Pomerance, Susan Vaupel
Designer: Joanne Janowiak
Illustration Planning: Ray Lowman
Production: Charles E. Zeller
Cover Design: Dan Pfisterer

Accurate indications, adverse reactions, and dosage schedules for drugs are provided in this book, but it is possible that they may change. The reader is urged to review the package information data of the manufacturers of the medications mentioned.

Printed in the United States of America

Library of Congress Cataloging-in-Publication Data

Dunnick, N. Reed.
   Textbook of uroradiology / N. Reed Dunnick, Ronald W. McCallum,
Carl M. Sandler.
      p.   cm.
   ISBN 0-683-02696-8
   1. Genitourinary organs—Radiography.   2. Genitourinary organs—
Diseases—Diagnosis.   I. McCallum, Ronald W. (Ronald William)
II. Sandler, Carl M.   III. Title.
   [DNLM: 1. Urography.   WJ 141 D924t]
RC874.D86   1991
616.6'0757—dc20
DNLM/DLC
for Library of Congress   89-70504
                                                               CIP

90 91 92 93 94
1 2 3 4 5 6 7 8 9 10

This book is dedicated to our residents who inspired us to undertake this project and to our families whose patience and understanding made it possible.

PREFACE

Our goal in producing *Textbook of Uroradiology* was to provide both the practicing radiologist and the radiology resident with a comprehensive, single-volume text that integrates all aspects of adult uroradiology. In order that the book be kept to a manageable size, the standard, "what one ought to know" rather than "what there is to know," was applied.

In any work of this type, there are many arbitrary decisions as to the material to be included and as to the placement of that material. We have presented the material on the anatomy, embryology, and congenital anomalies of the urinary tract as one unit because these topics are so interrelated that to disseminate this material in several different chapters would diminish the readers' ability to understand these important relationships. Chapter 3 provides an overview of the diagnostic imaging techniques that are discussed throughout the remainder of the book. Contrast material, which is fundamental to the practice of uroradiology, is included as Chapter 4. The remainder of the chapters have been divided into those dealing with various types of renal pathology (i.e., vascular disease, inflammatory disease, etc.), those dealing with anatomic regions of the urinary tract (i.e., adrenal gland, bladder, etc.), and topics that seemed best treated as a whole (i.e., trauma and transplantation).

The placement of material related to interventional uroradiology was especially problematic. For the most part, interventional topics have been placed adjacent to the material dealing with the underlying pathologic conditions for which the procedure is indicated. Thus, abscess drainage is discussed along with renal inflammatory disease, ureteral stenting with the ureter, and percutaneous stone extraction with stone disease. A separate interventional chapter has been included to provide a discussion of percutaneous nephrostomy and percutaneous biopsy as well as a general overview of these procedures.

This work represents the equal efforts of three practicing uroradiologists. Each of us reviewed and critiqued all of the material, and thus we decided not to assign authorship to any of the individual chapters.

Although *Textbook of Uroradiology* is intended to serve as a source of information about uroradiology for practicing radiologists and radiology residents, we believe that urologists, general surgeons, and nephrologists will also find the book useful. We hope it has been written in such a clear and succinct manner that it will not only be used as a reference source, but that it will also be read in its entirety.

ACKNOWLEDGMENTS

We gratefully acknowledge the many contributions of individuals at our respective institutions as well as the highly skilled professionals at Williams & Wilkins who made this book possible.

At Duke University, Drs. James Bowie, Richard Cohan, Kate Feinstein, Herman Grossman, Barbara Hertzberg, and Richard Leder provided valuable case material for illustration. Brady Lambert provided radiographic support by producing high quality prints for reproduction. Outstanding secretarial support was provided by Beverly Johnson Harris, who survived our impatience, typed much of the manuscript, and arranged the suggested readings.

The high quality images are due to a number of dedicated technologists. Although the efforts of numerous individuals contributed to the final text, the leadership roles of Carolyn Zakrzewski in Uroradiology, Debbie Disher in CT, and Michael Land in Angiography should be noted.

Many employees of the Department of Diagnostic Imaging at St. Michael's Hospital contributed to the successful production of this book. In particular, our sincere and appreciative thanks go to two imperturbable secretaries, Irene Silva and Judy Bibby, who translated hieroglyphic writing into the typed word. They showed no dismay at the number of revisions required over the past two years. For their help and energy we are much indebted.

Although this department does not have its own dedicated photography department, the hospital department of photography, under the direction of Sandy Collins, has been exemplary in its efforts to cope with the requests for print reproduction. Consultation with the photography department staff in highlighting the area of interest in each film produced superb prints, and we extend our gratitude to them. The efficiency of our film library quickly produced lists of films requested, and we are grateful to the film library staff and especially to their supervisor, Sandra Maraj.

Our well-trained radiologic technologists have consistently obtained excellent examinations. Although there are too many to name, we would especially like to thank our Chief Technologist, Lynn Mongeau, and Dorothy Moxley, our special procedure supervisor, who will express our thanks to all of our technologists. Many of the procedures shown in this volume required the help of our dedicated radiology nursing staff; to them we are most grateful, in particular to our head nurse, Julie Pradhan.

At the University of Texas Medical School at Houston the following faculty members provided case material for this work: Drs. Ruth G. Brush, Rodrigo Dominguez, Gregory Houston, Patricia A. Lowry, Nabil Maklad, Bharat Raval, Lawrence H. Robinson, Huyen Tran, and Elisabeth Ueberschar. Dr. Margot Rodriguez, of the Houston Veterans Administration Hospital and Baylor College of Medicine, also generously provided cases for illustration.

Drs. Andrew Kahn, Barry D. Kahan, and Janice Semenkovich offered many helpful comments and criticisms of portions of the manuscript. Kathleen Isch provided invaluable secretarial assistance and spent many hours typing portions of the manuscript and organizing the references. Millicent Williams, Radiology Librarian at the University of Texas Medical School, provided valuable research assistance. Sandra Moretti and Nancy Sacilowski, Senior Radiologic Technologists in the genitourinary section at Hermann Hospital consistently provided the high quality radiographs that which illustrate portions of the text. Jay Johnson and Keith Patricio, Department of Radiology, University of Texas Medical School at Houston, provided photographic support.

CONTENTS

ANATOMY AND EMBRYOLOGY

ANATOMY

Kidney

The kidneys are paired, retroperitoneal structures that parallel the psoas muscle on either side of the lumbar spine. The left kidney is usually slightly higher than the right and is slightly more medially located. The vertical axis of the kidneys, when compared with the midline, is approximately 20°. There is often considerable motility of each kidney, which varies with respiration and with body position; several centimeters of excursion may be demonstrated on deep inspiration or in the upright position.

The kidney is composed of a variable number of structural units known as the renal pyramids. Each pyramid consists of a minor calyx and its associated papillary ducts. The base of the pyramid is formed by its overlying renal cortex, and its apex is formed by the renal papilla which projects into the renal sinus. The papillae are cone-shaped structures that contain the openings of the distal collecting ducts (the ducts of Bellini), which empty into the minor calyces. The peripheral portion of the minor calyx is called the fornix and projects slightly above the central papillary portion; it is this appearance that is responsible for the cuplike configuration of a normal minor calyx. The minor calyces are arranged into three groups: an upper group, a middle or interpolar

group, and a lower group. Each group contains anterior and posterior calyces. On urography, anterior calyces are generally projected en face whereas the posteriorly located calyces are seen in profile. Four to six minor calyces come together to form a major calyx or infundibulum; these join together to form the renal pelvis.

On cut surface, the kidney may be divided into two discrete regions, the outer cortex and the inner medulla. The arcuate artery at the base of each pyramid marks the junction between the cortex and the medulla. The cortex overlying each pyramid is sometimes known as the *centrilobar cortex.* Columns of cortical tissue, however, may be found between each pyramid. These columns have been termed the septal cortex, but they are more commonly referred to as the columns of Bertin or Bertini. The minor calyces, the infundibulae, and the renal pelvis are jointly referred to as the *renal collecting system.* The renal sinus surrounds the collecting system and is filled with a variable amount of fat.

The kidneys and their surrounding fascial covering, Gerota's fascia, define the boundaries of the retroperitoneum (Fig. 1.1). The retroperitoneum is divided into three discrete compartments, the anterior pararenal space, the perirenal space, and the posterior pararenal space.

The anterior pararenal space extends from the posterior portion of the peritoneal cavity to the anterior layer of Gerota's fascia. The anterior pararenal space contains the pancreas, the second through fourth portions of the duodenum, the ascending and descending colon, and the hepatic and splenic arteries. Laterally, the posterior layer of peritoneum and the anterior layer of Gerota's fascia merge into the lateroconal fascia.

The perirenal space is defined by the anterior and posterior layers of the perirenal fascia. The two layers of perirenal fascia are usually fused in the midline, then open to surround the kidney, the adrenal gland, and the proximal ureter, and finally fuse again to merge into the

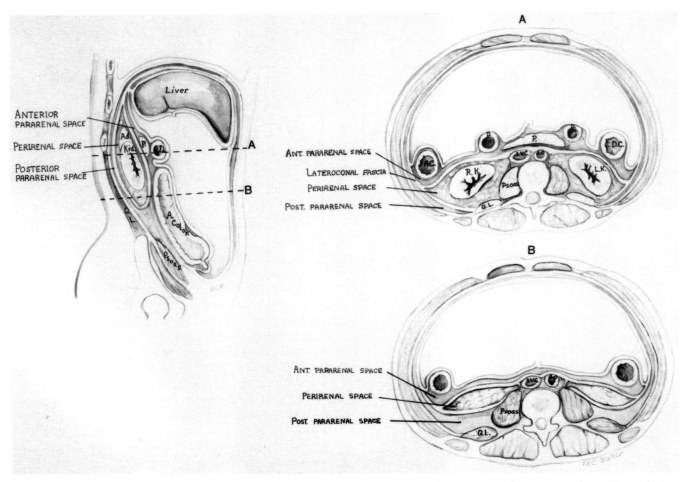

Figure 1.1. Cross-sectional anatomy of the retroperitoneum at **(A)** the level of the kidneys and **(B)** inferior to the lower pole of the kidneys. AC = ascending colon; Ad = adrenal; AP = aorta; D = duodenum; DC = descending colon; IVC = inferior vena cava; LK = left kidney; P = pancreas; QL = quadratus lumborum; RK = right kidney.

lateroconal fascia laterally. The perinephric space, as defined by the perirenal fascia, is cone shaped and filled with perinephric fat. The perinephric space is open at its top where it extends to the diaphragm and becomes progressively smaller inferiorly where it communicates through its open end with the pelvic extraperitoneal space. The ureter passes into the pelvic extraperitoneal space through this open end.

The posterior pararenal space is defined anteriorly by the posterior layer of the perirenal fascia (Zuckerkandl's layer) and posteriorly by the fascia that covers the psoas and quadratus lumborum muscles. The posterior pararenal space contains no organs. Laterally, it merges into the transversalis fascia; thus, the fat in the posterior pararenal space communicates with the properitoneal fat of the anterior abdominal wall. The fat between the lateroconal fascia and the transversalis fascia is continuous with the fat in the posterior pararenal space; laterally, it is known as the "flank stripe." The posterior space is quite small at the level of the kidneys as the posterior layer of Gerota's fascia inserts on the quadratus lumborum at this

level; inferiorly, it extends more medially to insert on the psoas muscle itself.

Unlike the retroperitoneum, the pelvic extraperitoneal space is not truly anatomically divided; however, it is often classified into four potential spaces for descriptive purposes: the space of Retzius (the anterior extraperitoneal space) between the symphysis pubis and the bladder, the retrovesicle space between the rectum and the bladder, the presacral space between the rectum and the sacrum, and the perirectal space that surrounds the rectum. The functional anatomy of the kidney is discussed in Chapter 4 and the vascular anatomy in Chapter 8.

Ureter

The ureter is a muscular conduit that transports urine from the renal pelvis to the bladder. It begins at the ureteropelvic junction, which is usually a gentle tapering of the pelvis to join the ureter. The ureter remains retroperitoneal throughout its course. It runs across the psoas muscle from lateral to medial. The most anterior portion is the point where it crosses anterior to the common or external iliac artery. The ureter then passes posteroinferiorly to enter the pelvis and courses laterally before entering the posterolateral aspect of the bladder wall. The ureters enter the bladder obliquely, tunneling for approximately 2 cm in the muscular wall before emptying into the bladder lumen at the trigone. The ureterovesical junction is the narrowest portion of the ureter.

The ureter is composed of mucosal, muscular, and adventitial layers. The mucosa is covered by transitional epithelium which is continuous with that of the renal pelvis proximally and the bladder distally. When the ureter is empty, the mucosa collapses into longitudinal folds.

The muscular layer has both circular and longitudinal muscle fibers separated by fibroareolar connective tissue. In the distal ureter longitudinal muscle fibers continue in the intravesical portion of the ureter and decussate with muscles of the trigone.

The distal ureter has not only a superficial but also a deep periureteral sheath that is derived from the bladder. A plane of cleavage containing loose connective tissue provides mobility for the intravesical ureter. The outer or adventitial layer is composed of fibrous tissue that blends with this outer sheath of the ureter.

The normal resting pressure of 8 to 15 mm Hg within the bladder compresses and closes the ureter. During peristalsis pressures of 20–35 mm Hg are sufficient to propel a bolus of urine from the ureter into the bladder. The length of the intramural ureter and the configuration of the longitudinal muscle that inserts onto the trigone are critical to the prevention of reflux.

The ureter receives arterial supply from many sources. The renal arteries provide branches to the renal pelvis and proximal ureter. The aorta, lumbar, gonadal, and iliac arteries supply the midportion of the ureter. The predominant vessel supplying the distal ureter is the inferior vesical artery. The uterine artery often sends branches to the ureter in females.

Urine is moved from the kidney to the bladder primarily by peristalsis, although gravity does play a small role as well. Contractions begin in the calyces and propel urine toward the renal pelvis. These contractions are propagated in the renal pelvis, although they contribute relatively little to urine flow. Most of the urine enters the ureter during the resting phase when the renal pelvis and ureter are in open communication.

Ureteral peristalsis results from the continuation of peristaltic waves in the renal pelvis. Stretching of the renal pelvis or ureteropelvic junction also contributes to the initiation of peristaltic activity. Increases in urine flow and ureteral distention increase the frequency of peristaltic contractions.

Bladder

The bladder is a hollow pelvic viscera consisting of smooth muscle, lamina propria, submucosa, and mucosa.

The muscle is the detrusor muscle and consists of three layers, an inner longitudinal, a middle circular, and an outer longitudinal layer. Each layer is closely applied to the other without separating laminae or fascia. The detrusor body is expandable and rises higher in the pelvis as it fills with urine. The three muscle layers condense inferiorly to form the trigone or bladder base plate. The ureters enter the bladder at the posterior aspect of the trigone. Between the ureteric orifices there is a muscular ridge, the interureteric ridge, at the posterior aspect of the trigone. Outer longitudinal muscle fibers extend inferiorly to the undersurface of the base plate and may contribute to the opening of the bladder neck when the detrusor muscle contracts during voiding. There is, however, a separate circular smooth muscle sphincter at the bladder neck, the internal sphincter.

The adult bladder lies deep in the pelvis when empty, but flexibility of the detrusor muscle fibers allows the bladder walls and dome to rise high in the pelvis when the bladder is full. The flexibility of the bladder is, however, limited since it is firmly fixed in position. The allantois obliterates to become the middle umbilical ligament. Obliterated umbilical arteries form lateral umbilical ligaments that attach the bladder to the anterior abdominal wall. The puboprostatic ligament extends from the pubic-bone to the prostate gland and contributes fibers to the anteroinferior aspects of the bladder. Posteriorly, the rectovesical ligaments represent condensations of Denonvilliers' fascia, which is a double-layered fascia separating the bladder and urethra from the rectum and anus. The external longitudinal smooth muscle fibers of the detrusor muscle contribute muscle fiber insertions into the puboprostatic and rectovesical ligaments. The trigone is triangular in shape with the base at the interureteric ridge and the apex anteriorly, extending around the urethral orifice or bladder neck to form the bundle of His.

The bladder dome and proximal third of the lateral walls are loosely covered by the peritoneum. When the bladder is empty, the peritoneum extends deep to the pelvis; when the bladder is full, the peritoneum is elevated. The male bladder is adjacent to the rectum posteriorly, the ampulla of the vas deferens and seminal vesicles posteroinferiorly, and the prostate base inferiorly. In the female, the uterus and vagina lie inferiorly and posteriorly to the bladder, and the fallopian tubes, fimbria, and ovaries lie laterally and superiorly to the empty bladder. Anteriorly, the space of Retzius lies between the anterior bladder wall and the posterior aspect of the symphysis pubis.

The blood supply of the bladder originates from the hypogastric arteries with branches that supply the bladder dome; the superior, posterior, and anterior parts of the walls (superior vesical artery); the middle parts of the lateral, posterior, and anterior walls (middle vesical artery); and the inferior, posterior, and lateral bladder walls and the trigone (inferior vesical artery). Additional arterial blood may come from branches of the obturator artery, the vas deferens artery, and the inferior gluteal artery. In the female, additional branches from the uterine and vaginal arteries may supply the lateral and inferior bladder walls. Capillaries from these supply arteries form a rich arterial network around the bladder. Consequently, there is a rich vesical venous plexus that surrounds the bladder and flows directly into the hypogastric (internal iliac) veins. There are also auxiliary veins connecting the vesical venous plexus to the hemorrhoidal veins that drain into the intervertebral venous plexus. This is the route of vesical venous drainage when the inferior vena cava is blocked. There is also a rich network of vesical lymphatics that drain into the internal and external iliac nodes with continued drainage into the common iliac and paraaortic nodes.

The nerve supply to the bladder is from the autonomic system. The parasympathetic nerves (the pelvic nerves) are motor to bladder function and are responsible for the micturition reflex arc (S2–S4) and for the emptying of the bladder. The sympathetic (hypogastric) nerves also supply the bladder and internal and intrinsic urethral sphincters. Sympathetic stimulation initiates α- and β-receptors within smooth muscle. Sympathetic stimulation of β-receptors causes smooth muscle relaxation whereas stimulation of α-receptors stimulates smooth muscle contraction.

The bladder body is rich in β-receptors. During bladder filling, receptor sympathetic stimulation causes detrusor relaxation. The internal sphincter at the bladder neck is rich in α-receptors, and causes contraction of the bladder neck sphincter. Consequently, bladder filling and retention of urine in the bladder is the result of sympathetic activity. When the bladder is fully stretched, receptors in the detrusor muscle stimulate the parasympathetic and micturition reflex arc to activity, causing motor activity in the parasympathetic pelvic nerves resulting in reciprocal reduction of sympathetic activity and relaxation of the smooth muscle sphincters to allow voiding. Voluntary relaxation of the striated external sphincter and pelvic floor muscles under the voluntary and reflex activity of the pudendal nerves (S2–S4) also allows normal voiding. Any abnormal activity of the parasympathetic, sympathetic, or pudendal nerves results in an abnormal voiding pattern such as that found in patients with a neurogenic bladder.

The bladder mucosa is composed of transitional cells and contains pain receptors. The mucosa is more sensitive to extreme temperature changes than to pain. The instillation of ice-cold water into the bladder stimulates detrusor contraction. Afferent pain and temperature impulses are conveyed via the parasympathetic (pelvic) and sympathetic (hypogastric) nerves. Consequently, pain and temperature stimulation result in detrusor contraction, which produces more frequent voiding.

Prostate

The normal prostate gland weighs up to 20 g and has a wider base (approximately 4.5 cm) than length (approximately 3.5 cm). Five prostatic lobes are present in the early fetus. By birth, the anterior lobe has atrophied and the lateral lobes have extended anteriorly to surround the urethra. Thus, there are four recognized lobes in the adult. The median lobe lies posterior and above the ejaculatory duct (Fig. 1.2), while the posterior lobe lies below the ejaculatory duct. The posterior lobe is fan-shaped and is the lobe palpated on rectal examination. The lateral lobes extend laterally and anteriorly. Through the posterior prostate pass the ejaculatory ducts that divide the median and posterior lobes. Microscopic studies of the prostate reveal an extensive fibrous tissue stroma more prominent in the transitional and central zone.

The prostate is fixed in position by two main attachments. The puboprostatic ligament extends from the posterior aspect of the pubis to the prostatic capsule and the bladder anteroinferiorly. The prostate is often represented diagrammatically as an upside-down pear with the apex resting on the superior fascia of the urogenital diaphragm and the base resting against the bladder trigone. Multiple microscopic studies of this region have not revealed any superior fascia of the urogenital diaphragm. The studies do reveal that the apex of the prostate is embedded in the striated muscle fibers of the external sphincter. True prostatic glands intermingle with these striated muscle fibers. Posteriorly, the prostate is sepa-

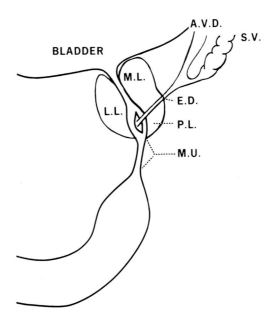

Figure 1.2. Diagram of normal prostate lobes in relation to bladder base, ejaculatory duct (ED), and membranous urethra (MU). AVD = ampulla of vas deferens; LL = lateral lobe; ML = medial lobe; PL = posterior lobe; SV = seminal vesicle. (From McCallum R: The adult male urethra. *Radiol Clin North Am* 27:227–244, 1979.)

rated from the rectum by Denonvilliers's fascia, which supplies posterior ligamentous fibers to the posterior bladder base. Thus, the prostate is firmly held in position by the puboprostatic ligament, bladder trigone, and external sphincter fibers at the urogenital diaphragm (which is not a true diaphragm).

In 1954, Franks described two separate types of glands and named them the inner and outer periurethral glands. The inner periurethral glands are mucosal and submucosal and are only present above the verumontanum. He attributed prostatic hypertrophy and hyperplasia to these glands. The outer periurethral glands are the true prostatic lobes and never undergo hypertrophy but are subject to carcinoma and infection.

In 1972, McNeal's anatomic dissections and microscopic studies emphasized the different types and sites of glandular tissue within the prostate. Rather than designating lobes, McNeal described three separate zones within the prostate. Corresponding to the inner periurethral glands of Franks, McNeal described a transitional zone that undergoes hypertrophy and hyperplasia to produce fibroadenomata. This zone represents only 5% of prostatic volume and is only seen above the veromontanum. McNeal's central zone is said to be true prostatic tissue centrally and above the verumontanum, the glands of which also undergo hypertrophy. The peripheral zone is true prostatic tissue, comprises the bulk of the prostate gland, and is subject to the development of carcinoma and infection. Hypertrophy of transitional zone glands centrally and posteriorly may result in an apparent intravesical filling defect, the so-called "lobe of Albarran."

Vas Deferens and Seminal Vesicles

Vas Deferens

The vas deferens arises from the tail of the epididymis, passes along the spermatic cord, and enters the pelvis through the internal spermatic ring. In the pelvis the vas deferens follows the lateral pelvic wall, curving inferoposteriorly and medially. It crosses superficial to the external iliac vessels, the vesical arteries, the obturator nerve and vein, and the ureter. As it crosses the ureter it becomes convoluted and dilated, increasing in diameter from 1 mm up to 1 cm. This is the ampulla of the vas deferens (Fig. 1.3). The diameter of the ampulla of the vas deferens varies from approximately 3 mm to 1 cm. The length of the vas deferens including the ampulla is 35–45 cm.

The beginning of the ampulla as it crosses the ureter is within 1.5 cm of the fundus of the seminal vesicle. The inferomedial course brings the vas deferens medial and adjacent to the seminal vesicle. As the ampulla courses to the midline it meets the excretory duct of the seminal vesicle. The distal ampulla and excretory duct join to form the ejaculatory duct. The ejaculatory duct is almost

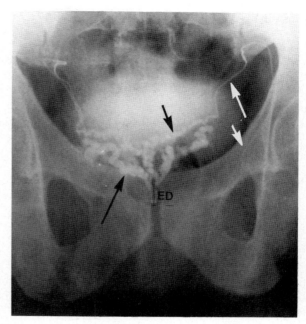

Figure 1.3. Normal seminal vesiculogram. Through scrotal incisions contrast medium is injected into the vas deferens and outlines the vas deferens (*white arrows*), the ampulla of the vas deferens (*black arrow*) the ejaculatory duct (ED), and reflux of contrast medium into the seminal vesicles (*long black arrow*). (From Putman C and Ravin C. *Textbook of Diagnostic Imaging,* Philadelphia, WB Saunders, 1988, Vol 2, p 1358.)

midline, coursing through the prostate posteriorly to empty into the verumontanum 1 mm lateral to midline. The ejaculatory duct is a continuation of the excretory duct with the ampulla contributing as a tributary in approximately 50% of males. In the other 50%, the ejaculatory duct is a confluence of both the excretory duct and the ampulla with equal contribution. The duct is approximately 1.5 cm in length, with a width of 1.5 mm.

The ejaculatory ducts are straight, parallel, and symmetric. Rarely, they are slightly curved or hooked. In normal males, the opening of the ejaculatory ducts into the verumontanum is 2–2.5 cm below the bladder neck. The vas deferens consists of three layers, an areolar layer externally, a smooth muscle layer, and a mucosal layer.

The muscle layer at the origin of the duct consists of three layers, an outer longitudinal, a middle circular, and an inner longitudinal layer. Shortly after the commencement of the duct, the inner longitudinal layer disappears leaving most of the length of the vas deferens with outer longitudinal and inner circular layers of smooth muscle. Most of the epithelial layer consists of one layer of columnar epithelium, which is not ciliated. Near its origin at the testicular end there is a double layer of columnar epithelium, the superficial layer of which is ciliated. The dilated convoluted ampulla of the vas deferens consists of the same structure as most of the length of the vas deferens. The ampullae of the vas deferens are generally symmetric in size and angulation.

Seminal Vesicles

Like the vas deferens, the seminal vesicles are paired structures that are usually symmetric. Each seminal vesicle is approximately 4.5–5 cm long and 2 cm wide when measured in its normal state. The seminal vesicle is a blind-ending tube, coiled on itself and convoluted, giving the appearance of numerous diverticula. The seminal vesicle is pyramidal in shape with the broader end directed laterally and posterosuperiorly. The lower end is funneled to form the excretory duct that joins with the distal end of the ampulla of the vas deferens to form the ejaculatory duct. The anterior surface of the seminal vesicle is in close contact with the posterior bladder wall and reaches to the fundus of the empty bladder. When the bladder is distended with fluid, the seminal vesicle reaches almost halfway up the posterior bladder wall. The posterior surface of the seminal vesicle lies on Denonvilliers's fascia, separating it from the rectum. The distal posterior surface is closely adjacent to the base of the prostate. The seminal vesicle lies at an angle of approximately 40° to the horizontal parallel and adjacent to the ampulla of the vas deferens. Laterally and posteriorly it reaches to the level of the pelvic ureter.

Like the vas deferens, the microscopic structure of the seminal vesicles consists of three layers enveloped in a dense fibromuscular sheath. The outer layer consists of fibroareolar tissue. The middle layer consists of two smooth muscle layers, an outer longitudinal and an inner circular layer. An internal mucosa consists of columnar epithelium. Within the pseudodiverticulae are numerous goblet cells that contribute to the seminal fluid. Arterial supply and venous drainage are from the middle and inferior vesical arteries and from the middle hemorrhoidal artery and vein. The nerve supply is autonomic, arising from the pelvic parasympathetic plexus.

Urethra

Anterior Urethra

The urethra consists of anterior and posterior portions, each of which is subdivided into two parts (Fig. 1.4). The anterior urethra extends from the external meatus to the inferior edge of the urogenital diaphragm. The penile (or pendulous) urethra extends from the external meatus to the penoscrotal junction inferiorly, and to the suspensory ligament superiorly. This is a relatively fixed point, although the suspensory ligament has some elasticity, allowing approximately 1 cm of inferior motion. The penile urethra has a slightly dilated segment approximately 1.5–2 cm proximal to the external meatus, which is known as the fossa navicularis and is approximately 1–1.5 cm in length.

The bulbous urethra extends from the penoscrotal junction to the inferior fascia of the urogenital diaphragm. There is a dilatation in the proximal half of the bulbous urethra, termed the bulbous urethral sump, where the diameter of the anterior urethra is greatest. The bulbous sump is approximately 2–3 cm long and is the most inferior part of the urethra.

The anterior urethra is lined by stratified columnar epithelium except at the external meatus where it

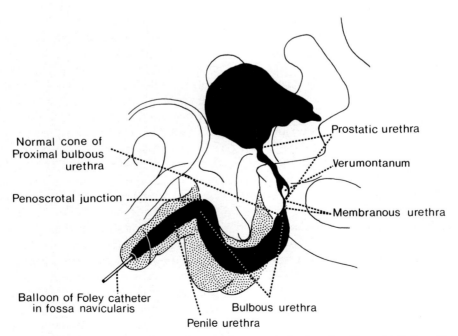

Figure 1.4.   Diagram of urethra with normal anatomic landmarks. (From McCallum R: The adult male urethra. *Radiol Clin North Am* 27:227–244, 1979.)

changes to stratified squamous epithelium, which covers the glans penis. Along the length of the anterior urethra are small mucus-secreting submucosal glands, termed the glands of Littre, which are more numerous in the bulbous sump and in the superior aspect of the penile urethra. They secrete mucus into the urethra during sexual stimulation. Two ductal openings empty into the sump of the bulbous urethra. These are the long ducts of the pea-sized glands of Cowper, which lie on either side of the membranous urethra, within the urogenital diaphragm. Cowper's glands also secrete mucus during sexual stimulation.

A small striated musculotendinous sling of the bulbocavernous muscle extends from the anterior and lateral surfaces of the proximal bulbous urethra. This structure is known as the musculus compressor nuda. (Fig. 1.5) and may indent the proximal bulbous urethra on dynamic retrograde urethrography or, rarely, on voiding urethrography. It should not be mistaken for stricture formation. The bulbocavernous muscle is involved in emptying the anterior urethra at the end of micturition. The levator ani muscles, the ischiocavernous muscles, and the superifical and deep transverse perineii are pelvic floor muscles involved in the active inhibition or interruption of micturition. Both anatomic dissections and dynamic retrograde urethrographic studies have shown a convex symmetric cone shape to the proximal bulbous urethra (Fig. 1.5). The tip of the cone shape is the point at which the bulbous urethra enters the urogenital diaphragm to continue as the membranous urethra.

Posterior Urethra

The posterior urethra extends from the bladder neck to the inferior aspect of the urogenital diaphragm and is divided into the prostatic and membranous portions.

The prostatic urethra is approximately 3.5 cm in length and passes through the prostate gland slightly anterior to midline. It continues as the membranous urethra, which is approximately 1–1.5 cm in length and ends at the inferior aspect of the urogenital diaphragm. A longitudinal ridge of smooth muscle extends from the bladder neck to the membranous urethra on the posterior wall of the posterior urethra. This longitudinal smooth muscle bundle swells about the midpart of the prostatic urethra to form an ovoid mound, which is the verumontanum (colliculus). The bulk of the verumontanum is posterior, is approximately 1 cm in length, and tapers distally in the prostatic urethra to continue as the urethral crest, which flattens in the membranous urethra.

The prostatic urethral mucosa is continuous with the bladder mucosa and is composed of transitional cells but changes to stratified columnar epithelium at the membranous urethra. The supracollicular prostatic urethra is the widest part of the prostatic urethra. During voiding the normal diameter of the bladder orifice and supracollicular prostatic urethra is approximately 1–1.5 cm. The submucosa in the supracollicular prostatic urethra differs from the submucosa at the verumontanum and inferiorly. Above the verumontanum, small mucosal and submucosal glands known as the inner periurethral glands that correspond to McNeal's transitional zone are present. These periurethral glands are only present above the verumontanum and are the glands that undergo hypertrophy and hyperplasia. Consequently, the supracollicular prostatic urethra may be compressed by prostatic adenomata that may enlarge to obstruct the bladder neck or indent the bladder base. Occasionally adenomata are so numerous and large that they may push the verumontanum inferiorly. Rarely do prostatic adenomata extend below the verumontanum. The inner periurethral glands or glands of the transitional zone empty into the supracollicular prostatic urethra and into the prostatic sulcus on both sides of the verumontanum.

There are three distinct orifices in the verumontanum. The most proximal orifice is central and represents the prostatic utricle, a vestigial remnant of the müllerian duct. On either side of the midline below the prostatic utricle are two openings of the ejaculatory ducts that are formed at the junction of the ampulla of the vas deferens

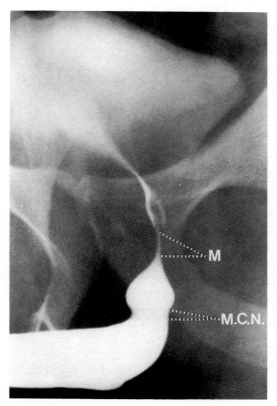

Figure 1.5. Dynamic retrograde urethrogram. M = membranous urethra; MCN = musculus compressor nuda. (From McCallum R: The adult male urethra. *Radiol Clin North Am* 27:227–244, 1979.)

and the short duct of the seminal vesicles. The verumontanum tapers inferiorly to continue as the urethral crest, which is longitudinal smooth muscle and continues to the membranous urethra. Within the submucosa of the posterior urethra is a network of blood vessels that predominate over the verumontanum and urethral crest. The verumontanum and urethral crest form a smooth muscle organ involved in lengthening the posterior urethra during voiding and shortening the urethra at the end of voiding. This muscular organ is also likely involved in contracting the posterior urethra during emission and ejaculation, directing the emission through the membranous urethra and into the bulbous urethra for ejaculation by contraction of the bulbocavernous muscle.

Urethral Sphincters

The internal urethral sphincter lies in the trigourethral area and is the primary muscle of passive continence (Fig. 1.6). There are two schools of thought regarding this complex area. Tanagho, Lapides, and Hutch are of the opinion that a true circular sphincter does not exist, and that the outer longitudinal muscle fibers from the detrusor muscle are inserted below the trigone. These investigators claim that detrusor contraction when the bladder is full pulls the base plate open from below, allowing the internal urethral orifice to open. This opinion is in direct contrast to the microscopic studies of McCallum and Colapinto as well as those of McNeal, Uhlenhuth, Woodburne, and Gil-Vernet, which found that compact circular smooth muscle fibers at the bladder neck (unlike detru-

sor muscle fibers) represent a true internal sphincter. In addition, physiologic studies by Kleeman have shown that the bladder neck sphincter can be made to contract under the action of sympathomimetic drugs, even while the detrusor muscle is contracting. There is sufficient evidence to state that there is a true circular internal sphincter at the bladder neck that acts as the primary muscle of passive continence. Detrusor external longitudinal smooth muscle fibers inserting into the inferior surface of the trigone are present and undoubtedly contribute to the opening of the bladder neck during voiding.

Below the mound of the verumontanum in the distal one-third of the prostatic urethra and surrounding the membranous urethra is a second smooth muscle sphincter, the intrinsic sphincter (Fig. 1.6). Microscopic cross-sections through the distal prostatic urethra show a longitudinal smooth muscle elevation in the posterior wall of the cross-section that is the urethral crest. Surrounding the distal prostatic urethra is a thick band of circular smooth muscle that continues inferiorly to surround the membranous urethra. The urethral crest flattens in the membranous urethra. Adjacent to the membranous urethra submucosa is a thick band of circular smooth muscle that constitutes the intrinsic sphincter surrounding the membranous urethra and distal prostatic urethra up to the inferior edge of the mound of the verumontanum. Only sparse circular or arcuate striated and smooth muscle fibers lie between the internal sphincter at the bladder neck and the intrinsic sphincter. Consequently, there appear to be two separate smooth muscle sphincters in the posterior urethra. Both of these sphincters function as muscles maintaining passive continence. If the internal sphincter at the bladder neck is ablated, as it is in any kind of prostatectomy, or as a result of trigourethral injury in pelvic fracture (rare), the intrinsic sphincter becomes the only and primary smooth muscle of passive continence. If both internal and intrinsic sphincters are damaged, the patient will be passively incontinent. The degree to which this condition is present usually depends on the extent of damage to the intrinsic sphincter.

The external sphincter is a striated voluntary muscle and is involved in active continence or the interruption of micturition. There is also reflex activity of the external sphincter, which contracts reflexly (along with the pelvic floor muscles) on increased intraabdominal pressure and inhibits stress incontinence. The external sphincter surrounds the membranous urethra peripheral to the intrinsic sphincter, and, in addition, sends arcuate fibers proximally beneath the prostatic capsule almost to the bladder base. The external striated sphincter plays no part in maintaining passive continence. Although the striated muscle fibers maintain tone, the resting tone of the striated muscle fibers is insufficient to maintain passive continence.

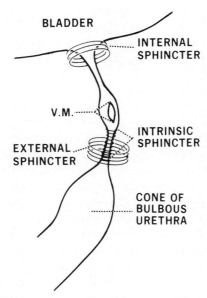

Figure 1.6. Diagram of the three urinary sphincters. The internal and intrinsic sphincters are smooth muscle while the external sphincter is striated voluntary muscle. (From McCallum R: The adult male urethra. *Radiol Clin North Am* 27:227–244, 1979.)

Microscopic studies through the membranous urethra and urogenital diaphragm clearly show that the external striated muscle fibers lie in close apposition to the smooth muscle fibers of the intrinsic sphincter and, in fact, intermingle with peripheral smooth muscle fibers. It is postulated that when micturition is physiologically necessary but socially unsuitable, voluntary contraction of the pelvic floor muscles including the external sphincter actively inhibits micturition by the transference of electrical impulses from the intermingling striated fibers of the external sphincter to the smooth muscle fibers of the intrinsic sphincter. Thus active continence becomes passive continence within a few minutes.

Contraction of voluntary muscles including the external sphincter can only be maintained for a few minutes after which striated muscle fibers tire. Consequently, when it is inconvenient to micturate but the urge to micturate is strong, micturition can be controlled by initiating active continence, maintained for a few minutes after which continence becomes passive and the immediate necessity to void passes.

The smooth muscle sphincters of the posterior urethra are rich in α-receptors that cause contraction with sympathetic stimulation. Consequently, passive continence is controlled by sympathetic (T11–L2) stimulation with reciprocal relaxation of the parasympathetic nerves to allow the bladder to fill. The filled bladder stimulates the parasympathetic (S2–S4) nerves to cause motor activity in the detrusor muscle and bladder contraction. Reciprocal sympathetic relaxation causes the smooth muscle sphincters to relax, allowing micturition to take place. The external striated sphincter and pelvic floor muscles also reflexly relax by reduced activity of the pudendal nerves (S2–S4), allowing good urinary flow.

The intrinsic sphincter has a second function that involves a milk-back action at the end of micturition. The milk-back action empties the posterior urethra at the end of micturition, projecting the 1–2 cm of urine in the posterior urethra back into the bladder. This function is likely the result of both the striated external sphincter and intrinsic sphincter. The bulbocavernous muscle empties the anterior urethra at the end of micturition, therefore, the whole urethra is empty of urine at the end of micturition.

The urethra is fixed at two points, the penoscrotal junction and the urogenital diaphragm. Consequently, the urethra normally maintains a reverse horizontal S-Shape. Thus, passage into the urethra of any straight metallic instrument that is maintained in position for a significant time may cause pressure necrosis at the fixed points, leading to scarring and stricture formation.

Penis

The penis is suspended superiorly from the pubic bone by the suspensory ligament. Inferiorly, the bulbous penis is longer and extends proximally between the testicles where the bulbocavernosus muscle covers the bulbous urethra. The penis consists of two separate bodies of cavernous tissue. The corpus spongiosum, through which the urethra passes, lies inferior to two parallel cavernous bodies, the corpora cavernosa. The corpus spongiosum is longer than the corpora cavernosa, and is bulbous at both ends. The distal end of the corpus spongiosum is formed by the glans penis, which fits like a cap on the blunt ends of the corpora cavernosa. The proximal end of the corpus spongiosum dilates as the bulbous penis, which is bound to the pubic arch by the inferior fascia of the urogenital diaphragm (i.e., the perineal membrane).

The corpora cavernosa are symmetric cavernous bodies capped distally by the glans penis. Proximally at the root of the penis, they become pointed and separated, and each is firmly connected to the rami of the pubic arch. Each corpus cavernosa is separated by a perforated septum, the septum pectiniform. Both corpora cavernosa and corpus spongiosum are bound together by a fibrous envelope, the deep (Buck's) fascia that is surrounded by the tunica albuginea. Within this fibrous tunica albuginea lies the deep dorsal vein, dorsal artery, and dorsal nerve of the penis. The tunica albuginea is surrounded by a loose areolar layer below the skin. The superficial dorsal vein of the penis lies within the areolar layer and drains the prepuce and skin of the penis.

The arterial supply to the penis is from the internal pudendal artery, which is a branch of the anterior division of the internal iliac artery. The four branches of the internal pudendal artery are the pelvic, gluteal, ischiorectal, and perineal. The dorsal penile artery usually arises from the perineal branch. Rarely, the dorsal penile artery arises from branches of the external pudendal artery, or from the inferior vesical artery. The deep dorsal artery extends to the glans penis and sends circumflex branches to the sinusoids of the spongy tissue of the three corpora. An increase in arterial blood flow to these sinusoids, as in sexual stimulation, results in erection.

The venous drainage of the penis is via the superficial and deep dorsal veins. The superficial vein drains the penile skin and prepuce, and drains into the external pudendal vein and saphenous vein. Circumflex veins interconnecting the superficial and deep dorsal veins are present and function when the penis is in the flaccid state. These circumflex veins are compressed during erection between tunica albuginea and the deep (Buck's) fascia and are temporarily obliterated, thus reducing venous drainage. The deep dorsal vein and circumflex veins of the penis have been shown to contain valves. These valves are closed during erection, further reducing venous drainage. The deep dorsal vein drains into the vesicoprostatic plexus. In the flaccid penis, cavernosography shows symmetric corpora cavernosa and shows the deep dorsal vein draining into the vesicoprostatic plexus. During erection, the valves in the deep dorsal vein are closed and may not be visualized during cavernosography in normal erection. The vesicoprostatic plexus should not be visualized nor should the superficial venous system. Because communications are temporarily obliterated during erection, these anatomic conditions are the basis for cavernosography in the assessment of impotence that may be due to venous leakage.

The dorsal nerve that lies within the deep fascia is a branch of the pudendal nerve and provides sensory input to the glans penis, penile skin, and urethra. Accompanying the dorsal nerve of the penis are the N. Erigentes, which are branches of the parasympathetic (pelvic) nerves. The parasympathetic nerves are the autonomic nerve supply that produces erection. Both the parasympathetic (pelvic nerve) and the pudendal nerves arise from the sacral segments S2–S4. The sympathetic nerve supply (i.e., hypogastic nerve) is responsible for emission of semen into the posterior urethra. The pudendal nerve supplying the bulbocavernous and pelvic floor muscles is responsible for ejaculation. Emission of semen and ejaculation are not yet fully understood since the bladder neck must remain closed to avoid retrograde ejaculation into the bladder, and the external and intrinsic sphincter (supplied by the pudendal nerve and sympathetic, respectively) must relax to allow the seminal emission to pass into the proximal bulbous urethra for ejaculation by the bulbocavernosus, which is supplied by the pudendal nerve. It is suspected that emission and ejaculation is a matter of precise timing and that the bladder neck is closed by contraction of the arcuate fibers of the external sphincter that pull the verumontanum up to the bladder neck to mechanically close the orifice. The emission then goes the route of least resistance and passes into the bulbous urethra.

Scrotum and Contents

The scrotum and contents are best considered as evaginations of the anterior abdominal wall produced by testicular descent through the inguinal canal and superficial inguinal ring. Consequently, the scrotal contents have eight different layers of tissue. By the time the testes and epididymis are ready for descent through the inguinal canal, they are already invested by the tunica albuginea, which is closely applied to the seminiferous tubules. The tunica albuginea extends septa between the seminiferous tubules that converge on the rete testis and divide the testis into seminiferous lobules. About the same time, a peritoneal fold on the anterior abdominal wall termed the saccus vaginalis, evaginates into the inguinal canal. Consequently, as the testicle descends through the inguinal canal and superficial inguinal ring, it becomes invested by three tunica. (1) The tunica albuginea is closest to the seminiferous tubules. (2) The tunica vasculosa consists of a plexus of blood vessels lining the tunica albuginea and interlobular septa, thereby allowing adequate blood supply to the testis. (3) The tunica vaginalis is a peritoneal layer continuous with the saccus vaginalis and surrounds both inner tunica. The tunica vaginalis is double layered, consisting of visceral and parietal layers with a cavity between them. The saccus vaginalis proximal to the testis obliterates so there is no connection between the testis and peritoneal cavity.

As the testis descends through the inguinal canal it takes with it the layers of the anterior abdominal wall including tunica vaginalis, subperitoneal fat, transversalis fascia, transversus, internal oblique and external oblique aponeurosis, subcutaneous fat, and skin. Within the subcutaneous fat layer extending to the scrotum is a layer of Colles fascia and the Dartos muscle.

The normal testis is 4–5 cm in length, 3 cm in width, and 2.5 cm in breadth. The testicular weight varies from 10 to 14 g. The epididymis lies along the lateral posterior border of the testis. The testicular appendix, a minute oval sessile body, lies at the upper end of the testis adjacent to the head of the epididymis. This is the hydatid of Morgagni, a vestigial remnant of the müllerian duct. The head of the epididymis also has a small appendix that is thought to be the result of detached efferent ducts. The internal structure of the testis consists of 250-400 lobules. Each lobule consists of several (one to five) convoluted tubules, supported by interstitial cells. From these convoluted tubules spermatogonia, spermatids, and spermatozoon develop. Cells of Sertoli are also present in the tubules and appear to be necessary for the progress of the spermatozoa along the tubules. Toward the hilum, the tubules become straight and coalesce to form 20–30 straight ducts that enter the fibrous tissue of the mediastinum testis. Here the tubules lose their walls and simply become channels through the fibrous tissue of the mediastinum, producing a fine network of channels called the rete testes. The channels of the rete testes progress to the proximal end of the mediastinum where a number of ducts develop for perforation of the tunica albuginea. These efferent ducts pass through the tunica albuginea in the head epididymis.

EMBRYOLOGY

Upper Urinary Tract

The human kidney develops in three discrete stages (Fig. 1.7). The first such stage, the *pronephros,* appears during the end of the third week of gestation and is so named because of its relatively cephalic position. The tubules of the pronephros drain into an excretory duct that terminates in the cloaca. After the third week of gestation, the pronephros involutes and is replaced by the *mesonephros,* which develops immediately caudal to the pronephros. The mesonephros consists of a series of

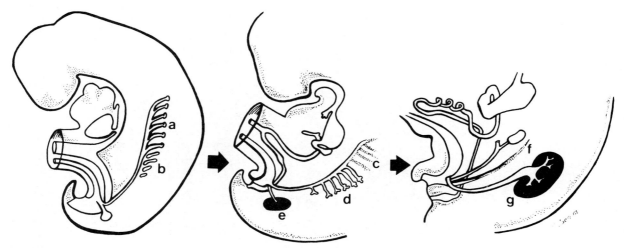

Figure 1.7 Embryogenesis of the Kidney. **A,** pronephros; **B,** early mesonephros; **C,** degenerating pronephros; **D,** me-sonephric duct; **E,** ureteral bud; **F,** degenerating mesonephros; **G,** metanephros.

uriniferous tubules, each of which is associated with a group of blood vessels to form primitive glomeruli. The uriniferous tubules develop from a pair of laterally placed mesodermal structures known as the nephrogenic cord. The tubules on each side drain into a medially located structure called the mesonephric or wolffian duct. The mesonephric duct in turn drains into the same excretory duct that had its origins in the pronephros stage. The mesonephric duct then begins to involute, however, remnants of this duct persist in both sexes into adulthood. In males, the mesonephric duct serves as the precursor of the vas deferens, the seminal vesicles, and the ejaculatory ducts. In females, remnants of the me-sonephric duct are vestigial.

Late in the fifth week of gestation, the final stage of development of the human kidney, the *metanephros,* be-gins. At the level of the 28th somite (the future site of the first sacral vertebra) a diverticulum forms from the me-sonephric duct. This outpocketing is known as the ure-teral bud. The tissue that surrounds the ureteral bud is known as the metanephric blastema and is derived from the caudal end of the nephrogenic cord. The me-tanephric blastema is induced to develop into nephrons under the influence of the ureteral bud, beginning at about the seventh week of gestation. The metanephric blastema will not develop nephrons unless the ureteral bud is present. The ureteral bud itself elongates and un-dergoes multiple divisions to form the renal tubules, the major and minor calyces (Fig. 1.8), the renal pelvis (Fig. 1.9), and the ureter. The divisions of the ureteral bud are dichotomous, however, more divisions occur in the polar regions of the kidney than in its midportion. For this reason, the renal parenchyma contains more nephrons and is thicker in its poles. This division process results in

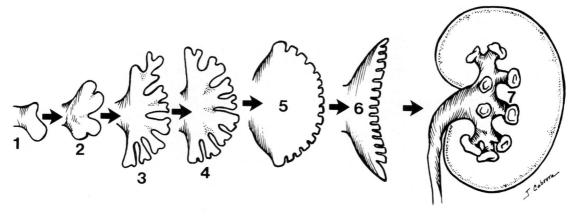

Figure 1.8. Development of calyx. New generations of branches are formed from the ureteral bud (1–3); early config-uration of calyx (4); progressive distention of the cavity (5); invagination of the cavity (6); cuplike structure or calyx is formed (7). (Modified from Potter EL: *Normal and Abnormal Development of the Kidney* Chicago, Year Book Medical Pub-lishers, 1972.)

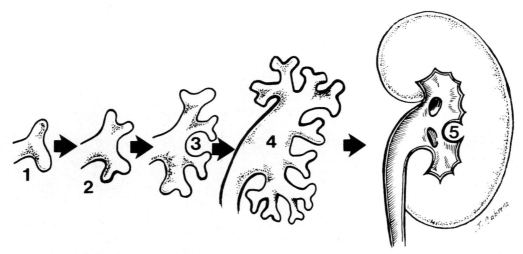

Figure 1.9. Development of renal pelvis. Divisions of ureteral bud (1), polar divisions (2), interpolar divisions (3), dilatation of individual branches (4), developed renal pelvis (5).

(Modified from Potter EL. *Normal and Abnormal Development of the Kidney.* Chicago, Year Book Medical Publishers, 1972.)

the formation of the renal pyramids. A pyramid together with its overlying cloak of renal cortex is known as a primitive renal lobe. The number of renal lobes formed thus depends on the number of calyces present. Also, between the fourth and eighth weeks, the developing kidneys migrate in a cephalic direction out of the pelvis to assume their adult position opposite the second lumbar vertebra. During the course of this migration, the kidneys rotate 90° about their longitudinal axis so that the renal pelvis lies in a medial position.

At the fourth month of gestation, there are classically 14 discrete renal lobes, seven anterior and seven posterior, separated by a fibrous longitudinal groove. Following the 28th week of gestation, assimilation of the boundary between these lobes occurs. Persistence of these grooves into adulthood results in a grooved appearance to the surface of the kidney known as persistent fetal lobulation. In addition, some of the calyces become fused so that the one-to-one relationship between the calyces and the papillae in the fetal kidney is lost in the adult kidney. This process is also more pronounced in the polar region of the kidney and results in the development of compound calyces each of which drains two to four papillae.

During this same period, there is assimilation of the septal cortex, which is also more pronounced in the polar regions of the kidney. When such fusion is complete, the medulla between adjacent lobes directly abut one another; where relatively little fusion is present, characteristically in the interpolar regions of the kidney, columns of cortical tissue may be found between adjacent medullary lobes. When these columns have a slightly bulbous appearance, an indentation on one of the major calyces or the renal pelvis may be produced, which simulates an intrarenal mass; such a renal "pseudotumor" is known as a hypertrophied column of Bertin.

Lower Urogenital Tract

The embryology of the lower urogenital tract is best considered as consisting of four separate developmental stages: (1) development of the cloaca; (2) separation of the cloaca into dorsal and ventral portions; (3) development of these into the bladder, allantois, and urogenital sinus; and (4) development of the ventral and vesicourethral portions of the bladder, and division of the urogenital sinus into pelvic and phallic portions.

The cloaca is a dilatation of the entodermal hindgut that is formed after fetal flexion and anterior movement of the allantois into the body stalk. Solid rods of cells form in the mesoderm of the lateral cell masses. These rods of cells move caudally to reach the ventral portion of the cloaca and become canalized to form the wolffian ducts. This process occurs at 4–5 weeks of gestation. Shortly after the formation of the wolffian ducts a second pair of ducts develop lateral to the wolffian ducts. These are the müllerian ducts that develop from coelomic evaginations. The cloaca is closed inferiorly from the exterior by the cloacal membrane, which consists of a thin entodermal layer and a thick ectodermal layer.

After the development and insertion of the wolffian and müllerian ducts into the ventral aspect of the cloaca, the cloaca is divided into dorsal and ventral portions by the cloacal septum (urorectal septum). The cloacal septum arises from the ridge separating the communication of the allantois with the intestine and the communication of the cloaca with the intestine. The dorsal portion of the cloaca becomes the rectum, and the ventral portion becomes the allantois, bladder, and urogenital sinus. The urogenital sinus divides into pelvic and phallic portions, and the allantois finally atrophies as the umbilical ligament.

The ventral bladder produces the bladder dome, the ventral bladder wall, and the urachus. The vesicourethral portion of the ventral bladder is the site of insertion of the wolffian and müllerian ducts. The lateral and posterior bladder walls, the bladder trigone, internal sphincter, and proximal urethra are formed from the vesicourethral portion of the ventral bladder. The two wolffian and two müllerian ducts develop into distinctive features that separate the sexes. In the male, the wolffian duct develops into the epididymis, the vas deferens, the seminal vesicles, the ejaculatory ducts, and the verumontanum. The proximal prostatic urethra and the proximal part of the prostate are also developed from the vesicourethral portion of the ventral bladder. The müllerian ducts atrophy but persist as a vestigial remnant as the prostatic utricle in the verumontanum and by appendices of the testes (the hydatid of Morgagni).

In the female, the müllerian ducts develop into the fallopian tubes and by fusing together produce the uterus, cervix, vagina, and proximal urethra while the distal wolffian ducts atrophy. The proximal wolffian ducts develop into long ducts, the ducts of Gartner.

The pelvic portion of the urogenital sinus also develops into the features differentiating the sexes. In the male, the pelvic portion produces the distal prostatic urethra, the membranous urethra, the distal prostate gland, and the urogenital diaphragm. In the female, the pelvic portion produces the distal urethra, the vestibule, and the greater vestibular gland.

In the male, the phallic portion of the urogenital sinus produces the bulbous and penile urethra, the glands and ducts of Cowper, the glands of Littre, the corpora cavernosa, and the corpus spongiosum. In the female, the phallic portion produces the clitoris, the labia major and minor, and the hymen.

Initially the development of the testes and ovaries is essentially the same in both sexes. Initial development consists of coelomic cavity epithelial thickening, which forms the genital ridge. Both ovaries and testes develop from this genital ridge. By the end of the seventh week sex distinction is apparent anatomically and microscopically.

The ovary develops from the genital ridge as a central mass of cells with a layer of surface epithelium, while ova develop from the central cell mass. Within the central cell mass is a connective tissue stroma. Each ova develops a covering of connective tissue resulting in rudimentary follicles, and these form an aggregate that becomes covered by a tunica albuginea. Caudal movement of the ovary to the uterus is effected by uterine adhesions that become the ovarian ligament.

The testis develops in a similar fashion to the ovary, arising as a central mass of cells. Within the central mass a series of epithelial cords arise from the surface epithelium, and aggregation of these epithelial cords covered by surface epithelium forms the rudimentary testes. The testis develops a tunica albuginea that separates the surface epithelium from these epithelial cords. The epithelial cords converge toward a hilum that becomes the rete testes, and the epithelial cords also develop peripherally into the seminiferous tubules. Residual mesonephros cells become the efferent ducts of the testis. The seminiferous tubules connect with these efferent ducts to form the functioning testis. At this stage the testis is attached to the posterior abdominal cavity by peritoneum. Peritoneal folds form the inguinal fold and inguinal crest. The gubernaculum testis develops within the inguinal crest and guides the testis and testicular vessels through the inguinal canal into the scrotum.

SUGGESTED READINGS

Anatomy

Bors ET, Commarr AE: *Neurological Urology.* Baltimore, University Park Press, 1971.

Chesbrough RM, Burkhard TK, Martinez AJ and Burks DD: Gerota Versus Zuckerkandl: the renal fascia revisited. *Radiology* 173:845, 1989.

Franks LM: Benign nodular hyperplasia of the prostate: Review. *Am R Coll Surg* 14:92, 1954.

Gil Vernet S: Morphology and function of vesico-prostato-urethral musculature. Canora, Treviso, p. 172, 1968.

Hunter DW: A new concept of urinary bladder musculature. *J Urol* 71:645, 1985.

Hutch JA and Rambo ON: A study of the anatomy of the prostate, prostatic urethra and the urinary sphincter system. *J Urol* 104:443, 1970.

Kaye KW, Reinke DB: Detailed caliceal anatomy for endourology. *J Urol* 132:1085, 1984.

Kleeman FJ: The physiology of the internal urinary sphincter. *J Urol* 104:549, 1970.

Lafortune M, Constantine A, Greton G, et al: Sonography of the hypertrophied column of Bertin. *AJR* 146:53, 1986.

Lapides J, Ajemian EP, Stewart BH, Breakey BA and Lichtwardt JR: Further observations on the kinetics of the urethrovesical sphincter. *J Urol* 84:86, 1960.

McCallum RW: The radiologic assessment of the lower urinary tract in paraplegics—a new method. *J Can Assoc Radiol* 25:34, 1974.

McCallum RW: The adult male urethra: normal anatomy, pathology and method of urethrography. *Radiol Clin North Am* 17:227, 1979.

McCallum RW, Colapinto V: *Urological Radiology of the Adult Male Lower Urinary Tract.* Springfield, IL, Charles C Thomas. 1975.

McCallum RW, Colapinto V: The role of urethrography in urethral disease: Part I. Accurate radiological localization of the membranous urethra and distal sphincters in normal male subjects. *J Urol* 122:607, 1979.

McNeal JE: The prostate and prostatic urethra: a morphological synthesis. *J Urol* 107:1008, 1972.

Mitty HA: Embryology, anatomy and anomalies of the adrenal gland. *Semin Roentgenol* 23(4):271, 1988.

Raptopoulos V, Kleinman PK, Marks S, Jr., et al: Renal fascial pathway: posterior extension of pancreatic effusions within the anterior pararenal space. *Radiology* 158:367, 1986.

Rifkin MD: *Diagnostic Imaging of the Lower Genitourinary Tract.* New York, Raven Press, 1985, pp 7.

Sampaio FJB and Aragao AHM: Anatomical relationship between the intrarenal arteries and the kidney collecting system. *J Urol* 143:679, 1990.

Tanagho EA, Smith DR: The anatomy and function of the bladder neck. *Br J Urol* 38:54, 1966.

Uhlenhuth E, Hunter DW and Loechel W: Problems in the Anatomy of the Pelvis. J.B. Lippincott, Philadelphia, 1953.

Woodburne RT: The structure and function of the urinary bladder. *J Urol* 84:79, 1960.

Embryology

Arey LB (ed): *Developmental Anatomy,* ed 7. Philadelphia, WB Saunders, 1966.

Potter EL: *Normal and Abnormal Development of the Kidney.* Chicago, Year Book Medical Publishers, 1972.

Sadler TW (ed): *Langman's Medical Embryology,* ed 5. Baltimore, Williams & Wilkins, 1985.

CHAPTER 2

CONGENITAL ANOMALIES

UPPER URINARY TRACT ANOMALIES

Renal Anomalies

Anomalies of Position

MALROTATION. Malrotation of a normally positioned kidney most commonly occurs as a result of failure of rotation of the kidney about its vertical axis. This results in an anterior position of the renal pelvis. In many cases, a partial malrotation is present with the renal pelvis located in an anteromedial position. The abnormality may either be bilateral or unilateral. Under rare circumstances, overrotation of the kidney may result in a laterally facing renal pelvis.

On urography, malrotation can be diagnosed when calyces are projected medial to the renal pelvis (Fig. 2.1). Rarely the appearance of malrotated kidney may be mistaken for a more significant renal abnormality such as the presence of a medially located renal mass. Occasionally, malrotation about the verticle axis of the kidney will be present. This is most commonly associated with a deformity of the spine and results in a foreshortened appearance of the affected kidney.

RENAL ECTOPY. As the fetal kidneys ascend from their pelvic position to meet the adrenal glands, each kidney acquires blood supply from the neighboring vessels. The initial supply from the external and internal iliac vessels is lost during this process and blood supply directly from the aorta is acquired around the eighth week of development. Any abnormality in acquiring such blood supply or an associated abnormality of the spine may prevent such cephalic migration from occurring. This will result in a condition known as renal ectopy or an abnormal position of the kidney. The most common form of simple renal ectopy is known as a *pelvic* kidney. In such cases, the kidney is located in the true pelvis or adjacent to the sacrum (sacral kidney). Occasionally the kidney may lie at the level of the iliac crest; such a position is termed abdominal ectopy. The reported incidence of renal ectopy varies between 1:500 and 1:1200. The exact incidence is difficult to determine as in many cases the condition is clinically silent. However, in nearly 50% of the cases, the pelvic kidney is associated with a pathologic process such as hydronephrosis or vesicoureteral reflux. These conditions may reduce renal function to such an extent that diagnosis by urography may be difficult or impossible.

Clinical symptoms related to the presence of a pelvic kidney are usually related to one of its associated conditions. These include pain related to obstruction or infection that may mimic the presence of gastrointestinal disease. Other genitourinary malformations commonly present in patients with pelvic kidneys include ureteropelvic junction obstruction, cryptorchidism or hypospadias in males, and the absence of a vagina in females. Extraurinary congenital anomalies including those of the skeleton (vertebral and rib abnormalities), heart (septal defects), gastrointestinal tract (malrotation, imperforate anus, and so forth) may be present. In nearly 50% of the patients with unilateral renal ectopy, an abnormality of the normally positioned kidney will also be present; in approximately 10% of the cases, the pelvic kidney will be solitary.

The findings on urography depend on the degree of renal function in the pelvic kidney and the presence of

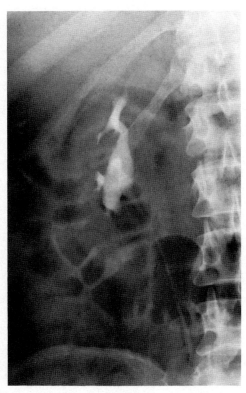

Figure 2.1. Malrotated kidney. The middle calyces are projected medial to the renal pelvis indicating failure of rotation of the right kidney.

associated abnormalities. When the ectopic kidney is small and no hydronephrosis is present, the kidney may be obscured by the bony pelvis. Tomography over the pelvis is frequently helpful in such cases (Fig. 2.2). Ultrasound (US) is the procedure of choice to demonstrate a small ectopic kidney that has not been demonstrated on

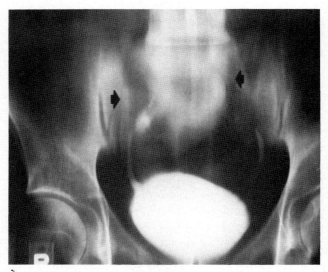

Figure 2.2. Pelvic kidney. Tomogram over the true pelvis shows that the right kidney (*arrows*) overlies the sacrum.

urography. On sonography, the reniform mass will be present in the pelvis with a characteristic pattern of renal sinus echoes. On computed tomography (CT), a functioning mass of renal parenchyma can usually be identified. Angiography is customarily employed prior to any contemplated surgical procedure on a pelvic kidney because of the highly variable nature of its blood supply.

INTRATHORACIC KIDNEY. This rare anomaly occurs when the kidney ascends to a position higher than the second lumbar vertebra. It has been assumed that the kidney may reach an intrathoracic location through a diaphragmatic aperture. The anomaly is more common in males and is more commonly found on the left side. The blood supply to an intrathoracic kidney generally arises from the abdominal aorta in its normal location. Intrathoracic kidney occurs in 1:15,000 births.

Anomalies of Number

RENAL AGENESIS. True renal agenesis is defined as the complete congenital absence of renal tissue. This condition is to be distinguished from acquired forms of agenesis in which renal tissue develops but atrophies either during development or during childhood because of an associated malfunction. Renal agenesis occurs in between 1:500 and 1:1500 births. It is thought to occur as the result of failure of formation of the ureteral bud or because of an inherent deficiency of the metanephric blastema. In the latter case, partial development of the ureter may be present. In true agenesis, a hemitrigone will be found in the bladder on cystoscopy. No renal artery is present. The colon occupies the renal fossa on the affected side, which may suggest the diagnosis on plain film examination or contrast studies of the colon. The ipsilateral adrenal gland is absent in 8–10% of the cases. Some investigators report a twofold increase in the incidence of congenital anomalies of the contralateral kidney in patients with unilateral renal agenesis.

Genital abnormalities may also be associated with unilateral renal agenesis and when present suggest an etiology that also affects the mesonephric duct. In males, such abnormalities include cysts of the ipsilateral seminal vesicle (Fig. 2.3), absence of the ipsilateral vas deferens, hypoplasia or agenesis of the testicle, and hypospadias. In females, renal agenesis may be associated with a unicornuate or bicornuate uterus, absence or hypoplasia of the uterus, and absence or aplasia of the vagina (Rokitansky-Kuster-Hauser syndrome).

Bilateral renal agenesis is extremely rare and incompatible with life. Males are affected in three-fourths of the cases. Infants with this abnormality exhibit the characteristic features of Potter's syndrome including low-set ears and a prominent palpebral fold.

SUPERNUMERARY KIDNEY. A supernumerary kidney is extremely rare. Cleavage of the metanephric blastema has

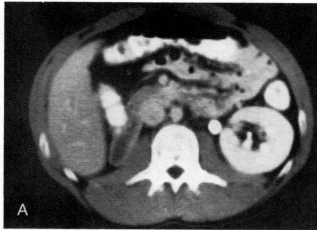

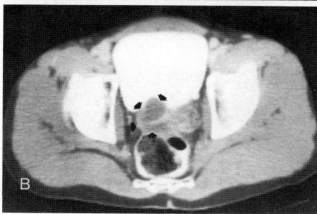

Figure 2.3. **A,** Computed tomography scan showing agenesis of the right kidney. Bowel loops occupy the right renal fossa and there is hypertrophy of the left kidney. **B,** Computed tomography scan through the pelvis demonstrates a cyst of the right seminal vesicle (*arrows*). (From Sandler CM, Raval B, David C: Computed tomography of the kidney. *Urol Clin North Am* 12(4):657–675, 1985.)

been suggested as the cause for this abnormality. Most supernumerary kidneys are caudally placed and are hypoplastic; they may be connected to the ipsilateral dominant kidney either completely or by loose areolar connective tissue. A separate collecting system in the supernumerary kidney is generally present.

Anomalies of Form

CROSSED ECTOPY.   Crossed ectopy is defined as a kidney that is located on the opposite side of the midline from its ureter. The crossed kidney usually lies below the normally situated kidney. In 90% of the cases, at least partial fusion between the kidneys is present (crossed fused ectopy). In the remainder, two discrete kidneys on the same side are present (crossed unfused ectopy). Other variations of crossed ectopy including solitary crossed ectopy and bilateral crossed ectopy have been described (Fig. 2.4). The anomaly is more common in males (2 : 1) and left-to-right ectopy is three times more common than

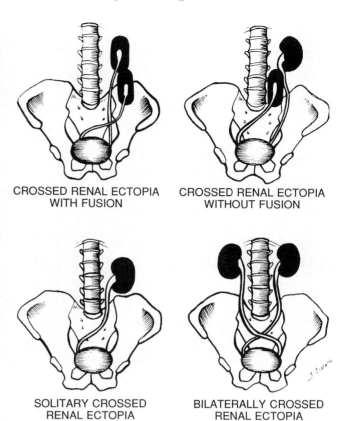

CROSSED RENAL ECTOPIA WITH FUSION

CROSSED RENAL ECTOPIA WITHOUT FUSION

SOLITARY CROSSED RENAL ECTOPIA

BILATERALLY CROSSED RENAL ECTOPIA

Figure 2.4. Schematic drawing showing the variations of crossed-renal ectopy.

is right-to-left. Crossed fused ectopy has been estimated to occur in approximately 1 : 1000 births.

The anomaly is thought to result because of an abnormally situated umbilical artery that prevents normal cephalic migration from occurring; in such cases the developing kidney takes the path of least resistance and crosses to the opposite side where cephalic migration resumes. Others have postulated that the abnormality occurs when the ureteral bud crosses to the opposite side where it induces nephron formation in the contralateral metanephric blastema.

In most cases of crossed renal ectopy, the ureters are not ectopic and cystoscopy reveals a normal trigone. The incidence of associated congenital anomalies is low. Clinically, symptoms of crossed renal ectopy are rare; these patients generally present in adulthood with abdominal pain, pyuria, or urinary tract infection. There is a slightly higher incidence of urinary tract calculi associated with crossed renal ectopy that is thought to be related to stasis. On urography, the abnormality is readily detected (Fig. 2.5) although differentiation of the fused from the unfused variety often requires additional imaging studies such as ultrasound or CT. On sonography, crossed-fused ectopy can be identified by a characteristic anterior or posterior "notch" between the two kidneys (Fig. 2.6). The blood supply to the crossed renal unit is generally anom-

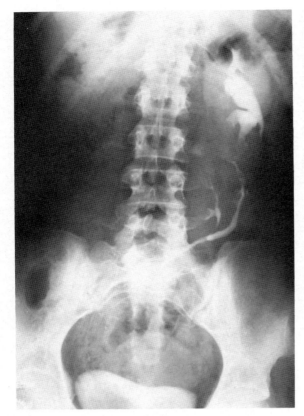

Figure 2.5.   Crossed ectopia. Both kidneys lie in the left abdomen and are malrotated.

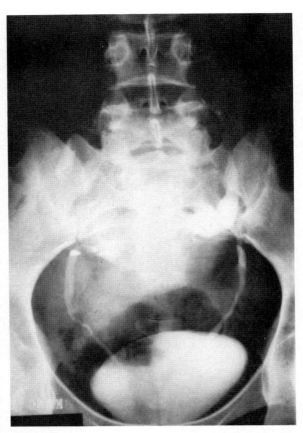

Figure 2.7.   Disc kidney. (Courtesy of Lawrence F. Bigongiari, M.D.)

alous; as is the case in pelvic kidney, angiography is usually recommended prior to surgical procedures.

OTHER FUSION ANOMALIES.   A variety of other fusion abnormalities may occur much less commonly than crossed renal ectopy. These include the *disc* or *pancake* kidney (Fig. 2.7), a kidney that is joined medially at its poles to

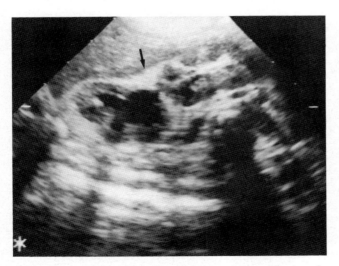

Figure 2.6.   Crossed-fused ectopy. Sonogram showing the notch (*arrow*) between the two kidneys. Mild dilatation of the collecting system of the upper kidney is present.

form a ring-like renal mass. The kidney is generally found overlying the sacrum; the collecting systems are separate with each ureter entering the bladder normally. The *lump* or *cake* kidney is a rare abnormality in which there is extensive fusion between the two renal masses. The kidney is found in the midline or slightly to one side, generally no higher than the sacral promontory. The renal pelves are anterior and generally drain separate portions of the kidney. The ureters generally do not cross.

HORSESHOE KIDNEY.   Horseshoe kidney is the most common anomaly of renal form, occurring in approximately 1:400 births. There is a 2:1 male predominance. The abnormality occurs when the two kidneys on either side of the midline are connected by an isthmus. The anomaly is thought to occur because an abnormal position of the umbilical artery results in disturbance of the normal pattern of cephalic migration. As a result, there is contact between the developing metanephric blastema on each side leading to partial fusion.

The isthmus of a horseshoe kidney usually consists of a band of parenchymal tissue which has its own blood supply. In some cases, the band consists merely of fibrous tissue (Fig. 2.8**A**). Usually, the band joins the lower poles of the kidney and prevents normal rotation from occurring, so that on each side the renal pelvis is in an

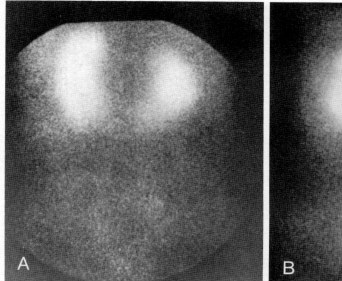

Figure 2.8.   Horseshoe kidney. **A,** Radionuclide examination using technetium-99m diethylenetriaminepentaacetic acid (^{99m}Tc DTPA) showing that the isthmus of the kidney is not composed of functioning renal tissue. **B,** Delayed image shows an accumulation of tracer within the pelvis of the left kidney consistent with an associated ureteropelvic junction obstruction.

anterior position. Rarely, the band connects the upper poles rather than the lower poles. The band is usually located anterior to the aorta and inferior vena cava, but behind the inferior mesenteric artery that is thought to prevent further cephalad migration from occurring. Alterations in this arrangement, however, are common so that the position of the kidneys, their blood supply, their relation to the major vessels, and even the size of the kidney on either side may be variable.

One-third of the cases of horseshoe kidney have an associated ureteropelvic junction obstruction (Fig. 2.8**B**), ureteral duplications occur in 10% and a smaller number have associated genital abnormalities. Approximately one-third of the patients have extraurinary congenital anomalies including anorectal malformations, cardiovascular abnormalities, and skeletal malformations.

One-third of patients with horseshoe kidney remain asymptomatic throughout their lifetime; in the remainder, symptoms of obstruction, infection, or a renal calculus bring the abnormality to medical attention. In some cases, symptoms referable to the gastrointestinal tract will be present. Some investigators report an increased incidence of renal malignancies in horseshoe kidneys; Wilms' tumor, in particular, has been reported to have a predilection to originate in the isthmus.

Several investigators report that a horseshoe kidney is more prone to suffer injury in patients suffering blunt abdominal trauma, presumably because of its relatively less protected, more anterior position.

The blood supply to a horseshoe kidney is quite variable. In one-third of the cases, a single renal artery to each kidney will be present. The remaining patients have multiple bilateral renal arteries (Fig. 2.9). The isthmus may be supplied by branches of the renal arteries or directly from the abdominal aorta, the inferior mesenteric artery, or the iliac arteries. The sonographic detection of a horseshoe kidney is made somewhat difficult because the lumbar spine will obscure the isthmus.

Urographic findings (Fig. 2.10) in patients with horseshoe kidneys include: (*a*) an abnormal axis for each kidney with their lower poles more medially located than their upper poles; (*b*) the kidneys are found in a somewhat more caudad position; and (*c*) there is bilateral malrotation with the renal pelves in an anterior position so that the lower calyces are projected in a more medial position than is the proximal ureter. The isthmus may be visualized if it is composed of functioning renal tissue.

On CT (Fig. 2.11), the isthmus of a horseshoe kidney is usually easily identified. The study also is helpful in defining the relationship of the kidney to the major vessels.

Anomalies of the Renal Pelvis and Ureter

Bifid Pelvis

In approximately 10% of individuals, the renal pelvis is split so that one pelvis drains the upper pole calyces, while a second pelvis drains the middle and lower pole calyces (Fig. 2.12). The two pelves join just proximal to the ureteropelvic junction. This abnormality is commonly viewed as an abortive attempt at ureteral duplication and generally carries no pathologic consequence.

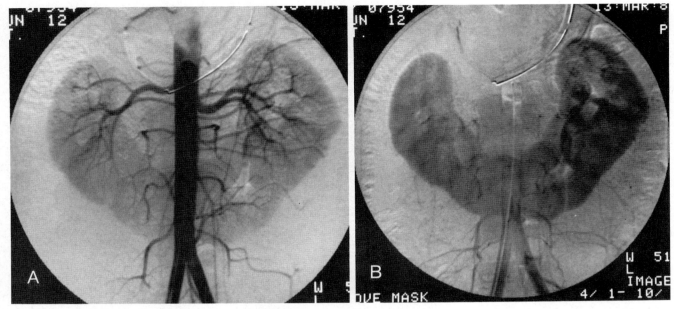

Figure 2.9. Horseshoe kidney. **A,** Intraarterial digital subtraction angiogram demonstrates that multiple renal arteries supply the kidney, all of which arise from the abdominal aorta.

B, Nephrogram phase showing persistent fetal lobulation in the kidney.

Ureteral Duplication

The commonly accepted explanation for the embryogenesis of complete ureteral duplication is that an additional ureteral bud arises from the mesonephric duct. The bud closest to the urogenital sinus becomes the ureter draining the lower pole of the kidney and is called the *orthotopic ureter*—the ureter that enters the bladder at or near the trigone. The higher ureteral bud rotates with the mesonephric duct medially and caudally to become the *ectopic ureter;* it drains the upper pole of the kidney

and ultimately enters the bladder in a more medial and inferior location with respect to the orthotopic ureter. This relationship between the two ureters in complete ureteral duplication has been termed the *Weigert-Meyer law* and is based on the descriptions of these two authors who studied the patterns of ureteral duplication nearly 75 years apart. Although exceptions to this law have been described, they are extremely rare.

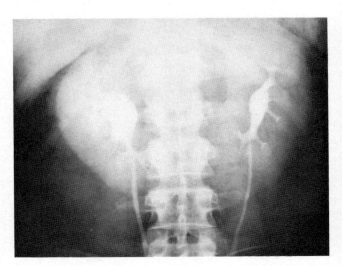

Figure 2.10. Horseshoe kidney. Typical urographic finding in a horseshoe kidney where isthmus is composed of functioning renal tissue.

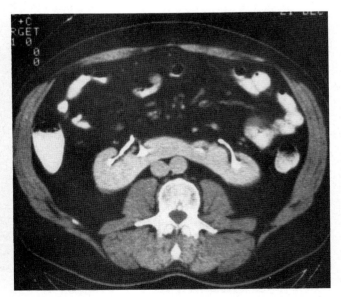

Figure 2.11. Horseshoe kidney. Computed tomography clearly demonstrates the isthmus.

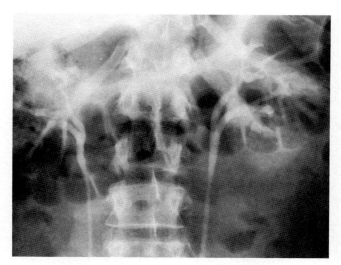

Figure 2.12.   Bilateral bifid renal pelves.

If there is premature branching of a single ureteral bud, before it reaches the metanephric blastema, a partial duplication of the ureter (also referred to as a bifid or **Y** ureter) (Fig. 2.13) will be present. In such cases, the kidney is drained by two separate ureters, however, they join to enter the bladder singly.

The incidence of duplication of the ureters has been derived both from clinical series and autopsy data. Ureteral duplication is the most common ureteral anomaly, occurring in between 1 : 100 and 1 : 150 births. Unilateral duplication occurs 6 times more commonly than does bilateral duplication. Although many clinical series indicate an increased incidence of the anomaly in females,

data from the autopsy series do not generally substantiate this impression. The incidence of partial duplications and complete duplications appears to be similar.

Partial duplications are usually clinically silent. Peristalsis from one ureter into the other ("yo-yo peristalsis") such that the peristaltic wave is reversed in one of the limbs of the duplication has been described, and has been implicated in the development of urinary tract infection. The phenomena is also thought to be responsible for the occasionally described dilatation of one or both renal collecting systems.

Complete ureteral duplication is associated with an increased incidence of urinary tract infection. In one series of more than 1100 children with pyuria, 27% were found to have duplication anomalies of the ureters. This high incidence of infection is associated with two complications of complete duplication, *obstruction* and *vesicoureteral reflux*. In adults, abdominal or flank pain may also be present as the predominant presenting symptom.

Although the lower pole ureter is referred to as the orthotopic ureter, it is not uncommon for both ureteral orifices to be displaced from their normal position in patients with complete duplications. If the lower segment ureter is displaced laterally with respect to the trigone, a shorter ureteral tunnel that is predisposed to vesicoureteral reflux will be present. Such reflux represents the most common source of acquired disease associated with duplication. Similarly, the ureter draining the upper pole moiety enters the bladder in an ectopic location according to the Weigert-Meyer law and its orifice may be stenotic leading to obstruction of this segment. Obstruction of the upper pole moiety may be present without reflux into the lower segment, reflux into the lower segment may be present without upper pole obstruction, or both abnormalities may be present concomitantly.

The radiologic findings in complete ureteral duplication depend on the extent to which complications of the abnormality are present. In uncomplicated duplication, the findings at urography are generally apparent, although it may be difficult to assess whether a complete or partial duplication is present because of variable filling of one of the ureters (Fig. 2.14). In such cases, the use of additional contrast material to ensure a good diuresis or prone radiographs may be helpful. In other cases, relatively subtle urographic findings may be present. Vesicoureteral reflux in the lower segment may produce dilatation that is apparent on urography. Rarely, dilatation of the lower segment will be present from incidental obstruction secondary to a calculus or ureteral stenosis. The presence of vesicoureteral reflux itself is best demonstrated on voiding cystourethrography.

Reflux into the lower moiety during childhood may produce marked scarring and deformity of the lower pole. When discovered in later life, such deformity may mimic a renal mass or infarct. The findings of a diminu-

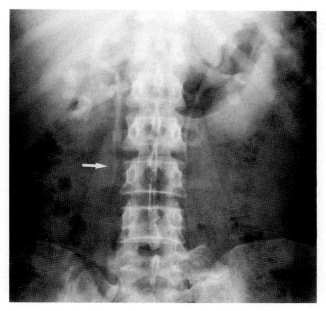

Figure 2.13.   Partial ureteral duplication. The point of junction of the two ureters is clearly demonstrated (*arrow*).

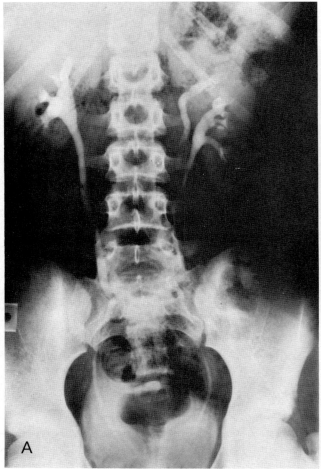

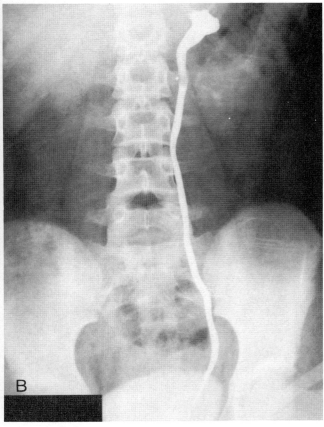

Figure 2.14. Complete duplication. **A,** Urogram demonstrates duplication of the left renal collecting system, however, because of variable filling of the ureters it is not possible to determine whether the duplication is complete. **B,** Retrograde pyelogram shows complete duplication. An air bubble has been inadvertently introduced and produces a filling defect in the proximal ureter.

tive lower pole in a patient with a duplex collecting system has been termed the "nubbin" sign and may be demonstrated by urography, US, or CT.

On sonography, a duplication may be demonstrated on longitudinal scans as two distinct groups of renal sinus echoes. Some investigators have reported, however, that this finding may be absent in a significant number of cases. Uncomplicated duplication may be difficult to demonstrate on CT because of the cross-sectional nature of the technique. Often, the two ureters may be demonstrated on caudal sections, but no one section will demonstrate both renal pelves. Scans obtained through the junction of the upper and lower pole moieties (Fig. 2.15), however, will demonstrate an absence of collecting system elements or renal sinus fat; this feature has been termed the "faceless kidney" and may help identify duplication even in the absence of contrast enhancement.

An obstructed upper pole moiety may be difficult to diagnose because it may be confused with an upper pole

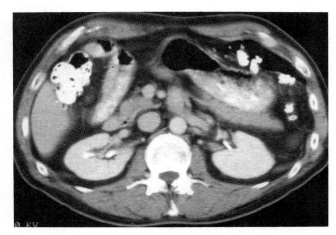

Figure 2.15. Duplicated collecting system. A CT scan between the two renal pelves has been described as a "faceless kidney."

renal mass. On urography, the kidney will retain its reniform shape, but the hydronephrotic upper pole collecting system may not opacify. It may be difficult, at times, to recognize that the nondilated lower calyces, in fact, represent only a portion of the collecting system (Fig. 2.16). With massive hydronephrosis of the upper pole, the lower pole calyces may appear to be displaced downward. This finding has been called the "drooping lily" sign. Recognition of the possibility that the "mass" represents an obstructed duplication should suggest to the examiner that delayed films be obtained. Such radiographs will often demonstrate sufficient opacification to allow the diagnosis to be established.

On sonography the "mass" can often be seen to be connected with a dilated renal pelvis and ureter, thus establishing the correct diagnosis. When there is superimposed infection, however, or the mass cannot clearly be connected with the pelvis, confusion with an upper pole complex mass or even a simple cyst may occur. Computed tomography will also demonstrate the true nature of the mass and may demonstrate contrast material excretion in the upper pole insufficient to be visualized with urography. The dilated but unopacified ureter may be followed to its termination in the bladder in nearly every case. In addition, CT allows a reliable assessment of the amount of renal parenchyma that remains in the upper pole prior to possible renal-sparing surgery.

Antegrade or retrograde pyelography is the method of choice to demonstrate the true extent of a suspected upper moiety obstruction. Percutaneous nephrostomy drainage may be utilized to temporize patients who present with infection prior to definitive surgery.

Ureteral Triplication

Ureteral triplication (Fig. 2.17) is a very rare anomaly that may be present in a variety of different forms. When there are three complete ureters, the anomaly is thought to occur when three ureteral buds arise from the mesonephric duct. In such cases, the segment draining the most caudad segment of the kidney inserts at the trigone while the remaining two are ectopic. In other instances, the anomaly can occur when there are two ureters, one of which is itself bifid or when there are three separate ureters that join to enter the bladder singly. Ureteral triplication is reported to be associated with a high incidence of anomalies of the contralateral kidney.

Blind-ending Ureter

Blind-ending ureter occurs when the ureteral bud fails to associate with the metanephric blastema so that the ureter does not drain any portion of the renal parenchyma. Blind-ending ureter can occur in association with renal agenesis or in association with the formation of a second ureteral bud such that one ureter is present and drains a normal kidney while the second ureter is blind-ending and enters the bladder in an ectopic location. More commonly, the anomaly is found in association with early branching of a single ureteral bud such that a bifid ureter is present, one of which is blind-ending. In such cases, the blind-ending segment is considered to represent a *congenital ureteral diverticulum* (Fig. 2.18). The abnormality can usually be diagnosed by excretory urography because to and fro peristalsis causes filling of the blind-ending segment. In other instances, retrograde pyelography will be required for diagnosis.

Anomalous Termination of the Ureter

The most common anomaly of termination of the ureter, ureterocele, is discussed with anomalies of the bladder.

An *ectopic ureter* is defined as a ureter that does not terminate in the normal location at the trigone of the bladder. By convention, however, the term is used to define a ureter that opens outside the urinary bladder. Eighty percent of ectopic ureters are found in association with complete duplication of the ureter. The anomaly is more common in females by a 6:1 ratio. In males, however, the majority of ectopic ureters drain single systems. With unilateral single ectopia, a hemitrigone will be found in the bladder. In the very rare instance of bilateral single ureteral ectopia, the bladder fails to completely develop and there is no trigone.

Embryologically, the anomaly results when the ureteral bud fails to separate from the mesonephric duct, and, therefore, its orifice opens in a structure that originates either from the urogenital sinus or the wolffian duct (the bladder neck (Fig. 2.19), urethra, seminal vesicles (Fig. 2.20), vas deferens, or ejaculatory duct in males and the bladder neck, vestibule, or urethra in females). In females, ureteral ectopy may also be associated with the uterus, the vagina, or the cervix. Such cases are difficult to explain as these structures are of müllerian origin, however, it has been assumed that some wolffian remnants must be incorporated into the müllerian system for these anomalies to occur.

Clinically, ectopic ureters are associated with urinary infection, obstruction, and, in females, urinary incontinence. In many cases, the abnormalities are not diagnosed until adulthood, particularly when incontinence is absent. In males with ectopic orifices that terminate in the genital tract, symptoms may be delayed until after the onset of sexual activity.

In almost all cases associated with duplication, the orifice of the ectopic ureter is stenotic, resulting in upper moiety obstruction. Thus, the findings on urography will be similar to those described in association with ureteral duplication. If the ectopic orifice terminates within the urinary tract, the diagnosis is usually confirmed during careful cystoscopy and retrograde pyelography. In other cases, sonography or CT may suggest the correct diagno-

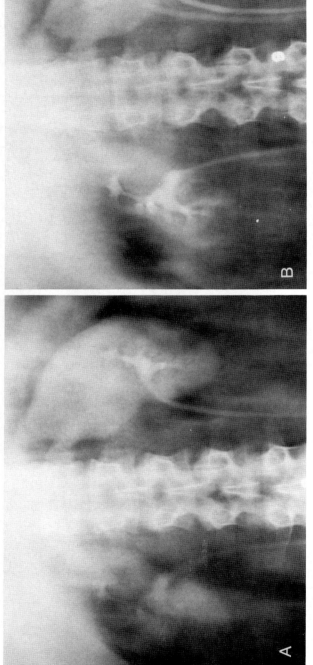

Figure 2.16. Obstructed duplication. **A,** Tomogram demonstrates an apparent "mass" in the upper pole of the left kidney. A small fleck of calcification is seen that was present on the scout film. **B,** Delayed tomogram shows that the "mass" represents an obstructed duplication containing a small calyceal calculus.

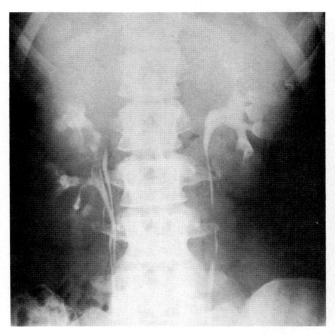

Figure 2.17. Ureteral triplication. Three separate ureters can be seen draining the right kidney.

sis. In cases where ureteral ectopia is associated with a single ureter, a nonfunctioning dysplastic kidney is present on the affected side.

Ureteropelvic Junction Obstruction

Congenital obstruction of the ureteropelvic junction (UPJ) is the most common congenital anomaly of the urinary tract. The disorder produces caliectasis and marked pelviectasis as a result of a functional narrowing of the UPJ. Secondary UPJ obstruction due to an acquired disorder of the renal pelvis or vesicoureteral reflux will not be considered in this section.

The lesion is usually caused by either an intrinsic or extrinsic abnormality of the UPJ. The intrinsic form accounts for 80% of the cases. The precise etiology of intrinsic UPJ obstruction is not known, but many authors postulate that a defect in the circular muscle bundle of the renal pelvis leads to an inability to transmit peristalsis normally. Some authors have considered the abnormality as representing an exaggerated form of an extrarenal pelvis. In other cases, abnormal folds or a kink of the UPJ are present, however, as these findings can be seen without significant UPJ obstruction, their role in the pathogenesis of this disorder has been questioned. Extrinsic lesions are usually caused by aberrant renal vessels that cross anterior to the renal pelvis or proximal ureter; such cases are thought to account for no more than 15–20% of the total (Fig. 2.21).

Congenital UPJ obstruction is the most common cause of an abdominal mass in a neonate. The disorder is being increasingly discovered in the antenatal period because

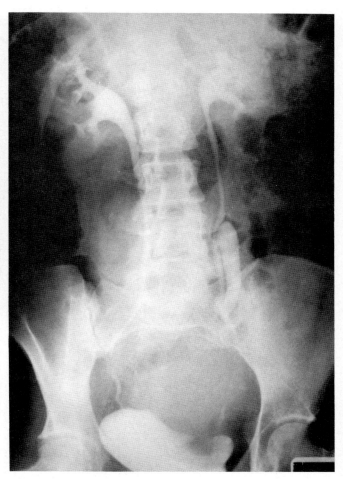

Figure 2.18. Ureteral diverticulum. Oblique film demonstrates origin of a ureteral diverticulum from the junction of the middle and distal thirds of the left ureter.

of the almost routine use of obstetric ultrasound. In a significant number of cases, however, the abnormality is clinically silent until adulthood, when symptoms of flank pain, fever, or, rarely, hypertension cause the patient to seek medical attention. Cases in which presentation has been delayed well into the sixth or seventh decade have been reported. Bilateral UPJ obstruction is present in 10–40% of the cases. Males are affected more often than females by a 2 : 1 ratio and the left side is more commonly affected than the right for unknown reasons. A familial tendency toward the disorder has also been reported.

In some cases, symptoms may only be present in the setting of a sustained diuresis, a condition that has become known as "beer-drinker's hydronephrosis." Such cases have been attributed to a very mild form of UPJ obstruction such that under conditions of normal diuresis the UPJ is compensated. Urograms made while such a patient is asymptomatic may show only an extrarenal pelvis; the use of a diuretic renogram or a urographic study during acute symptoms has been advocated to demonstrate the underlying abnormality.

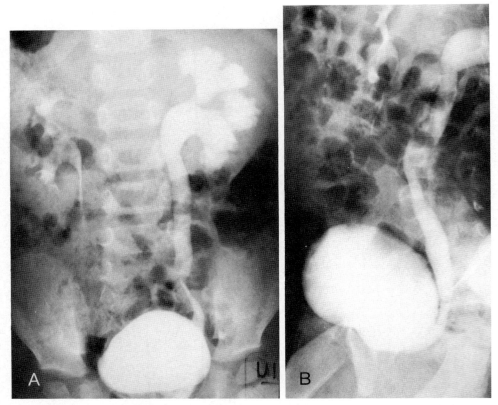

Figure 2.19.   Ectopic ureteral insertion. Anteroposterior **(A)** and oblique **(B)** radiographs in a male child demonstrating an ectopic single left ureter which terminates in the bladder neck.

On urography, a dilated renal pelvis and calyces will be demonstrated. Because of the dilatation, slow opacification of the affected side is the rule and delayed radiographs are usually necessary to demonstrate that the UPJ is, in fact, the point of obstruction (Fig. 2.22). With long-standing or very high-grade obstruction, a virtually non-functioning kidney may be present. The renal pelvis may be markedly dilated (more than 10 cm in diameter) with a ballooned appearance. The UPJ itself may be difficult to visualize; in some cases it appears to join the renal pelvis in a higher or more medial position. Care must be taken to differentiate a true UPJ obstruction from a large ex-

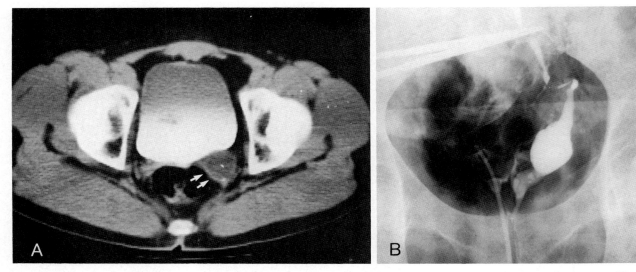

Figure 2.20.   Ectopic ureteral insertion. **A,** Computed tomography scan at the level of the bladder shows a dilated seminal vesicle (*arrows*). **B,** Operative radiograph after injection of contrast material into the ureter (clamped) showing filling of the seminal vesicle and drainage into the posterior urethra.

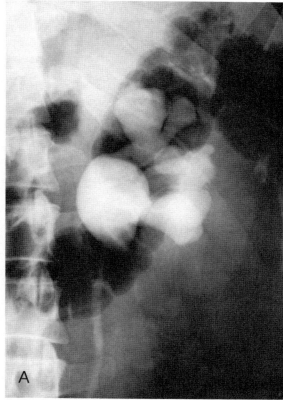

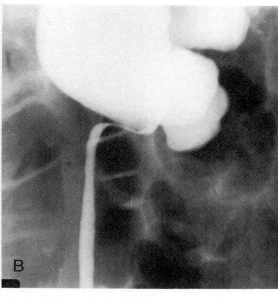

Figure 2.21. UPJ obstruction. Radiograph from an IVP **(A)** demonstrates a dilated renal pelvis and caliectasis. On retrograde pyelography **(B)** a "kink" in the proximal ureter is clearly demonstrated. At surgery, an aberrant lower-pole renal artery was found.

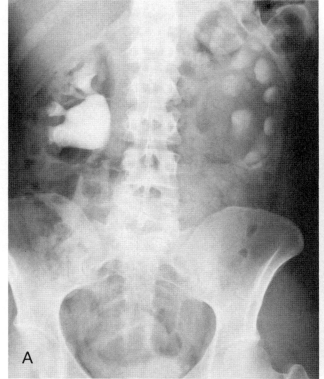

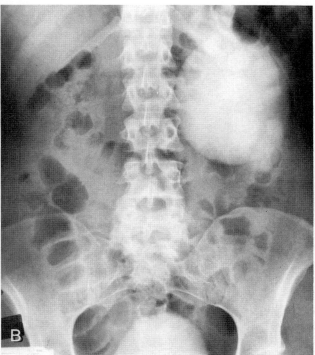

Figure 2.22. Ureteropelvic junction obstruction. **A,** Ten-minute film from an IVP demonstrating dilated calyces with delayed opacification of the remainder of the collecting system. **B,** Twenty-four-hour delayed radiograph shows a markedly dilated renal pelvis.

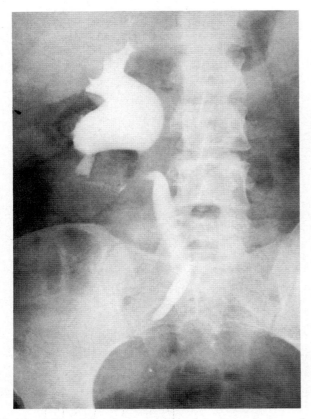

Figure 2.23. Dilated extrarenal pelvis. Retrograde pyelogram showing a dilated extrarenal pelvis. Note that the calyces are not dilated, which helps to differentiate this condition from true UPJ obstruction. Mild fullness of the ureter secondary to pregnancy dilatation is also present.

trarenal pelvis (Fig. 2.23); in the latter case, the renal pelvis may appear quite dilated, however, in the absence of caliectasis, the diagnosis of UPJ obstruction should not be entertained. There may be variable filling of the ureter distal to the UPJ. In the past, it has been suggested that the absence of ureteral filling is an important criterion for determining whether significant obstruction is present; most authorities agree, however, that such an assessment is not reliable. When there is significant kinking of the UPJ, the possibility that the obstruction is secondary to an aberrant vessel should be considered.

When there is insufficient contrast excretion on urography or the ureter itself is not visualized, the diagnosis may be established by either antegrade or retrograde pyelography. The former is preferred as a predecessor to percutaneous nephrostomy; the later may be performed to confirm the diagnosis prior to a contemplated surgical procedure. Most authorities suggest that voiding cystourethrography be performed in all patients with suspected UPJ obstruction to exclude vesicoureteral reflux as a cause of the renal pelvic dilatation.

On sonography (Fig. 2.24), hydronephrosis associated with a very dilated renal pelvis may be readily identified. This finding in association with the inability to demonstrate a dilated ureter suggests the diagnosis of UPJ obstruction with a high degree of certainty. The diagnosis may also be suggested by CT, however, such studies are rarely indicated or necessary in uncomplicated UPJ obstruction.

In patients with equivocal UPJ obstruction, or in cases where there is a discrepancy between the patient's clini-

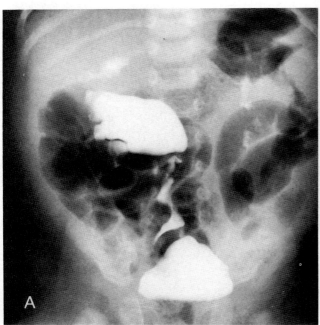

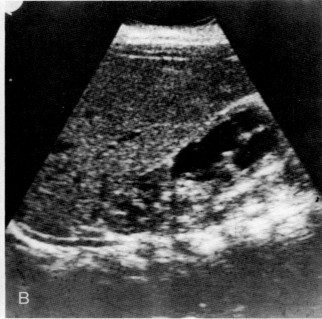

Figure 2.24. Ureteropelvic junction obstruction. Excretory urogram (IVP) **(A)** and sonogram **(B)** demonstrate a UPJ obstruction in the lower-pole moiety of a duplicated renal collecting system.

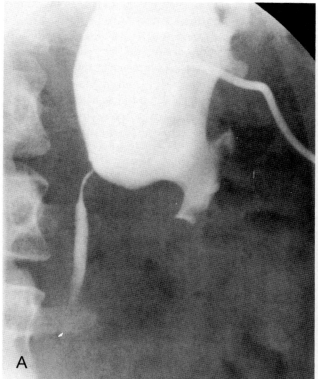
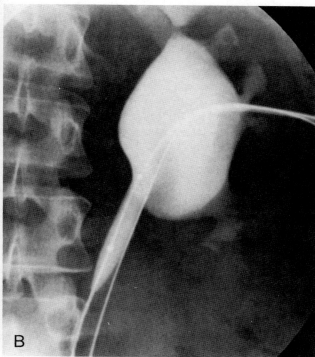

Figure 2.25. Balloon pyeloplasty. **A,** Nephrostogram demonstrates typical appearance of UPJ obstruction. **B,** Balloon catheter has been inflated in the UPJ to perform pyeloplasty.

cal symptoms and the radiologic findings, diuresis renography or the Whitaker procedure may be employed to assess whether functionally significant obstruction is present (see Chapter 14).

Pyeloplasty utilizing one of a number of surgical techniques has been considered the treatment of choice for UPJ obstruction. Recently, however, the use of percutaneous nephrostomy followed by either balloon pyeloplasty (Fig. 2.25) or by endoscopic endopyelotomy has been reported both as a primary procedure and as a secondary procedure in patients in whom surgical therapy has failed. Success rates of 85% have been reported, however, long-term follow-up studies have yet to be completed. The procedure probably should not be used in small infants and has a higher failure rate in patients with extremely redundant renal pelves. Neither technique should be attempted when there is clinical suspicion that the obstruction is secondary to an aberrant vessel unless angiography is first performed to exclude this possibility.

PRUNE BELLY SYNDROME

Prune belly syndrome (Eagle-Barrett syndrome) is a rare congenital syndrome characterized by the classical triad of absent abdominal musculature, undescended testicles, and urinary tract abnormalities initially described in the late 19th century. Although absence of abdominal

musculature has been described in females, the full syndrome including the urinary tract abnormalities only develops in males.

Clinically, the syndrome is recognizable at birth because of the characteristic features produced by the absent abdominal musculature (Fig. 2.26). The deficiency typically affects the lower abdominal wall; the upper abdomen has a normal appearance. In some cases, the muscular defect is either partial or asymmetric. The overlying skin has a wrinkled appearance reminiscent of a prune; in older children the wrinkling tends to disappear and is replaced by a "potbelly" appearance. The precise cause of the syndrome has been a matter of dispute; some authorities believe that the muscular defect is secondary to the distended urinary system that prevents abdominal muscle development. Others have postulated that prostatic dysgenesis and transient neonatal ascites are responsible; still others feel that both the urinary tract abnormalities and the abdominal wall defect are secondary to a mesodermal deficiency.

The urinary tract abnormalities affect the kidneys, the ureters, the bladder, and the urethra. Although the kidneys may be normal, either renal dysplasia or hydronephrosis is often described. The findings in the kidneys tend to be asymmetric with a normal renal unit on one side while the opposite kidney is dysplastic. The ureters tend to be tortuous and dilated (Fig. 2.27), most often in a

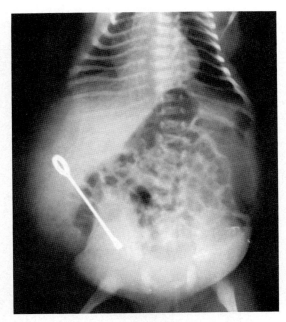

Figure 2.26. Prune belly syndrome. An abdominal radiograph of a newborn with prune belly syndrome shows bulging of the flanks as a result of the absence of abdominal musculature.

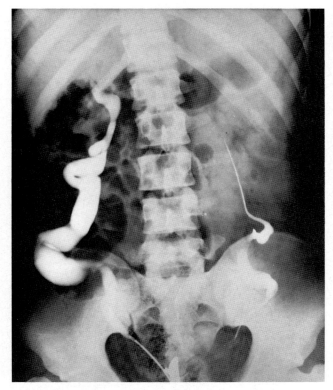

Figure 2.27. Prune belly syndrome. Bilateral retrograde pyelograms show a segmentally dilated, tortuous ureter on the *right*. On the *left,* the ureter is tortuous, dilated, and blind-ending. (Courtesy of Marc Banner, M.D.)

segmental distribution. Vesicoureteral reflux is common. The ureteral abnormalities have been attributed to a deficiency of smooth muscle. The bladder is typically very large and may be associated with a patent urachus. The prostatic urethra is characteristically dilated and tapers rapidly at the membranous urethra in a fashion resembling posterior urethral valves. The dilated urethra is believed secondary to prostatic hypoplasia. The anterior urethra is usually normal, although an association with megalourethra has been described. The testes are cryptorchid, usually in an abdominal location.

Extraurinary abnormalities that may be present include intestinal malrotation, congenital heart defects, and musculoskeletal deformities.

Patients with urinary tract abnormalities characteristic of the prune belly syndrome, but who have normal abdominal musculature, have been described. Such cases are thought to represent an incomplete or variant manifestation of the syndrome.

LOWER URINARY TRACT ANOMALIES

Bladder

Extrophy

The most common congenital bladder lesion is extrophy. It is the result of a deficiency in development of the lower abdominal wall musculature, so that the bladder is open and the mucosa of the bladder is continuous with the skin. There is associated epispadias in which the urethra is open dorsally and urethral mucosa covers the dorsum of a short penis. The condition occurs in one in 50,000 births and has a male/female ratio of 2:1.

Skeletal and gastrointestinal anomalies are commonly associated with extrophy. Diastasis of the symphysis pubis correlates well with the severity of the extrophy-epispadias complex (Fig. 2.28). Over 60% of cases of separation of the symphysis are associated with the extrophy-epispadic anomaly. Approximately 25% are associated with the epispadic anomaly alone. The extrophy-epispadic anomaly is often associated with ureteric obstruction and unilateral or bilateral pelvicaliectasis due to either ureterocele formation or fibrosis at the ureterovesical junction. Umbilical and inguinal hernias are frequently present. The diagnosis is clinical, and management includes ureteral diversion, bladder augmentation, and skin grafting. Radiologic assessment is done in the postoperative period to exclude adenocarcinoma that may develop at the anastomosis years after ureterosigmoidostomy is performed. This complication is not uncommon and radiologic monitoring is mandatory.

Bladder Duplication

Bladder duplication is rare and may be complete or incomplete. Variations include bladder septum, which

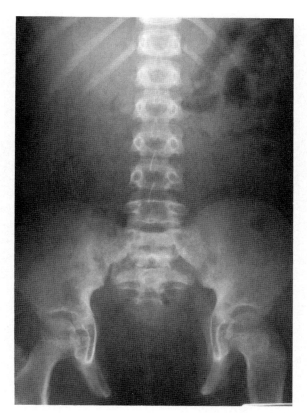

Figure 2.28. Bladder extrophy. Diastasis of the symphysis pubis is commonly associated with bladder extrophy.

may be multiple and which divides the bladder into two or several compartments. The embryogenesis of bladder duplication is not clearly understood. Complete duplication may result from a bifurcation of the cloacal septum resulting in two ventral bladders and urogenital sinuses. In complete duplication both bladders lie side by side, separated by a peritoneal fold. Each bladder has normal musculature and mucosa and the ipsilateral ureter drains into each bladder. Each bladder has separate urethral orifices that may drain into a common urethra with a single penis, or there may also be complete duplication of the urethra and penis. Lower gastrointestinal anomalies are commonly associated.

Incomplete duplication is less common and is not associated with duplication of the external genitalia. Both bladders drain into a common urethral orifice. A bladder septum may divide the bladder into two equal or unequal chambers. Each chamber has a ureteric orifice but the septum may have the distal insertion to one side of the urethral orifice, leading to obstruction of one side. This leads to unilateral intrauterine obstruction resulting in a aplastic or hypoplastic kidney.

Agenesis of the bladder is usually incompatible with life, death resulting from obstruction and renal failure. A few cases of bladder agenesis have been reported in children who lived long enough for a diagnosis to be made. Most of these were females.

Ureterocele

Ureteroceles are classified as either simple or ectopic. A simple ureterocele is commonly an incidental finding on excretory urography and rarely results in clinical symptoms. It is the result of prolapse of ureteric mucosa into the bladder. The prolapsing ureteric mucosa takes with it a layer of bladder mucosa, so that the ureterocele consists of a cavity covered by two layers of mucosa. It is said that the probable cause of the ureterocele is persistence of Chawalla's membrane, which should atrophy in the fetus.

The typical radiologic appearance on excretory urography is that of a cobra head (Fig. 2.29). This is due to the ureterocele containing contrast medium, the double layer of mucosa that is radiolucent, and contrast medium in the bladder. Excretory urography is usually sufficient radiologic assessment for simple ureterocele, but US also shows the ureterocele. Simple ureteroceles are usually small, but if large (Fig. 2.30), they may be complicated by stones within the ureterocele (Fig. 2.31) or by pyelonephritis.

An ectopic ureterocele is a more complex problem and is usually associated with a double collecting system. The upper moiety of a double collecting system has the ureter, which is inserted ectopically. Ectopic sites include the bladder, the seminal vesicles (Fig. 2.32), the prostatic urethra in the male, and the vagina or urethra in the female. The most common ectopic site is within the bladder.

Ectopic ureteroceles are usually large by the time of presentation. Obstruction of the upper moiety of a double collecting system is commonly the result of an ectopic ureterocele (Fig. 2.33). The lower moiety of the double collecting system is more often subject to ureteral reflux.

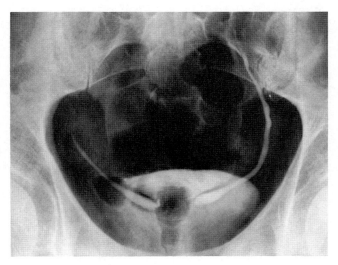

Figure 2.29. Excretory urogram showing bilateral simple ureteroceles with classic cobra head appearance.

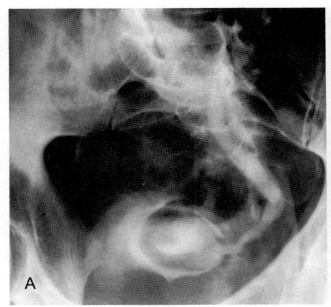

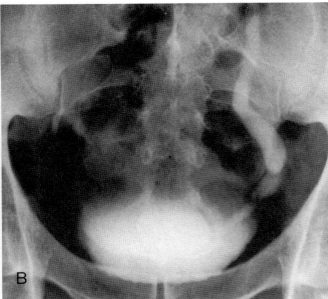

Figure 2.30. **A,** Oblique supine view of excretory urogram showing large simple ureterocele containing contrast medium. The distal one-third of the left ureter is slightly dilated. **B,** Same patient. Upright prevoid film showing ureterocele has filled with contrast medium. The double layer of mucosa compressing the wall of the ureterocele is radiolucent.

The upper moiety of a double collecting system may be seen as having dilated blunt calyces, an intrarenal mass, or the upper moiety collecting system may not be seen at all. In all cases of obstruction of the upper moiety collecting system, the ureter is dilated. The ureterocele is seen as a filling defect in the bladder. Contrast medium is seen within the ureterocele and the double mucosal wall is seen as a radiolucent round or crescentic defect. Occasionally the ureterocele is large enough to obstruct the bladder outflow. When no ureterocele is recognized within the bladder, an extravesical site should be suspected. Clinical assessment for urethral or vaginal ectopic ureterocele is mandatory when an atypical upper pole cystic mass is demonstrated without visualization of an intravesical ureterocele. A vaginogram with injection of

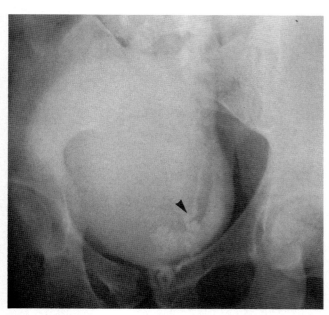

Figure 2.31. Excretory urogram in a patient with left renal colic. A simple ureterocele with ureteric dilatation is seen. The small radiolucent defect at the ureterocele orifice is a small stone (*arrowhead*).

Figure 2.32. Excretory urogram in a patient with lower abdominal and perineal pain. Ectopic insertion of the left ureter into the left seminal vesicle is seen. The ejaculatory duct and refluxing contrast medium into the ampulla of the vas deferens (*arrowhead*) is seen.

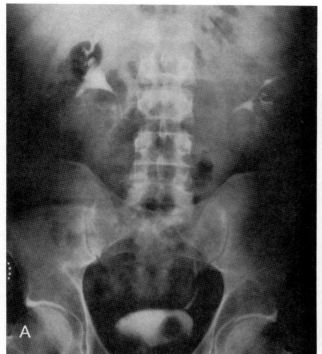

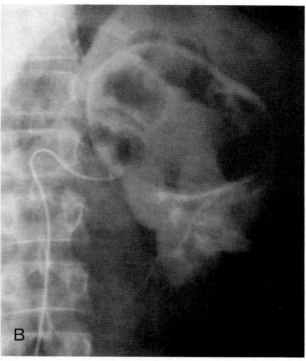

Figure 2.33.   **A,** Excretory urogram showing a left upper pole mass displacing the upper visualized calyx laterally and downward. A filling defect within the bladder represents an ectopic

ureterocele. **B,** Same patient. Selective renal arteriogram showing a large cystic area with thick irregular walls representing the obstructed upper moiety of a double collecting system.

contrast medium into the vagina may reveal the ureterocele. Ultrasound has been shown to be an excellent method of assessing an ectopic ureterocele (Fig. 2.34). Dilated upper pole calyces, a cystic mass in the upper pole, a dilated ureter, and the ectopic ureterocele within the bladder may all be demonstrated. Ureterocele stones

can be clearly seen as bright echoes with acoustic shadowing.

Excretory urography and ultrasound are usually sufficient to make the diagnosis. Computed tomography shows calyceal dilatation or a cystic mass (Fig. 2.35), and transaxial views through the pelvis reveal the ureterocele as a bladder filling defect containing contrast medium.

It is to be emphasized that an upper-pole mass is the most common presentation of an obstructed double col-

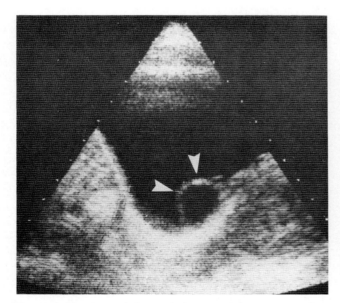

Figure 2.34.   Transabdominal ultrasound showing typical appearance of ectopic ureterocele. (From Weiser WJ, Montanera W: Ultrasonographic demonstration of a ureterocele in an adult: a case report. *Medical Ultrasound* 8:160–161, 1984.)

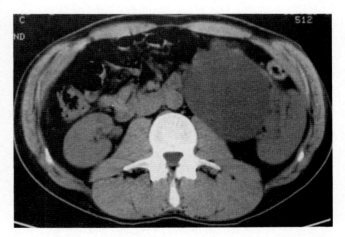

Figure 2.35.   Computed tomography performed for examination of the spine in a patient with back pain. An incidental finding was the large cystic mass which extended from the left upper pole to the pelvis. The cystic mass proved to be an obstructed upper collecting system due to a ureterocele.

lecting system, but it is possible that an obstructed upper pole moiety of a double collecting system may have atrophied, so that no mass effect is present. Most calyceal systems are symmetric. In a symptomatic patient when an unobstructed double collecting system is seen on one side and a single collecting system is seen on the other side without the presence of an upper pole mass, every effort must be made to exclude a double collecting system on the side where a single collecting system is visualized. This includes a urologic search for the ectopic ureterocele, which may not be in the bladder.

Urachal Anomalies

The allantois is the attachment of the bladder dome to the umbilicus. Initially the bladder is an abdominal organ but then descends into the pelvis. As this happens, the bladder dome narrows to form the urachus, which elongates with bladder descent. Normally this umbilical attachment of the bladder becomes completely obliterated as the umbilical ligament in approximately 50% of adults, but a small 1-mm lumen persists in the remainder. Anomalous regression of normal closure of the umbilical ligament includes a patent urachus in which the urachus and ligament are patent and urine can flow from the bladder to the abdominal exterior via the umbilicus. The male:female ratio of patent urachus is 3:1. Failure of closure of the urachus at the bladder attachment results in a urachal cyst. Failure of closure at the umbilical attachment results in an umbilical cyst. Urachal cyst (Fig. 2.36) is usually clinically silent until infection supervenes, consequently the clinical presentation is usually in the adult. Calculi are reported within urachal cysts and may be seen on plain film as small punctate calcifications above the bladder outline. Cystography is usually sufficient to make the diagnosis, oblique views being most helpful.

Müllerian Duct and Prostatic Utricle Cysts

Normal müllerian duct atrophy occurs about the sixth week in the fetus. The vestigial remnants of this ductal obliteration are the prostatic utricle and the appendix of the testis. Nonatrophy of the müllerian duct may produce cystic dilatations along the route of the vas deferens from the scrotum to the ejaculatory ducts. Müllerian duct cysts are rare but most commonly occur deep in the pelvis close to the prostate and not in the midline. They present clinically in the 20- to 40-year age group, and may attain a large size causing obstructive symptoms. If infection supervenes, suprapubic and rectal pain occur. Fluid aspirated from a müllerian duct cyst may be serous, mucoid, purulent, or hemorrhagic. No spermatozoa are present in these cysts.

Prostatic utricle cysts are commonly associated with hypospadias and incomplete testicular descent. The normal prostatic utricle is 8–10 mm in length, narrow at its orifice (2 mm) in the verumontanum, and bulbous at its blind end. These cysts are midline, and congenital cystic dilatation with the above associated findings of hypospadias (Fig. 2.37) and absence of a scrotal testis raises the possibility of intersexuality. Clinical presentation is in the first and second decade as opposed to müllerian duct cysts, which clinically present later.

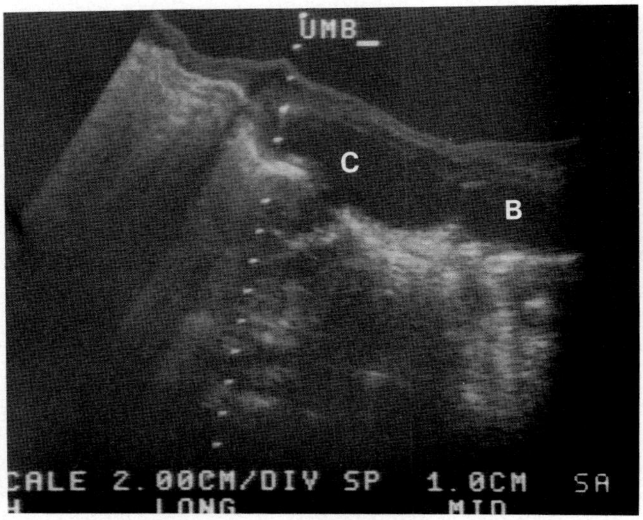

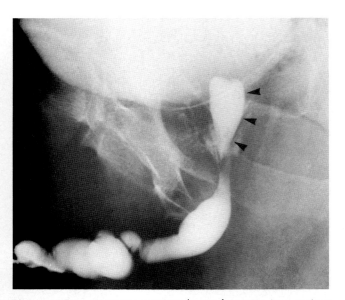

Figure 2.36. Transabdominal US longitudinal scan in a 3 year-old boy with a palpable abdominal mass. The study shows a urachal cyst (C) with clear definition of space between the cyst and the bladder (B). (Courtesy of A. Daneman, M.D.)

Figure 2.37. Dynamic retrograde urethrogram in a patient with hypospadias and multiple postoperative anterior urethral strictures. Congenital cystic dilatation of the prostatic utricle (*arrowheads*) is demonstrated. (From McCallum RW, Colapinto V. *Urologic Radiology of the Adult Male Lower Urinary Tract.* Springfield, IL, Charles C Thomas, 1976, p 55.)

Seminal Vesicles

Congenital seminal vesicle anomalies result from interruption or failure of the normal development of the mesonephric duct. The mesonephric duct develops ureteric buds dorsomedially after 5 weeks of gestation. The ureteric buds grow cranially and dorsally to meet the nephrogenic ridge and form the metanephros, which becomes the normal kidney. As fetal growth continues, the ureters derive separate openings into the bladder, and the mesonephric duct moves caudally and ends as the ejaculatory duct. Small buds develop in the distal mesonephric duct that become the seminal vesicles.

Any deviation of the development of the ureteric bud or seminal vesicle bud results in a congenital anomaly. When both buds fail to develop, the ipsilateral kidney, ureter, hemitrigone, and seminal vesicle are lost. Failure to develop the normal ureteric bud results in renal agenesis and a normal seminal vesicle. Failure to develop a normal seminal vesicle bud results in a normal kidney, ureter, and hemitrigone and absent seminal vesicle. Abnormal development of the distal mesonephric bud may result in atresia of the seminal vesicle duct, resulting in seminal vesicle obstruction producing a seminal vesicle cyst (Fig. 2.38). Seminal vesicle cyst is commonly associated with ipsilateral absence of the kidney and ureter. Rarely, the anomaly involves delay in the origin of the ureteric bud such that the seminal vesicle bud gives rise to the ureteric bud resulting in ectopic insertion of the ureter into the seminal vesicle. Seminal vesicle cysts rarely enlarge enough to be of clinical significance. They most commonly present in the third decade but have

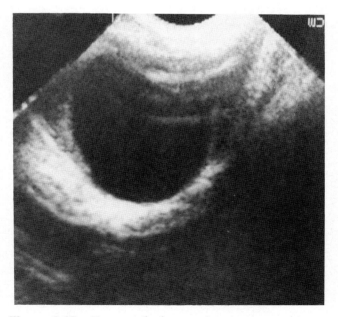

Figure 2.38. Transrectal ultrasound in a 50-year-old man with lower abdominal pain. A 4-cm cyst is seen arising from the left seminal vesicle.

been reported up to the age of 60 years. When large, patients present clinically with urgency, frequency, and dysuria. Pelvic and perineal pain are common.

Urethra

Congenital Lesions

Most congenital urethral lesions are obstructive and consequently produce vesical and ureteric dilatation. Severe obstruction results in gross hydronephrosis with renal obstructive atrophy. Because the lower urinary tract has completely formed by the end of the fourth month of gestation and fetal micturition also occurs at this time, complete obstruction may lead to intrauterine death. Incomplete obstruction may be compatible with a live birth, but failure to thrive and vomiting in the neonate or early life are symptoms of renal failure, which raises the possibility of outlet obstruction from a urethral anomaly.

Posterior Urethral Valves

The continuation of the inferior aspect of the verumontanum is the urethral crest, which is a mucosal fold that is originally midline but divides into two to four fins (plicae colliculi) that take a spiral course to end inferiorly in the membranous urethra, anteriorly and midline. These plicae colliculi are vestigeal remnants of the migrating wolffian duct orifices. When the origin of the wolffian duct orifice is too far anterior, normal migration is altered leading to abnormal fusion and insertion of the plicae colliculi and resulting in thick valve cusps.

In 1919, Young classified urethral valves into three types. Type 1 is the most common and produces clinical manifestations (Fig. 2.39) that are present in the bulbomembranous urethra. Type 2 posterior urethral valves are mucosal folds extending proximally from the verumontanum to the bladder neck. These are rare and there is controversy as to whether their presence is primary or secondary in outlet obstruction. Type 3 posterior urethral valves are also rare and unrelated to the verumontanum. They occur in the membranous urethra as a disc-like membrane with a central pinhole orifice.

CLINICAL PRESENTATION. Posterior urethral valves are the most common cause of obstructive symptoms and occur only in males. The condition may cause complete obstruction leading to renal failure, oligohydramnios, and intrauterine death. The massive hydrostatic pressure on the calyx may cause calyceal rupture leading to fetal intracapsular, perirenal, or intrarenal urinomas. Fetal urine ascites may also occur. Neonatal clinical diagnosis therefore includes palpable kidneys and bladder, abdominal distention, ascites, straining to void, absence of a urinary stream, and dribbling. Blood urea nitrogen and creatinine levels are usually elevated, indicating renal impairment. Commonly renal function returns to normal after

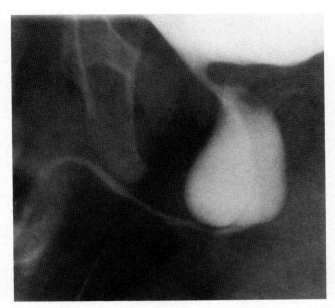

Figure 2.39. Voiding cystourethrogram in a 2-year-old boy. The posterior urethra is dilated down to the membranous urethra. The valves are visible. (Courtesy of A. Daneman, M.D.)

the obstruction is relieved. Occasionally, chronic renal failure progresses in spite of surgical intervention to relieve obstruction.

Young children may present with symptoms of urinary tract infection. Fever, vomiting, and hematuria lead to an investigation of the urinary tract when some degree of outlet obstruction is demonstrated. Vesicorenal reflux may result in pyelonephritis that can become chronic and lead to failure to thrive.

The degree of obstruction due to posterior urethral valves may be so mild that investigation is delayed until superimposed infection occurs. This is the case in older children and young adults when urinary tract investigation leads to the diagnosis. The variability of the degree of obstruction may lead to dilemmas of diagnosis and management. Children and young adults have been mistakenly diagnosed as neurogenic bladder. It is therefore mandatory to include posterior urethral valves in the differential diagnosis of urinary tract infection or outlet obstruction in male infants, children, and young adults.

Radiology

PRENATAL DIAGNOSIS. Urinary tract anomalies and their effects can be demonstrated early in fetal life by US. The incidence of urinary tract anomalies demonstrated by US is 0.2%. The kidneys and bladder are recognizable and functioning by 14–16 weeks of gestation, and the bladder size should vary by partially emptying every hour. Failure of intrauterine micturition results in oligohydramnios, which results in pulmonary hypoplasia and a small thorax. The prenatal ultrasonic demonstration of dilated renal pelves, dilated tortuous ureters, and distended bladder with oligohydramnios are indicative of fetal outlet obstruction. The prenatal demonstration of outlet obstruction is an indication for intrauterine surgery or early fetal delivery, to reduce the incidence of chronic renal failure in infants. The pelvicalyceal dilatation may be reduced or absent if decompression has occurred by the rupture of a calyceal fornix producing an intracapsular, perirenal, or intrarenal urinoma. Careful examination of the bladder may reveal an open bladder neck and dilated posterior urethra, an almost pathognomonic finding in outlet obstruction due to posterior urethral valves.

POSTNATAL DIAGNOSIS. Neonates with impaired renal function are best examined by ultrasound. Excretory urography is less useful in impaired renal function and is contraindicated in severe renal function impairment. Renal function and the degree of renal damage can be best evaluated by renal isotope studies. Technetium -99m diethylenetriaminepentacetic acid (^{99m}Tc-DTPA) or technetium -99m glucoheptonate (^{99m}Tc-GH) are the isotopes of choice. The degree of hydronephrosis and differential renal function can be assessed and, in addition, pinpoint the site of obstruction causing the hydronephrosis. ^{99m}Tc-DTPA can be followed by furosemide (Lasix), causing a diuresis and a differentiation of obstruction from nonobstructive hydronephrosis.

In older children and young adults with normal renal function, excretory urography provides an estimation of the degree of hydronephrosis, a comparison of function of the kidneys, and an evaluation of the bladder. Voiding cystourethrography at the end of the urogram may demonstrate the posterior urethral valves.

Posterior urethral valves are best demonstrated in children and young adults by voiding cystourethrography (Fig. 2.39). There is no difficulty with the insertion of a catheter into the bladder in type 1 valves, but catheter insertion may be difficult in type 3 valves. If a dynamic retrograde study is used to fill the bladder, the retrograde study is usually normal. Bladder filling demonstrates a large-capacity bladder, bladder trabeculation and diverticula, vesicoureteral reflux, and occasionally a Hutch diverticulum (periureteric in the presence of reflux). Reflux is present in 50% of cases presenting in the first year of life. The voiding study demonstrates a dilated posterior urethra and a linear radiolucent defect in the bulbomembranous urethra representing the posterior urethral valves. There is also commonly a hypertrophied posterior bladder lip causing relative narrowing of the bladder neck. The urinary stream is usually reduced distal to the demonstrated valves in the membranous urethra.

Type 2 posterior urethral valves are not true valves and may be seen extending proximally from the verumontanum in any patient with outlet obstruction distal to the verumontanum. These hypertrophied mucosal folds have been demonstrated in adult patients with urethral stricture, resulting from trauma or infection.

Transrectal voiding sonourethrography may be useful in young adults suspected of having posterior urethral valves. Transrectal ultrasound with the patient voiding can demonstrate the bladder abnormalities and the dilated prostatic urethra. The obstruction can be pinpointed to the membranous urethra but it is doubtful that the valves can be visualized.

Fibromyoma

Fibromyoma in the urethra is rare and is of embryonic origin, usually originating in the prostate and projecting into the urethra. It occurs in infancy and presents with difficulty in micturition or intermittent stream stoppage that may progress to retention. These symptoms are usually present from birth. Unlike a fibrous polyp, the fibroma has no stalk and on cystourethrography is seen as a filling defect in the prostatic urethra, generally at the level of the verumontanum.

Atresia Ani-urethralis

Anal atresia in the male may produce a fistulous tract between the bowel and posterior urethra, resulting in increased angulation of the posterior urethra so that catheter passage into the bladder may be difficult. If the fistulous tract is untreated, recurrent urinary tract infection may result in reflux nephropathy and renal failure. Treatment of the anal atresia by colostomy is insufficient since urine passes along the fistulous tract into the bowel forming "bowel calculi," the result of urinary crystalloids combining with colonic mucous.

Anterior Urethral Anomalies

MEATAL STENOSIS. Congenital meatal stenosis can account for severe outlet obstruction in the male and can produce the same degree of hydronephrosis, bladder dilatation, and trabeculation as urethral valves. Meatal stenosis of this degree is a much less common cause of hydronephrosis than is posterior urethral valves. Catheter insertion through the external meatus is difficult or impossible. The stenosis may be dilated as a temporizing procedure but requires a meatal urethroplasty for complete cure. There may be an associated wide-necked diverticulum arising from the urethra within the glans penis. Voiding cystourethrography through a suprapubic cystostomy tube demonstrates dilatation of the entire urethra, and an associated diverticulum may be demonstrated. Meatal stenosis in female infants is less common than in males and is usually managed by simple dilatation.

HYPOSPADIAS. In hypospadias, the external urethral meatus is found on the ventral surface of the penis anywhere from just proximal to the glans penis to the penoscrotal junction (Fig. 2.37). It is usually asymptomatic until bladder training has been completed after which the urinary stream is found to be difficult to direct and may be a

sprayed stream. Urethroplasty is required with the formation of a new urethra passing through the glans.

EPISPADIAS. Epispadias is less common than hypospadias. The external urethral orifice opens onto the dorsum of the penis, and urethroplasty as for hypospadias is required for correction.

Congenital Urethral Diverticulum

Congenital urethral diverticulum is said to occur only in male infants and children and to arise from the ventral surface of the anterior urethra. Urethral diverticulum in the adult female is thought to be acquired. However, there is no way of knowing that a female urethral diverticulum has not been present since birth and only presents in later life when superimposed infection occurs. In the male, anterior urethral diverticulum is the result of either failure of closure of urethral folds or an abortive attempt at urethral duplication. When the latter is the cause, there are usually associated anterior urethral valves in the region of the penoscrotal junction. The diverticulum has a narrow neck and fills slowly during voiding. As the diverticulum fills, it increases in size and narrows the true urethra. This may cause obstruction resulting in incomplete bladder emptying and bladder infection. At the end of micturition, the diverticulum causes dribbling. Removal of the diverticulum requires urethroplasty to repair the defect in the urethral floor.

Urethral Duplication

No satisfactory embryologic explanation has been suggested to explain duplication that may be complete or incomplete.

In complete duplication in the male, the anomalous urethra may be anterior or posterior to the true urethra and has a separate opening into the bladder and a separate external meatus. It may be accompanied by either bladder or penile duplication or both. The two urethras lie one above the other in males, but may be side by side in females. When the anomalous urethra lies outside the control of the internal and distal sphincter mechanism, urinary incontinence is the presenting symptom. The anomalous urethra has either an epispadiac or hypospadiac external meatus and is subject to recurrent infection. Indications for removal of the anomalous urethra are urinary incontinence and urethritis in the anomalous urethra.

In incomplete duplication there may be two external meati with the two urethras joining in the region of the penoscrotal junction (Fig. 2.40). A double urethra may have formed in the bulbous urethra with the anomalous urethra having a hypospadiac opening inferiorly at the penoscrotal junction. An accessory urethra is an incomplete duplication with an external meatus but no communication with the bladder or proximal urethra. The accessory urethra is subject to infection and may present

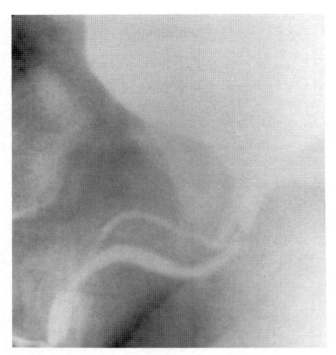

Figure 2.40. Incomplete urethral duplication. The two urethras join in the proximal bulbous urethra. The incomplete duplication is epispadic. (Courtesy of M. Asch, M.D., and D. Marcuzzi, M.D.)

as a purulent discharge from the epispadiac or hypospadiac meatus. Retrograde injection of contrast medium into the abnormal orifice will delineate the accessory urethra. Persistent recurrent infection requires surgical removal of the accessory urethra.

Congenital Urethral Stricture

Congenital urethral stricture has been reported in children but not in neonates or infants. It is questionable whether urethral stricture is ever congenital. More likely they are the result of some form of trauma. The classic site for congenital urethral stricture is in the bulbous urethra adjacent to the penoscrotal junction.

Retention Cyst of Cowper's Duct or Accessory Cowper's Glands

Cowper's glands are two pea-sized glands lying within or at the inferior fascia of the urogenital diaphragm. The ducts of these glands are long and extend from the urogenital diaphragm inferiorly and pass through the corpus spongiosum to enter the midbulbous urethra on both sides of midline. Rarely the ducts join before entering the urethra as a single opening. Small accessory Cowper's glands are multiple small projections of glandular tissue arising from the distal end of the ducts adjacent to the bulbous urethra. Cowper's glands secrete mucin that is a lubricator for semen and adds coagulation to spermatozoa during ejaculation. Cowper's duct or accessory gland

cysts have been reported in newborn infants and are thought to be the result of a congenital malformation of the ostia producing ductal or glandular obstruction resulting in retention cyst swelling. The retention cyst projects into the bulbous urethra and may cause minor urinary symptoms such as frequency or strangury, and large retention cysts may cause obstructive symptoms. Retention cysts of Cowper's ducts may burst spontaneously into the urethra without causing symptoms and may be more common than appreciated. Retention cysts in adults are generally the result of an inflammatory process such as infection or trauma.

On urethrography, a retention cyst of Cowper's duct or accessory gland is seen as a filling defect in the floor of the mid- or distal bulbous urethra or as an indentation in the floor of the bulbous urethra.

Scrotal Contents

The undescended testicle commonly occurs as an isolated phenomenon or it may be associated with other urogenital anomalies such as renal agenesis or ectopia, prune belly syndrome, and epispadias. Up to 20% of premature and preterm males are born with undescended testes. In most of these infants normal descent into the scrotum occurs within the first few weeks to months of life. Less than 3% of all males have persistent undescended testes, more commonly unilateral.

The undescended testicle is often smaller than the normal descended testis. In a small number of these patients there is testicular agenesis. The most common ectopic position for the undescended testicle is in the inguinal canal. However, arrested descent of the testes may occur in the abdomen, pelvis, or high in the scrotum after passage through the inguinal canal. Failure of normal testicular descent into the scrotum is due to either hormonal dysfunction or mechanical obstruction. The hormonal stimulus for testicular descent is testosterone, the production of which by the fetus is dependent on adenohypophyseal gonadotrophin. Abnormality in the secretion of either hormone may result in arrested descent of the testes. Gonadotrophin secretion is commonly normal, but the normal response of the gubernaculum in guiding the testes into the scrotum is lacking.

The testis itself may be abnormally formed resulting in a lack of testosterone production. When secretion of gonadotrophin and testosterone are normal, arrested descent is due to mechanical obstruction. Since the most common site for undescended testicle is in the inguinal canal, one can assume that hormonal secretion has been normal in order to get the testes so far descended, and that the lack of further descent is mechanical, either due to obstruction of the process vaginales or to the formation of a septum at the scrotal neck. Complications of the undescended testicle include malignant change, sterility, and testicular torsion. A testis arrested in the inguinal canal is also subject to accidental injury. The incidence of malignant change in the undescended testicle is high. In the normal male population the incidence is approximately 2:100,000. This increases to 10:100,000 in inguinally placed undescended testis and the rate is even higher in arrested descent in the pelvis or abdomen.

Imaging modalities that have been used in the detection of undescended testicle include excretory urography, ultrasound, CT, isotope studies, angiography, spermatic venography, and herniography. Ultrasound is useful in the detection of the undescended testicle when the arrest is in the inguinal canal. It is of little value in the detection of arrested descent in the abdomen or pelvis unless malignant change has occurred producing a mass. High-frequency transducers can successfully define the undescended inguinal testis in most cases. Both sides should be examined for symmetry. An asymmetric mass in the inguinal region with the echogenic characteristics of the normal testes is the common finding. However the mediastinum testes must be identified. Rarely, the pars infravaginales gubernaculi (PIG) can present a similar echogenic appearance to the testis and may be distant from the undescended testis that may be in the pelvis. The PIG does not show the characteristic mediastinum testes. The undescended testis that is atrophic is more difficult to identify since the echogenicity of the atrophic testis may be variable and, unlike the normal testis, the epididymis may not be seen. Malignant change in the undescended testis is seen on US as a mass of indefinable echogenicity in the inguinal canal.

Computed tomography accurately identifies the undescended testicle in any position adjacent to the inguinal canal (Fig. 2.41). Tomographic cuts are obtained every 5 mm from the scrotum up to the iliac crest. Normally structures in this region are symmetric. In undescended testes there is asymmetry with the presence of a small

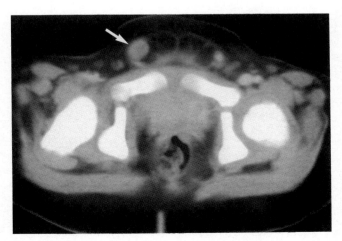

Figure 2.41.   Underscended testicle. A CT scan through the level of the symphysis pubis demonstrates the right testis (*arrow*) in the inguinal canal.

mass on the affected side corresponding to the undescended testicle. An asymmetric mass larger than the expected testicular size raises the possibility of malignant change. Since an undescended testicle may be as small as 1 cm in size, oral and transrectal contrast medium is necessary to delineate bowel. Intravenous contrast medium may be administered to produce an increase in density in the undescended testicle.

The normal spermatic cord may be identified low in the inguinal canal medial and anterior to the femoral vessels. The cord usually contains fat and is a little larger than the femoral vessels. If the undescended testis lies in the inguinal canal, the spermatic cord of the undescended testicle is not seen at the level of the normal spermatic cord. As sequential cephalad images are obtained, a mass representing the undescended testicle will be demonstrated. In such a case the spermatic cord may be seen in the inguinal canal due to normal evolution of the vas deferens.

Spermatic venography is useful in identifying the nonpalpable undescended testicle. Localization of the abdominal or pelvic undescended testicle is demonstrated by visualization of the pampiniform plexus, which is seen as a collection of linear coalescing vessels. Agenesis of the testis is demonstrated when no pampiniform plexus is seen and the spermatic vein exhibits a blind end. In film interpretation, care should be taken not to mistake the epididymal veins for the pampiniform plexus. The epididymal veins are commonly much lower in the abdomen or pelvis than the pampiniform plexus, since the vas deferens and epididymis descend ahead of the testes. Successful demonstration of the pampiniform plexus is approximately 80% on the left. Because of more difficult catheterization of the right spermatic vein and the fact that valves are more common in the right spermatic vein, successful demonstration of the right pampiniform plexus is reduced to 60%. Spermatic arteriography is a difficult procedure to perform, causes significant patient discomfort, and is rarely required.

Herniography may be of value in locating an undescended testis. The method includes the injection of dilute water-soluble contrast medium into the peritoneal cavity. The amount of contrast medium injected varies between 10 and 60 ml depending on the patient's weight. Radiographs are obtained in the prone position with the head of the table elevated 35°. Eighty percent of boys with undescended testis are said to show a patent processus vaginalis or hernia sac, and the undescended testis can be identified within the inguinal canal as a filling defect in the contrast medium-filled hernia sac.

SUGGESTED READINGS

Upper Urinary Tract Anomalies

Blair D, Rigsby C, Rosenfield AT: The nubbin sign on computed tomography and sonography. Urol Radiol 9:149, 1987.

Cronan JJ, Amis ES, Zeman RK, et al: Obstruction of the upper pole moiety in renal duplication in adults: CT evaluation. *Radiology* 161:17, 1986.

Curtis JA, Pollack HM: Renal duplication with a diminutive lower pole: The nubbin sign. *Radiology* 131:327, 1979.

Curtis JA, Sadhu V, Steiner RM: Malposition of the colon in right renal agenesis ectopia, and anterior nephrectomy. *AJR* 129:845, 1977.

Fallat ME, Skoog SJ, Belman AB, Eng G and Randolph JG: The prune belly syndrome: a comprehensive approach to management. *J Urol* 142:802, 1989.

Gay BB, Jr, Dawes RK, Atkinson GE, et al: Wilms' tumor in horseshoe kidneys: Radiologic diagnosis. *Radiology* 146:693, 1983.

Goodman JD, Norton KI, Carr L, et al: Crossed fused renal ectopia: Sonographic diagnosis. *Urol Radiol* 8:13, 1986.

Hadar H, Gadoth N, Gillon G: Computed tomography of renal agenesis and ectopy. *J Comput Assist Tomogr* 8:137, 1984.

Horgan JG, Rosenfield NS, Weiss RM, et al: Is renal ultrasound a reliable indicator of a nonobstructed duplication anomaly? *Pediatr Radiol* 14:388, 1984.

Young HH, Frontz WA and Baldwin JC: Congenital obstruction of the posterior urethra. *J Urol* 2:298, 1919.

Hulnick DH, Bosniak MA: "Faceless Kidney": CT sign of renal duplicity. *J Comput Assist Tomogr* 10(5):771, 1986.

Lee WJ, Badlani GH, Karlin GS, et al: Treatment of ureteropelvic strictures with percutaneous pyelotomy: experience in 62 patients. *AJR* 151:515, 1988.

Macpherson RI: Supernumerary kidney: typical and atypical features. *J Can Assoc Radiol* 38:116, 1987.

Mascatello VJ, Smith EH, Carrera GE, et al: Ultrasonic evaluation of the obstructed duplex kidney. *AJR* 129:113, 1977.

Perlmutter AD, Retic AB, Bauer SB: Anomalies of the upper urinary tract. In Walsh PC, Gittes RF, Perlmutter AD, Stamey TA (eds): Campbell's Urology. Philadelphia, WB Saunders, 1986, p 1665.

Prune Belly Syndrome

Berdon WE, Baker DH, Wigger JH, et al: The radiologic and pathologic spectrum of the prune belly syndrome. Radiol Clin North Am 15(1):83, 1977.

Greskovich FJ, Nyberg LM: The prune belly syndrome: a review of its etiology, defects, treatment and prognosis. J Urol 140:707, 1988.

Lower Urinary Tract Anomalies

Amins M, Wheeler CS: Selective venography in abdominal cryptorchidism. *J Urol* 115:760, 1976.

Lee JKT, McClennan BL, Stanley RJ, et al: Utility of computed tomography in localisation of the undescended testicle. *Radiology* 135:121, 1980.

Rifkin MD: *Diagnostic Imaging of the Lower Genitourinary Tract.* New York, Raven Press, 1985, p 253.

Weiser WJ, Montanera W: Ultrasonographic demonstration of a ureterocele in an adult: a case report. *Medical Ultrasound* 8:160, 1984.

White JJ, Shaker IH, Oh JS, et al: Herniography: a diagnostic refinement in the management of cryptorchidism. *Am Surg* 39:624, 1973.

CHAPTER 3

EXAMINATION TECHNIQUES

CONTRAST-DEPENDENT TECHNIQUES

Excretory Urography

Excretory urography, despite recent declines in its popularity, remains the cornerstone of radiologic diagnosis of the urinary tract. The strength of the urogram lies in its ability to provide an overall survey of the urinary tract, superb anatomic information about the kidney, and information about renal function. Thus, a disease process that is primarily manifested by an acute impairment of renal excretion, e.g., unilateral ureteral obstruction, without much change in renal anatomy, may be readily diagnosed by urography. The strength of the urogram is also its greatest limitation; when the ability of the kidneys to excrete the contrast is impaired, the information obtained from the study is markedly reduced.

The decline in the number of urograms being performed is a result of increased availability of other imaging studies of the urinary tract, the need for cost containment, a hesitancy to expose certain patients to contrast material, as well as the elimination of urography as a screening study for patients with nonspecific complaints. However, for patients with specific complaints related to the urinary tract i.e., flank pain, hematuria, urinary retention, and other such complaints, urography remains a highly efficacious and cost-effective examination. One recent review of more than 3000 patients demonstrated that to detect 95% of the patients who have some abnormality, 90% of patients would have had to be studied. This is a higher efficacy rate than for other common radiologic studies, i.e., upper gastrointestinal series, barium enema, and cranial CT. In the preceding studies, the detection of any abnormality was considered a "positive" study.

Other authors have approached the study of urographic efficacy in a different fashion. If one looks at the therapeutic implication of specific findings, rather than the detection of any abnormality as a "positive" examination, a different result is obtained. Both Donker and Bauer demonstrated that routine urography prior to prostatectomy did not significantly alter the therapy in the group of patients they studied. Similarly, routine urograms in patients with recurrent urinary tract infection has been shown to yield little information that directly affects the patient's therapy. The value of urography in selected patients with urinary tract infection, however, remains unquestioned (see Chapter 7). Other situations in which the value of routine urography has been questioned include patients with stress urinary incontinence, patients undergoing hysterectomy, and as a screening study to exclude a renovascular cause for hypertension.

Routine Urogram

It is incumbent on the radiologist to monitor closely the technical factors employed during urography to optimize the diagnostic information obtained from the study. A film screen combination with a relatively long gray scale should be employed. Close attention should be paid to positioning and collimation, and the films should be free from artifacts and not degraded by respiratory motion. To optimize the subject contrast, a KvP no higher than 60–75 with the MAS varying with the patient's size should be employed.

The advisability of routine bowel preparation with laxatives prior to urography remains unsettled. Many radiologists feel that if routine tomography is employed, there is no necessity to "cleanse" the bowel prior to urography. Others feel that this procedure, although uncomfortable for the patient, may improve the quality of the study and should be employed when urography is performed on an elective basis. This is particularly true when renal calculi are suspected because fecal material in the colon may obscure their presence.

When bowel preparation is desired, we prefer the use of an oral laxative administered 12–18 hours prior to the examination, supplemented by a rectal suppository on the morning of the examination. Care should be exercised that the patient does not become inadvertently dehydrated as a result of the bowel preparation.

When symptoms are acute, there is little justification to deny urography merely because the patient has not received bowel preparation. It is not advisable to employ cleansing enemas in this situation, as a large quantity of air inadvertently introduced during the enema may obscure detail further. Solid food should be withheld for several hours prior to the examination so that the patient's stomach will be empty if emesis should occur after injection of the contrast material, but dehydration should be avoided.

There is no universally accepted filming sequence for an excretory urogram. Perhaps in no other radiologic study is there such variability in both the number and sequence of films that are made as part of a "routine" urogram. "Optimal" urography is most likely to be obtained if the study is monitored by the radiologist and modified to answer the clinical question posed. Certain essential features include the following:

THE SCOUT FILM. The preliminary or scout radiograph is an indispensable part of every excretory urogram. This is usually performed as a single radiograph that includes the upper abdomen and pelvis. If the patient is too large to fit on a single film, a second collimated radiograph of either the kidneys or the pelvis to include the symphysis pubis should be obtained. A preliminary tomogram should also be made to evaluate the technique and the level of tomographic cuts to be obtained after the contrast material is injected.

Scout films may reveal errors in positioning or radiographic technique that must be corrected prior to the injection of contrast material. Calcifications within the urinary tract must also be detected prior to contrast injection, as they are often obscured after the contrast administration. Oblique scout films or tomograms of the kidneys may be obtained to help distinguish renal from overlying calcifications. Oblique films, however, to determine whether a calcification lies in the urinary tract, but outside the kidney, are of no value as the precise course of the ureter cannot be determined until after contrast material is injected. The detection of calcification in the lower urinary tract (i.e., the bladder or ureter) is equally important. Faintly opaque bladder stones may be easily overlooked, and their subsequent discovery may be a source of embarrassment to the responsible radiologist.

Another use of the scout radiograph is to detect abnormal soft tissue densities. The presence of unilateral or even bilateral small kidneys may be a clue to the nature of the underlying pathology. Enlargement or displacement of an organ can often be detected while loss of the psoas silhouette may represent underlying pathology in the retroperitoneum.

Detection of abnormal gas collections is also an important role of the scout radiograph. The presence of free intraperitoneal air or gas within the biliary tree or gallbladder may be important evidence that the gastrointestinal tract rather than the urinary tract is the source of the patient's complaints. Detection of air within the urinary tract almost always signals important underlying pathology, including the presence of infection or a fistulous communication between the urinary tract and the gastrointestinal tract. The presence of a small amount of air in the urinary bladder in a patient with a Foley catheter, however, may be normal as air can be introduced during placement of the catheter.

Bone abnormalities may also indicate the presence of underlying urinary tract pathology. Characteristic osteoblastic metastases from carcinoma of the prostate may be the first indicator of this disease. The presence of an abnormal spinal column may be the clue to urinary tract dysfunction on the basis of a neurogenic bladder.

EARLY NEPHROGRAM FILMS. The rate of excretion of the contrast material is directly related to the level of the plasma concentration of the contrast material. Therefore, the nephrogram is at its peak intensity with maximum concentrations in the nephron 30 seconds to 1 minute after the injection of contrast material (Fig. 3.1). An immediate postinjection coned view of the kidneys or a tomogram of the kidneys will allow the best visualization of the renal parenchyma. For this reason, masses that distort the renal parenchyma are most readily evaluated on such early films.

TOMOGRAPHY. The routine use of tomography increases the detection of renal masses and thereby increases the sensitivity of the urogram. This is obtained at a relatively small cost (i.e., the increased radiation exposure to the patient and increased film costs). Lloyd, in a prospective study, determined that only 29% of renal masses observed would have been detected without the routine use of tomography. In a study from the Mayo Clinic, only one-third of renal masses less than 2.5 cm in

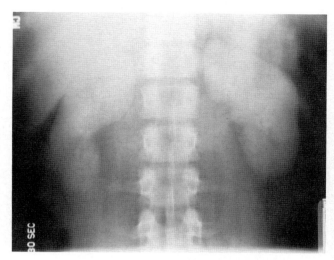

Figure 3.1. Early nephrogram film. A 30-sec tomogram shows the renal margins to be sharply demarcated with intense enhancement of the renal parenchyma. Faint early opacification of the calyces is evident.

diameter would have been detected without the aid of tomographic sections. Routine tomograms are also used in evaluating abnormalities of the collecting system, particularly subtle changes in calyceal anatomy and the presence of filling defects within the collecting system.

Almost all available tomographic-urographic tables employ linear tomographic motion. An arc of 25° provides adequate blurring yet covers the thickness of an average kidney with three exposures. This angle is, therefore, recommended for screening tomography. A tomographic angle of 40° will increase the amount of blurring and decrease the thickness of each slice, but to cover the entire thickness of the kidneys, multiple slices must be obtained. A tomographic cut of 5° provides insufficient blurring for routine use.

The optimal level for the tomographic cuts of the kidneys is most highly correlated with the anteroposterior thickness of the patient (Table 3.1). The midcoronal plane of the kidney can often be determined in the scout

Table 3.1.
Tomographic Levels for Nephrotomography[a]

Anteroposterior Diameter (cm) Including Table Pad	Tomographic Levels
cm	
14–17	6, 7, 8
18–22	7, 8, 9
23–26	8, 9, 10
27–29	9, 10, 11
>30	10, 11, 12

[a] From Newberg AH, Mindell HJ: Predicting tomographic levels for urography. *Radiology* 118:460, 1976.

tomogram when the pedicles of the L_2 vertebral body are in sharpest focus. Sections 1 cm above and 1 cm below this level are usually sufficient.

The optimal timing for the tomographic sections is a matter of preference. Many authorities argue that since the major value of the tomogram lies in the detection of renal masses, the tomograms should be carried out immediately after injection. However, if tomographic evaluation of the collecting system is also desired, they are best performed approximately 5 miuntes after the initial injection (Fig. 3.2).

ABDOMINAL COMPRESSION. The purpose of the compression device is to assure that adequate filling of the pelvocalyceal system and ureters are adequately filled. In the uncompressed patient, normal peristaltic activity, as well as layering of the contrast material in the dependent portions of the collecting system, frequently results in underfilling of one or more portions of the collecting system. This may be a special problem with the use of low osmolar or nonionic contrast materials that produce an inherently smaller diuresis than do the older ionic contrast agents. To be effective, the abdominal compression device must be placed so that it will compress the ureters where they cross the pelvic brim (Fig. 3.3). We prefer the use of a device around the patient rather than a device that attaches to the x-ray table. The device must be placed tightly enough that the patient is not able to tense the abdominal musculature and overcome the pressure exerted by the compression. In addition, if the device is improperly positioned, i.e., too high or too low, effective compression will not be achieved.

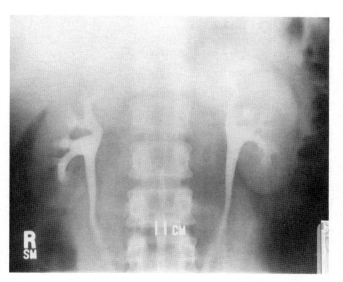

Figure 3.2. A tomographic section 11 cm above the tabletop made approximately 5 min after contrast material injection demonstrates the midcoronal plane of the kidney. The minor calyces are sharply focused in the right kidney. Both renal outlines are well demonstrated.

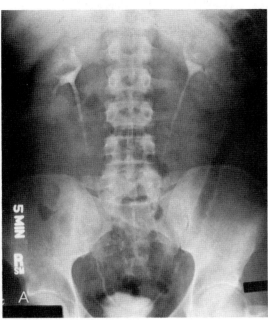

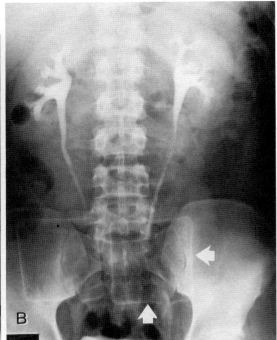

Figure 3.3. Effect of abdominal compression. **A,** In the uncompressed patient, the calyces and proximal ureters are poorly distended. **B,** After application of the compression device (*arrows*), the calyces and proximal ureter are much better demonstrated.

Contraindications to the use of abdominal compression include an abdominal aortic aneurysm, ureteral obstruction, recent abdominal surgery, and the presence of an ostomy. As with the routine use of tomography, the use of abdominal compression aids in the diagnostic utility of the urogram without appreciable cost to the patient.

EXCRETION FILMS. A series of two or three films should be made between 5 and 15 minutes after the injection of the contrast for an overall evaluation of the urinary tract. Some radiologists prefer one of these films to be collimated to the kidneys, particularly if tomograms are not made. The exact choice and timing of the radiographs is a matter of preference.

Additional Views

In addition to the standard views obtained routinely during the urogram, many additional views should be utilized to evaluate specific clinical problems. Some of these views may, by preference, be incorporated into the "routine" urogram. *Oblique plain films* or *oblique tomograms* more precisely localize a suspected defect within the collecting system and are useful to define the presence of a mass in the renal parenchyma. These are preferably performed on films collimated to the kidney. Both oblique views are frequently necessary to completely evaluate a filling defect or pseudofilling defect due to a crossing vessel. The *prone radiograph* is useful to evaluate the ureters when routine supine films do not adequately demonstrate their course. This radiograph is particularly helpful in a patient in whom acute ureteral obstruction is present, but the exact point of obstruction has not been demonstrated. Because contrast material is heavier than unopacified urine, in the prone position the contrast and nonopacified urine will exchange, and thus, the point of obstruction may be demonstrated without resorting to further delayed radiographs. A film made with the patient in the *upright* position after release of abdominal compression is very useful in assessing the effect of gravity on the "drainage" of the upper urinary tract. This is especially helpful when there is equivocal dilatation of one or both of the ureters (Fig. 3.4); drainage of the contrast material from the collecting system on the upright radiograph indicates that the dilatation is not on the basis of obstruction. The upright radiograph also allows the contrast material to optimally demonstrate the base of the bladder. The routine use of such a radiograph will indicate the presence of such bladder abnormalities as cystoceles, pelvic floor relaxation, and bladder hernia that might not be appreciated on routine supine views. The upright radiograph may also be useful in patients with ureteral obstruction in that the most distal extent of the contrast column can more readily be identified.

Traditionally, the *postvoid film* has been utilized to evaluate the patient's ability to empty the bladder. This is a frequent concern, especially in older males with suspected bladder outlet obstruction. It must be remem-

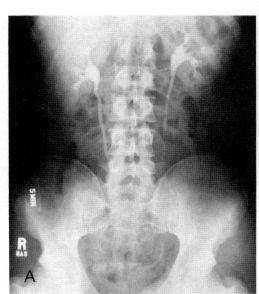
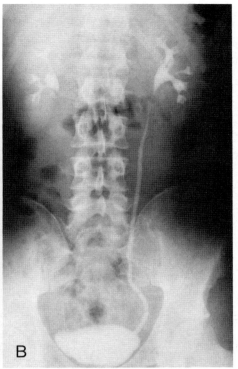

Figure 3.4.   Value of the upright film. **A,** A 5-min radiograph demonstrates equivocal dilatation of the distal left ureter. **B,** The upright film made a few moments later shows poor drain-

age of the left collecting system as a consequence of a partially obstructing distal left ureteral calculus.

bered, however, that a postvoid radiograph that shows residual contrast opacified urine does not mean that the patient could not empty his bladder but only indicates that he did not. Conversely, a nearly empty bladder may be demonstrated, but only after considerable effort on the part of the patient. An important use of the postvoid radiograph, however, is to evaluate the distal ureters that are frequently hidden behind the distended bladder on the prevoiding radiographs. This is especially important in patients with suspected distal ureteral calculi. *Oblique postvoid radiographs* may also be very useful in this regard. The postvoid radiograph allows evaluation of the bladder mucosa (Fig. 3.5) and may be the only radiograph on which small filling defects or other urothelial lesions of the bladder are demonstrated.

DELAYED RADIOGRAPHS.   In patients with acute ureteral obstruction, delayed filling of the collecting system and ureter is the rule. The amount of delay is highly variable and depends on both the acuity and the degree of obstruction. In this situation, delayed radiographs are frequently necessary to demonstrate the precise point of obstruction, and these should be obtained until this point is demonstrated. The precise timing for these delayed films varies from department to department, but a reasonable schedule would include films at 1, 3, 6, 12, and 24 hours after injection or until the point of obstruction is demonstrated.

The Normal Excretory Urogram

Analysis of the excretory phase of the urogram begins with the kidneys.

SIZE.   There is a wide variation in the size of "normal" kidneys. As determined radiographically, renal size varies according to a number of factors unrelated to intrinsic

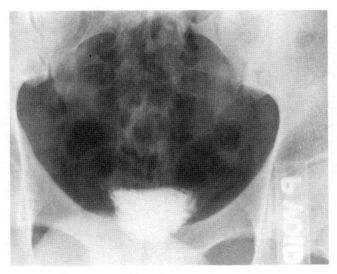

Figure 3.5.   Postvoid film. The normal mucosal pattern of the bladder is demonstrated.

renal pathology. Such factors include the degree of magnification, the amount of diuresis that is induced by the contrast material, and the patient's state of hydration. Ordinarily, the left kidney is approximately 0.5 cm larger than the right kidney. This discrepancy has usually been explained because blood flow to the left kidney is slightly greater than the right owing to the shorter length of the left renal artery. Thus, there should be no greater discrepancy in length of the two kidneys greater than 1.5 cm if the right kidney is larger than the left or no more than 2 cm if the left kidney is larger than the right.

Because the size of the kidneys varies with the size and sex of the individual, an average renal length of three to four vertebral bodies is normal. Simon evaluated 100 kidneys that were normal on autopsy and found a range of 9.4–13.7 cm with the mean length being 11.7 cm on standard abdominal radiographs. He found that two standard deviations of normal would yield a measurement of 2.6–3.6 times the height of the L_2 vertebral body and its interspace. As a practical matter, experienced radiologists can usually visually inspect the kidneys and determine whether or not the renal size falls within the range of normal.

POSITION. The kidneys lie in the retroperitoneum with their long axis parallel to the outer border of the psoas muscle. In heavier individuals the kidneys may assume a more vertical configuration. The renal hilus usually sits at the level of the L_2–L_3 vertebral body. Abnormal position of the kidneys may be related to a variety of processes including patient habitus, the presence of spinal abnormalities, such as rotoscoliosis, developmental failures, such as a failure of ascent and/or rotation, and/or displacement of the kidney by a variety of pathologic processes either in the kidney or adjacent to it.

ABNORMALITIES OF CONTOUR. The normal kidney should be sharply marginated and smooth in contour. The normal shape of the kidney is usually referred to as "reniform." Occasionally, in very asthenic individuals whose investment of perinephric fat is thin, the superior margins of the kidneys may be in contact with other intraabdominal organs. For example, the superior border of the right kidney may contact the liver, and its margins may be difficult to appreciate even on tomographic sections. With this aside, failure to completely visualize the renal outlines segmentally should be considered to represent an abnormality until proven otherwise (Fig. 3.6).

Indentations on the contour of the kidney are frequently seen. A lobulated contour of the renal margin either in its entirety or segmentally representing fetal lobulation (Fig. 3.7) may be present. These indentations represent incomplete fusion of the embryologic renal lobules. They are usually differentiated from pathologic scarring by their smooth contour and regular spacing. A pyelonephritic scar, for example, is usually deeper than a renal lobulation and is always located adjacent to an underlying abnormal calyx. Renal infarcts tend to occur randomly without the regular spacing associated with renal lobation (Fig. 3.8). Especially prominent grooves may sometimes be seen in the superior or inferior margins of the kidneys. This also represents a residua of the fetal renal anatomy and is sometimes termed the sulcus interpartialis superior or inferior, respectively.

A prominent bulge on the superior lateral border of the left kidney is sometimes appreciated. This has been called a dromedary hump (Fig. 3.9) and represents a normal variation that is due to molding by the spleen. Occasionally, enlargement of either the liver or spleen may compress the kidney anteriorly, producing the appearance of the unilaterally enlarged kidney.

THE PELVOCALYCEAL SYSTEM. The average human kidney contains 12–15 calyces although this number may vary considerably and still fall within the normal range. The

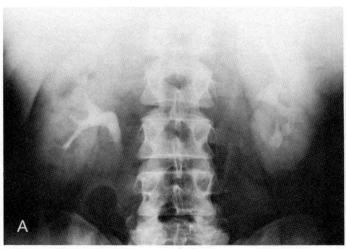
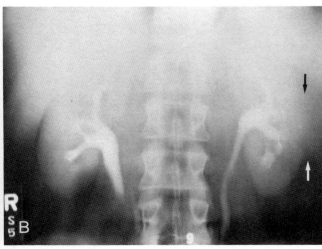

Figure 3.6. **A,** The left renal margin is incompletely visualized along its lateral margin. **B,** Tomogram demonstrates typical findings of a simple cortical cyst (*arrows*).

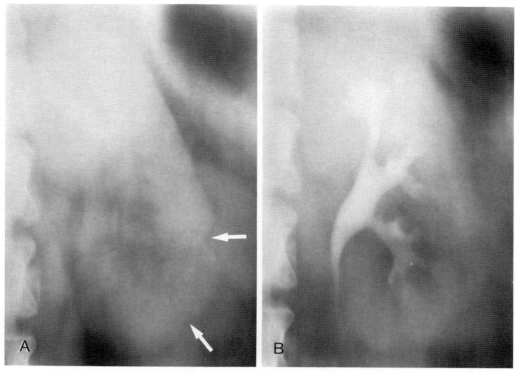

Figure 3.7. Fetal lobation. **A,** Nephrotomogram at 1-min demonstrates two cortical indentations (*arrows*). **B,** A film dur- ing excretion phase shows that the calyces are normal and that the identations occur between calyces.

calyceal systems are roughly divided into upper, middle, and lower calyceal groups. Calyces in the polar regions, in particular, the right upper pole, may be compound, i.e., two or more calyces may share a common infundibu- lum. The calyces, themselves, should be deeply cupped and delicate in appearance without blunting or distor- tion. The infundibulae should be straight with no bowing or displacement. Occasionally, a small blush of contrast may be noted in the renal papilla just outside the calyx,

which is related to a relatively high concentration of con- trast material in the distal collecting ducts as they enter the minor calyces. This appearance is quite normal. In older patients, especially, the calyces and renal pelvis may be compressed by an accumulation of fat in the renal sinus. This condition, termed renal sinus lipomatosis (Fig. 3.10), may produce a spidery and attenuated appear- ance of the collecting system and may prevent calyceal

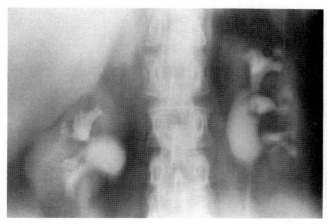

Figure 3.8. Multiple cortical infarcts. Multiple irregular scars, most pronounced in the right kidney, are now present as a result of multiple cortical infarcts.

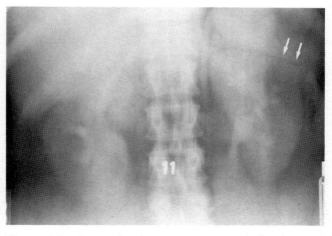

Figure 3.9. Dromedary hump. A prominent bulge (*arrows*) is present on the superior border of the left kidney produced by compression of the renal margin by the spleen.

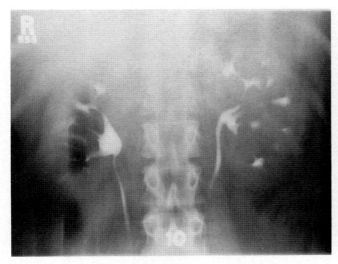

Figure 3.10. Renal sinus lipomatosis. The calyces have a compressed appearance because of an accumulation of fat in the renal sinus. This fat appears relatively radiolucent on the tomographic section.

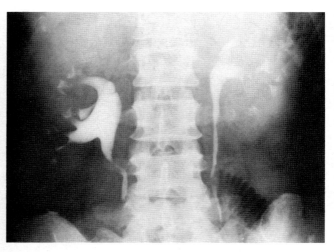

Figure 3.12. Hypertrophied column of Bertin. There is bowing of the upper pole infundibulum and an impression on the renal pelvis of the right kidney secondary to hypertrophy of a column of Bertin.

adequate distention, but otherwise carries no pathologic significance. Frequently, impressions are present on the infundibula of the major or minor calyces produced by either segmental arteries or by veins (Fig. 3.11). The defects are sharply marginated and when produced by a crossing vein may occasionally be eliminated with tight abdominal compression. An extrinsic impression on the infundibulae or renal pelvis may be produced by a hypertrophied column of Bertin. This is most common at the junction of the upper and middle thirds of the kidney (Fig. 3.12).

The major calyces come together to form the renal pelvis, which can be extremely variable in appearance. In some patients, the renal pelvis is intrarenal in location

(i.e., surrounded by renal sinus fat) whereas in others it appears to be outside the confines of the kidneys and has a ballooned appearance (the extrarenal pelvis). If the calyces are normal in appearance, significant obstruction is not present even though the renal pelvis may appear to be quite large in relation to the calyces. There is usually a smooth transition between the renal pelvis and the proximal ureter.

Although there is a tendency toward symmetry of the collecting systems in the two kidneys, there may be considerable variation in any individual. A lack of symmetry should not be considered abnormal, as it has been said that renal morphology may be as distinctive as an individual's fingerprints.

THE URETER.   The ureters generally exit the renal pelvis at the level of the second lumbar vertebra and descend through the cone of renal fascia duct lateral to the transverse processes of the upper lumbar vertebra. The middle third of the ureter usually overlaps the transverse processes of the lower lumbar vertebra to the level of the pelvic brim. The ureter is at its most anterior location where it crosses the iliac vessels; it then descends into the pelvis taking a more lateral course before finally entering the bladder at the trigone. The course of the ureter generally parallels that of the psoas muscle. The degree to which the ureters are visualized depends on the level of renal function; however, even in patients in whom renal function is normal, the ureters may be only fractionally visualized on any single radiograph. The degree to which the ureters are normally filled is highly variable, and lack of filling of a particular segment of the ureter is not necessarily pathologic. An attempt should be made to visualize as much of the entire course of the ureter as possible by utilizing the additional views described

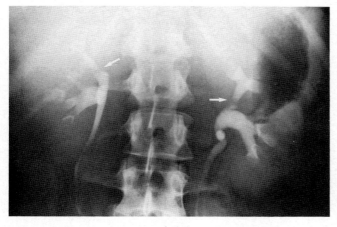

Figure 3.11. Crossing vessel defects. Extrinsic compression (*arrows*) on the upper pole infundibulae bilaterally produced by crossing segmental arteries.

above. One or more slight constrictions of the ureter sometimes may be visualized at the level of the uretero-pelvic junction (Fig. 3.13). These are transverse folds that represent physiologic indentations of the ureter rather than true anatomic sphincters. They are frequently more prominent in infants and young children. Normal indentations on the course of the ureter that may be present include an impression at the level of the L_3–L_4 interspace caused by hypertrophy of the ovarian vessels in women, and tortuosity of the ureter as it crosses the iliac vessels, particularly in older patients. In younger male patients, the ureters may appear to have a more medial course in their middle and distal third due to hypertrophy of the psoas muscles (Fig. 3.14).

BLADDER. The size and contour of the bladder vary with the degree of filling. In its usual state of distention it has a roughly spherical or oblong shape with the superior portion indented by the overlying viscera. The normal bladder is smooth in contour with rounded borders. Any straightening or deformity of one of the contours of the bladder should be considered a sign of bladder pathology until proven otherwise. On the postvoid radiograph the mucosal pattern of the bladder should be identified without evidence of mass or filling defect.

Retrograde Pyelography

Retrograde injection of contrast material directly into the ureter or ureteral orifice allows visualization of the collecting system and ureter without relying on the kidneys ability to excrete contrast media. In addition, the degree of opacification and the degree of distention of the collecting system can be controlled by varying the amount and concentration of the contrast material that is injected. To perform retrograde pyelography, the ureteral orifice in the bladder is cannulated cystoscopically.

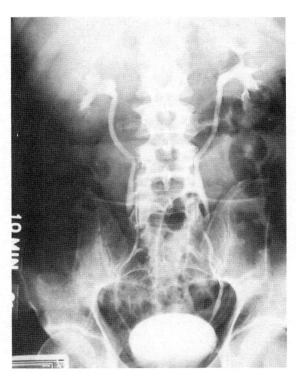

Figure 3.14. Psoas hypertrophy. The ureters have a more medial course secondary to hypertrophy of the psoas muscles in this young male patient.

The catheter may be advanced to the level of the renal pelvis or the contrast material may be injected into the lower ureter and filling of the ureter and the collecting system monitored fluoroscopically. In other instances, a bulb-shaped catheter is wedged in the ureteral orifice and the contrast material injected from this location. This technique is sometimes referred to as a bulb pyelogram. If the room is so equipped, spot filming and positioning may be done directly in the cystoscopy suite, or as an alternative, the catheter may be placed in the cystoscopy suite and the patient brought to the Radiology Department where the injection of contrast and the filming is performed. When a urothelial lesion is suspected on the basis of the film studies, brushing of the lesion for cytologic evaluation may be accomplished at the same time.

The advisability of performing bilateral retrograde pyelograms has been debated by urologists for many years. The obvious danger of bilateral retrograde pyelography is the introduction of infection into a previously uninfected renal unit. With modern urography, however, bilateral retrograde pyelograms are very rarely necessary.

Care must be exercised in filling the collecting system since inadvertent overdistention of the calyces can occur easily. This overdistention may result in pyelovenous extravasation in which contrast material escapes from the collecting system into the veins, pyelosinus extravasation which results from rupture of a fornix and extravasation

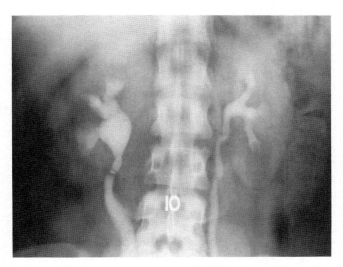

Figure 3.13. Transverse ureteral folds. Several band-like constrictions are present in the right proximal ureter which have no physiologic or pathologic consequence.

of the contrast material into the renal sinus, pyelolymphatic extravasation which results in filling of the perirenal lymphatics, and pyelotubular back flow in which there is retrograde filling of the distal collecting ducts at the level of the renal papilla.

The primary use of retrograde pyelography is the evaluation of suspected ureteral obstruction in the patient in whom the ability of the kidney to excrete contrast material is significantly impaired or to evaluate possible filling defects in either the collecting system or the ureter where urography has failed to adequately demonstrate a suspected lesion. In addition, on rare occasions retrograde pyelography may be useful in localizing a suspected calculus or in the evaluation of a duplicated collecting system.

Retrograde pyelography should not be used as a primary diagnostic procedure as it offers no evaluation of the renal parenchyma and is relatively invasive as cystoscopy is required for placement of the catheters. It should be used as an adjunctive technique when conventional imaging studies fail to adequately demonstrate the suspected pathology.

A variation of retrograde pyelography termed air pyelography is occasionally useful. In such instances, air rather than opaque contrast material is injected in the collecting system. This technique can be utilized when the suspected filling defect, such as a stone, is obscured with the injection of conventional contrast media.

Antegrade Pyelography

Antegrade pyelography is a study of the collecting system of the kidney and ureter made via the direct injection of contrast material into the collecting system. As a diagnostic study, antegrade pyelography is usually performed when urography fails to demonstrate the desired information about the collecting system and retrograde pyelography is either hazardous or cannot be performed.

Antegrade pyelography is usually performed via a direct puncture of one of the calyces or the renal pelvis using a 20- or 22-gauge needle. The collecting system may be localized using fluoroscopy, ultrasonography or, rarely, CT. Fluoroscopic guidance is usually preferred as this facilitates filming after the collecting system is opacified. If ultrasonic or computed tomographic guidance is utilized, the patient is generally transferred to a fluoroscopy room following placement of the needle or catheter.

Indications

The indications for antegrade pyelography are listed in Table 3.2. The antegrade approach to opacification of the urinary tract for the study of suspected urinary tract obstruction may be preferable in patients with ileal conduits and patients in whom ureteroneocystostomy has

Table 3.2.
Indications for Antegrade Pyelography[a]

Morphologic (Pathologic Anatomy)
  Confirmation and evaluation of hydronephrosis
  Determination of resting pressure
  Urinalysis: cystologic study, culture, biochemical analysis
  Site and etiology of obstruction
Urodynamic (perfusion, pressure-flow)
  Assessment of ureteral resistance
    Congenital and acquired dilatation
    Following corrective treatment
    Effect of bladder distention
Assessment for percutaneous nephrostomy and other interventional procedures
  Drainage
  Dilatation of stenosis
  Stenting
  Balloon occlusion
  Stone removal
  Biopsy

[a] From Pfister RC, Papanicoulaou N, Yoder IC: Diagnostic morphologic and urodynamic antegrade pyelography. *Radiol Clin North Am* 24(4):561–571, 1986.

been performed. In both instances the ureteral orifice may be very difficult to catheterize from a retrograde approach. In addition, the antegrade study is preferred in male children in whom cystoscopy and the introduction of a catheter is often technically very difficult and hazardous because of the child's small urethra and the small size of the instruments that must be used.

Ureteral perfusion studies to assess the functional integrity of the collecting system and ureter have been proven to be a useful adjunct in the evaluation of anatomic abnormalities of the upper urinary tract. Antegrade pyelography is also commonly performed as a prelude to percutaneous nephrostomy and other percutaneous interventional procedures in the urinary tract.

Technique

To perform antegrade pyelography, the patient is placed prone on the fluoroscopy table and the soft tissues of the back and flank are prepared and draped as for any sterile procedure. It is prudent to evaluate bleeding parameters and to discontinue anticoagulation therapy prior to the procedure. If infection in the upper urinary tract is suspected and is the prime indication for the procedure, the use of prophylactic broad-spectrum antibiotics should be considered as the distention that may accompany antegrade pyelography in the face of a distal obstruction may place the patient at risk for the development of sepsis.

After the appropriate site is selected for the puncture, the skin and soft tissues of the flank are anesthetized with 1 or 2% procaine and the needle puncture accomplished during suspended respiration. When urine is aspirated from the kidney, the correct needle placement is confirmed via the injection of contrast material. The calyces and ureter are filled to the point of obstruction. A tilting table is somewhat helpful so that gravity may be utilized to carry the contrast material to the most dependent portion of the urinary tract. If this is not available, contrast may be instilled directly into the collecting system, the needle removed, and filming then accomplished in supine, prone, and upright positions. If there is any suspicion of infection, urine should be aspirated and sent for bacteriologic studies.

Complications

In general, antegrade pyelography is a safe and easily performed procedure. Complications of the procedure, include bleeding, sepsis, and the inadvertent puncture of an adjacent organ. Pneumothorax may occur if the pleural space is traversed during the introduction of the needle. This complication can be minimized when a direct posterior approach is utilized as the costophrenic sulcus is generally shallower in the direct posterior position than in an approach from the posterior axillary line. Virtually every patient in whom antegrade pyelography is performed will develop at least microscopic hematuria which is usually transient and not considered a complication.

Cystography

Static cystography is performed to assess low-pressure vesicoureteral reflux or to assess bladder rupture. However, static cystography does not exclude high-pressure vesicoureteral reflux nor does it always exclude bladder rupture.

Voiding Cystography

The bladder is filled with water-soluble contrast medium via a urethral catheter. This may be done by the drip method connected to the bladder catheter or by direct injection of contrast medium via a 50-ml syringe filled with contrast medium. The filled bladder may show low pressure vesicoureteral reflux, radiolucent filling defects, such as tumor or radiolucent stone, bladder diverticulum or vesicocolic fistula. The bladder should be filled until the patient is certain he or she can void when the catheter is removed and voiding cystography is performed with fluoroscopy. A cine or video recording of bladder emptying may be obtained, and the procedure can be recorded by spot films, or 100-mm cut film or continuous 105-mm film. High-pressure reflux, bladder extravasation, or a small necked diverticulum may not be apparent until the voiding study is obtained.

Air Contrast Cystography

Coating of the bladder wall with barium followed by the injection of air through the bladder catheter may be required for visualization of small bladder lesions. After the insertion of 100 ml of barium, the patient rotates so that a contrast medium coating is applied to the complete bladder wall. The barium is then drained from the bladder. The bladder is distended with air, carbon dioxide, or nitrous oxide and supine, prone, oblique, upright, and decubitus views are obtained. Small bladder lesions and lesions in a bladder diverticulum may best be visualized by this method.

Retrograde Urethrography and Voiding Cystourethrography

The bladder can be filled to capacity via a Foley catheter with the balloon of the catheter positioned in the fossa navicularis and inflated with 1 ml of saline. This avoids the insertion of the catheter into the bladder, (always desirable) and therefore the possibility of introducing infection or catheter irritation of the bladder mucosa which may result in early bladder contraction. The Foley catheter with the balloon in the fossa navicularis is connected to a 50-ml syringe and contrast medium injected directly by hand or the catheter may be connected to a drip, in which the rate of flow of contrast medium can be controlled. This technique opacifies the urethra and bladder. When the patient's bladder is filled, the catheter is removed and a voiding study obtained. This method is only applicable to males.

Cystography in Male Patients with Neuromuscular Bladder Dysfunction

The method used is as described above. A Foley catheter balloon is inserted into the fossa navicularis and the bladder is filled by dynamic retrograde urethrocystography. Unlike dynamic urethrocystography for the assessment of urethral stricture or urethral trauma, the catheter remains in position during the voiding study so that voiding occurs into the catheter and syringe in the operator's hand. This is the method of choice to assess vesicoureteral reflux, sphincter dyssynergia, and bladder abnormality in neurogenic bladder patients. When low-pressure reflux is demonstrated, a compression band, as is used in excretory urography, is applied to stop vesicoureteral reflux reaching the kidneys.

Ileal Conduit Studies

Following cystectomy, an ileal conduit is commonly constructed for supravesicle urinary diversion. One end of an isolated segment of ileum is brought to the skin as an ileocutaneous stoma. The ureters are implanted in the opposite end of the loop which is closed off and placed retroperitoneally, if possible. As the ureters are anastomosed to the loop in an end-to-side fashion, there is generally ready reflux from the conduit into the ureters. Therefore, contrast material instilled into the ileal loop may be used to demonstrate the ureters and the renal collecting systems. Such a study is called an ileal conduit study or a "loopogram."

To perform a loopogram, an appropriate Foley catheter (generally between 20 and 26 French) is inserted into the stoma and the balloon inflated to a volume of 5–8 ml within the stoma. Contrast material is then instilled into the Foley catheter either by gravity infusion or by hand injection. Gravity infusion is generally preferred, as the pressure is limited by the height of the bottle of contrast material. Under fluoroscopic observation, contrast material fills the loop and will usually reflux into the ureters. The study is especially useful in patients with impaired renal function, and serves in lieu of retrograde pyelography to exclude ureteral obstruction.

Urethrography

The urethra may be visualized either in a retrograde or antegrade fashion. Retrograde and antegrade urethrography may be done separately, but the best method for assessing urethral disease is combined dynamic retrograde urethrography immediately followed by voiding cystourethrography.

Static Retrograde Urethrography

This method of assessing the urethra is inadequate even to assess the anterior urethra. Nevertheless, it is still performed by urologists. The method consists of injecting contrast medium into the urethra, placing a clamp (such as a Cunningham clamp) over the glans penis, and exposing a film while the contrast is static within the urethra. This examination gives limited information about the penile and bulbous urethra but no information about the proximal bulbous urethra or posterior urethra. The membranous urethra cannot be localized, and any contrast medium which has passed into the posterior urethra has been milked-back (by the distal sphincters) into the bladder, therefore, the posterior urethra is not visualized.

Dynamic Retrograde Urethrography

Dynamic retrograde urethrography is the method of choice for retrograde study of the urethra. Contrast medium flowing through the urethra by retrograde injection will visualize the whole urethra if the film is exposed during injection, so that a continuous flow of contrast medium is visualized. Two main methods are in use.

1. *The Foley catheter method* in which a 12 or 14 French Foley catheter is inserted 2–3 cm into the penis and the balloon of the catheter is dilated in the fossa navicularis. The balloon is inflated with 1–1.5 cc of saline, enough to keep the balloon fixed in position but insufficient to tear the urethral mucosa. The catheter is connected to a 50-ml syringe filled with water-soluble contrast medium. Injection of contrast medium outlines the

whole urethra and films are exposed during retrograde injection.

2. *The Brodny clamp method.* The Brodny clamp consists of a clamp apparatus containing an external meatal plug through which contrast medium can be injected from a syringe attached to the apparatus. The plug is held in position by a clamp which is fitted over the glans penis. Injection of contrast medium outlines the whole urethra if films are exposed during retrograde injection. Either method is successful in obtaining dynamic retrograde urethrography. The Foley catheter method has some advantages.

1. The operator's hands are farther away from the x-ray beam.
2. Both methods require gentle traction on the penis to straighten the urethra at the penoscrotal junction. Traction on the Brodny clamp may be painful and injure the mucosa of the glans penis.
3. The Foley catheter method provides more control of the injection, as well as penile and patient positioning.

Both methods are best done with fluoroscopic control, but both may be done using an overhead tube, instructing the technician to expose the film while the operator is injecting. Both methods can also be done with portable equipment, either as an emergency or in the patient's bed. After obtaining two or three dynamic retrograde films, the bladder should be filled via the same Foley catheter or Brodny clamp to obtain a voiding cystourethrogram. The catheter or clamp should then be removed and voiding films obtained. During the retrograde and voiding studies the patient should remain obliqued 40° to the right. The retrograde study is usually obtained with the patient supine; the voiding study is usually obtained with the patient in the semierect or erect position. In both dynamic retrograde and voiding studies, the patients' thighs should be separated as far as possible to minimize the thigh soft tissue shadow's reduction of urethral visibility. The dynamic retrograde and voiding cystourethrogram can be completed in 15–20 minutes.

Excretory Voiding Cystourethrography

This method advocates the acquisition of a voiding cystourethrogram at the end of excretory urography. The method involves either obtaining the excretory urogram before the patient voids so that the bladder is full at the end of the urogram or giving the patient water to drink to fill the bladder after the urogram films are obtained. There are several flaws in this method.

1. It is commonly time-consuming, and entails the patient intermittently occupying a room when the patient thinks he or she is ready to void and is not.
2. It usually involves extended patient time in the department, which is not always convenient for the patient.
3. Most importantly, voiding cystourethrography alone

may provide misleading information on the extent of urethral disease, and does not demonstrate paradoxical dilatation of softly scarred urethral tissue proximal to hard primary scars or strictures. It has been shown that 95% of patients with a primary hard scar in the proximal bulbous urethra with an abnormal cone to the proximal bulbous urethra on dynamic retrograde urethrography, have scarring extending into the membranous urethra. Sixty percent of such patients show paradoxical dilatation of the scarred membranous urethra. This is due to the very high hydrostatic pressure proximal to a primary hard scar in the proximal bulbous urethra. The high hydrostatic pressure is capable of dilating the membranous urethra which is involved with softer scarring, hence the designation "paradoxical dilatation."

Cavernosography

Corpus cavernosography has been traditionally performed for the evaluation of Peyronie's disease, penile fracture, or for the assessment of priapism. The technique of the examination is straightforward. The skin on the dorsal lateral shaft of the penis just proximal to the glans is infiltrated with 1% Xylocaine for local anesthesia and a 21-gauge scalp vein needle is inserted into one of the corporal bodies with a sharp thrusting motion which facilitates puncture of the tunica albuginea. Test injection of diluted contrast material will confirm the intracorporeal location of the needle tip. Under fluoroscopic guidance, additional diluted contrast material is injected until the body of the corpora is filled with contrast material. Injection of one of the corpora fills both because there are multiple anastomoses between the two corporeal bodies. Anteroposterior (AP) and oblique film studies are generally obtained.

Recently, there has been increased interest in corpus cavernosography for the evaluation of organic impotence. Current thinking suggests that approximately 50% of the cases of organic impotence are vasculogenic in origin. Vasculogenic impotence is, in turn, subdivided into arterial (i.e., an inadequate in-flow of flood to the corpora) and venous (due to a defect in venoocclusive mechanism of the corpora cavernosa, such that rapid blood flow out of the corpora prevents an erection from occurring or being maintained despite adequate inflow). Failure of this venoocclusive mechanism of the corpora is commonly referred to as a venous leakage. Cavernosography in such cases is usually combined with corpus cavernosometry so that correlation of the images with intracorporeal pressure measurements can be obtained.

The technique of cavernosography is similar to that used for standard cavernosography except that two needles are placed, one in each corpora. The first needle is used to infuse diluted contrast material or saline at standard infusion rates, while the second needle is used to monitor intracorporeal pressure during these infusions. Most authorities now use supraphysiologic infusion rates (up to 400 ml/min) in an attempt to produce an artificial erection is not valid, and therefore, cavernosography should only be performed after injection of pharmacologic agents designed to activate the corporeal venoocclusive mechanism. Therefore, between 40 and 60 mg of papaverine, a smooth muscle dilator, is injected intracorporeally prior to the start of the infusion. Some authorities recommend the addition of phentolamine 0.5–1 mg intracorporeally as well. The drugs are diluted in 10 ml of saline and infused slowly over a period of 4–5 minutes. Infusion of normal saline is then performed at an initial rate of 30–40 ml/min and, if necessary, to a maximum of 120 ml/min. If infusion at these rates does not produce an artificial erection, the study is terminated and no conclusion about the relative contribution of venous leakage to the patient's impotence can be drawn. If, however, a rigid erection occurs, the infusion is terminated and the fall in corporeal pressure monitored. If intracorporeal pressure falls precipitously, the presence of a venous leak is inferred. The infusion is then repeated with diluted contrast material in order to ascertain the sites of venous leak during full erection. Film studies are generally performed in the AP and both oblique projections. Common sites of venous leakage include the deep crural veins, the glans penis, and the deep and superficial dorsal veins of the penis. If, however, only slow detumescence is present following cessation of the saline infusion, no evidence of venous leakage is present and, therefore, injection of contrast material is not necessary.

Vasography

A seminal vesiculogram is an operative procedure in which the vas deferens is cannulated after making a small incision in the scrotum. Injection of contrast medium into the vas outlines the course of the vas and the ampulla. The ejaculatory duct is visualized and reflux of contrast medium into the seminal vesicle occurs. Contrast medium passing into the prostatic urethra is normally retrogradely propelled into the bladder. In patients who have had transurethral prostatectomy or in patients who have had severe urethral and prostatic infection, dynamic retrograde urethrography and voiding urethrography occasionally shows the ejaculatory ducts, the seminal vesicles, and the vas deferens. This results from reflux of contrast medium into the ejaculatory ducts due to patency of these ducts from infection or operation.

CROSS-SECTIONAL IMAGING

Ultrasonography

The physical principles of ultrasonography are beyond the scope of this book, however, sonography offers a method of visualizing soft tissue structures within the urinary tract, which is painless, noninvasive, and does not require the use of contrast agents or ionizing radiation. Real-time sonography has essentially replaced the older static gray-scale images for the evaluation of the urinary tract. Real time equipment allows the physician to closely monitor the examination and allows constant observation of the anatomy from section to section. The resolution of real-time units now surpasses that of the older static units.

Renal Sonography

The forte of ultrasonography is its ability to differentiate fluid-filled structures and solid tissue. For this reason, one of the earliest applications of sonography in the urinary tract was its use in differentiating solid renal mass lesions from renal cysts. This remains a primary use of this modality whose accuracy in differentiating a solid mass from a cyst has been reported as high as 98% in the hands of an experienced sonographer. In practical terms, the spatial resolution of modern equipment for detection of renal masses is approximately 2 cm. Completely sonolucent masses and exophytic masses of somewhat smaller dimension may be detected.

The uses of sonography in the urinary tract have expanded to include the evaluation of a wide variety of morphologic diseases of the kidney, including the evaluation of renal cystic disease, medical renal disease, perirenal fluid collections, renal transplants, and nonfunctioning kidneys. In patients in whom urography demonstrates a poorly visualized kidney or shows a questionable abnormality, US is often the next imaging study. Ultrasound has become the imaging method of choice for the initial evaluation of the azotemic patient. It may also be used as a primary imaging method in patients with severe contrast allergies, for the evaluation of the urinary tract in infants, and in children with palpable abdominal masses.

Ultrasound has been particularly useful in evaluation of hydronephrosis, especially when it is of a long-standing duration. Both opaque and nonopaque renal calculi may be detected by sonography because of their highly echogenic nature and characteristic acoustic shadow caused by the attenuation of the sound beam behind the stone. Intraoperative sonography may facilitate complete stone removal in patients undergoing operative pyelolithotomy. Ultrasound is also utilized as a guidance technique for a variety of invasive procedures, including antegrade pyelography, percutaneous nephrostomy, percutaneous renal biopsy, and percutaneous abscess drainage. Ultrasound may also be used in the evaluation of pregnant patients because, to date, no adverse biologic effects of the technique have been demonstrated.

As with any diagnostic technique, the limitations and disadvantages of US should be recognized. The technique offers a purely anatomic demonstration of the morphology in a single plane. The technique is much more operator-dependent than virtually any other method of diagnostic imaging, and therefore, the results often depend on the experience of the operator, as well as the quality of the equipment. The right kidney is generally better imaged than the left because the liver can be used as a sonographic window. Sound waves are completely reflected by gas and completely absorbed by bone. For this reason the bony pelvis and intestinal gas often pose significant limitations within the abdomen. The lower pole of the left kidney, in particular, can be difficult to image because of overlying intestinal gas. The technique is difficult to use to evaluate the ureter as it is impossible to distinguish a nondistended ureter from its surrounding retroperitoneal fat. In addition, since the transducer must be directly applied to the patient's skin, recent surgery, bandages, or ostomies may pose significant limitations. With obese patients, greater deflection of the sound waves is apparent which significantly distracts from the resolution of the images.

Bladder Sonography

The full bladder is well visualized by several ultrasonographic approaches.

1. The transabdominal approach is the most commonly used, but requires a full bladder. This is best done by waiting until the patient's bladder naturally fills with urine, or if there is renal impairment or suspected bladder trauma, the bladder may be filled with normal saline via a urethral catheter. Transverse and longitudinal views are essential. The transducer is placed in the suprapubic area adjacent to the pubic bone and angled inferiorly toward the bladder trigone. For visualization of structures on the right side of the bladder the transducer should be placed to the left of midline and angled obliquely toward the right, and the opposite for visualization of structures on the left side of the bladder. Gain control adjustment may be necessary to make the bladder content echofree at the beginning of the procedure. The filled bladder was initially used to provide an acoustic window for the visualization of the uterus and ovaries in females and for prostate visualization in males. However, intrinsic bladder lesions are relatively well seen. Bladder stones that move with alteration of patient position are seen as a hyperechoic area with acoustic shadowing. Isoechoic lesions without acoustic shadowing generally represent bladder tumors which remain fixed in position. Bladder foreign bodies may be hyperechoic if calcified or isoechoic if not calcified but usually move with the patient. Bladder diverticula are well seen on transabdominal ultrasound. Extravesical fluid collections are demonstrated as hypoechoic areas adjacent to the bladder. These can represent urine, urachal cystic fluid, or lymph. Old hemorrhage is mixed echogenicity and usually contains numerous bright echoes without acoustic

shadowing. Bladder residual volumes can be estimated by transabdominal ultrasound. Measurements in the transverse and longitudinal planes give width, length, and depth measurements. Using the empirical formula, bladder volume may be calculated as follows:

$$\text{Bladder volume Vc} = 0.7(W \times H \times D)$$

Such estimation of bladder residual volume is accurate within approximately 20%, which is considered acceptable.

2. Transrectal ultrasound, more commonly used for assessment of the prostate can also be used to examine the bladder. The bladder must be distended with fluid. The length of the transrectal probe is designed for prostatic assessment, and consequently, it may be difficult to visualize the dome of the bladder. Separate radial head and linear array transducers may be used. Sector transrectal probes are available allowing transverse and longitudinal visualization without changing the probe. Transrectal probes vary between 3.5 and 7.5 MHz, ranging from 1 to 7 cm from the edge of the transducer. The examination is well tolerated but mildly uncomfortable. The patient is placed in the left lateral fetal position. Cranial and caudal, right and left positioning of the monitor may initially be confusing but clarifies with practice.

3. *Transurethral Ultrasound.* Specialized transurethral probes have been recently developed and provide excellent assessment of the bladder. Unlike transabdominal and transrectal ultrasound, transurethral ultrasound usually requires heavy sedation or anesthesia, particularly in males. The transurethral ultrasound transducer is large enough to require a 24 French cystoscope for passage into the bladder and the examination performed at the time of cystoscopy. The bladder must be fluid-filled after removal of the cystoscope light. The transducer is passed through the cystoscope into the bladder and progression of the transducer into the bladder monitored as it progresses toward the bladder dome. Half-centimeter-spaced transverse images are obtained from the bladder dome to the bladder trigone. This method provides excellent detail of the bladder wall.

Prostate Sonography

Initially, a 3-MHz transducer was able to use the full bladder as an acoustic window for visualization of the prostate. Prostate size, shape, and the effect of the prostate on the bladder base could be assessed. However, transrectal ultrasound has become the method of choice for prostate assessment. A transducer with a radial head is used to obtain transverse images of the prostate and a linear array transducer with a varying number of transducers (between 64 and 120) is used to visualize the prostate in longitudinal fashion. The importance of transrectal US is in the assessment of carcinoma of the prostate. Approximately 85% of prostatic carcinomas are inoperable at the time of clinical diagnosis. It is, therefore, important to find a method of diagnosing carcinoma of the prostate while it is stage A carcinoma, i.e., not palpable to the urologist's finger and within the prostatic capsule. Transrectal US is at present the most promising method to make the diagnosis of operable carcinoma. The method consists of covering the transrectal transducer with a water-filled condom and inserting it under real-time US to the appropriate depth for prostate visualization.

The method is not difficult for the operator or the patient. However, proper positioning and assessment of echogenicity is time-consuming, difficult and requires considerable experience for accurate assessment. There is still a discrepancy of opinion among expert ultrasonologists as to the appearance of prostate carcinoma by transrectal ultrasound. There is general agreement that hypoechoic areas within the prostate should be biopsied and that operable prostatic carcinoma is more commonly hypoechoic. However, transrectal ultrasound usually clearly delineates the central zone from the peripheral zone. Prostatic carcinoma arises in the peripheral zone. Any hypoechoic or hyperechoic area in the peripheral zone requires biopsy since hyperechoic areas in the peripheral zone have also been shown to be carcinoma by biopsy.

Biopsy of hypoechoic and hyperechoic areas is guided by transrectal US. Attached to the handle of the transrectal transducer is a fitting which takes the biopsy needle for transrectal or perineal biopsy and this can be guided to the appropriate hypoechoic area during the transrectal study. Prostatic carcinomas which have gone through the capsule or are locally invasive are not so readily distinguished by echogenicity from prostatic hypertrophy.

Seminal Vesicle Sonography

On transabdominal US, the seminal vesicles are visualized, using the filled bladder as an acoustic window, as hypoechoic linear or crescentic areas. They are not quite as hypoechoic as the bladder. On longitudinal views, the seminal vesicle echogenicity approaches that of the prostate and they appear as proximal extensions of the prostate.

The seminal vesicles are well seen on transrectal ultrasound which is usually performed as a method of assessing the prostate gland. The patient administers a Fleet enema to himself or herself to empty the rectum following which the transrectal probe is gently passed into the rectum. If the probe is inserted up to the base of the prostate and bladder trigone, the seminal vesicles are well seen. The transverse views show the seminal vesicles as hypoechoic with a bowtie or crescentic shape. Longitudinal views show the seminal vesicles as linear hypoechoic areas adjacent to the base of the prostate where they present as beak shaped in normal patients. Absence of the beak appearance on longitudinal transrectal scan raises the possibility of invasion from prostatic carcinoma.

Scrotal Sonography

Over the past several years, the development of high-resolution, short-focused 7.5–12 MH$_z$ real time transducers has allowed detailed resolution of the scrotal contents. The normal testis has a homogeneous echo texture and can easily be differentiated from the epididymis which is located superior and posterior to the testicle itself.

The most common indication is for scrotal enlargement and to differentiate such benign conditions of the testis as hydroceles from solid tumors of the testis. The accuracy of scrotal sonography in differentiating solid lesions of the testis from cystic lesions and in differentiating intratesticular disease from extratesticular disease has been reported to approach 100% in some series.

Scrotal sonography may also be of value in finding the cause of male infertility in that varicoceles may readily be detected. Cryptorchid testes below the inguinal ligament may be evaluated by sonography.

Computed Tomography

Computed tomography uses the same ionizing radiation as conventional radiography. With CT, the data from multiple planar projections are mathematically recombined to produce a cross-sectional image. Images can be reformatted into coronal, sagittal, or oblique projections, but this is seldom needed. Although the spatial resolution of CT is less than conventional film-screen radiography, the contrast resolution is far superior. Thus, fat is easily distinguished from other soft tissues of muscle or organ density, and contrast enhancement is an important diagnostic feature.

There have been several generations of CT equipment, but the basic process of image generation remains the same. A series of exposures from different projections is made. The image is formed by back-projecting the relative densities into a matrix which assigns a value to each element. These back-projections are then filtered to eliminate star artifact. The result is a matrix of numbers corresponding to the attenuation of volume elements (voxels) of the patient. A water phantom is used to calibrate the scanner and allow conversion of the relative tissue densities to Hounsfield units (HU) which range from −1000 to +1000. Air measures −1000, water should be 0, and bone approaches +1000 HU.

The CT image consists of a matrix, usually 512 × 512 picture elements (pixels), of numbers ranging from −1000 to +1000. Although the computer image contains 2000 levels, the human eye can perceive only 16 to 20 gray levels. Thus, the computer data are combined into 16 displayable levels.

The display can be varied in both width and level. A wide window allows visualization of the greatest amount of tissue but minimizes the differences of density. A narrow window accentuates subtle differences and is useful for carefully examining a relatively homogeneous organ such as the liver. Wider windows are used when tissues with a broad range of densities are examined.

The optimal window level depends upon the tissue density. Pulmonary parenchyma for instance must be viewed at a low level such as −700, but the mediastinum will be completely white at this level. The mediastinum is better imaged near 0, while bony structures are often best at +100 to +200.

Current CT scanners are either third or fourth generation. Third-generation scanners use a system of parallel detectors in which the x-ray tube and detectors rotate in unison. Fourth-generation scanners have a complete ring of stationary detectors such that only the x-ray tube moves. Resolution is a function of the number, size, and efficiency of the detectors and their distance from the x-ray source.

In addition to these conventional CT scanners, an electron beam sweep with a fixed detector array has been designed by Imatron to provide ultrafast scans and eliminate motion artifact. Scans as fast as 50 msec can be used to image dynamic structures such as the heart. It may also prove useful in examining uncooperative patients such as children or trauma victims, as the rapid scan speed prevents motion artifact.

The many advantages of CT scanning have made a dramatic impact on genitourinary radiology. Computed tomography is essential in the examination of the adrenal glands and is an important modality for the kidney and retroperitoneum. Although it is seldom used to directly image the bladder, prostate, or testes, it is commonly employed to stage tumors arising in those organs.

There are, however, some disadvantages to CT scanning. Computed tomography remains an expensive modality which results in relatively expensive examinations. The CT table has highly accurate incrementation under normal weight loads. However, when large patients (over 300 lb) are scanned the incrementation is not accurate and very large patients may even have to be pushed as the table may not move. Biopsy procedures may also be limited by the size of the patient opening in the gantry. Very few interventional procedures can be performed under CT guidance because the time required for image reconstruction slows needle and catheter manipulation.

Magnetic Resonance Imaging

Magnetic resonance imaging (MRI) is another form of CT. Whereas conventional transmission computed tomography yields an image whose pixel value is the mean attenuation of the x-ray beam normalized to water, MRI yields an image whose pixel value represents the amount of radiosignal that was received from the voxel of tissue.

The physics of image production from magnetic resonance is complicated and beyond the scope of this text, but a simplified model can explain the phenomena of imaging. Protons within the patient can be thought of as small spinning bar magnets. Hydrogen molecules have a single proton. When a patient is placed in a large magnetic field, the hydrogen protons within the body align, and this alignment leads to the formation of a net magnetic vector within the patient. By applying radiofrequency (RF) pulses to the patient, this vector can be made to spin. A wire (the antenna) lying outside the patient will have a current induced within it by the spinning bar magnet. This current radiosignal from the tissues, and its magnitude is related to the intensity of the pixel in the magnetic resonance image.

The intensity of the signal from the tissues is related to both tissue and system parameters. The tissue parameters are the number of protons that have aligned within the voxel (initial magnetization, MO), the T_1 relaxation time, the T_2 relaxation time, the affects of flow and motion in the tissues, as well as local changes to the magnetic field. T_1 and T_2 are time constants that describe decay mechanisms of the spinning bar magnet. System parameters that affect the intensity of the signal from the tissue include the manner in which the RF pulses are applied to the patient and the time between the application of these RF pulses.

Images can be created with contrast between tissues dependent primarily on the T_1 values of tissues (T_1-weighted images), or the T_2 values of the tissues (T_2-weighted). One of the most common ways to do this is to use a sequence of RF pulses known as the spin echo pulse sequence. Timing parameters in the spin echo pulse sequence are TR and TE. An image of which the contrast is primarily due to the differences of T_1 values in the tissues is produced by a relatively short TR (approximately 250–600 msec), and a relatively short TE (approximately 12–25 msec). T_2-weighted images have a long TR (TR = 2000–4000 msec), and a relatively long TE (TE = 40–120 msec). Values of TR and TE between these ranges produce images with a mix of T_1 and T_2 contrast. Other pulse techniques are available that will allow adjustment of contrast between the soft tissues depending on either their MO, T_1, or T_2, or techniques that will accentuate blood flow within vessels.

The advantages that MRI has over CT include the lack of ionizing radiation and much greater potential contrast available between soft tissues. Furthermore, this contrast between tissues can be prospectively adjusted by the radiologist. MRI also allows multiplanar acquisition. This enables high-resolution images to be obtained in either the coronal, sagittal, or axial plane, as well as oblique planes. MRI can also determine vessel patency without intravenous contrast administration.

The primary disadvantage of MRI is the high cost amounts. MRI is also relatively insensitive to small amounts of calcification and may even displace ferromagnetic materials within the patient. Current contraindications to MRI include patients with pacemakers, intraoccular foreign bodies, ferromagnetic foreign bodies, intracranial aneurysmal clips, otic implants, and neurostimulators. However, some of these contraindications may change over time.

Three basic magnet types are currently being used for imaging. Resistive magnets operate up to the field strength of 0.15 Tesla (T). They are the least expensive to build and do not require cryogens. However, there is a significant cost in electrical energy and only lower field strengths are available.

Permanent magnets allow field strengths up to approximately 0.35 T. These units do not require cyrogens and use only a moderate electric current. However, they are permanent magnets, are very heavy, and cannot be disabled.

Clinically used superconductive magnets operate with a field strength up to 2.0 T. This higher field strength results in improved contrast resolution and is essential for spectroscopy. Although the electrical requirements are not high, the basic unit is quite expensive and the use of cryogens adds to the continuing operating expense. Furthermore, shielding requirements may add significantly to the cost and space needed for installation.

There are many exciting areas of MR research that will begin to have great clinical impact in the next few years. These include the use of intravenous contrast agents (gadopentetate dimeglumine), projectional angiograms, and spectroscopy. Spectroscopy can either measure relative amounts of fat and water within a tissue or look at the energy status of the tissue by assaying high-energy phosphate compounds versus low-energy phosphate compounds. Further work will be necessary to determine the use of these advancements in imaging the genitourinary system.

INVASIVE TECHNIQUES

Angiography

Despite advances in noninvasive imaging modalities, both arteriography and venography remain important techniques in genitourinary radiology.

Arteriography

Diagnostic arteriography may be used to define either the renal arteries or mass lesions. The renal arteries are most commonly studied for suspected renovascular hypertension where the stenosis is usually in the main renal artery, and often at the origin from the aorta. Smaller renal arteries may be studied in patients with a vasculitis, such as polyarteritis nodosa, in which the renal arteries are commonly affected. However, renal arteriography may also be used to identify an embolus or renal infarction.

Arteriography may be needed to define the organ of origin of an abdominal mass or to delineate the vessels in a variety of clinical situations. When a mass becomes large, it compresses adjacent structures and obliterates fat planes. When other organs are distorted it may not be possible to determine the tissue of origin of the mass. This is especially true in the upper abdomen where an adrenal mass may be indistinguishable from an exophytic renal mass, liver mass, or even primary retroperitoneal tumor. By defining the vessels supplying these large tumors it may be possible to predict the tissue type.

Arterial access is usually gained via the right femoral artery, but the left femoral artery, left brachial or even the right brachial artery may be used if necessary. Most angiographers prefer working with 5 French catheters. Thin-walled catheters allow high flow rates while preserving the small outer diameter. Larger catheters may be required for some interventional procedures and smaller catheters (3 or 4 French) may be used with digital techniques.

If evaluation of the main renal arteries is desired, a flush aortogram should be performed as the initial run. This allows visualization of the origin of the renal arteries, although oblique views are occasionally needed to see the renal origin in profile. The flush aortogram also provides visualization of the renal arteries before a catheter or guidewire are introduced into the renal artery, as this manipulation may cause vascular spasm.

Abdominal aortography may be performed with either pigtail or straight end and side hole catheters. The straight catheter has a slight advantage, as it avoids the potential problem of uncoiling and unwanted selective vessel catheterization that can occur with a pigtail catheter. However, this is a rare complication, and most angiographers feel the tighter bolus obtained with the pigtail configuration more than compensates for this potential problem.

The position of the catheter tip in the abdominal aorta depends on the specific indication for the arteriogram, however, it is usually placed just above or just below the renal arteries. If the pigtail is placed just below the renal arteries, contrast injection will reflux 2 or 3 cm cephalad and provide opacification of the renal arteries. This avoids reflux into the celiac and superior mesenteric arteries, which may obscure portions of the renal arteries by opacifying overlying vessels.

There are a variety of catheters available for selective catheterization of the renal arteries. A simple J hook is all that is required but a specific renal curve, the Mikaelson curve, or the visceral cobra curve are the most popular catheter shapes. The choice of catheter depends on personal preference and what other maneuvers may be needed during the arteriogram.

Selective adrenal arteriography is much more demanding as the adrenal arteries are small. Flush aortography may be useful but the adrenal arteries are often difficult to identify due to the many overlying vessels. The easiest adrenal artery to opacify is the superior adrenal artery which arises from the inferior phrenic artery. Selective injection of the ipsilateral inferior phrenic artery usually provides adequate opacification of the superior adrenal artery. The inferior adrenal artery arises from the renal artery and injection of the renal artery usually results in sufficient visualization of the inferior aspects of the adrenal gland. The smallest of the adrenal arteries is the middle adrenal artery which arises directly from the aorta. Unless this artery is enlarged, it is difficult to catheterize and seldom worth the time required and possible damage to the vessel.

Diagnostic arteriography of the other genitourinary structures is seldom required, although there has been increased interest in the arterial supply and venous drainage of the penis for problems of impotence. Selective injection of the internal iliac arteries with an oblique projection will demonstrate medium-sized vessels supplying the dorsal penile artery. A flush aortogram may also be useful to see if a common iliac artery stenosis might be amenable to percutaneous transluminal angioplasty.

Digital Subtraction Angiography

Digital subtraction techniques may be used to image either arteries or veins, but is most often applied to procedures to screen for abnormalities of the renal arteries and to guide interventional procedures. In digital subtraction angiography (DSA), the analog information obtained with fluoroscopy is digitized. Similar digital information from a mask obtained before contrast injection is subtracted from the frames obtained during contrast injection. Digital computers capable of making these subtractions at very high speed allow visualization of the subtracted images during the procedure. The technique has very high contrast sensitivity but does not have the spatial resolution of conventional film screen angiography.

Since contrast sensitivity is high, less contrast is needed to adequately image the vessel. Thus, DSA may be used to image arteries after an intravenous injection. This may be done to screen patients for renovascular hypertension or to look for anomalies of the renal arteries in potential renal transplantation donors. With a peripheral injection of 40 ml of 60% iodinated contrast material at 10 ml/sec, the renal arteries can be imaged. An alternative approach injecting contrast into the inferior vena cava or right atrium require a caval catheter. However, both of these are intravenous injections and avoid the potential complications of arterial catheterization.

If the contrast is injected directly into the artery studied, adequate images can be obtained with much less contrast material than conventional arteriography. This may be desired in a patient with renal failure in whom the contrast load should be minimized to decrease the risk of contrast nephropathy. It is important to dilute the contrast material to 30–50% of the conventional concentration rather than decrease the volume, as a small volume will not replace blood flow and produce artifacts.

During lengthy interventional procedures such as embolization or angioplasty, DSA may save time. The digital image is available for immediate viewing, as film loading and processing is not required.

Venography

Access to the venous system is usually through the right femoral vein, although the left femoral vein or a vein in the antecubital fossa may be used if needed. The most common use of venography in GU radiology is collection of blood samples from the renal veins for renin assay in patients suspected of having renovascular hypertension.

When blood samples are obtained from a large vein, such as the renal vein, a side hole near the catheter tip is often helpful, as the end hole of a downward-directed catheter tip may be occluded by the wall of the vein. It is important to be aware of the location of veins such as the inferior phrenic vein or left gonadal vein which drains into the renal vein, as inadvertent catheterization of these vessels will result in a spurious result. The use of a small amount of contrast material to confirm location of the catheter tip does not affect the blood sample if the catheter is flushed and blood reaspirated to avoid dilution. If there is suspicion of a branch artery stenosis, narrowing of an accessory renal artery or a renin producing tumor, samples should be taken from smaller renal vein branches to reflect the upper and lower poles as well as the central portion of the kidney.

Adrenal venography is occasionally needed to identify an autonomous hyperfunctioning adrenal tumor. Selective catheterization of the left adrenal vein may be accomplished via the femoral and left renal veins. The left adrenal vein joins the inferior phrenic vein which enters the superior aspect of the left renal vein just to the left of the vertebral body. This vein can usually be catheterized with a variety of catheters but a double-curved catheter specifically designed for this purpose is available.

The right adrenal vein is more difficult to catheterize due to its small size and variable entrance directly into the inferior vena cava (IVC). A down-pointing tip with a secondary curve which reaches the opposite wall of the IVC is needed. This can be accomplished by forming a catheter to fit the expected shape or using a preformed catheter such as a Mikaelson or sidewinder configuration. In either case, heparin irrigation is useful to prevent clot formation in either the small adrenal veins partially occluded by the catheter or in the catheter itself. Adrenal venous sampling can be a slow and tedious process and should be performed by experienced angiographers.

Gonadal venography is used either in preparation for occlusion therapy for a varicocele or to identify the pampiniform plexus of an undescended testis. Catheterization of the left gonadal vein is accomplished with a variety of catheters but a visceral cobra is often used. Since the left gonadal vein enters the inferior surface or the left renal vein, it is usually easy to find. The right gonadal vein enters the inferior vena cava below the level of the renal veins, usually at L_2 or L_3. Since a variety of catheters can be used, the choice of the specific catheter should be determined by the other goals of the procedure.

Lymphography

Lymphography was introduced for use in human beings in 1952 and subsequently gained widespread acceptance to evaluate the retroperitoneal lymph nodes. Although it has largely been replaced by CT, lymphography can identify smaller metastatic foci by detecting alterations in internal architecture. The injected contrast material remains within lymph nodes 1–2 years providing visualization of opacified nodes on surveillance abdominal radiographs.

Superficial lymphatic vessels, usually in the dorsum of the foot, are cannulated and an iodinated oily contrast material infused. Much of this contrast is retained in the draining lymph nodes resulting in prolonged opacification. Contrast that is not taken up by the lymph nodes is trapped by pulmonary capillaries. This creates multiple small pulmonary emboli that result in a predictable impairment of pulmonary function. The diffusion capacity is most severely affected although a decrease in vital capacity has also been shown. The maximum impairment is seen about 36 hours after contrast infusion and recovery is usually complete in 3–5 days. Thus, significant impairment of pulmonary function is a contraindication to lymphangiography. If any doubt exists, pulmonary function tests should be obtained.

The presence of normal lymphaticovenous shunts will increase the pulmonary embolic load if they are present prior to the lymph nodes, as the shunts decrease the extent of lymph node uptake of contrast. These lymphaticovenous communications are undesirable, but still keep the oily contrast material on the right side of the heart. However, the presence of a right-to-left shunt is an absolute contraindication to lymphography, as the contrast will bypass the lung and become a systemic embolus, possibly leading to stroke or other neurologic dysfunction.

Although technically more challenging, lymphography may be performed in children as well as adults. In a review of 1079 cases from three institutions, Castellino et al. reported successful bilateral studies in 90% of children 15 years of age or under. An additional 8.7% had successful unilateral lymphograms so that the bilateral failure rate was only 1.3%. Ketamine anesthesia is recommended in younger children and care should be taken to limit proportionately the amount of contrast infused.

The interpretation of lymphograms in patients with solid tumors differs from the interpretation of those with malignant lymphomas. Metastases to lymph nodes from solid tumors tend to produce peripheral filling defects. As criteria for metastases, these defects are most reliable if they are greater than 1 cm in diameter and multiple. It is important to check the 2-hour channel films to be sure that lymphatic channels do not traverse these filling defects, as channels will not pass through a metastatic deposit. Small filling defects are much less reliable even if they are multiple, as they may be due to a variety of etiologies, such as fat, fibrosis, or an irregularly shaped lymph node. If the metastasis becomes large, it may totally obstruct the lymphatic channel and prevent opacification of a lymph node or group of nodes. Although this is a reliable criteria, it is often difficult to be sure that lymphatic obstruction is present. Persistent filling of lymphatic channels at 24 hours or evidence of an unopacified mass seen on other studies such as CT help to confirm this impression.

In each case, the lymphogram should be interpreted with knowledge of the pertinent clinical information. The type, location, and extent of the tumor are important, as lymphatic metastases follow the normal lymphatic drainage routes. Testicular neoplasms metastasize to the high paraaortic regions while prostatic tumors are usually first seen in the iliac chains. If, however, the tumor has locally invaded beyond the fascial confines of the gland, it may take alternate pathways and the usual drainage patterns are no longer reliable. Finally, the presence of an unopacified mass recognized by other means, such as CT or US, may indicate a lymph node or group of nodes that are not filled on the lymphogram.

Percutaneous Biopsy

Although exquisite images can be provided by a variety of radiographic modalities, the precise nature of the abnormal tissue is seldom certain. Pathologic proof, in the form of histology or cytology, is often required. Percutaneous needle biopsy guided precisely into the area of abnormality by an imaging modality has achieved a high level of success. Pathologic diagnoses can be made without subjecting the patient to the morbidity, mortality, or long recovery time associated with open surgery. These techniques are now commonly used for masses in the adrenal glands, kidney, and prostate gland, as well as other sites which may represent metastatic disease.

Adrenal

The adrenal glands are a common site of metastases from a variety of primary malignancies. Proof of the nature of an adrenal mass may be critical in determining the most appropriate therapy for such patients. Magnetic resonance may be used to distinguish an adrenal metastasis from a benign nonhyperfunctioning adenoma, but 21–31% of patients will fall into an "overlap" or indeterminate group. Thus, percutaneous biopsy may be needed, especially if an adrenal mass is the only site suspicious for metastatic disease.

The adrenal glands are centrally located within the torso and may be approached anteriorly, posteriorly, or through the liver. The anterior approach uses a needle tract through a variety of tissues and often results in difficult needle positioning because of respiratory motion. The posterior route is preferred as it traverses only the paraspinal muscles and the perirenal fat. However, in many patients the posterior pulmonary sulcus lies between the adrenal gland and the skin. In such cases, a triangulated approach may be used. The needle is inserted below the diaphragm and angled cephalad toward the adrenal mass. This technique avoids the lung but is cumbersome to use. The transhepatic route is a convenient compromise for right adrenal masses. The liver is a vascular organ, but bleeding complications are rare.

Although 22-gauge Chiba needles were most commonly employed for adrenal biopsy, they are difficult to maintain on a steady course to a target as deep as the adrenal gland. Most interventionalists prefer a 20-gauge biopsy or aspiration needle and some routinely use 18-gauge needles. Complications are uncommon, with insignificant periadrenal bleeding seen most often. A pneumothorax may be seen if the pulmonary sulcus is traversed, but these can be treated successfully with a small chest tube if they are clinically significant.

Renal

There are many indications for biopsy of a renal mass, but relatively few are actually performed. A renal mass suspicious for primary renal adenocarcinoma is usually staged radiographically and taken to surgery on the assumption that it is malignant. Percutaneous aspiration is performed if metastases are suspected and tissue confirmation is needed to avoid surgery. However, even when metastatic disease is present, nephrectomy may be performed to treat or prevent complications of the tumor, such as pain, hematuria, or a paraneoplastic syndrome.

Since a negative aspiration does not necessarily exclude malignancy, few oncologists are willing to forego possible curative surgery on the assumption that a suspicious renal mass is not malignant. Similarly, aspiration of indeterminate or cystic renal masses can only provide further support for a benign etiology but cannot exclude cancer. Thus, surgery is often performed on the assumption that a lesion is a renal adenocarcinoma. If the lesion is found to be benign, a confident diagnosis will have been made by providing optimal tissue for evaluation.

The needle size and route are seldom a problem when biopsying a renal mass. Aspirating needles, usually 20- or 22-gauge, are routinely used. The approach is dictated by the location of the mass in the kidney. If possible, normal renal parenchyma and hilar structures should be avoided. Larger cutting needles can be employed, but since renal carcinomas are usually hypervascular, bleeding complications are more likely.

Serious complications are uncommon but include local bleeding, hematuria, arteriovenous fistula, or false aneurysm formation and, rarely, tumor seeding along the needle tract.

Prostate

Prostate biopsy is an integral part of the endorectal ultrasound examination of the prostate gland (Chapter 17). Since sonography is used to guide the needle into the most abnormal portion of the gland, the approach depends on the equipment available. If a rectal biopsy probe is used, an 18-gauge needle can fit into a biopsy guide and be advanced into the suspicious area. Since the rectal mucosa is not sterile, antibiotics are often given to the patient prior to the biopsy to prevent or minimize bacterial seeding.

Transperineal biopsies are performed after sterilizing the skin and are considered a sterile procedure. Since the perineum is a sensitive area, care must be taken to thoroughly infiltrate the needle tract. A variety of needles, including 20- or 22-gauge aspirating needles and 14- or 18-gauge-cutting needles, have been used with good results. In general, the sensitivity of the aspirating needles has been slightly less than with the larger needles used to obtain histologic specimens, but this must be weighed against the greater patient discomfort and hematuria associated with use of the larger needles.

Metastatic Sites

Genitourinary malignancies, such as tumors of the bladder and prostate, may spread by local extension to the pelvic sidewall or via lymphatics or vessels to distant sites. Testicular carcinoma typically follows the lymphatic drainage and spreads to the high paraaortic lymph nodes. Primary renal or adrenal malignancies spread to regional lymph nodes but may also have distant hematogenous metastases. Percutaneous fine-needle aspiration biopsy may be appropriate to confirm metastases to any of these as well as other, less common sites.

In general, these lesions are best approached using CT guidance which both identifies the target and defines the

needle tract. Since 20-gauge needles are easier than 22-gauge needles to direct into a distant mass, they have become the most popular biopsy needle. Complications from abdominal aspirations are sufficiently rare that these procedures are often performed on outpatients.

Renal Cyst Puncture

During the early 1970s renal cyst puncture gained great popularity as the definitive procedure, short of surgery, for the diagnosis of a renal cyst, and was advocated in some quarters in virtually every case. By the late 1970s and early 1980s, however, there was widespread acceptance of CT and US as studies that could approach the accuracy of cyst puncture. The role of cyst puncture has, therefore, changed so that it is now primarily a procedure that is utilized to evaluate renal masses not adequately characterized by these noninvasive studies. In addition to its use as a diagnostic procedure, renal cyst puncture may be utilized as a therapeutic maneuver in selected patients.

Indications

The current diagnostic indications for cyst puncture have recently been summarized by Sandler (Table 3.3). Approximately 5–8% of all renal lesions will not be adequately characterized by either US or CT. In addition, when there is a discrepancy between the imaging studies or between the radiographic appearance of the lesion and the clinical symptoms for which the initial studies were obtained, renal cyst puncture may be quite helpful. For example, patients that have unexplained fever or hematuria might be placed in this category.

Technique

Ultrasound, CT, or fluoroscopic guidance may be utilized. With the fluoroscopic technique, intravenous contrast material is needed to identify the lesion. For larger cysts, the fluoroscopic technique is preferred so that radiographic evaluation of the cyst is facilitated. During

Table 3.3.
Indications for Cyst Puncture[a]

Diagnostic
  Indeterminate mass
  Ultrasound and CT inconclusive
  Ultrasound and CT results conflicting
  Unexplained hematuria—apparent cyst
  Unexplained fever—apparent cyst
  Calcification within cyst wall (?)
Therapeutic
  Local symptoms
  Hydronephrosis
  Hypertension—renin-dependent

[a] From Sandler CM, Houston GK, Hall JT, et al.: Guided cyst puncture and aspiration. *Radiol Clin North Am* 24(4):527–537, 1986.

suspended respiration a 22-gauge Chiba needle is advanced percutaneously into the cyst. The depth of the lesion is usually estimated from a preceding CT or US examination. Once the tip of the needle is in the lesion, an aliquot of fluid is aspirated and sent for analysis. The remainder of the fluid is then aspirated and exchanged for contrast material and air on an equal volume basis. Under ideal circumstances, approximately 25% of the volume of the cyst should remain as cyst fluid, approximately 25% as contrast material and approximately 50% as air. Once the air and contrast material have been injected into the lesion, the needle is withdrawn and radiographs are obtained in multiple horizontal beam projections so that all of the walls of the cyst can be demonstrated with double contrast images (Fig. 3.15).

If after needle placement either no fluid or only grossly bloody fluid can be aspirated, and it has been verified that the needle is in the proper location, it can be presumed that the mass is solid. A small amount of contrast material may be injected to verify the needle position. This will result in a "tumorogram" which will demonstrate extravasation of the contrast material within the interstices of the lesion (Fig. 3.16).

If complete aspiration of the cyst fluid is necessary prior to therapeutic sclerosis of the cyst, a pigtail catheter is placed into the lesion over a guide wire. In this fashion, complete evacuation of the renal cyst fluid is possible.

Radiographic Features

The radiographic assessment of the renal cystogram begins with a comparison of the size of the lesion as demonstrated by the cystogram to the mass that has been discovered on the preceding imaging examination. If the exact dimensions of the mass are not entirely explained by the cyst, either the presence of an additional cyst or a cyst adjacent to another mass must be considered.

The walls of a simple renal cyst should be entirely smooth without evidence of nodules or masses. On the horizontal beam radiographs a sharp demarcation between the injected air and the contrast material should be demonstrated. Any irregularity of this surface should suggest the possibility that the lesion does not represent a simple cyst. Occasionally, internal septations may be demonstrated within the lesion that may explain the presence of internal echoes that may have been present on a preceding ultrasound examination.

Fluid Analysis

Analysis of the fluid aspirated from a renal cyst includes: (*a*) the appearance, (*b*) the laboratory evaluation,

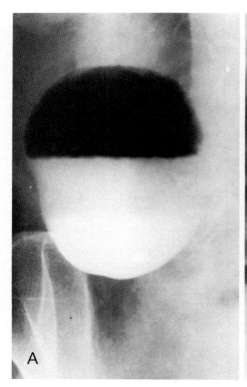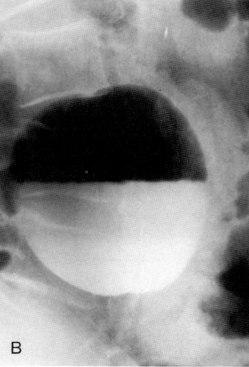

Figure 3.15. Double-contrast renal cyst study. **A,** Anteroposterior and **B,** lateral horizontal beam radiographs showing a large simple cyst. The walls of the cyst are smooth. Air outlines the upper margin of the cyst, while contrast material outlines the dependent portion. A rippled appearance is present at the air-fluid interface produced by standing waves as a result of transmitted arterial pulsations. (From Sandler GM, Houston GK, Hall JT, Morettin LB: Guided cyst puncture and aspiration. *Radiol Clin North Am* 24(1):527–537, 1986.)

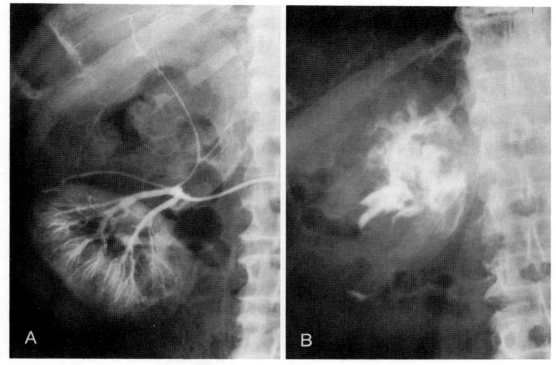

Figure 3.16. **A**, Angiographic examination demonstrates an avascular mass in the upper pole of the right kidney. **B**, Contrast material was injected after diagnostic aspiration failed to reveal fluid and is present within the interstices of this proven renal cell carcinoma. (From Sandler CM, Houston GK, Hall JT, Morettin LB: Guided cyst puncture and aspiration. *Radiol Clin North Am* 24(1):527–537, 1986.)

and (*c*) the histology of the cellular content (Table 3.4). A clear, straw-colored cyst aspirate is strongly correlated with an entirely benign cyst. Thus, some authorities have felt that cytologic and biochemical examination of clear cyst fluid is unnecessary.

Traumatic puncture of a benign cyst will occasionally occur and give rise to an initially bloody aspirate. In this case, however, progressive clearing of the aspirate should occur. If hemorrhagic fluid persists or the fluid appears xanthochromic, a hemorrhagic cyst may be diagnosed.

Inflammatory and neoplastic lesions characteristically reveal fluid demonstrating a spectrum ranging from turbid to frankly bloody. As a rule, inflammatory cysts tend to have a turbid to murky fluid, whereas neoplasms will generally be frankly bloody.

Routine microbiologic studies should be obtained whenever the cyst fluid does not meet the criteria of a simple cyst. Cytologic examination should also be obtained in these instances. The hallmark of malignant disease is the identification of tumor cells on cytology, however, the absence of tumor cells does not exclude

Table 3.4.
Analysis of Fluid Obtained at Cyst Puncture[a]

Mass	Color	Wall	Fat	Protein	LDH	Smear	Cell Block
Benign cyst	Clear yellow	Smooth	None	Low	Low	Negative	Negative
Inflammatory lesion	Clear ± turbid to bloody	Smooth, slightly irregular fibrin deposits	None to trace	High	Very high	Negative, occasionally indeterminate secondary to cellular atypia	Negative
Tumor	Murky to bloody	Nodules, mass shaggy but occupying entire space of lesion in question	High	High	Low to normal	Positive or negative	Positive

[a] From Sandler CM, Houston GK, Hall JT, Morettin LB: Guided cyst puncture and aspiration. *Radiol Clin North Am* 24(4):527–537, 1986.

malignancy and solid appearing masses should be explored despite a negative cytologic report.

The accuracy of diagnostic renal cyst puncture for the exclusion of malignancy approaches 100%. In the series of cyst punctures reported by Lang, the double-contrast cystogram combined with fluid analysis was accurate in 199 of 208 cases (96%).

Therapeutic Applications of Cyst Puncture

In the occasional patient, diagnostic puncture and therapeutic sclerosis may be indicated. Patients in this category include those with unexplained pain, hydronephrosis as a result of compression of the collecting system by the cyst, and rarely the presence of renin dependent renal hypertension caused by the renal cyst. Occasionally, infection in a preexisting renal cyst will be suspected, and if confirmed, percutaneous drainage may be established for therapy.

The majority of symptomatic cysts can be treated by percutaneous drainage or a combination of percutaneous drainage and sclerosis. Drainage without scleral therapy will result in a recurrence of 30–78% of cases. A number of sclerosing agents have been used to prevent cyst fluid reaccumulation. The two most commonly used are iophendylate (Pantopaque) (Fig. 3.17) and 95% ethanol. With alcohol sclerosis, a minimum of 25% of the original cyst volume should be replaced with 95% ethanol. The patient is then placed in the prone, supine, and decubitus positions for a minimum of 5 minutes to allow adequate contact of the alcohol with all areas of the cyst. Following instillation, the alcohol is aspirated through the pigtail catheter. Using this technique, Bean has shown a 0.5% incidence of recurrence in 34 cysts followed for 3 months.

Radionuclide Evaluation

The biodistribution of a small amount of radiotracer injected intravenously and detected with an external scintillation counter forms the basis for radionuclide evaluation of the urinary tract. The evaluation of the kidney is one of the oldest techniques in nuclear medicine. Initially, because of limitations in radiopharmaceuticals and radiation dose considerations, only functional information about the distribution of the tracer was available from such studies. With the development of newer radiopharmaceuticals, functional and limited anatomic information about the urinary tract can now be obtained. Modern radiopharmaceuticals often provide information about the urinary tract at a radiation dose well below a number of common radiologic procedures. Because the information is quantifiable and can be acquired by computer, the information can be stored, manipulated, and analyzed in detail. The most common scintillation detector utilized today is the gamma camera fitted with a

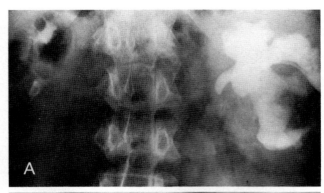
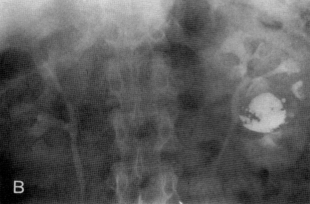

Figure 3.17. **A,** A large left parapelvic renal cyst causing moderate caliectasis is present. **B,** Following aspiration and instillation of Pantopaque, the caliectasis has resolved. (Courtesy of M. P. Banner, M.D.) (From Sandler CM, Houston GK, Hall JT, Morettin LB: Guided cyst puncture and aspiration. *Radiol Clin North Am* 24(1):527–537, 1986.)

crystal that is large enough that both kidneys may be analyzed simultaneously.

Radiopharmaceuticals

A number of radiopharmaceuticals have proven useful in evaluation of the urinary tract (Table 3.5). Unlike contrast materials used for conventional radiologic studies, radiopharmaceuticals are remarkably free of adverse reactions.

Eighty percent of an injected does of I-131-labeled *Hippuran* is excreted by tubular secretion. The primary use of this agent is in the radioisotopic evaluation of renal excretion, particularly in patients with diminished renal function. Because of the relatively long half-life of I-131 and its associated radiation dose, only relatively small amounts of this isotope (microcuries) can be utilized. Therefore, this agent is unsuitable for an evaluation of renal perfusion. However, because such a high percentage is excreted by tubular secretion, the isotope may be utilized to calculate effective renal plasma flow. I-123-labeled Hippuran has the same chemical and physiologic

Table 3.5.
Radiopharmaceuticals for Urinary Tract Imaging

Radiopharmaceutical	Physical Half-life	Principle Gamma Energy (keV)	Usual Dose
[131I]Orthoiodohippurate (hippuran)	8 days	364	300 μCi
[123I]Orthoiodohippurate (hippuran)	13.3 hr	160	1–2 μCi
99mTechnetium- diethylenetrianine pentacetic acid (DTPA)	6 hr	140	10–20 μCi
Glucoheptonate			10–20 μCi
Dimercaptosuccinic Acid (DMSA)			1–5 μCi
Mercaptoacetyltriglycine (MaG$_3$)			5 μCi

properties as the I-131-labeled variety, but has a much shorter half-life and as a consequence, a lower radiation dose. In addition, its gamma emission is much better suited to imaging than is the energy of I-131. Unfortunately, it is expensive to produce and has a very short shelf-life, which limits utility and it is, therefore, not in widespread clinical use.

99mTc-DTPA is useful for evaluation of renal perfusion as well as for imaging the kidneys and the urinary tract. A small percent of this radiopharmaceutical is protein-bound, but the majority is excreted by glomerular filtration without significant tubular resorption or secretion. About 90% of an injected dose of DTPA is excreted within 4 hours. Because it can be administered in relatively large (millicurie) amounts, the arrival of the tracer can be documented on camera images made every two or three seconds. In this fashion, a "radionuclide angiogram" can be obtained (Fig. 3.18). Since DTPA is cleared so rapidly from the kidneys, it is not suitable as a cortical imaging agent.

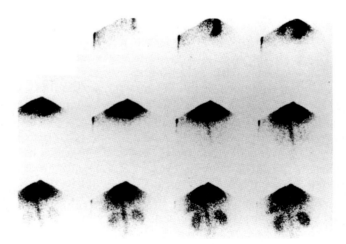

Figure 3.18.   Radionuclide angiogram. A bolus of 99mTc-DTPA has been injected. The activity can be seen circulating through the heart (*top row*), the lungs (*middle row*), and into the abdominal aorta and kidneys (*bottom row*).

99mTc-Glucoheptonate is a labeled carbohydrate that, in contrast to DTPA, is excreted very slowly by the kidney. Approximately 50% of this agent is protein-bound and while about 40% is excreted within the first hour, approximately 15% of the injected agent is retained within the renal cortex. The primary use of glucoheptonate, therefore, is as a cortical imaging agent when anatomic information about the kidney is desired in addition to information about perfusion and excretion.

Technetium-99m-dimercaptosuccinic acid (99mTc-DMSA) is cleared from the kidney even more slowly than is glucoheptonate. Approximately 50% of the injected dose remains in the renal cortex 6 hours after the injection. DMSA is of particular value when high-resolution images of the renal cortex are needed and little information about the excretion of the material is desired. Only about 15% of the dose of DMSA is excreted in the urine and there is significant excretion of this agent by the liver as well. Because there is so much binding of this agent to the renal cortex, the radiation dose is higher than with other technetium-labeled isotopes. Thus, unlike the other technetium agents, DMSA is not suitable for perfusion studies.

Technetium-99m-mercaptoacetyltriglycine (99mTc-MAG$_3$) is a new radiopharmaceutical not yet approved for clinical use which has a very high rate of clearance from the plasma (similar to Hippuran), but has the advantage of having the imaging characteristics of a technetium labelled compound. In the future, MAG$_3$ may replace Hippuran as the agent of choice for imaging patients with reduced renal function.

The Radioisotope Renogram

The major radionuclide tool for evaluation of renal function is called the radioisotope renogram. Such a renogram represents a curve demonstrating the radioactivity within the kidney plotted against the time after injection of the radiopharmaceutical. This is also referred to as a time-activity curve. Renogram curves may be constructed for studies performed with either DTPA or Hippuran. Analysis of the shape of the renogram curve can be used to suggest the diagnosis of many pathologic conditions of the kidney, including acute tubular necrosis, suspected urinary tract obstruction, and renal transplant rejection. A modification of the standard radioisotope renogram, called the *diuretic renogram,* is useful in differentiating functionally insignificant urinary tract dilatation from that caused by urinary tract obstruction. With this technique, a diuretic, commonly furosemide, is injected shortly after the radiopharmaceutical appears in the collecting system and the effect of the diuretic on the shape of the renogram curve is analyzed. In patients with functionally insignificant urinary tract dilatation, the diuretic will cause a prompt reduction in the amount of activity in the renal collecting system, whereas, in those with true urinary tract obstruction, the amount of activity in the collecting system will increase after the diuretic is administered (see Chapter 14).

Radionuclide Renal Imaging Studies

RENAL PERFUSION. A renal perfusion study may be obtained following the intravenous administration of 10–20 μCi of ^{99m}Tc-DTPA or glucoheptonate given as a compact bolus. Images are obtained on the gamma camera every 2–5 seconds for the first 1 minute following the injection and demonstrate the arrival of the bolus of activity in the abdominal aorta and the iliac vessels, as well as the arrival of the tracer in the kidneys. On the early images, the circulation of the radiopharmaceutical in the liver and spleen is also visualized. The camera should be positioned posterior to the patient when native kidneys are being evaluated and anterior to the iliac fossa for the evaluation of a transplanted kidney. Data from the perfusion study (first minute after injection) may be acquired in a computer and a time activity curve generated for each kidney. Such a curve will demonstrate the relative perfusion of each kidney. Data acquired between 1 and 3 minutes may also be used to generate a time activity curve which can be utilized to calculate the relative contribution of each kidney to total renal function (also known as split renal function studies) (Fig. 3.19). Static images are normally obtained 3–5 minutes following the injection as well.

RENAL CORTICAL IMAGING. Renal cortical imaging may be performed following intravenous administration of 10–20 μCi ^{99m}Tc-glucoheptonate or 1–5 μCi of ^{99m}Tc-DMSA. One of the more common uses of these agents is in the evaluation of renal pseudotumors, normally functioning renal tissue which simulate a renal mass lesion. The uptake of the radiopharmaceutical by such pseudotumors differentiates them from pathologic renal masses which will not accumulate any activity. This technique is frequently used to evaluate such conditions as a "hilar lip," a hypertrophied column of renal tissue medially that may

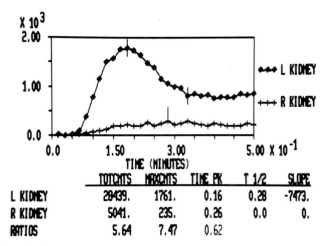

	TOTCNTS	MAXCNTS	TIME PK	T 1/2	SLOPE
L KIDNEY	28439.	1761.	0.16	0.28	-7473.
R KIDNEY	5041.	235.	0.26	0.0	0.
RATIOS	5.64	7.47	0.62		

Figure 3.19. Split renal function studies performed using ^{99m}Tc-DTPA. Computer generated curves of activity (*x*-axis) plotted against time after injection (*y*-axis) for each kidney. The activity in the right kidney is demonstrated to represent 15% of the total renal function (activity left kidney plus activity right kidney divided into activity right kidney).

impress the renal pelvis; a "dromedary hump" or splenic impression on the lateral portion of the left kidney; or a hypertrophied column of Bertin, an invagination of the cortex into the medullary portion of the kidney which may simulate an intrarenal mass.

RENAL FUNCTIONAL IMAGING. Renal functional imaging may be carried out following intravenous administration of 300 μCi of I-131-labeled Hippuran. Sequential images are frequently obtained every 2–3 minutes for a period of 20–30 minutes. Such studies will demonstrate the excretion of the radionuclide by the kidney into the bladder. Because relatively small amounts of activity are utilized, no radionuclide angiogram is possible. Unless obstructed, the collecting system and the ureter are also not visualized on such images. A renogram curve is frequently obtained simultaneously when imaging with Hippuran is performed. Delayed functional imaging may be performed with ^{99m}Tc-DTPA, as well.

RENAL TRANSPLANT EVALUATION. A major use of radionuclides in the urinary tract is the evaluation of the status of a renal transplant. Many different radiopharmaceuticals are utilized for this purpose. Most typically, renal perfusion studies using ^{99m}Tc-DTPA (Fig. 3.20) and delayed images of the kidney are performed. In some institutions, a combination of ^{99m}Tc-DTPA perfusion and I-131 Hippuran images are obtained. The combination of these two studies frequently is helpful in evaluating such complications of transplantation as obstruction of the renal artery, acute tubular necrosis, rejection, perirenal fluid collections, cyclosporine nephrotoxicity, and various mechanical complications such as ureteral obstruction and urinary extravasation.

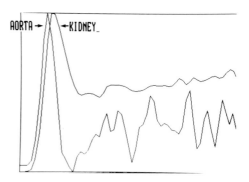

Figure 3.20. Renal perfusion curve of a transplant obtained with ^{99m}Tc-DTPA. The arrival of the bolus activity into the kidney as compared to the aorta is demonstrated in the first 1 min after injection. Relative activity is plotted on the x-axis and time is plotted on the y-axis.

Radionuclide Renal Function Studies

GLOMERULAR FILTRATION RATE. A radionuclide estimation of glomerular filtration, while not as accurate as an inulin clearance performed under strict laboratory conditions, nonetheless, provides a reasonable method for estimation of the glomerular filtration rate (GFR). ^{99m}Tc-DTPA is usually utilized for radionuclide calculation of the GFR. Three to five blood samples drawn over a 2- to 4-hour period after the injection of a known dose of the radiopharmaceutical are obtained and a plasma disappearance curve for the DTPA is calculated.

EFFECTIVE RENAL PLASMA FLOW. Effective renal plasma flow can be calculated using I-131-labeled orthoiodohippurate. Many methods for this determination, which is qualitatively similar to that used for determination of GFR, have been described. Both blood and urine samples are usually required. Modification of the technique which requires only a single blood sample has also been described.

Nonrenal Imaging Studies

RADIONUCLIDE CYSTOGRAPHY. Radionuclide cystography can be performed in children to follow the course of vesicoureteral reflux. 0.5–1 μCi of technetium pertechnetate is instilled via a Foley catheter into the bladder and diluted with an appropriate amount of saline. While the method offers considerably less spatial resolution than conventional voiding cystourethrography made with fluoroscopic spot films, it has the significant advantage of offering a lower radiation dose. Although it has a lower spatial resolution than the radiologic techniques, the sensitivity of a scintigraphic voiding cystourethrogram is said to be the same or greater than the radiologic study for the detection of vesicoureteral reflux greater than grade 1. When an initial radiographic study shows that reflux is present, this technique provides a relatively sensitive method for following the course of the reflux in children

with minimal radiation exposure. If the radionuclide study suggests that an increased amount of reflux is present, repeat radiographic studies should then be obtained.

The amount of reflux that is present on the radionuclide study can be quantitated by evaluating specific regions of interest over the distal ureters.

SCROTAL IMAGING. Radionuclide techniques have been utilized extensively to evaluate patients who present with acute, painful scrotal swelling. The primary purpose of these techniques is to differentiate patients with epididymoorchitis from those with testicular torsion or a testicular abscess. Scrotal imaging is performed as a perfusion study centered over the pelvis following intravenous administration of 10–20 μCi of technetium pertechnetate. Dynamic scintiphotos made at 2- to 3-second intervals followed by static images are utilized for this purpose.

ADRENAL IMAGING. A resurgence in interest in radionuclide imaging of the adrenal gland has occurred as the result of the introduction of I-131-labeled metaiodobenzylguanidine (MIBG). This compound is taken up by the adrenal medulla and is capable of demonstrating adrenal medullary hyperplasia and pheochromocytomas.

Adrenal cortical imaging with I-131- or I-123-19-iodocholesterol has never achieved great clinical popularity because of relatively low uptake of the precursor by the adrenal and the fact that delayed imaging for up to 15 days is required. I-131-iodomethyl 19-norcholesterol (NP 59) has been somewhat more successful in its evaluation of patient's with Cushing's syndrome in differentiating patients with adrenal hyperplasia from those with functioning adenomas and contralateral adrenal suppression.

SUGGESTED READINGS

Excretory Urography

Banner, MP, Pollack HM: Evaluation of renal function by excretory urography. *J Urol* 124:443, 1980.

Bauer DL, Garrison RW, McRoberts JW: The health and cost implications of routine excretory urography before transurethral prostatectomy. *J Urol* 123:386, 1980.

Daughtridge TG: Ureteral compression device for excretory urography. *AJR* 95(2):431, 1965.

Donker PJ, Kakisilatu F: Preoperative evaluation of patients with bladder outlet obstruction with particular regard to excretory urography. *J Urol* 120:685, 1978.

Doubilet P, McNeil BJ, Van Houten FX, et al.: Excretory urography in current practice: evidence against overutilization. *Radiology* 154:607, 1985.

Dure-Smith P, McArdle GH: Tomography during excretory urography: technical aspects. *Br J Radiol* 45:896, 1972.

Eklof O, Ringertz H: Kidney size in children. *Acta Radiol Diagn* 17(5):617, 1976.

Gillespie HW, Maile WBD: Routine tomographs with excretion urography. *Br J Radiol* 27:344, 1954.

Goldwasser B, Cohan RH, Dunnick NR, Andriani RT, Carson CC and Weinerth JL: The role of linear tomography in evaluation of patients with nephrolithiasis. *Urology* 23:253, 1989.

Hattery RR, Williamson B Jr, Hartman GW, et al.: Intravenous urographic technique. *Radiology* 167:593, 1988.

Lloyd LK, Witten DM, Bueschen AJ, Daniel WW: Enhanced detection of asymptomatic renal masses with routine tomography during excretory urography. *Urology* 11:523, 1978.

Mellins HZ, McNeil BJ, Abrams HL, et al.: The selection of patients for excretory urography. *Radiology* 130:293, 1979.

Newberg AH, Mindell HJ: Predicting tomographic levels for urography. *Radiology* 118:460, 1976.

Pollack H: Some limitations and pitfalls of excretory urography. *J Urol* 116:537, 1976.

Pollack HM, Banner MP: Current status of excretory urography a premature epitaph? *Urol Clin North Am* 12(4):585, 1985.

Sandler CM, Conley SB, Fogel SR: Splenic compression of the left kidney simulating pathologic unilateral renal enlargement. *J Comput Assist Tomogr* 4(2):248, 1980.

Simon AL: Normal renal size and absolute criterion. *AJR* 92(2):270, 1964.

Antegrade Pyelography

Hare WS, McOmish: Skinny needle pyelography. *Med J Aust* 2:123, 1981.

Pfister RC, Newhouse JH: Interventional percutaneous pyeloureteral techniques: I. Antegrade pyelography and ureteral perfusion. *Radiol Clin North Am* 17:341, 1979.

Pfister RC, Papanicolaou N, Yoder IC: Diagnostic morphologic and urodynamic antegrade pyelography. *Radiol Clin N Am* 24(4):561, 1986.

Urethrography

McCallum RW: The radiologic assessment of the lower urinary tract in paraplegics: a new method. *J Can Assoc Radiol* 25:34, 1974.

McCallum RW: The adult male urethra: normal anatomy, pathology and method of urethrography. *Radiol Clin North Am* 17:227, 1979.

McCallum RW, Colapinto V: *Urological Radiology of the Adult Male Lower Urinary Tract.* Springfield, IL, Charles C Thomas, 1976.

McCallum RW, Colapinto V: The role of urethrography in urethral disease: I. Accurate radiological localization of the membranous urethra and distal sphincters in normal male subjects. *J Urol* 122:607, 1979.

Cavernosography

Bookstein JJ, Valji K, Parsons L, et al.: Penile pharmacocavernosography and cavernosometry in the evaluation of impotence. *J Urol* 137:772, 1987.

Bookstein JJ: Cavernosal veno-occlusive insufficiency in male impotence: Evaluation of degree and location. *Radiology* 164:175, 1987.

Lue TF, Hricak H, Schmidt RA, et al.: Functional evaluation of penile veins by cavernosography in papaverine-induced erection. *J Urol* 135:479, 1986.

Ultrasonography

Amis ES, Jr, Hartman DS: Renal ultrasound 1984: a practical overview. *Radio Clin North Am* 22(2):315, 1984.

Chang VH, Cunningham JJ: Efficacy of sonography as a screening method in renal insufficiency. *J Clin Ultrasound* 13:414–417, 1985.

Coleman B: Ultrasonography of the upper genitourinary tract. *Urol Clin North Am* 12(4):633, 1985.

Fowler RC, Chennells PM, Ewing R: Scrotal ultrasound: a clinical evaluation. *Br J Radiol* 60(715):649, 1986.

Haller JO, Cohen HL: Pediatric urosonography: an update. *Urol Radiol* 9:99, 1987.

Rifkin MD: Scrotal ultrasound. *Urol Radiol* 9:119, 1987.

Taylor KJ, Burns PN: Duplex Doppler scanning in the pelvis and abdomen. *Ultrasound Med Biol* 11(4):643, 1985.

Taylor KJ, Burns PN: Duplex Doppler scanning in the pelvis and abdomen. *ULtras Med Biol* 11(4):643, 1985.

Computed Tomography

Dunnick NR, Korobkin M: Computed tomography of the kidney. *Radiol Clin North Am* 22(2):297, 1984.

Love L, Churchill RJ, Reynes CJ, Moncada R, Demos T: CT of the kidney and perinephric space. *Semin Roentgenol* 16(4):277, 1981.

McClennan B, Lee JKT, Peterson RR: Anatomy of the perirenal area. *Radiology* 158:555, 1986.

Sandler CM, Raval B, David CL: computed tomography of the kidney. *Urol Clin North Am* 12(4):657, 1985.

Wadsworth DE, McClennan BL, Standley RJ: CT of the renal mass. *Urol Radiol* 4:85, 1982.

Magnetic Resonance

Gore JC, Emery EW, Orr JS, Doyle FH: Medical nuclear magnetic resonance imaging: I. physical principles. *Invest Radiol* 16:269, 1981.

Hendee WR, Hendrick RE: Magnetic Resonance, In Putman CE, Ravin CE (eds): *Textbook of Diagnostic Imaging.* WB Saunders, Philadelphia, 1988, pp. 82–90.

Papanicolaou N, Hahn PF, Edelman RR, Newhouse JH, Pfister RC, Stark DD, Yoder IC, Brady TJ: Magnetic resonance imaging of the kidney. *Urol Radiol* 8:139, 1986.

Pykett IL, Newhouse JH, Buonanno FS, Brady TJ, Goldman MR, Kistler JP, Pohost GM: Principles of nuclear magnetic resonance imaging. *Radiology* 143:157, 1982.

Angiography

Ekelund L: Pharmacoangiography of the kidney: an overview. *Urol Radiol* 12:9, 1980.

Harrington DP, Levin DC, Garnick JD, Davidoff A, Bettmann MA, Kuribayashi S, Torman HA: Compound angulation in the angiographic evaluation of renal artery stenosis. *Radiology* 146:829, 1983.

Johnsrude IS, Jackson D, Dunnick NR: A Practical Approach to Angiography. Little, Brown, Boston, 1987.

Levin DC, Schapiro RM, Boxt LM, Dunham L, Harrington DP, Ergun DL: Digital subtraction angiography: principles and pitfalls of image improvement techniques. *AJR* 143:447, 1984.

Robertson PW, Dyson ML, Sutton PD: Renal angiography: a review of 1,750 cases. *Clin Radiol* 20:401, 1969.

Saddekni S, Sos TA, Sniderman KW, Srur M. Bodner LJ, Kneeland JB, Cahill PT: Optimal injection technique for intravenous digital subtraction angiography. *Radiology* 150:655, 1984.

Lymphography

Dunnick NR: The radionuclide evaluation. In Javadpour N (ed): *Principles and Management of Urologic Cancers.* Edited by Javadpour N. Baltimore, Williams & Wilkins, 1979.

Dunnick NR, Castelino RA: Pediatric lymphography. *AJR* 129:639, 1977.

Dunnick NR, Javadpour N: Value of CT and lymphography: Distinguishing retroperitoneal metastases from nonseminomatous testicular tumors. *AJR* 136:1093, 1981.

Percutaneous Biopsy

Bernardino ME: Percutaneous biopsy. *AJR* 142:41, 1984.

Haaga JR, LiPuma JP, Bryan PJ, Balsara VJ, Cohen AM: Clinical comparison of small- and large-caliber cutting needles for biopsy. *Radiology* 146:665, 1983.

Wittenberg J, Mueller PR, Ferrucci JT Jr, Simeone JF, van Sonnenberg E, Neff CC, Palermo RA, Isler RJ: Percutaneous core biopsy of abdominal tumors using 22 gauge needles: further observations. *AJR* 139:75, 1982.

Yankaskas BC, Stabb EV, Craven MB, Blatt PM, Sokhandan M, Carney CN: Delayed complications from fine-needle biopsies of solid masses of the abdomen. *Invest Radiol* 21(4):325, 1986.

Renal Cyst Puncture

Amis ES Jr, Cronan JJ, Yoder IC, et al.: Renal cysts: curios and caveats. *Urol Radiol* 4:199, 1981.

Bean WJ: Renal cysts: Treatment with alcohol. *Radiology* 138:329, 1985.

Lang EK: Renal cyst puncture and aspiration: a survey of complications. *AJR* 128:723, 1977.

Pollack HM, Banner MP, Arger PH, et al.: The accuracy of gray-scale renal ultrasound in differentiating cystic neoplasms from benign cysts. *Radiology* 143:741, 1982.

Raskin NM, Roen SA, Serafini AN: Renal cyst puncture: combined fluoroscopic and ultrasonic technique. *Radiology* 113:425, 1974.

Sandler CM, Houston GK, Hall JT, et al.: Guided cyst puncture and aspiration. *Radiol Clin North Am* 24(4):527, 1986.

Radionuclide Evaluation of the Urinary Tract

Blaufox MD, Kalika V, Scharf S, et al.: Applications of nuclear medicine in genitourinary imaging. *Urol Radiol* 4:155, 1982.

Doubovsky EV, Russel CD: Quantitation of renal function with glomerular and tubular agents. *Semin Nucl Med* 12:308, 1982.

Kirchner PT, Rosenthal L: Renal transplant evaluation. *Semin Nucl Med* 12:370, 1982.

Lutzker LG: The fine points of scrotal scintigraphy. *Semin Nucl Med* 12(4):387, 1982.

Mettler FA Jr, Guiberteau MJ: *Essentials of Nuclear Medicine Imaging,* ed 2. Orlando, FL, Grune & Stratton, 1986.

Taux WN, Dubovsky EV, Kidd T, et al.: New formulas for the calculation of effective renal plasma flow. *Eur J Nucl Med* 7:51, 1982.

CHAPTER 4

FUNCTIONAL RENAL ANATOMY, RENAL PHYSIOLOGY, AND CONTRAST MATERIAL

FUNCTIONAL RENAL ANATOMY AND RENAL PHYSIOLOGY

The principal function of the kidney is to maintain the homeostasis of body fluids. A number of specialized tasks are involved in this homeostasis. These include the excretion of metabolic end products and toxins, the regulation of body fluid volume, blood pressure regulation, and the regulation of mineral and acid-base balance. Body fluids are divided into two discrete compartments. Approximately two-thirds of the fluid is located within cell membranes and this is termed the *intracellular fluid*. The remaining one-third is contained in the extracellular compartment (ECF). Approximately one-third of the volume of the ECF is contained within the vascular space and two thirds is in the interstitium. The regulatory function of the kidney directly effects the fluid that is located in the vascular compartment, however, because there is free movement of water between the intracellular and extracellular fluid compartments, the effect of this function is to regulate the composition of all body fluids.

Functional Renal Anatomy

On gross inspection, a bisected kidney can be divided into two major regions (Fig. 4.1): (*a*) the inner renal medulla, and (*b*) outer renal cortex.

The functional unit of the kidney is the nephron (Fig. 4.2). Each kidney contains approximately one million nephrons. Each nephron consists of a specialized capillary vascular network called the *glomerulus* which is surrounded by Bowman's capsule, a balloon-like structure into which the capillary tufts of the glomerulus protrude. Each glomerulus is connected to a series of specialized

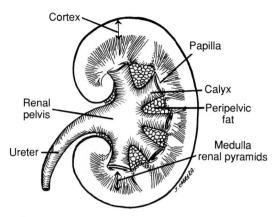

Figure 4.1. Bisected section of the kidney showing the relationship of the cortex, the medulla, and the renal collecting system. Fat in the renal sinus surrounds the calyces and the renal pelvis.

epithelial segments which collectively is known as the *renal tubule.*

The tubule, in turn, is divided into several segments. The first segment is called the proximal tubule which in turn is subdivided into a convoluted and a straight portion; the second segment, the loop of Henle, is subdi-

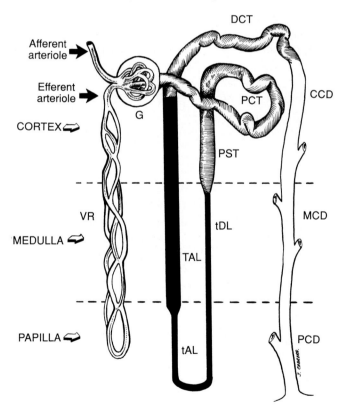

Figure 4.2. The nephron. G = glomerulus; TAL = thick ascending limb of the loop of Henle; tAL = thin ascending limb of the loop of Henle; PST = proximal straight tubule; PCT = proximal convoluted tubule; DCT = distal convoluted tubule; CCD = cortical collecting duct; MDC = medullary collecting duct; PCD = papillary collecting duct; A = afferent arteriole; E = efferent arteriole; VR = vasa recta.

vided into the thin descending, the thin ascending, and the thick ascending limbs; and the third segment, the distal tubule, is subdivided into the distal convoluted tubule and the cortical, medullary, and papillary collecting ducts. The cortex contains the glomeruli, the proximal tubule, the distal tubule, and the cortical collecting duct. The medulla is made up of the loops of Henle, the medullary and papillary collecting ducts, and renal pyramids, the apices of which project into the minor calyces. The nephrons that are located close to the corticomedullary junction have larger glomeruli and their loops of Henle descend deeper into the renal papilla than those located more superficially in the renal cortex.

The main renal artery branches into interlobar arteries which give off the arcuate arteries located at the corticomedullary junction. These, in turn, give off the interlobular arteries and finally the afferent arterioles each of which leads to a glomerulus. The glomerulus is drained by an efferent arteriole which subdivides to form a peritubular capillary network known as the *vasa recta.* The vasa recta then anastomose to form venous channels. This unique arrangement in the kidney in which the glomerulus is located between two resistive capillary networks, as opposed to the arteriole-capillary-venule arrangement of the other tissues of the body, helps to maintain constant hydrostatic pressure at the level of the glomerulus despite changes in blood pressure (Fig. 4.3) and is the driving force for glomerular filtration.

The *macula densa* is a distinctive portion of the tubule between the ascending loop of Henle and the distal convoluted tubule which courses between the afferent and efferent arterioles. The macula densa represents the tubular component of a specialized area of the nephron

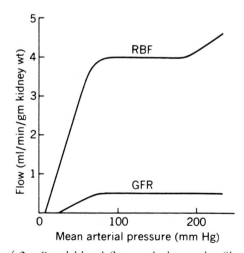

Figure 4.3. Renal blood flow and glomerular filtration remain constant over a wide range of blood pressure. This helps to maintain a constant level of glomerular filtration. (From Gottschalk CW, Lassiter WE: Mechanisms of urine formation. In Mountcastle VD (ed): *Medical Physiology,* Vol 2, ed 14. St. Louis: CV Mosby, 1980.

called the *juxtaglomerular apparatus* (JGA). The JGA is the site of renin synthesis and plays a major role in the blood pressure regulation function of the kidney.

Basic Renal Physiology

The homeostatic functions of the kidney are achieved through two simultaneous processes: (*a*) glomerular filtration, and (*b*) tubular resorption/secretion. Glomerular ultrafiltration occurs as a result of the net Starling forces across the glomerular capillary wall. The net filtration pressure (NFP) is equal to the sum of the glomerular hydrostatic pressure and the colloid osmotic pressure in Bowman's capsule (which favors fluid movement from the capillary space into Bowman's space) minus the sum of the mean glomerular capillary oncotic pressure and the hydrostatic pressure in Bowman's space (the principal forces opposing ultrafiltration). Because protein is not filtered by the glomerulus, the fluid in Bowman's space is protein-free and thus the colloid osmotic pressure in Bowman's space is negligible. The glomerular filtration rate (GFR) is determined by the NFP and the surface area available for filtration as well as the permeability of the glomerular capillary bed. Thus, GFR can be expressed as

$$GFR = K_f \times NFP$$

where K_f is a constant expressing the product of the capillary permeability and the surface area of the capillary bed and NFP is the net filtration pressure. The glomerular filtration rate in a normal patient is approximately 125 ml/min which is equal to 180 liters/day or approximately 12 times the volume of the ECF.

Although 180 liters of fluid is filtered in a day, only 1–2 liters of urine is produced per day in which wastes and toxins may be concentrated 100- to 200-fold above their plasma concentration. This concentration of the final urine product is the result of tubular reabsorption and secretion. Under normal conditions, approximately two-thirds of the ultrafiltrate volume is reabsorbed by the proximal tubule by a process linked to the active secretion of hydrogen ions and the active reabsorption of sodium, glucose, amino acids, and other solutes. Isotonicity of the fluid in the proximal tubule with the plasma is maintained as the cells of the proximal tubule are freely permeable to water.

In the loop of Henle, which begins at the corticomedullary junction, differential absorption of sodium chloride occurs so that the fluid in the tubular lumen, initially isotonic with the interstitium, becomes progressively more concentrated in the descending limb reaching its maximum concentration at the bend of the loop and then progressively more hypotonic with respect to plasma as it reaches the thick ascending limb of the loop. This differential absorption of sodium chloride occurs because the cells in the descending limb have a high permeability for water, but a low permeability for salt; whereas, in the thick ascending limb, the cells are impermeable to water, but have a high permeability for salt which is actively reabsorbed. This process, known as the *renal countercurrent mechanism,* results in progressive interstitial hypertonicity in the medulla and is required for final concentration of the urine by the distal tubules.

The distal tubule continues the water dilution of urine through the active transport of sodium and chloride coupled with relative water impermeability. The collecting ducts are the primary site of action of antidiuretic hormone (ADH). It is in the collecting ducts that the final 15% of water absorption is achieved. The collecting ducts are virtually impermeable to water in the absence of ADH, but when ADH is present, water passes freely across the tubular wall allowing the tubular fluid to achieve the same tonicity as the fluid in the surrounding interstitium. Thus, a hypertonic urine is produced without the active transport of water. The distal nephron also reabsorbs sodium and secretes hydrogen ions and potassium under the influence of aldosterone. Parathyroid hormone also acts on the distal tubule to conserve calcium.

Clearance

The rate at which a substance is removed from the plasma in a given period of time is termed the *clearance* of that substance. For a substance that is freely filtered and not reabsorbed or secreted by the tubule, the rate of clearance of that substance is equal to the GFR. The rate of clearance is expressed as the urinary volume per unit time, multiplied by the urine concentration of that substance, divided by the plasma concentration of the substance. Thus

$$GFR = \frac{U \times V}{P}$$

where U is the urine concentration of the substance, V is the urine volume produced per unit time, and P is the plasma concentration of the substance.

The polysaccharide, inulin, meets the criteria expressed above and therefore can be used to determine GFR. Creatinine, an endogenous product of muscle metabolism, is produced by the body in relatively constant amounts per day, is present in the plasma and is excreted by glomerular filtration. Measurement of creatinine clearance is therefore convenient, although it is not as exact as the inulin clearance because a small amount of creatinine is secreted by the tubules.

Renal Plasma Flow

If a substance were freely filtered and removed from the blood completely in one pass through the kidney, then clearance of that substance should represent the renal plasma flow. The substance paraminohippurate (PAH) is freely filtered and that portion that is not filtered is virtually completely secreted by the proximal tubule, so that at low plasma concentrations of PAH, all plasma supplying nephrons is completely cleared of the substance. The clearance of PAH, therefore, should represent the renal plasma flow (RPF), however, since 10–15% of renal blood flow supplies non-nephron-bearing portions of the kidney (i.e., the renal capsule and the peripelvic fat), the clearance of PAH is referred to as the effective renal plasma flow (ERPF). The normal value for ERPF is 650 ml/min/1.73 m² in males and 600 ml/min/1.73 m² in females. Once the ERPF has been calculated, the effective renal blood flow (ERBF) can be calculated by the formula

$$ERBF = \frac{ERPF}{1 - hematocrit}$$

The filtration fraction is the ratio of the clearance of inulin to that of PAH or C_{inulin}/C_{PAH}. In humans this ratio is normally 0.2.

CONTRAST MEDIA—HISTORICAL BACKGROUND

Attempts at radiography in the urinary tract began with the retrograde insertion of rigid metal stylets into the ureters to demonstrate their course shortly after Roentgen's discovery of x-rays in 1895. In 1905, the techniques of retrograde cystography and pyelography using Kollargol, a colloidol preparation of silver, were introduced by Voelcker and Von Lichtenberg. The first report of opacification of the urinary tract via excreted contrast material came in 1923 when Osborne, Sutherland, Scholl, and Rowntree, from the Mayo Clinic in Rochester, Minnesota reported that there was discernible opacification of the bladder on abdominal radiographs in patients who had received a 10% solution of sodium iodine, either orally or intravenously, for the treatment of syphilis. This report represented the initial discovery that iodine could be utilized as a radioopaque contrast agent. Successful opacification of the urinary tract using sodium iodide, however, was not routinely possible because it proved to be far too toxic in sufficient quantities to achieve diagnostic opacification.

The next significant breakthrough came in 1925 and 1926 when the German chemists Kurth Rath and Arthur Binz synthesized several organic pyridine compounds containing a single atom of iodine per molecule. They had been seeking to devise therapeutic agents that would be useful in the treatment of bacterial infections of the kidney and gallbladder. One of these pyridine compounds was found to be excreted by both the kidney and the liver and was called Selectan neutral (Fig. 4.4).

Clinical therapeutic trials of Selectan neutral were performed in Hamburg, Germany under the direction of Professor Leopold Lichtwitz. Dr. Moses Swick, a young American urologist, was working with Professor Lichtwitz and became interested in the potential of Selectan neutral for imaging the urinary tract. Professor Lichtwitz was

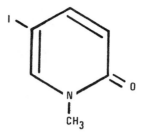

Figure 4.4.   Selectan—neutral.

so impressed with Swick's preliminary investigation that he suggested the investigation be continued in Berlin with Professor Von Lichtenberg, the eminent German urologist, who several years earlier had described retrograde pyelography and cystography. Von Lichtenberg had also been working on developing a satisfactory contrast agent for intravenous injection that would allow visualization of the urinary tract. After several discussions among Von Lichtenberg, Binz, and Swick, modifications of Selectan neutral designed to increase its water solubility and decrease its neurotoxicity were proposed. This collaboration resulted in the synthesis of Uroselectan (Iopax) (Fig. 4.5) which contained 42% iodine. Swick found that Uroselectan was the first agent to produce reliable opacification of the urinary tract after intravenous administration and that it was much better tolerated than the previously available compounds. Shortly thereafter, a further modification of the compound was made by Binz that was known as Uroselectan B in Europe and as Neo-Iopax (Fig. 4.6) in the United States. Neo-Iopax represented a significant improvement over Iopax in that it contains two iodine atoms per molecule and, therefore, the radioopacity of the compound was significantly greater. In addition to Neo-Iopax, Binz and Rath also synthesized an additional diiodo compound known as iodopyracet which was marketed as Diodrast (Fig. 4.7). These two products (Neo-Iopax and Diodrast) became the radiologic contrast media of choice and were used successfully for the next 20 years.

In 1933, Swick, who by then was working as a urologist at Mt. Sinai Hospital in New York, proposed that the six-carbon benzene ring serve as the carrier of iodine instead of the heterocyclic five-carbon atom and one-

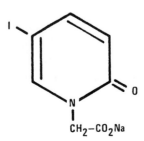

Figure 4.5.   Uroselectan.

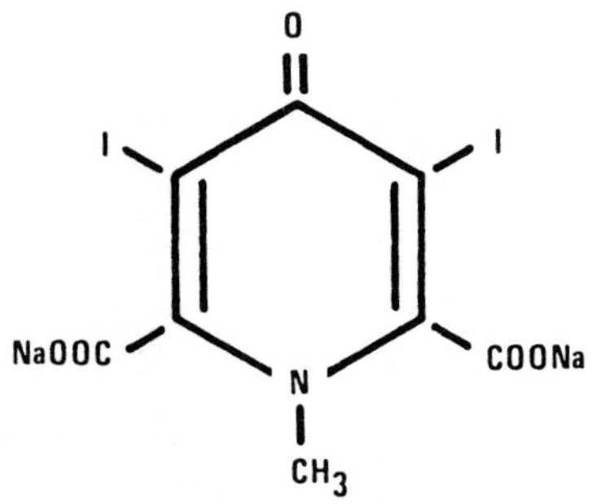

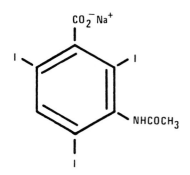

Figure 4.6. Sodium iodomethamate (Neo-Iopax).

Figure 4.9. Sodium acetrizoate (Urokon).

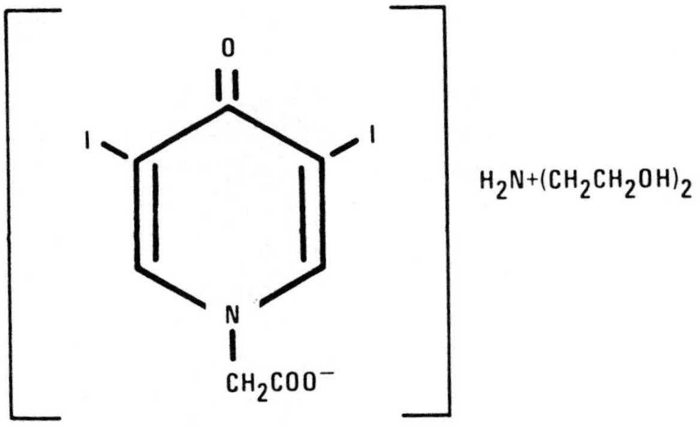

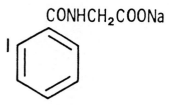

Figure 4.7. Iodopyracet (Diodrast).

nitrogen-atom pyridine ring as had been used by Binz and Rath. The product that was introduced, sodium monoiodo hippurate (Fig. 4.8) did not prove, however, to be a significant improvement over Diodrast or Neo-Iopax. However, the principle of using the six-carbon benzene ring as the carrier of iodine was established by this investigation.

It was not for approximately another 20 years that the six-carbon molecule was perfected as a contrast agent. In the late 1940s, Wallingford et al. at the Mallinckrodt Chemical Works of St. Louis synthesized acetrizoate which became the first triiodo derivative of benzoic acid to have proven clinical efficacy. This product, marketed as Urokon (Fig. 4.9), contained 65.8% iodine, and showed distinct advantages over the diiodo products because of its improved radioopacity, decreased toxicity,

and high water solubility. Initial physiologic studies indicated that it was excreted principally by glomerular filtration and thus better urinary tract opacification was achieved.

In 1955, Hoppe et al. at Sterling Winthrop Research Institute produced further modification of the triiodo benzoic acid ring by the addition of an additional side chain in the five position. This compound was known as sodium diatrizoate and was given the brand name Hypaque (Fig. 4.10). This product and its derivatives, including sodium/meglumine diatrizoate (Fig. 4.11) and meglumine iothalmate (Fig. 4.12) became the standard urographic contrast agents for the next 30 years.

It was realized during this period that while these ionic contrast media were much safer than the previously used materials, a great portion of the remaining toxicity of the compounds was related to their high osmolality (greater than 1500 mosm/kg of water or approximately 5 times greater than plasma). In 1968, Torsten Almen of Malmo, Sweden, a radiologist, theorized that the high osmolality of ionic contrast could be reduced by synthesizing a product that would be nondissociating. He suggested that the ionizing carboxal group of conventional contrast be replaced with a nondissociating group such as an amide. This would theoretically reduce the osmolality by 50% by reducing the number of particles in solution without loss of iodine content. Almen's hypothesis was pursued by a Norwegian company, Nyegaard AS and

CONHCH₂COONa

Figure 4.8. Sodium monoiodo hippurate.

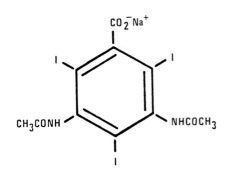

Figure 4.10. Sodium diatrizoate (Hypaque).

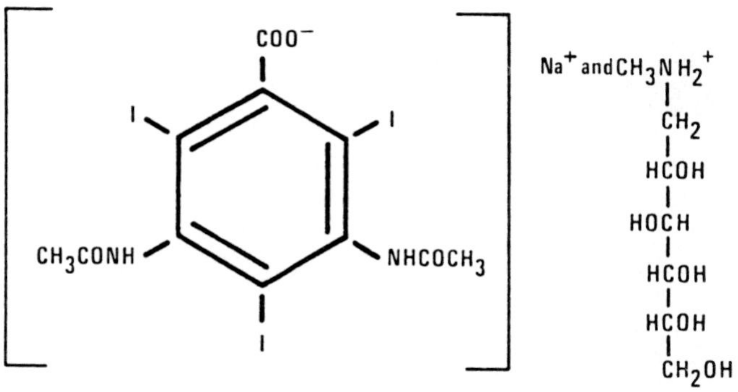

Figure 4.11. Sodium/meglumine diatrizoate (Renografin 60).

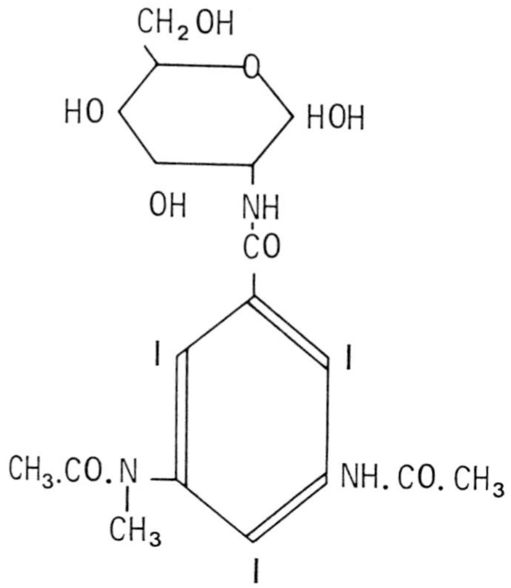

Figure 4.13. Metrizamide.

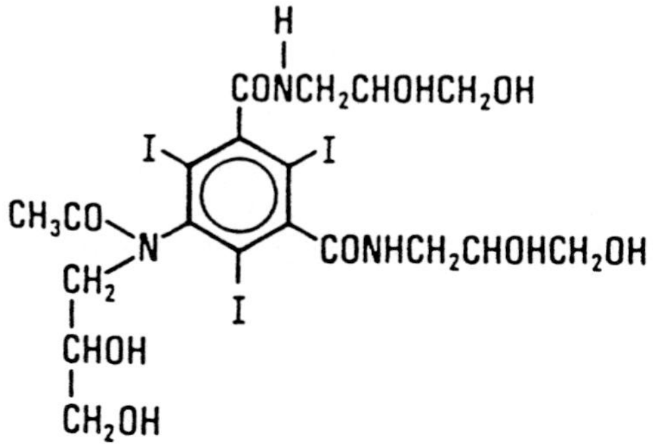

Co., which produced the first nonionic contrast medium, metrizamide (Fig. 4.13). Metrizamide, itself, while readily excreted by the kidneys was never utilized in the United States as a urographic agent. This was, in part, due to its considerable cost and the inability to sterilize the product by autoclave. It was necessary to package the material as a freeze-dried lypholized powder which needed to be reconstituted with water immediately before use.

Several years after the introduction of metrizamide, second-generation low-osmolality contrast agents were introduced into clinical practice. These products developed along two general lines. In the first group, hydrophilic nonionizing radicles are introduced in positions one, three, and five of the benzene ring, while positions two, four, and six remain the position of the iodine atoms. Because the number one position does not dissociate, the number of iodine atoms relative to the number of particles in solution is increased from 1.5 to 3 as compared to ionic contrast media. Compounds in this category that have been approved for clinical use include iohexol (Omnipaque) (Fig. 4.14), iopamidol (Isovue) (Fig. 4.15), and ioversol (Optiray) (Fig. 4.16). These products are generically known as nonionic monomers. The second line of development of low osmolality contrast has been directed toward the linkage of two triiodinated benzene rings sharing one ionizing carboxal group.

Figure 4.14. Iohexol (Omnipaque).

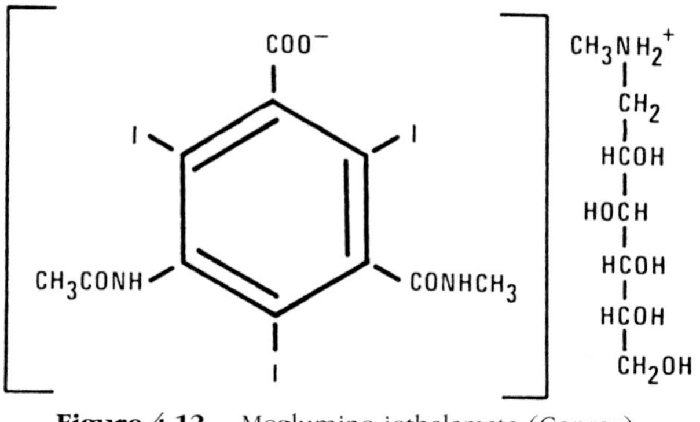

Figure 4.12. Meglumine iothalamate (Conray).

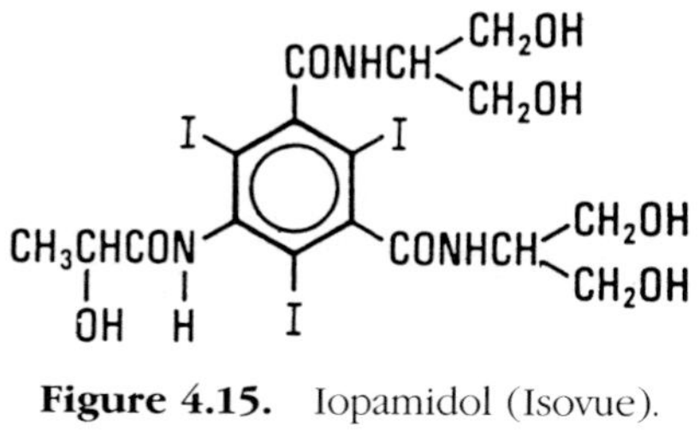

Figure 4.15. Iopamidol (Isovue).

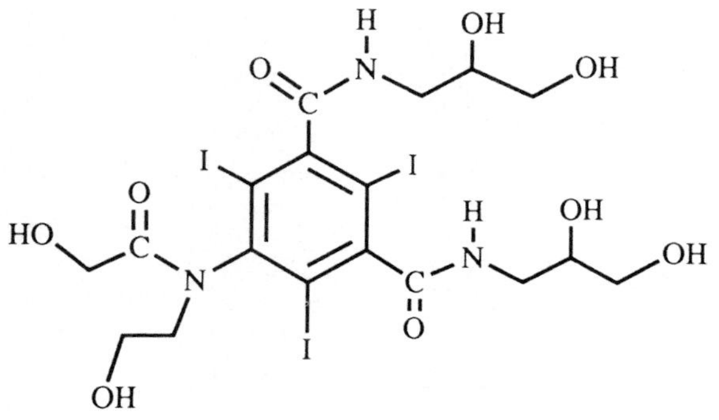

Figure 4.16. Ioversol (Optiray).

These compounds have a ratio of six iodine atoms to two molecules in solution and therefore also produce a ratio of 3. They are generally known as *monoacidic dimers.* Sodium-meglumine ioxaglate (Hexabrix) (Fig. 4.17) is a monoacidic dimer and has been introduced into clinical practice within the past several years.

The next obvious line of development for contrast agents will be the development of nonionic monoacidic dimers which will have a ratio of six iodine atoms to one particle in solution and will represent, therefore, ratio six compounds. This modification will, theoretically, reduce the osmolality of the contrast agent close to that of plasma.

PHYSIOLOGY OF CONTRAST EXCRETION

A knowledge of the basic physiology of contrast material excretion is crucial to the optimal performance of the urogram and its interpretation.

In 1960, Woodruff and Malvin demonstrated that the modern triiodobenzoic acid derivative contrast agents were excreted by glomerular filtration without a significant component of tubular secretion. This is in contrast to the diiodo pyridone–based contrast agents (Diodrast and Neo-Iopax) in which a significant component of tubular secretion is present.

In 1964, Schwartz et al. described using a "double dose" of contrast material to perform urography in patients with impaired renal function. The authors theorized that if contrast material is excreted by glomerular filtration excretion of the contrast should be governed by its plasma concentration. They reasoned that with de-

pressed renal function (i.e., a depressed glomerular filtration rate), raising the plasma concentration of contrast by increasing the administered dose would compensate for the depressed renal function and therefore improve the quality of the urogram that could be obtained in patients with azotemia. Their study demonstrated the efficacy of such an approach and was the first attempt to improve the quality of urography using basic physiologic principles. This report thus became the first description of "high-dose" urography.

In the same year, Schenker, popularized the technique of drip infusion pyelography in which a large volume (150 ml) of contrast material diluted with an equal volume of dextrose and water was infused by gravity through an 18-gauge needle. This technique was touted as a method of achieving better visualization of the collecting system. Schenker theorized that the majority of improvement in opacification of the collecting system was due to a diuretic effect achieved by mixing the contrast material with the dextrose and water. He felt that this would obviate the need for abdominal compression and dehydration and that better visualization would be achieved by "flooding the collecting system from above."

In the late 1960s, Purkiss et al. developed an ultraviolet spectrographic absorption technique by which plasma and urine contrast concentrations could be directly measured. In 1967, Cattel et al. at St. Bartholomew's Hospital in London utilized the technique to perform the first direct physiologic studies of contrast excretion in humans. They showed that there was a direct relationship between the plasma concentration of contrast and the dose of contrast administered (Fig. 4.18). In addition, they reported that the urinary contrast concentration is directly related to its rate of glomerular filtration. They further demonstrated that after intravenous injection of contrast material, there is a rapid rise followed by a rapid fall in plasma concentration of contrast, however, only 12% of the fall in plasma concentration in the first 10 minutes after injection of contrast is due to renal excretion; the remainder (88%) of the rapid fall is due to equilibration of the contrast throughout the ECF.

These studies were later amplified by Dure-Smith who emphasized that while only 12% of the fall in contrast concentration was due to excretion of the contrast by the kidneys, this 12% represents the critical amount of con-

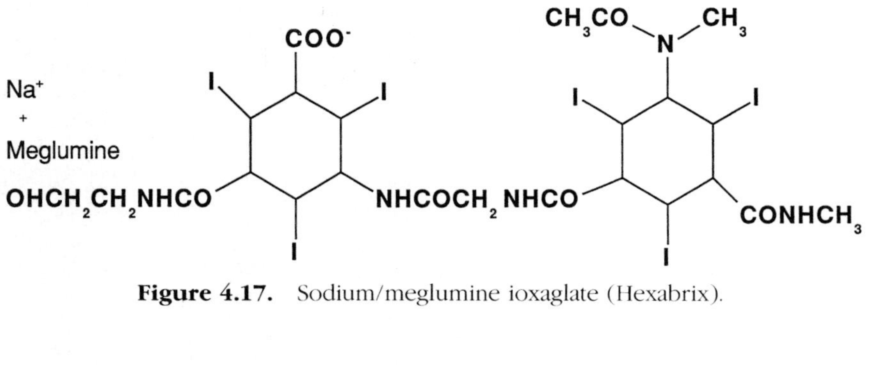

Figure 4.17. Sodium/meglumine ioxaglate (Hexabrix).

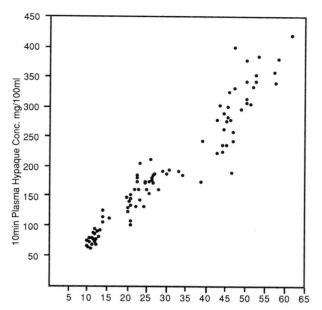

Figure 4.18. Graph showing that a linear relationship between plasma contrast concentration normalized to body surface area and administered dose is present 10 min after intravenous injection. (From Cattell WR, Fry IK, Spencer AG, et al.: Excretory urography I: Factors determining the excretion of Hypaque. *Br J Radiol* 40(476):561–571, 1967.)

trast that produces the diagnostic opacification of the urinary tract during urography since it is during this period that glomerular filtration of the contrast is at its maximum (Fig. 4.19). It is therefore within the first few moments after injection that the nephrogram, representing contrast within the renal tubules, is at its peak intensity. Dure-Smith also pointed out that the degree of opacification of the urinary tract is not a function of the concentration of the contrast material in the urine alone, rather it is the total amount of contrast (urinary contrast concentration times the volume of urine produced) upon which opacification depends. Thus, it is the total number of iodine atoms in the path of the x-ray beam rather than their concentration in their urine on which opacification depends. Both authors demonstrated that there is a dose-related rise in urine flow rate which occurs after contrast administration related to the fact that the contrast material acts as an osmotic diuretic (Fig. 4.20).

As we previously noted, the formula for glomerular filtration is

$$GFR = \frac{U_cV_c}{P_c}$$

Opacification of the urinary tract can be described by rearranging the equation so that

$$U_cV_c = GFR \times P_c$$

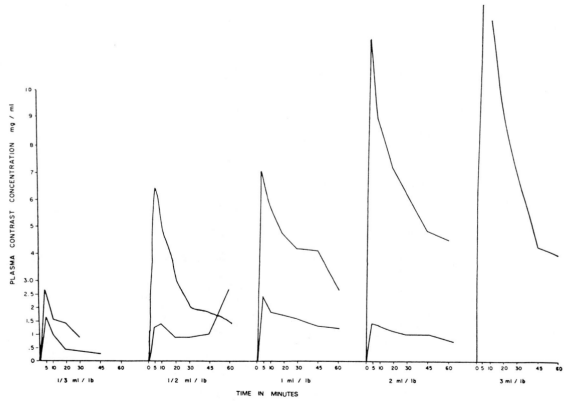

Figure 4.19. Minimum and maximum plasma concentration of contrast material at various dose levels plotted against the time after injection. Approximately 12% of the rapid fall is due to excretion of the contrast in the urine. (From Dure-Smith P, Simenhoff M, Zimskind PD, et al.: The bolus effect in excretory urography. *Radiology* 101:29–34, 1971.)

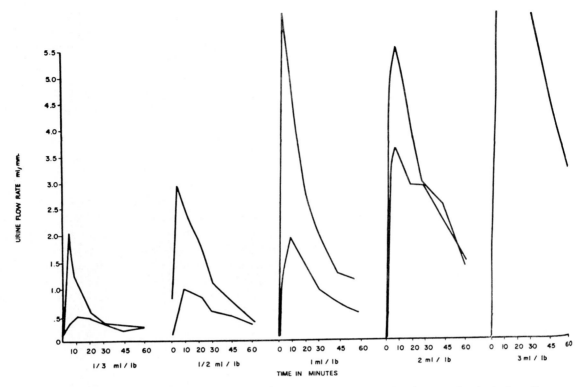

Figure 4.20. Minimum and maximum urine flow rates following varying doses of contrast material. (From Dure-Smith P, Simenhoff M, Zimskind PD, et al.: The bolus effect in excretory urography. *Radiology* 101:29–34, 1971.)

where U_c is the urinary contrast concentration, V_c is the volume of urine produced, P_c is the plasma concentration of contrast, and GFR is the patient's GFR. The product, U_cV_c, therefore, represents the total amount of contrast material in the urine. It becomes apparent that since the GFR is fixed in any given patient, the only factor over which the radiologist has control is the plasma concentration and this is directly related to the dose of contrast material administered. As a corollary, in a patient with a reduced GFR, P_c must be raised proportionately to achieve the same U_cV_c that would give satisfactory opacification in a patient with normal renal function. Therefore, the improvement in opacification described by Schenker with the drip infusion technique was not related to the method of administration of contrast, but rather to the total dose of contrast administered (Fig. 4.21). While the rate of excretion of contrast material is greatest in the first 10 minutes after injection, it falls logarithmically thereafter. With increasing time, the contrast that had equilibrated with the ECF, returns to the vascular space and is excreted. Approximately 24 hours is required to excrete 100% of the administered dose (Fig. 4.22).

It has been shown that the sequential change in CT attenuation value for the renal cortex that occurs following bolus administration of contrast material intravenously directly correlates with the amount of iodine administered. Indeed, a plot of CT number against time (Fig. 4.23) produces a curve similar in appearance to the

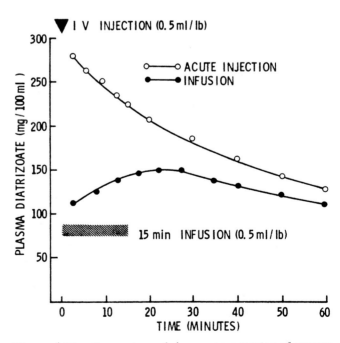

Figure 4.21. Comparison of plasma concentration of contrast from equivalent doses of diatrizoate administered by infusion and by bolus injection. The bolus injection produces a higher contrast concentration throughout the entire study. (From Cattell WR: Excretory pathways for contrast media. *Invest Radiol* 5(6):473–497, 1970.)

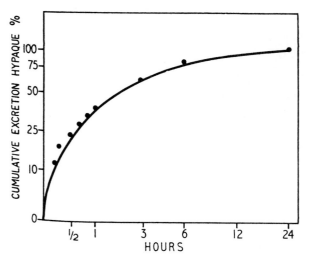

Figure 4.22.   Graph demonstrating cumulative excretion of Hypaque. (From Cattell WR, Fry IK, Spencer AG, et al.: Excretory urography 1—factors determining the excretion of Hypaque. *Br J Radiol* 40(476):561–571, 1967.)

plot of plasma contrast concentration against time. Therefore, the change in CT number in the renal cortex following contrast administration accurately reflects the physiology of contrast excretion.

Physiologic Considerations

Body Size and Dose

It is apparent from the foregoing that the dose of contrast administered is the greatest single factor affecting the quality of opacification achieved during excretory urography. It is generally useful to relate the dose administered to the body weight of the patient and to quantitate the dose in terms of the amount of iodine that is administered. In this fashion, contrast materials of varying concentrations can be equated. In an average patient with normal renal function, a dose of 15–20 g of iodine will generally produce a satisfactory study. In patients who are obese, a proportionately larger dose is customarily employed; however, when a rapid bolus technique is used, obesity is a less important consideration as the vascular compartment is unrelated to body weight and

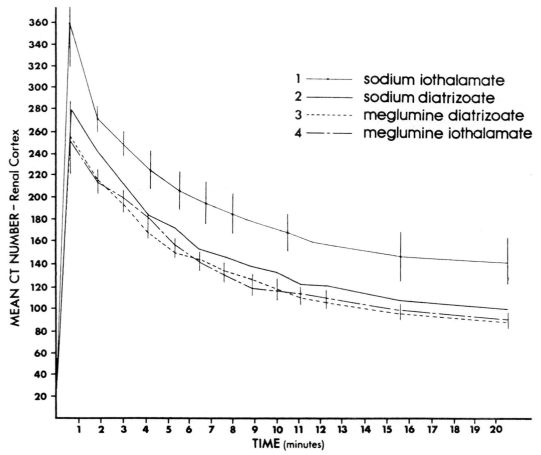

Figure 4.23.   The sequential change in CT numbers measured in the renal cortex following an acute injection of contrast material shows a rapid decline similar to that shown in Figure 4.18. (From Brennan RE, Curtis JA, Pollack HM, et al.: Sequential changes in the CT numbers of the normal canine kidney following intravenous contrast administration. I. The renal cortex. *Invest Radiol* 14(2):141–148, 1979.)

Table 4.1.
Contrast Dose Schedule for Excretory Urography[a]

Adults	
Less than 40 years of age	100–150 mg I₂/lb (⅓–½ ml/lb)
40–55 years	150–200 mg I₂/lb (½–¾ cc/lb)
55 years and older	200–300 mg I₂/lb (¾–1 ml/lb up to a maximum initial dose of 125 ml)
Pediatric patients	
Infancy	400 mg I₂/lb (1½ ml/lb)
Childhood	300 mg I₂/lb (1 ml/lb)
Adolescence	150–200 mg I₂/lb (½–¾ ml/lb)

[a] *Note:* Dosage in parentheses is calculated using standard urographic media containing 300 mg I₂/ml.

since the majority of radiographs in a routine urogram are made in the first 10 minutes after injection before complete mixing of the contrast with the ECF has occurred.

Age and Dose (Table 4.1)

There is a progressive decrease in GFR with age; this is a particular problem in the elderly male patient where the fall in GFR has been attributed to nephron loss as a result of prostatic hypertrophy. This nephron loss may not be reflected in the serum creatinine level as there is a corresponding loss of muscle mass, as well. In addition, atheromatous disease results in nephron loss from multiple small cortical infarcts. As a result, it is prudent to administer a higher dose of contrast material to patients in an older age group.

Correspondingly, in the pediatric age group, there is an inverse relationship between age and the GFR; at birth, the absolute GFR is under 5 ml/min which when corrected for body surface area represents a GFR of 20–30 ml/min/1.73 m². By the age of 1 year, however, the GFR corrected for body surface area has reached a level comparable to that of the adult patient, but the absolute GFR in children remains diminished until adolescence. It is customary, therefore, to use a larger dose related to body weight in the pediatric age group than is commonly used for adult examinations.

It is customary in adult patients to round off the administered dose to the nearest 25 ml; for children, except infants, the dose is usually rounded off to the nearest 5 ml.

Other Considerations

TYPE OF CONTRAST.   With conventional ionic contrast media, the various anions in use are all derivatives of benzoic acid and the differences in these anions usually does not significantly impact the renal handling of the agent. Iodamide (Renovue), which differs from diatrizoate only by the addition of an additional carbon atom on one of the side chains, has been shown by some authorities to have a greater rate of clearance than diatrizoate and this was thought to be evidence of active tubular secretion for

this agent. This claim, however, has been disputed and clinical trials have suggested that while a slightly greater density of the pyelogram may be present, there is little overall difference between iodamide and diatrizoate.

The cations, either sodium or methylglucamine, however, do affect the physiologic property of the contrast. The sodium-based media result in a higher urinary contrast concentration because the sodium is resorbed actively by the tubules. Some authors have suggested that this factor results in a detectably greater density in the pyelogram when compared to studies performed with methylglucamine. Methylglucamine, on the other hand, is not resorbed by the tubules and therefore contributes to the osmotic diuresis that is obtained following contrast administration. Theoretically, this should result in slightly improved distention of both the renal tubules and the collecting system. This increased distention, therefore, may result in slightly denser opacification of the nephrogram. In practice, however, the differences between sodium and methylglucamine are very slight and in the vast majority of patients do not significantly affect urographic quality.

With low osmolar agents, a significantly higher urinary contrast concentration is produced accompanied by a significantly reduced osmotic diuresis as compared to ionic contrast agents. Total iodine excretion rates, however, are similar (Fig. 4.24). It has been demonstrated that urography with low osmolar contrast agents produce perceptibly greater opacification of the collecting system, but that abdominal compression is required to achieved satisfactory distention. There is little perceptible difference in the quality of the tubular phase (nephrogram) of the urogram.

STATE OF HYDRATION.   In the past, overnight fluid restriction was often recommended to improve the diagnostic quality of urograms. The rationale of this approach was based on solid physiologic principles—namely, that in a dehydrated state ADH production is stimulated and this results in a more concentrated urine. At the same time, however, a lower urine volume is produced. Experimental studies in animals show that with dehydration the urinary contrast concentration is indeed increased as

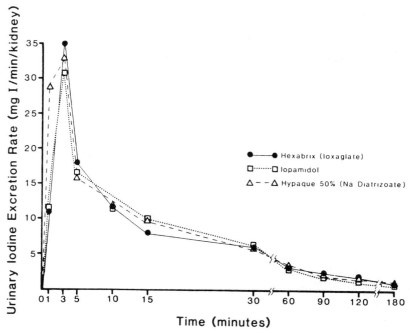

Figure 4.24. The total excretion rates for nonionic, ionic low osmolar, and conventional contrast media are similar. (From Spataro RF, Fischer HW, Boylan L: Urography with low-osmolal- ity contrast media: comparative urinary excretion of iopamidol, Hexabrix, and diatrizoate. *Invest Radiol* 5(17):494–500, 1982.)

compared to the nondehydrated state. However, when higher doses of contrast medium are used, the relative contribution of increased urinary concentration to total opacification is diminished. Furthermore, it has been shown that the usual period of overnight fluid restriction is ineffective in producing a statistically significant change in preinjection urinary osmolality. In addition, the increment of increased contrast concentration that is needed to be visible radiographically at the usual contrast concentrations in the collecting system approaches 80–100%. This level of increase is unlikely to be approached by fluid restriction alone.

While these data demonstrate little evidence in support of the practice of fluid restriction before urography, there is little doubt that inadvertent dehydration may occur as a result of bowel preparation, the diuresis that occurs from the contrast material itself, and overnight fluid restriction. This inadvertent dehydration may pose an increased risk to the patient, particularly, the so-called high-risk debilitated patient or the patient with multiple myeloma. Whether dehydration plays a role in contrast-induced nephrotoxicity remains an open question and this will be discussed in the section on contrast-induced renal dysfunction. For all these reasons, however, deliberate fluid restriction prior to contrast administration cannot, therefore, be recommended.

It is clear, however, that deliberate overhydration may have an adverse effect on pyelographic density when the hydration is sufficient in and of itself to produce a sustained diuresis. It is unlikely that such a diuresis could be achieved in the average patient with routine oral hydra-

tion, but in patients being hydrated with intravenous fluids, a "washout" of the pyelogram can occur. The quality of the nephrogram, however, is usually unaffected.

The ideal patient for urography, therefore, is one in a state of euhydration and this is probably best achieved by giving the patient or the referring physician no specific instructions on fluid intake prior to a urographic study.

TYPE OF EXAMINATION. Much of the foregoing discussion has centered on the physiologic factors affecting the quality of opacification in excretory urography. As has been discussed, the greatest single factor affecting the quality of the urogram is the dose of contrast administration and it is usually necessary to increase the dose of contrast in patients with reduced renal function. The same considerations, however, do not apply when the contrast is to be administered for other types of examinations. When the purpose of contrast administration is to achieve generalized organ opacification in head or body CT, patients with depressed renal function, should receive a proportionately lower dose of contrast as there will be less renal excretion. With angiographic examinations, the type of contrast utilized and the dose administered is usually governed by the type of examination and by the maximum dose of contrast that may be safely administered.

The optimal method of contrast administration for body CT has been studied extensively. After contrast administration, three distinct phases of contrast enhancement can be identified: (*a*) a bolus phase, (*b*) a non-equilibrium phase, and (*c*) an equilibrium phase. Studies have suggested that enhancement and thus tissue differentiation is greatest in all three phases for body CT when the contrast is administered as a bolus rather than by infusion technique.

Extrarenal (Vicarious) Excretion

In patients with normal renal function, less than 1% of a dose of injected contrast material is excreted via a nonrenal route. The primary routes of nonrenal excretion are through the biliary tract and the small bowel. Under normal circumstances, this excretion is not detectable on plain radiographs even when a high dose of contrast medium is employed. Contrast may be visible, however, in the gallbladder on CT scans made 15–48 hours after a large dose of contrast is administered. This visibility is presumed to be related to the high contrast sensitivity of CT and is not a manifestation of either renal or hepatic disease.

In patients with depressed renal function, however, excretion of the contrast via the biliary and small bowel routes is markedly increased and may be visible on plain films. Such excretion has been termed *vicarious excretion*. The exact mechanism for this phenomenon is not certain, but it is speculated that in such patients protein binding of the contrast material occurs and this results in increased hepatic excretion. It is for this reason that contrast administration is felt to be contraindicated in patients with both hepatic and renal disease. In addition to the biliary excretion, there is evidence that there is direct transmural excretion of the contrast through the small bowel. Such excretion is usually not visible until the contrast reaches the colon where water absorption increases its radioopacity. Direct colon excretion of the contrast material is not thought to occur.

The phenomenon of vicarious excretion may occasionally be seen in patients with unilateral ureteral obstruction, but an otherwise normally functioning opposite kidney, and in whom overall renal function is normal. These cases are thought to result from a decreased total renal blood flow and prolonged recirculation of the contrast material.

CONTRAST MEDIA—PHYSICAL PROPERTIES

A variety of physical and chemical properties may be used to describe the contrast agents in general use in the United States. With the older, ionic contrast agents, the strength of the contrast is frequently expressed in terms of percent concentration. This number represents the number of grams of the contrast per 100 ml of water. For example, Hypaque 50 is 50 g of sodium diatrizoate in 100 ml of water. This designation does not, per se, describe the amount of iodine in solution, but in general the higher the percent concentration the more radioopaque the contrast agent. Some contrast agents use the numerical designation to denote the amount of iodine in milligrams per milliliter of the contrast material. Thus, Conray

325 contains 325 mg of iodine per milliliter of solution.

The osmolality of the contrast is determined by the concentration of disolved solute per unit of solvent and the molecular size of the compound. In general, the larger the molecular weight of the agent, the lower the osmolality. The osmolality of a particular contrast must be compared with respect to other agents of similar iodine content.

Another physical property of contrast agents is *viscosity*. This property describes the relative adhesiveness of the molecules of the contrast for one another and is important because the viscosity of the contrast determines how rapidly the contrast may be injected. The viscosity of contrast agents decreases with increasing temperature. The unit of viscosity is the poise; the commonly used unit is the centipoise (CPS) which is equal to 0.01 poise.

A list of several of the contrast agents commonly utilized in uroradiology in the United States is presented in Table 4.2.

Drug Incompatibilities

Conventional ionic contrast material forms a precipitate when mixed with some antihistamines. Ioxaglate has recently been reported to be incompatible with vasodilators such as papaverine. To prevent such incompatibilities, it is important that intravenous lines or catheters be thoroughly flushed prior to injecting pharmacologic agents after contrast material has been injected.

ADVERSE REACTIONS TO CONTRAST MEDIA

Significant reactions to contrast media, while uncommon, continue to constitute a significant hazard to patients despite considerable research into their nature, incidence, and mechanism. Minor side effects including flushing, a metallic taste in the mouth, and tachycardia are common; they usually resolve within a few minutes and should not be considered reactions in the usual sense.

Adverse effects of contrast media can generally be divided into two groups: (*a*) idiosyncratic or anaphylactoid reactions, those which mimic an allergic response to contrast media, and (*b*) chemotoxic effects, those thought to be secondary to a direct toxic effect of the contrast material. Since many of the known reactions of contrast material mimic those produced by known allergens, i.e., urticaria or bronchospasm, but are not mediated by immunoglobulins, these reactions are sometimes referred to as *anaphylactoid*.

Idiosyncratic Reactions

Idiosyncratic reactions are generally classified as: (*a*) mild, (*b*) moderate, (*c*) severe, and (*d*) death. Mild reac-

Table 4.2.
Commonly Used Contrast Media in Uroradiology

Trade Name	Generic Name	Manufacturer	Percent Solution	Iodine (mg/ml)	Osmolality (mOsm/kg)	Viscosity at 25°C (CPS)
Conventional Ionic Contrast Media						
Cysto-Conray II	Meglumine iothalamate	Mallinckrodt	17.2	81	NA	1.5
Cystografin Dilute	Meglumine diatrizoate	E.R. Squibb	18	85	349	1.4
Conray-30	Meglumine iothalamate	Mallinckrodt	30	141	600	2.0
Hypaque 30%	Meglumine diatrizoate	Winthrop	30	141	633	1.92
Reno-M-Dip	Meglumine diatrizoate	E.R. Squibb	30	141	566	1.9
Urovist Meglumine DIU/CT	Meglumine diatrizoate	Berlex	30	141	640	1.9
Angiovist 282	Meglumine diatrizoate	Berlex	60	282	1400	6.1
Conray	Meglumine iothalamate	Mallinckrodt	60	282	1400	6.0
Reno-M-60	Meglumine diatrizoate	E.R. Squibb	60	282	1500	4.6
Angiovist 292	Sodium 8% meglumine 52% diatrizoate	Berlex	60	292	1500	5.9
Renografin-60	Sodium 8% meglumine 52% diatrizoate	E.R. Squibb	60	292	1420	5.9
Hypaque 50%	Sodium diatrizoate	Winthrop	50	300	1550	3.43
Renovue-65	Meglumine iodamide	E.R. Squibb	65	300	1558	8.7
Urovist Sodium 300	Sodium diatrizoate	Berlex	50	300	1550	3.3
Conray 325	Sodium iothalamate	Mallinckrodt	54.3	325	1700	4.0
Angiovist 370	Sodium 10% meglumine 66% diatrizoate	Berlex	76	370	2100	13.8
Hypaque 76	Sodium 10% meglumine 66% diatrizoate	Winthrop	76	370	2016	13.34
Renografin 76	Sodium 10% meglumine 66% diatrizoate	E.R. Squibb	76	370	1940	13.8
Conray 400	Sodium iothalamate	Mallinckrodt	66.8	400	2300	7.0
Vascoray	Sodium 26% meglumine 52% iothalamate	Mallinckrodt	78	400	2400	10.7
Hypaque-M 90%	diatrizoate	Winthrop	90	462	2938	34.7
Low-osmolality Contrast Media						
Omnipaque	Iohexol	Winthrop	51.8	240	504	4.43
Isovue 300	Iopamidol	E.R. Squibb	64.7	300	616	8.8
Omnipaque	Iohexol	Winthrop	64.7	300	672	10.35
Optiray 320	Ioversol	Mallinckrodt	67.8	320	702	9.9
Hexabrix	Sodium 19.6% meglumine 39.3% ioxaglate	Mallinckrodt	58.9	320	600	15.7
Omnipaque	Iohexol	Winthrop	75.5	350	844	18.50
Isovue 370	Iopamidol	E.R. Squibb	76	370	796	20.9

tions are defined as those having physiologic side effects requiring no therapy. Moderate reactions are those that are transient and not life-threatening, but usually require therapy. Severe reactions are defined as those that are life-threatening and that require intensive therapy. The symptoms of these reactions are listed in Table 4.3.

In separate studies, Shehadi (1975) and Ansell (1970) cite an overall incidence of 4.7% of contrast reactions with conventional ionic contrast in unselected series after intravenous injection. Of these, mild reactions represent the great majority (3.3%). Moderate reactions comprise 1–2%. Severe reactions occur in only 0.009% of patients following intravenous contrast injection. The reported incidence of death after intravenous injection ranges from 1 in 14,000 to 1 in 75,000.

Lalli, in a survey based on data reported by manufacturers involving contrast media deaths, found that the majority of deaths involved a cardiovascular event including acute myocardial infarction, ventricular fibrillation, or pulmonary edema. The initial symptoms in patients who subsequently had a fatal contrast reaction was frequently nausea and vomiting or respiratory distress. Other common initial symptoms include hypotension, cardiac arrhythmia, seizures, restlessness, and chills. In only one patient in this series was urticaria the initial manifestation of a subsequently fatal reaction.

Objective data on the incidence of contrast reactions with low-osmolality contrast media (LOCM) have mostly been based on trials outside the United States. Katayama evaluated more than 300,000 patients who received intravenous contrast agents for a variety of examinations in Japan. The overall incidence of an adverse drug reaction was 12.7% in those who received ionic contrast; in the nonionic group, the overall incidence was 3.1%. More importantly, the incidence of severe and very severe contrast reactions was 0.26% for ionic media and 0.04% for the nonionic group. Katayama estimated that nonionic media could be considered safer by a factor of 6 compared to conventional contrast. In another study, Palmer reviewed a total of 106,000 patients for the Royal Australian College of Radiology. Their patients were stratified into high- and low-risk categories and were given ionic or nonionic contrast at the discretion of the attending radiologist. Adverse reactions occurred 5 times more commonly in low-risk patients who received ionic media compared to those who received nonionic contrast. Reactions were 3 times more common in low-risk patients who received ionic contrast when compared to high-risk patients who received nonionic contrast. Severe reactions were 4.5 times as common in the ionic group for all patients. While the methodology of this study has been criticized, the results are generally consistent with the findings of other large-scale trials.

The death rate in patients who receive non-ionic contrast has been difficult to estimate. There were only two deaths in Palmer's study (both in the ionic group) and only one death in each group in the Katayama study. These data suggests that with modern methods of resuscitation, the death rate among all patients who receive contrast media is very low. McClennan, based on manufacturers' statistics, estimates that the death rate with LOCM will be no greater than one in 250,000. In Europe, many of the fatalities associated with LOCM have been in very ill patients or those with significant cardiovascular disease.

Risk Factors

Factors that may predispose a patient to developing an idiosyncratic reaction to contrast material have been extensively studied. In general, the population at greatest risk are in the older age groups and have significant preexisting disease.

Patients with a history of allergy to food, drugs, and ragweed (i.e., hayfever) or asthma have an increased chance of having a contrast reaction but, the magnitude of this increased risk varies somewhat in the reported series (Table 4.4). Witten et al. indicate a minimal increased risk for most types of allergies when compared to the overall 4.7% incidence of reactions in the general public, while Shehadi indicates that the risk may be increased as much as three-fold. The data are of special interest with respect to seafood allergy which is popularly believed to correlate highly with a sensitivity to con-

Table 4.3.
Symptoms of Contrast Material Reactions

Minor
  Nausea
  Mild vomiting, retching
  Heat sensation
  Mild urticaria
  Flushing
  Arm pain
  Tachycardia
  Sneezing

Intermediate
  Faintness, mild hypotension
  Severe vomiting
  Generalized urticaria
  Bronchospasm, laryngospasm (mild)
  Dyspnea
  Facial edema
  Vasovagal reaction

Severe
  Hypotension (systolic blood pressure < 70 mm Hg)
  Loss of consciousness
  Pulmonary edema
  Epiglottic edema, severe bronchospasm
  Cardiac arrest
  Sustanied cardiac arrhythmia

Table 4.4.
Incidence of Reactions Related to Type of Allergic History[a]

Type of Allergy	Incidence of Reaction (%)	
	Witten	Shehadi
Asthma	6	11.2
Hayfever	4	10.3
Seafood	6	15
Other food	6	14
Other allergies	7	13
Penicillin, sulfa	—	7.5

[a] Data from Witten, DM Hirsch, FD and Hartman, GW: Acute reactions to urographic contrast medium. *AJR* 119:832–840, 1973; Shehadi, WH: Adverse reactions to intravascularly administered contrast media. *AJR* 124:145–152, 1975.

trast. Using Shehadi's (1975) data, 85% of such patients will undergo a contrast examination without an adverse reaction.

A history of a previous reaction to the administration of contrast material is the greatest single predictor of an untoward reaction. In Witten et al.'s series, 20% of patients giving a history of mild or moderate reaction to contrast on reexamination suffered a contrast reaction; in Shehadi's (1975) series, the number varied between 16 and 22%. No patient in Witten's series experienced a reaction that was more serious than was the case on the prior exposure to the contrast material, although this occurrence has been reported by others. A history of prior exposure to contrast material without difficulty in the past does not confer immunity to a subsequent contrast reaction. There are multiple cases reported in which patients suffered a contrast reaction after several prior studies without difficulty. In Shehadi's most recent report (1982) from the cooperative study of the International Society of Radiology, approximately 1% of the reactions reported occurred in patients with a history of no reaction to a prior examination. It can be concluded that a history of prior mild or moderate reaction to contrast material should not be taken as an absolute contraindication to reexamination when a repeated study is grounded on sound medical indications. At worst, only 20% of such patients will experience a contrast reaction on rechallenge. A history of a severe reaction to contrast material, on the other hand, is considered a contraindication to reexamination in all but the most urgent cases.

Other Factors

Sex

The incidence of reactions is virtually identical overall in men and women.

Age

The incidence of moderate and severe reactions is approximately equal in all age groups. The data do not validate the commonly held notion that reactions are virtually unknown in the pediatric population. Ansell's (1980) data indicate that the majority of deaths, however, occur in the older (greater than 50 years) age group. Most of the deaths occur in patients with significant pre-existing cardiac or vascular disease.

Dose

The incidence of reactions is unrelated to the dose for mild and moderate reactions; for severe reactions the incidence appears to be slightly higher when larger doses (greater than 20 g of iodine) are used. In fact, Ansell (1980) reported the incidence of reactions to be 3 times greater when infusion pyelography was compared to conventional urography.

Ethnicity

Data from the United Kingdom suggest patients of Indian and Mediterranean extraction carry an increased risk when compared to those of Northern European extraction. Comparable data from the United States are not available.

Rate of Administration of the Contrast

Several studies have shown no difference in the rate of reactions when rapid administration of the contrast was compared to slow injection. These data contrast with the popular opinion that rapid administration of the contrast increases its side effects.

Type of Examination

Intraarterial contrast injection appears to reduce the overall incidence of reactions by approximately one-half to an incidence of 2.3%. With nonvascular examinations, e.g., retrograde pyelography, the exact incidence of reactions is very difficult to determine, but anaphylactoid reactions and deaths have been reported. In these cases, it is assumed that a small amount of contrast has been absorbed into the vascular system.

Type of Contrast

There appears to be little difference among the high-osmolality contrast media (HOCM) in the overall rate of reactions. Ansell (1970) reports, however, that bronchospasm appears to be 4 times as common when the methylglucamine salts are used as compared to the pure sodium salts. The data for LOCM have been described in the previous section. Ioxaglate (Hexabrix), however, appears to produce nausea and vomiting with frequency comparable to that of HOCM. This is in contrast to the nonionic media in which the incidence of nausea and vomiting is less than 1.5%.

Timing of Reactions

Most contrast reactions occur within the first 10 minutes after injection of the contrast material; some patients have symptoms almost immediately, while in others, the reaction is not noted until the end of the examination. A few patients report the development of arm pain or urticaria several hours after the examination has been completed.

Mechanism of Contrast Reactions

At present there is no universally accepted mechanism that acceptably explains the diverse manifestations of idiosyncratic contrast reactions.

Brasch has been the principal proponent of an antigen-antibody mediated mechanism. There are a few case reports in which either IgE or IgM antibodies to contrast have been reported in patients suffering severe contrast reactions. Brasch has also demonstrated significantly greater binding of serum immune globulins in patients who have had contrast reactions when compared to nonreactors. Analogues of contrast material, when chemically linked to a carrier protein, can act as a haptene and induce antibodies in rabbits. Indeed, the most suggestive evidence, albeit indirect, in support of the antigen-antibody hypothesis is the immune-like nature of some contrast reactions and thus the designation anaphylactoid.

Despite these data, there is overwhelming evidence that in the majority of cases, contrast reactions are not mediated by the immune system. The fact that some patients react on their first exposure to contrast (and thus prior to any sensitization) and that most repeat reactions are not progressive militate against the immune theory. In addition, no circulating antibody can be demonstrated in the sera of the vast majority of patients studied after contrast reactions. Finally, rats immunized with diatrizoate conjugated to albumin do not manufacture anitcontrast immunoglobin (IgE).

Lalli has proposed that anxiety, mediated through the hypothalamus, plays a significant role in the pathogenesis of contrast reactions. He believes that small amounts of contrast material cross the blood-brain barrier and in the presence of anxiety on the part of the patient or the patient's perception of anxiety on the part of radiology personnel provokes a contrast reaction by activation of the limbic system. In support of this hypothesis are data that show that diazepam, which depresses the limbic system, significantly increases the LD_{50} of iothalmate (see definition of LD_{50} under Chemotoxic Effects, below).

Histamine release has been implicated in the pathogenesis of contrast reactions. It is known that contrast can induce histamine release from mast cells and basophils, but whether this can occur in sufficient quantities to produce the type of reaction seen with contrast sensitivity has been questioned. Activation of the complement system has been shown to occur following contrast administration and this mechanism is implicated by other authorities. Whether a cause-and-effect relationship between complement activation and the clinical syndrome of contrast sensitivity exists remains in doubt, however.

Recently, attention has been directed toward the contact system as a cause of contrast material reactions. This system begins with activation of clotting factor XII (possibly by local disruption of the vascular endothelium as a result of the needle puncture and the introduction of the contrast material) and continues as a cascade involving the activation of kallikrein from prekallikrein and kinins from high-molecular-weight kinogens. Lasser (1980) has demonstrated a higher rate of prekallikrein-kallikrein transformation in patients who have suffered contrast reactions than in non-reactors.

Still other factors have been implicated. Clustering of reactions has at times suggested that these adverse effects are the result of contamination of the contrast material itself rather than as the result of an untoward reaction to the contrast on the part of the patient. Chemical tests of contrast material from the same lot of contrast that was implicated in a contrast reaction, however, have almost always proven fruitless. It has been suggested that such clustering may be the result of contamination of the contrast material by lubricants or other contaminants in the rubber seals of the plastic syringes used to inject the contrast. This observation prompted the recommendation that contrast materials be drawn into the syringe immediately prior to use rather than in advance as is done in many departments. It is further recommended that contrast material be stored upright so as to avoid contamination from the rubber stoppers used to seal the contrast vials. Finally, additives, preservatives, or chelators added to the contrast material by the manufacturers have been implicated as a possible source of untoward contrast reactions.

Iodism, an acute reaction to the iodine itself, is a syndrome characterized by sialadenitis, diarrhea, and occasionally pulmonary edema that has been reported following contrast administration. Such cases are referred to as "iodine mumps." Contact allergy to iodine containing products is thought to be unrelated to contrast sensitivity.

Prevention of Anaphylactoid Contrast Reactions

Attempts to predict or modify anaphylactoid reactions to contrast material have been attempted with varying degrees of success for a number of years. Prediction of those who will have an adverse reaction to contrast material have largely centered around the use of a test dose of contrast. At various times, intradermal, subcutaneous, intraoccular, and intravenous test doses of contrast have been utilized. The most widely used procedure has been the intravenous test dose, however, it has not been shown to reliably predict a subsequent adverse reaction to the full dose of contrast material, and its use has largely been abandoned. In Lalli's (1980) series of fatal contrast reactions, 29 of 32 patients given a test dose showed no adverse affect, but subsequently died after administration of the full dose; the remaining 3 patients died after the test dose itself. In Witten's series, the test alone induced nausea and vomiting in 28 patients; in all 28 individuals the administration of the full dose of contrast continued after the initial symptoms subsided. In only six of these patients did the full dose of contrast produce additional nausea and vomiting.

The routine use of antihistamines, either mixed with the contrast or administered immediately prior to the contrast study, was initially described more than 40 years ago. There are no data, however, that show that this technique in any way modifies the overall incidence of adverse reactions to contrast material and it does not prevent severe reactions from occurring. This practice has also been largely abandoned.

Because of the anaphylactoid-like nature of idiosyncratic reactions, the empirical use of corticosteroids to prepare "high-risk" patients for contrast studies has been utilized for many years. The scientific basis for this practice, however, has until recently been scanty. Lasser (1977) has presented theoretical and limited experimental evidence in an animal model that pretreatment with steroids is of benefit in preventing some minor contrast reactions, when the steroids were administered more than 12 hours prior to the contrast study.

More recently, a multinstitutional randomized prospective study has shown two doses of orally administered coricosteroids (methylprednisolone, 32 mg) at 12 and 2 hours prior to a contrast examination significantly reduced the incidence of contrast reactions of all types in a group of patients who received conventional ionic media. There was no such protective effect in a group of patients who received a single dose of steroids two hours before examination. In this study, Lasser (1987) felt that the incidence of contrast reactions using conventional ionic media with steroid pretreatment approached the overall incidence of reactions using nonionic media without pretreatment. In another study, Wolf, Arenson, and Cross, using an identical protocol to the one used by Lasser, found an overall incidence of reactions of 4.4% in those who received ionic contrast, 4.0% in those who received ionic contrast and steroid premedication, and 0.6% in those who received iohexol. The data in this study indicated a reduced risk factor for iohexol of at least 25-fold for severe reactions when compared to either ionic regimen.

Greenberger has presented data on clinical trials of pretreatment with corticosteroids in patients who have a history of a prior contrast reaction. In this study, 10 of 150 patients experienced mild reactions on rechallenge with contrast material, an incidence well below that would have been predicted if no pretreatment regimen had been utilized. There were no serious contrast reactions in this series. The regimen they utilized consisted of prednisone, 50 mg orally, every 6 hours, for three doses ending 1 hour before the contemplated examination and diphenhydramine, 50 mg intramuscularly, 1 hour before the study. In an expanded series, Greenberger reports that a pretreatment regimen consisting of prednisone, diphenhydramine, and ephedrine reduced the overall rate of reaction on re-challenge to 5%. Ephedrine should be withheld in patients with hypertension or unstable angina.

Severe reactions have been reported despite pretreatment regimens. In Lalli's (1980) series of contrast associated deaths, 3 of the 140 patients who died during urography had received pretreatment with corticosteroids.

Only limited data are available concerning the efficacy of LOCM in patients who have suffered a previous reaction to HOCM. Holtas found no reactions occurred using iohexol without premedication in 17 patients that suffered a previous reaction to HOCM. Fischer (1990) has presented data demonstrating that when nonionic contrast media is used in patients with a prior history of reaction to ionic contrast, only 4 percent of such patients experienced a repeat reaction. This is well below the expected rate of 20%. On theoretical grounds, the use of LOCM in previous contrast reactors seems justified in view of the overall increased safety of LOCM. Siegle (1986) has recommended that both a steroid preparation and LOCM be utilized when a contrast examination is necessary in a patient who has experienced a previous reaction to HOCM. The Committee on Drugs and Contrast Media of the American College of Radiology has also recommended that LOCM be used in patients requiring reexamination after a previous significant contrast reaction.

Chemotoxic Effects

Chemotoxic effects are those effects of the contrast thought to be due to direct organ toxicity of the contrast material. The LD_{50} is a number commonly used in toxicology to describe the dose of a compound that will kill 50% of the affected test animals. The LD_{50} for various contrast media in mice are given in Table 4.5.

In humans, the primary manifestation of contrast overdosage is neurotoxicity, including the induction of seizures. The exact dose in humans at which this occurs is not known, but systemic doses of contrast material exceeding 5–6 ml/kg should be exceeded only in extreme circumstances. The neurotoxicity of nonionic contrast agents has been shown to be less than that produced by ionic media in in vitro experiments. In addition, the sec-

Table 4.5.
LD$_{50}$ of Various Contrast Agents[a]

Contrast Agents	LD$_{50}$ g I/kg
Sodium/meglamine diatrizoate	7.6
Sodium iothalmate	8.0
Ioxaglate	10.2–13.5
Metrizamide	18.1
Iopamidol	21.8–22.1
Iohexol	24.3

[a] Modified from McClennan BL: Low osmolality contrast media: premises and promises. *Radiology* 162:1–8, 1987.

ond-generation nonionic agents (iohexol and iopamidol) show less neurotoxicity than does metrizamide, perhaps because there is less interference with glucose metabolism in the brain with these agents.

Hyperosmolar Effects

Conventional ionic media (HOCM) cause vasodilatation, vascular spasm, hemodilution, changes in red cell morphology, and changes in vascular permeability, all of which are related to their high osmolality. Changes in the permeability of the blood-brain barrier are also likely related to osmolality and may be responsible for some of the neurotoxicity of HOCM. As would be expected, LOCM markedly reduce these effects in both human and animal studies.

Cardiovascular Effects

Several studies have demonstrated that significant electrocardiographic abnormalities may occur during the intravenous administration of contrast material. These changes which consist of tachycardia, minor or major cardiac arrhythmias, and ischemic changes, are transient and may occur in a small number (5%) of patients with normal baseline electrocardiograms (EKGs) and in up to 25% of patients with preexisting cardiac abnormalities. These changes are usually asymptomatic and are only discovered if electrocardiographic monitoring is employed. These abnormalities have been attributed to a direct toxic effect of the contrast on the heart, but whether these changes play a role in the development of hypotensive contrast reactions is not known. Recent studies using LOCM have demonstrated a marked reduction in the frequency of such changes and for this reason the use of LOCM in patients with significant underlying cardiac disease has been advocated.

Ionic contrast media have been demonstrated to cause a fall in free ionic calcium levels which is followed by an immediate increase in serum parathormone levels. The decrease in serum calcium levels is presumed to be caused by divalent cation chelators that are added by the manufacturers to the contrast. The magnitude of the fall

in serum calcium is so small as to be clinically insignificant except in a small number of patients with preexisting cardiac disease in whom the contrast is administered for coronary angiography. In these patients this mechanism has been implicated in the development of cardiac arrhythmias.

HOCM are known to exert negative inotropic and chronotropic actions on the heart; both of these effects are diminished with LOCM.

Hematologic Effects

HOCM inhibit platelet aggregation and cause a prolognation of the thrombin time by inhibition of fibrin monomer polymerization. These anticoagulant properties have a beneficial effect in angiography by helping to prevent thrombus formation in catheters and syringes. In addition, red cell deformation has been reported after incubation with HOCM. This phenomenon may explain the pulmonary hypertension that occasionally complicates pulmonary angiography. In patients with sickle cell anemia, contrast material is known to provoke sickling and occasional development of sickle cell crisis. LOCM cause less inhibition of platelet aggregation than do HOCM. Caution must be exercised when using LOCM in angiographic procedures because clots may form in contrast containing syringes and may be inadvertantly injected into patients.

Thrombophlebitis

A chemical phlebitis may develop after injection of contrast material, particularly when it is used for lower-extremity venography. This complication has been reported in up to 30% of patients when 60% contrast is utilized and is most likely the result of prolonged contact of the contrast with the venous endothelium as the result of slow flow. The clinical syndrome can be markedly reduced by using diluted contrast material and other measures including a heparinized saline flush following the procedure. It may rarely be seen in patients in whom the contrast has been injected in the upper extremity for other imaging studies.

Extravasation of Contrast Material

Subcutaneous or intradermal extravasation of some contrast material is not an uncommon occurrence. Such extravasation may result in local pain, erythema, and swelling, but these symptoms usually resolve with local therapy and without any sequelae. Rarely, significant tissue necrosis and dermal sloughing can occur with even very small amounts of extravasation. In some cases, the extravasation may be so small as to be inapparent until the complication develops. When severe sloughing and local necrosis develops, the extremity may turn cold with severe ecchymosis and edema. The pulses in the extremity may vanish. These features are typical of a compartment syndrome and may require extensive releasing incisions and subsequent skin grafting. Most of the reported cases in which this extensive reaction develops are in children or in the elderly and it is more common for it to occur when the injection was made either in the hand or in the foot. This phenomenon may occur with either LOCM or HOCM.

Indications for the Use of Low-Osmolality Contrast Material

Accumulated data indicate that LOCM have a significantly lower incidence of adverse drug reactions than HOCM. Overall, the rate of reactions following intravenous use is reduced by a factor of at least 4, the death rate is reduced by a factor of at least 6, and the chemotoxic effect of contrast is significantly lowered. For urography, physiologic studies indicate a higher excretion rate for LOCM and urographic quality that is at least as good as that obtained with HOCM. In addition, there is a marked improvement in patient tolerance for LOCM, particularly for previously painful angiographic procedures.

These data would seem to indicate that LOCM should completely replace HOCM for most imaging studies. In parts of Canada and Europe, this has largely been the case. In the United States, two schools of thought have been developed. The first group has argued that the available data justify a complete switch to LOCM, at least for intravenous use. The second group of authorities have advocated a policy of "selective use" of LOCM largely because LOCM costs 10–25 times more than HOCM. Wolf has estimated that approximately 5.2 million contrast-assisted procedures are performed in the United States per year and that a total switch to LOCM will increase the yearly expenditures for contrast in this country to over 300 million dollars. Others have placed this cost to be in excess of one billion dollars. Assuming a sixfold decrease in the death rate associated with contrast administration, this translates into a contrast cost of $650,000 for each death prevented using Wolf's data. These calculated costs may well be lowered when factors such as increased hospital stay, rehabilitation costs, and especially litigation costs for contrast reactions are considered. The argument that such costs may in and of themselves justify a complete switch to LOCM has been advanced, however, a recent study has shown that a complete switch to LOCM cannot be justified on an economic basis alone.

Those who advocate "selective use" of LOCM suggest that these contrast materials be used only in those patients who are at "high risk" for an adverse reaction to conventional contrast material and that LOCM should, therefore, be used only for specific indications. However, agreement on what constitutes "high risk" cannot be made without a certain amount of subjectivity. Furthermore, if too many factors are judged to place the patient at high risk, there comes to be little justification in not using LOCM in every patient. Among the indications that have been suggested are the following: (*a*) a prior history of sensitivity to contrast material, (*b*) age less than 1 year or greater than 65 years, (*c*) patients with significant ischemic cardiovascular disease or a history of cardiac arrhythmia, (*d*) asthma, and (*e*) examination in which a high dose (greater than 60 g of iodine) will be required, and (*f*) patients with certain blood dyscrasias such as multiple myeloma, sickle cell disease, or paroxysmal nocturnal hemoglobinuria. In addition, LOCM should be used in every examination in which a significant element of patient discomfort with HOCM is present. A slightly different list of indications for the use of LOCM has been proposed by Bettmann for the Society of Cardiovascular and Interventional Radiology.

The preferential use of LOCM in patients with preexisting renal insufficiency (serum creatinine greater than 2 mg/dl) has been advocated by some authorities, but is difficult to justify on the basis of currently available data.

CONTRAST—INDUCED ACUTE RENAL DYSFUNCTION

Reports linking contrast material with the development of acute renal failure began to appear with increasing frequency in the early 1970s. In one of the initial studies, Krumlovsky et al. reported eight patients in whom acute renal dysfunction (ARD) developed following exposure to radiographic contrast materials that were identified during a period in which 7125 contrast procedures were performed at their institution, an incidence of 0.112%. In other reported series, the incidence of contrast-induced renal failure has ranged from 0 to 100%, when only selected patients who were retrospectively identified as being at high risk for the development of this complication are considered.

At least part of this discrepancy in incidence is related to varying definitions of what constitutes ARD and to reports based on poorly controlled retrospective data. There is no doubt that contrast material has been held responsible for ARD in some cases that are multifactorial in etiology. This impression is substantiated in a report by Cramer in which patients undergoing cranial CT were evaluated for the presence of ARD. Their data included three patients who experienced ARD following head CT, but who had not received contrast material.

The definition of ARD has varied widely in the reported series. Most authors define ARD as a rise in blood urea nitrogen (BUN) of 50% or 20 mg/dl and/or an increase in serum creatinine of 50% or 1 mg/dl within 48 hours of the procedure. Others have required an absolute rise in creatinine of 1 mg/dl or have required the rise to occur within 24 hours of the administration of the contrast. In some series, when GFR has been measured, ARD has been defined as a 25% change in GFR.

ARD associated with contrast material is usually nonoliguric and in the typical case, the serum creatinine peaks in 3–5 days and returns to baseline values within 7–10 days. In the rare case, the renal failure is oliguric and in these cases the damage is more likely to be permanent.

Most studies have identified specific risk factors for the development of contrast-induced ARD. In virtually every case, conflicting data are present in other studies.

Risk Factors

Preexisting Renal Insufficiency

Preexisting renal insufficiency has been identified as a major risk factor by a number of authors. In most studies, the higher the baseline level of serum creatinine, both the risk for developing ARD and the magnitude of the renal compromise that was present were increased. D'Elia et al. in a study of 378 patients undergoing angiography defined the risk of ARD as 33% for patients with baseline serum creatinine levels over 1.5 mg/dl or serum BUN levels over 30 mg/dl; for the remainder of the patients in their series, the incidence was 2%. An even higher incidence of ARD (41.7%) in patients with preexisting azotemia was cited by Martin-Paredero et al. Of their patients, 8.3% required dialysis.

Preexisting renal insufficiency has not been found to predispose patients to ARD in other studies. Parfrey et al., in a prospective study, concluded that there was little risk of clinically important nephrotoxicity following use of contrast material in patients with preexisting renal insufficiency. Mason studied 120 patients who underwent angiography and found an overall incidence of ARD of 31%, however, there was no difference between those with preexisting renal insufficiency and those without. Cruz et al. studied 125 patients, including 11 with baseline creatinine values greater than 4 mg/dl, and did not find a single case of ARD. Preexisting renal insufficiency, when secondary to obstructive uropathy, has not been associated with an increased risk of contrast-induced ARD.

These data are of particular interest because prior to 1960, renal dysfunction was considered a contraindication to the use of contrast material. In 1963, Schwartz et al. introduced "high-dose" urography specifically for the purpose of identifying those patients in whom there was a correctable cause of renal insufficiency. They concluded that contrast administration was both safe and efficacious in patients with renal insufficiency. Other early studies by Gup, MacEwan, and others showed no deleterious effect of contrast material on renal function. These conclusions were summarized in a review by Grainger published in 1972. The precise factors that have contributed to the apparent dramatic change in the appreciation of the nephrotoxic potential of contrast material are not known.

Diabetes Mellitus

Harkonen et al. found that 76% of 29 diabetic patients with baseline creatinines greater than 2 mg/dl had deterioration of renal function after exposure to contrast material; in 9 of these patients the deterioration was irreversible. He found the risk of nephrotoxicity to be greatest in patients with long-standing diabetes (particularly of juvenile onset) and in those requiring insulin. VanZee et al. found the presence of diabetes to be a major risk factor with regard to contrast-induced ARD. There was deterioration of renal function in 50% of diabetics with baseline creatinine values of 1.5–4.5 mg/dl and in 100% of the small number studied with baseline creatinine values greater than 4.5 mg/dl. In neither series were diabetic patients without renal insufficiency at greater risk than the general population for development for ARD.

Conflicting data on the risk of diabetes for the development of contrast-induced ARD can also be found. In the study of Mason et al., diabetics were at no increased risk as compared to the remainder of the study group, and Parfrey et al.'s prospective study concluded that the risk for diabetic patients with preexisting renal insufficiency for ARD was 9%, much lower than previously reported.

Dehydration

Some authors speculate that dehydration either from the contrast study itself or from the preparation for the study may play a role in the development of contrast induced ARD. Harkonen et al. found that the state of hydration did not appear to play a role, however. Eisenberg et al. believed that vigorous hydration with normal saline could prevent the development of ARD. In his series of 537 patients in whom hydration was maintained before and during angiography, there were no patients in whom ARD could be identified. Other authors, however, have reported conflicting data. Martin-Paredero and Gomes both report that hydration during and after a contrast study did not prevent the development of ARD in their patients. Others have reported that volume expansion with mannitol or the use of furosemide may be beneficial in protecting high-risk patients from the development of ARD.

Dose of Contrast

Lang et al. felt that the dose of contrast administered was a major factor in the development of ARD. In his series, the incidence of ARD increased with increasing dose of contrast material. In other series, however, ARD has been described in patients receiving contrast containing as little as 30 g of iodine. Cruz et al. did not find an increased incidence of ARD in the subgroup of their study who received a dose of contrast material containing greater than 48 g of iodine. Hayman et al. found no difference in the incidence of ARD following contrast-enhanced cranial CT when a dose of 43 g of iodine was compared to a dose of 80 g. Miller et al. reported no consistent effect on renal function with increasing doses of either ionic or nonionic contrast material.

Other Factors

A multitude of other factors have been implicated in the development of other contrast-induced ARD. These include advanced age, hypertension, the presence of peripheral vascular disease, digitalis requiring congestive heart failure, proteinuria, and liver dysfunction. Multiple contrast studies within a short interval (72 hours or less) have also been implicated.

Patients with multiple myeloma have long been held as being at increased risk for ARD thought to be related to precipitation of myeloma proteins in the renal tubules. This mechanism for renal dysfunction associated with myeloma after contrast administration has recently been questioned and most authorities now feel that contrast studies in patients with myeloma can be performed with safety provided dehydration is avoided.

The mechanism for contrast-induced ARD remains obscure and our understanding of the pathogenesis of this disorder is hampered by the lack of a reproducible animal model. Speculation has centered around structural changes in the proximal tubule epithelium, contrast-induced vasoconstriction of renal blood vessels, and increased tubular pressure caused by the osmotic diuresis associated with contrast material. Other workers have demonstrated that contrast material can cause lysis of proximal tubule cells in vitro in the presence of ischemia and further that this damage is reduced when nonionic contrast material is used.

Still other investigators have focused on intratubular obstruction perhaps caused by contrast-induced precipitation of Tamm-Horsfall proteins, or by other causes. In support of this theory, Older el al. report that a persistent nephrogram will be seen 24 hours after the contrast has been administered in approximately 50% of the patients subsequently shown to develop contrast-induced ARD. A similar phenomenon has recently been reported on CT. Several studies have shown that contrast material acts as a powerful uricosuric agent and this mechanism has been implicated in the development of acute urate nephropathy in patients with hyperuricemia. This syndrome may also be encountered in patients with myeloproliferative disorders or leukemia following chemotherapy. The role of the uricosuric effect of contrast in other cases of ARD is probably small.

The effect of LOCM on renal function is still unclear. Some authorities have speculated that because of lower osmolality, lower chemotoxicity will be observed. Indeed, LOCM have been shown to cause less of an effect on renal blood flow, reduced proteinuria, and less damage to proximal tubular epithelial cells in vitro compared to HOCM. In addition, LOCM can experimentally be shown to produce less nephrotoxicity than HOCM in several animal models. However, in virtually every clinical trial, no difference in nephrotoxicity between HOCM and LOCM has been demonstrated.

TREATMENT OF ADVERSE REACTIONS TO CONTRAST MEDIA

Every physician utilizing contrast materials must be prepared to deal with a contrast-induced emergency. These preparations should be thorough, but not so extensive as to cause undue alarm on the part of the patient. An organized plan to deal with the emergency, so that the physicians and technical staff work together in a coordinated fashion, is desirable. All personnel in the department must be familiar with the location of emergency drugs and equipment.

A common sense approach to dealing with the emergency should be utilized, as overtreatment may be as disastrous as undertreatment. Familiarity with the basic principles of cardiopulmonary resuscitation (including A—airway, B—breathing, C—circulation) is mandatory. The physician responsible for the contrast study must be immediately available for at least 10 minutes after the injection and generally available for the next 30 minutes. Equipment for resuscitation including blood pressure monitoring equipment, ventilatory equipment, cardiac monitors or electrocardiograph machines, defibrillators, drugs, and oxygen must be immediately available. It is prudent to inject the contrast through a secure intravenous line which is then left in place for the first several minutes after the injection so that immediate venous access is available should the need arise.

The radiologist should be prepared to deal with mild and moderate reactions as well as the initial therapy of severe reactions. However, life-threatening reactions occur so infrequently in the career of an average radiologist that it is prudent to have available the assistance of physicians who deal with resuscitative emergencies on a more frequent basis. Therefore, only general principles for the initiation of therapy will be offered here.

At the first sign of a significant reaction, the patient's pulse and blood pressure should be assessed. It is also prudent to perform chest auscultation to assess the adequacy of ventilation.

Minor Reactions

Minor reactions, by definition, are not serious and for the most part do not require therapy. Occasionally, limited urticarial reactions may benefit from the administration of antihistamines primarily for their antipuritic effect. Caution should be exercised when using antihistamines, particularly in outpatients, because of their tendency to cause drowsiness. Some authors have found that the H$_2$ antagonist, cimetidine, is of value in the treatment of contrast-induced urticarial reactions and have recommended their use either in addition to or in place of the H$_1$ antagonist, diphenhydramine.

More extensive dermal reactions usually respond to antihistamines (diphenhydramine 50 mg intravenously given over 1 or 2 minutes). Epinephrine (1 : 1000) 0.1–0.3 ml administered subcutaneously may be necessary if the urticaria is so extensive that generalized edema is present.

Respiratory Reactions

Bronchospasm and mild laryngospasm should be treated with epinephrine (1 : 1000) 0.3–0.5 ml administered subcutaneously. For mild reactions, a lower dose of 0.1–0.3 ml may be employed. The dose of epinephrine may be repeated in 15 minutes if no response is obtained. In severe cases it may be necessary to add aminophylline, 5–6 mg/kg intravenously infused over 20–30 minutes. Aminophylline, however, may accentuate hypotension and should only be used if the bronchospasm fails to respond to epinephrine, or in patients in whom epinephrine is contraindicated. Corticosteroids (hydrocortisone 500 mg intravenously) probably have no immediate impact on respiratory distress, but can be administered as a supplemental agent to prevent a secondary recurrence of the clinical symptoms.

Vasovagal Reactions

It is crucial to distinguish hypotensive bradycardia from hypotensive tachycardia. Vasovagal reactions are characterized by sinus bradycardia and may be present with or without hypotension. If the reaction is vagal in origin, atropine 0.5 mg intravenously should be administered. An additional dose of 0.5 mg may be administered every 5 minutes until a heart rate of 60 beats/min is achieved or a maximum dose of 2 mg has been given.

Hypotensive Tachycardia

The vast majority of patients experiencing hypotensive anaphylactoid contrast reactions will have hypotensive tachycardia. Supportive measures such as placing the patient in the Trendelenburg position or elevating the legs as well as the administration of oxygen should begin immediately. In addition, electrocardiographic monitoring should be started.

vanSonnenberg et al. have recently shown that patients experiencing hypotensive tachycardia are manifesting circulatory hypovolemia resulting from a variety of factors including decreased venous return, decreased cardiac filling, peripheral vasodilatation, and most importantly sequestration of fluid in nonvital compartments. In this circumstance, an effective circulatory hypovolemia ensues. Administration of large volumes of intravenous fluid has been shown to be a highly effective therapy. They recommend either isotonic saline or lactated Ringer's solution (500–1000 ml or more) be administered intravenously as quickly as possible. The use of a second intravenous line may facilitate this therapy.

In younger patients, epinephrine (1 : 1000) 0.3 ml subcutaneously or 1–3 ml of 1 : 1000 diluted in 10 ml of saline (1 : 10,000) intravenously can be utilized if the hypotension is severe and if it fails to respond to fluid therapy alone. vanSonnenberg feels that the use of epinephrine in older patients, especially those with significant underlying cardiovascular disease, is fraught with hazard because of the tendency of this drug to produce cardiac arrhythmias. If an older patient fails to respond to fluid therapy alone, dopamine 10–20 mg/kg/min may be added. The rate of infusion should be titrated to the blood pressure response. Dopamine should also be used in younger patients who fail to respond to epinephrine.

The use of older pressor agents, such as levarterenol (Levophed) and metaraminal (Aramine) as first-line agents should probably be avoided.

Patients taking β-adrenergic blocking agents (i.e., propranolol) may present a special problem in diagnosis should hypotension develop during the course of a contrast reaction. β-blockers produce a sinus bradycardia which may not vary in the face of shock, making the distinction of a vasovagal reaction from an anaphylactoid reaction difficult. In addition, since epinephrine is both an α- and a β-adrenergic agonist, the β-blocker may successfully neutralize the β-effect of epinephrine, leaving its α-effect unopposed. This combination of circumstances can result in a precipitous rise in blood pressure. In such cases, fluid therapy alone should probably be utilized until more specialized help becomes available. Calcium channel blocking agents such as nifedipine and diltiazem are potent peripheral vasodilators and this may also complicate the therapy of a contrast reaction.

Ventricular Arrhythmias

In the event that significant ventricular arrhythmias such as multifocal premature ventricular contractions, couplets, or ventricular tachycardia develop, immediate consultation with a qualified specialist should be obtained. A loading dose of lidocaine of 1 mg/kg may be administered followed by an infusion at the rate of 1–4 mg/min. If sustained ventricular tachycardia with hypotension or ventricular fibrillation develops, electrical defibrillation will be necessary.

Cardiac Arrest

If a full-scale cardiac arrest develops, cardiopulmonary resuscitation should immediately be instituted.

SUGGESTED READINGS

Functional Renal Anatomy and Renal Physiology

Andreoli TE, Culpepper RM, Thompson CS, Weinman EJ: Essentials of normal renal function. In Andreoli TE, Carpenter CCJ, Plum F, Smith LH (eds): *Cecil's Essentials of Medicine.* WB Saunders, Philadelphia: 1986.

Gottschalk CW, Lassiter WE: Mechanisms of urine formation. In Mountcastle VB (ed): *Medical Physiology,* vol 2, ed 14. St. Louis: CV Mosby. 1980.

Meschan I: Background physiology of the urinary tract for the radiologist. *Radiol Clin North Am* 3(1):13, 1965.

Vander AJ: *Renal Physiology,* ed 3. New York: McGraw-Hill, 1985.

Contrast Media—Historical Background

Almén, T: Development of nonionic contrast media. *Invest Radiol* (Suppl) 20:S2, 1985.

Elkin M: Stages in the growth of uroradiology. *Radiology* 175:297, 1990.

Grainger RG: Intravascular contrast media—the past, the present and the future. *Br J Radiol* 55(649):1, 1982.

Physiology of Contrast Excretion

Becker JA, Gregoire A, Berdon W, Schwartz D: Vicarious excretion of urographic media. *Radiology* 90:243, 1968.

Benamor M, Aten EM, McElvany KD, et al: Ioversol clinical safety summary. *Invest Radiol* 24(1):S67, 1989.

Benness GT: Urographic excretion study. *Invest Radiol* 11:261, 1967.

Benness GT: Urographic contrast agents: a comparison of sodium and methylglucamine salts. *Clin Radiol* 21:150, 1970.

Brennan RE, Curtis JA, Pollack HM, Weinberg I: Sequential changes in the CT numbers of the normal canine kidney following intravenous contrast administration. I. The renal cortex. *Invest Radiol* 14:141, 1979.

Brennan RE, Curtis JA, Pollack HM, Weinberg I: Sequential changes in the CT numbers of the normal canine kidney following intravenous contrast administration. II. The renal medulla. *Invest Radiol* 14:239, 1979.

Brennan RE, Rapoport S, Weinberg I, et al: CT determined canine kidney and urine iodine concentrations following intravenous administration of sodium diatrizoate, metrizamide, iopamidol and sodium ioxaglate. *Invest Radiol* 17:95, 1982.

Purkiss P, Lane RD, Cattel WR, et al: Estimation of sodium diatrizoate by absorption spectrophotometry. Invest Radiol 3:271, 1968.

Cattell WR: Excretory pathways for contrast media. *Invest Radiol* 5:473, 1970.

Cattell WR, Fry IK, Spencer AG, Purkiss P: Excretory urography I: factors determining the excretion of Hypaque. *Br J Radiol* 40(476):561, 1967.

Chamberlain MJ, Sherwood T: The extrarenal excretion of diatrizoate in renal failure. *Br J Radiol* 39:765, 1966.

Dure-Smith P: The dose of contrast medium in intravenous urography: a physiologic assessment. *AJR* 108(4):691, 1970.

Dure-Smith P, Simenhoff M, Brodsky S, Zimskind PD: Opacification of the urinary tract during excretory urography: concentration vs. amount of contrast medium. *Invest Radiol* 7:407, 1972.

Dure-Smith P, Simenhoff MB, Zimskind PD, Kodroff M: The bolus effect in excretory urography. *Radiology* 101:29, 1971.

Fry IK, Burgener FA, Hamlin DJ: Contrast enhancement in abdominal CT: bolus vs. infusion. *AJR* 137:351, 1981.

Lautin EM, Friedman AC: Vicarious excretion of contrast media. *JAMA* 247(11):1608, 1982.

Schencker B: Drip infusion pyelography. *Radiology* 83:12, 1964.

Schwartz WB, Hurwit A, Ettiger A: Intravenous urography in the patient with renal insufficiency. *N Engl J Med* 269(6):277, 1963.

Sherwood T, Doyle FH: Value of fluid deprivation in large dose urography. *Lancet* 2:754, 1968.

Spataro RF: Newer contrast agents for urography. *Radiol Clin North Am* 22(2):365, 1984.

Spataro RF: Fischer HW, Boylan L: Urography with low osmolality contrast media: comparative urinary excretion of iopamidol, Hexabrix and diatrizoate. *Invest Radiol* 17(5):494, 1982.

Woodruff MW, Malvin RL: Localization of renal contrast media excretion by stop flow analysis. *J Urol* 84(5):677, 1960.

Adverse Reactions to Contrast Media

Ansell G: Adverse reactions to contrast agents: scope of problem. *Invest Radiol* 5:374, 1970.

Ansell G, Tweedie MCK, West CR, et al: The current status of reactions to intravenous contrast media. *Invest Radiol* 15(6 Suppl):S32, 1980.

Bettmann MA: Guidelines for use of low-osmolality contrast agents. *Radiology* 172:901, 1989.

Bettmann MA: Ionic versus nonionic contrast agents for intravenous use: are all the answers in? *Radiology* 175:616, 1990.

Bettmann MA, Holzer JF, Trombly ST: Risk management issues related to the use of contrast agents. *Radiology* 175:629, 1990.

Brasch RC: Allergic reactions to contrast media: accumulated evidence. *AJR* 134:797, 1980.

Brasch RC: Evidence supporting an antibody mediation of contrast media reactions. *Invest Radiol* 15(6 Suppl):S29, 1980.

Carr DH: Contrast media reactions: experimental evidence against the allergy theory. *Br J Radiol* 57:469, 1984.

Cohan RH, Dunnick NR: Intravascular contrast media: adverse reactions. *AJR* 149:665, 1987.

Cohan RH, Leder RA, Bolic D, et al: Extravascular extravasation of radiographic contrast media: effects of conventional and low-osmolar agents in the rat thigh. *Invest Radiol* 25:504, 1990.

Cohen JC, Roxe DM, Said R, Cummins G: Iodide mumps after repeated exposure to iodinated contrast media. *Lancet* 1(8171):762, 1980.

Fareed J, Walenga JM, Saravia GE, Moncada RM: Thrombogenic potential of nonionic contrast media? *Radiology* 174:321, 1990.

Fischer HW: Occurrence of seizure during cranial computed tomography. *Radiology* 137:563, 1980.

Fischer HW, Siegel R: Value of non-ionic contrast medium in previous reactors. Experience thus far. *AJR* 154:195, 1990.

Greenberger PA, Patterson R, Simon R, et al: Pretreatment of high-risk patients requiring radiographic contrast media studies. *J Allergy Clin Immunol* 67(3):185, 1981.

Greenberger PA, Patterson R, Tapio CM: Prophylaxis against repeated radiocontrast media reactions in 857 cases. *Arch Intern Med* 145:2197, 1985.

Hartman GW, Hattery RR, Witten DM, Williamson B Jr: Mortality during excretory urography: Mayo Clinic experience. *AJR* 139:919, 1982.

Holtas S: Iohexol in patients with previous adverse reactions to contrast media. *Invest Radiol* 19:563, 1984.

Jacobsson BF, Jorulf H, Kalantar MS, et al: Nonionic versus ionic contrast media in intravenous urography: clinical trial in 1,000 consecutive patients. *Radiology* 167:601, 1988.

Jensen N, Dorph S: Adverse reactions to urographic contrast medium: rapid versus slow injection rate. *Br J Radiol* 53:659, 1980.

Johenning PW: Reactions to contrast material during retrograde pyelography. *Urology* 16(4):442, 1980.

Katayama H, Yamaguchi K, Kozuka T, et al: Adverse reactions to ionic and nonionic contrast media: a report from the Japanese committee on the safety of contrast media. *Radiology* 175:621, 1990.

Katzberg RW, Morris TW, Schulman G, et al: Reactions to intravenous contrast media. *Radiology* 147:327, 1983.

Lalli AF: Contrast media reactions: data analysis and hypothesis. *Radiology* 134:1, 1980.

Lalli AF, Greenstreet R: Reactions to contrast media: testing the CNS hypothesis. *Radiology* 138:47, 1981.

Lasser EC: A coherent biochemical basis for increased reactivity to contrast material in allergic patients: a novel concept. *AJR* 149:1281, 1987.

Lasser EC, Berry CC, Talner LB, et al: Pretreatment with corticosteroids to alleviate reactions to intravenous contrast material. *N Engl J Med* 317(14):845, 1987.

Lasser EC, Lang JH, Lyon SG, Hamblin AE: Changes in complement and coagulation factors in a patient suffering a severe anaphylactoid reaction to injection of contrast material: some considerations of pathogenesis. *Invest Radiol* 15(6 Suppl):S6, 1980.

Lasser EC, Lang J, Sovak M, et al: Steroids: theoretical and experimental basis for utilization in prevention of contrast media reactions. *Radiology* 125:1, 1977.

Leung PC, Cheng CY: Extensive local necrosis following the intravenous use of x-ray contrast medium in the upper extremity. *Br J Radiol* 53:361, 1980.

Lieberman P, Siegle RL: Complement activation following intravenous contrast material administration. *J Allergy Clin Immunol* 64(1):13, 1979.

Love L, Lind JA, Olson MC: Persistent CT nephrogram: significance in the diagnosis of contrast nephropathy. *Radiology* 172:125, 1989.

Madowitz JS, Schweiger MJ: Severe anaphylactoid reaction to radiographic contrast media: recurrence despite premedication with diphenhydramine and prednisone. *JAMA* 241(26):2813, 1979.

McClennan BL: Low osmolality contrast media: premises and promises. *Radiology* 162:1, 1987.

Palmer FJ: The RACR survey of intravenous contrast media reactions. Final report. *Australas Radiol* 32:426, 1988.

Panto PN, Davies P: Delayed reactions to urographic contrast media. *Br J Radiol* 59:41, 1986.

Pfister RC, Hutter AM Jr: Cardiac alterations during intravenous urography. *Invest Radiol* 15(6 Suppl):S239, 1980.

Powe NR, Steinberg EP, Erickson JE, et al: Contrast medium-induced adverse reactions: economic outcome. *Radiology* 169:163, 1988.

Rine J, Rothenberger KH, Clauss W: Prevention of anaphylactoid reactions after radiographic contrast media infusion by combined histamine H_1- and H_2-receptor antagonists: results of a prospective controlled trial. *Int Arch Allergy Appl Immunol* 78:9, 1985.

Robertson HJF: Blood clot formation in angiographic syringes containing nonionic contrast media. *Radiology* 163:621, 1987.

Shehadi WH: Adverse reactions to intravascularly administered contrast media. *AJR* 124:145, 1975.

Shehadi WH: Contrast media adverse reactions: occurrence, recurrence, and distribution patterns. *Radiology* 143:11, 1982.

Shehadi WH: Death following intravascular administration of contrast media. *Acta Radiol (Diagn)* 26:457, 1985.

Shehadi WH, Toniolo G: Adverse reactions to contrast media. *Radiology* 137:299, 1980.

Siegle RL: Current problems of contrast materials. *Invest Radiol* 21(10):779, 1986.

Siegle RL, Lieberman P, Jennings BR, Rice MC: Iodinated contrast material: studies relating to complement activation, atopy, cellular association and antigenicity. *Invest Radiol* 15(6 Suppl):513, 1980.

Spataro RF, Katzberg RW, Fischer HW, McMannis MJ: High dose clinical urography with the low osmolality contrast agent Hexabrix: comparison with a conventional contrast agent. *Radiology* 162:9, 1987.

Stadalnik RC, Vera Z, DaSilva O, et al: Electrocardiographic response to intravenous urography: prospective evaluation of 275 patients. *AJR* 129:825, 1977.

Steinberg EP, Anderson GF, Powe NR, et al: Use of low-osmolality contrast media in a price-sensitive environment. *AJR* 151:271, 1988.

White RI, Halden WJ Jr: Liquid gold: low osmolality contrast media. *Radiology* 159:559, 1986.

Witten DM, Hirsch FD, Hartman GW: Acute reactions to urographic contrast medium. *AJR* 119:832, 1973.

Wolf GL: Safer, more expensive iodinated contrast agents: how do we decide? *Radiology* 159:557, 1986.

Wolf GL, Arenson RL, Cross AP: A prospective trial of ionic vs. nonionic contrast agents in routine clinical practice: comparison of adverse effects. *AJR* 152:939, 1989.

Wolf GL, Mishkin MM, Arenson R, et al: Adverse reactions to intravenous contrast media in routine clinical practice. Presented at the 75th Annual Meeting and Scientific Session of the Radiological Society of North America, Chicago IL, November 1989.

Contrast-induced Acute Renal Dysfunction

Cramer BC, Parfrey PS, Hutchinson TA, et al: Renal function following infusion of radiologic contast material. *Arch Intern Med* 145:87, 1985.

Cruz C, Hricak H, Samhouri F, et al: Contrast media for angiography: effect on renal function. *Radiology* 158:109, 1986.

D'Elia JA, Gleason R, Alday M, et al: Nephrotoxicity from angiographic contrast material. A prospective study. *Am J Med* 72:719, 1982.

Eisenberg RL, Bank WO, Hedgock MW: Renal failure after major angiography can be avoided with hydration. *AJR* 136:859, 1981.

Gomes AS, Baker JD, Martin-Paredero V, et al: Acute renal dysfunction after major arteriography. *AJR* 145:1249, 1985.

Gomes AS, Lois JF, Baker JD, et al: Acute renal dysfunction in high-risk patients after angiography: comparison of ionic and nonionic contrast media. *Radiology* 170:65, 1989.

Grainger RG: Renal toxicity of radiological contrast media. *Br Med Bull* 28(3):191, 1972.

Gup AK, Fischman JI, Aldridge G, Schlegel JU: The effect of drip infusion pyelography on renal function. *AJR* 98:102, 1966.

Harkonen S, Kjellstrand CM: Exacerbation of diabetic renal failure following intravenous pyelography. *Am J Med* 63:939, 1977.

Hayman LA, Evans RA, Fahr LM, Hinck VC: Renal consequences of rapid high dose contrast CT. *AJR* 134:553, 1980.

Krumlovsky FA, Simon N, Santhanam S, et al: Acute renal failure. Association with administration of radiographic contrast material. *JAMA* 239(2):125, 1978.

Lang EK, Foreman J, Schlegel JU, et al: The incidence of contrast medium induced acute tubular necrosis following arteriography. *Radiology* 138:203, 1981.

MacEwan DW, Dunbar JS, Nogrady MB: Intravenous pyelography in children with renal insufficiency. *Radiology* 78:893, 1962.

Martin-Paredero V, Dixon SM, Baker JD, et al: Risk of renal failure after major angiography. *Arch Surg* 118:1417, 1983.

Marx M, Bettmann MA: Contrast induced renal failure. *Postgrad Radiol* 5:343, 1985.

Mason RA, Arbeit LA, Giron F: Renal dysfunction after arteriography. *JAMA* 253(7):1001, 1985.

Miller DL, Chang R, Wells WT, et al: Intravascular contrast media: effect of dose on renal function. *Radiology* 167:607, 1988.

Myers GH Jr, Witten DM: Acute renal failure after excretory urography in multiple myeloma. *AJR* 113:583, 1971.

Older RA, Korobkin M, Cleeve DM, et al: Contrast-induced acute renal failure: persistent nephrogram as clue to early detection. *AJR* 13:339, 1980.

Parfrey PS, Griffiths SM, Barrett BJ, et al: Contrast material-induced renal failure in patients with diabetes mellitus, renal insufficiency, or both. *N Engl J Med* 320(3):143, 1989.

Postlethwaite AE, Kelley WN: Uricosuric effect of radiocontrast agents: a study in man of four commonly used preparations. *Ann Intern Med* 74:845, 1971.

Schwab SJ, Hlatky MA, Pieper KS, et al: Contrast nephrotoxicity: a randomized controlled trial of a nonionic and ionic radiographic contrast agent. *N Engl J Med* 320(3):149, 1989.

Schwartz WB, Hurwit A, Ettinger A: Intravenous urography in the patient with renal insufficiency. *N Engl J Med* 269(6):277, 1963.

Stacul F, Carraro M, Magnaldi S, et al: Contrast agent nephrotoxicity: comparison of ionic and nonionic contrast agents. *AJR* 149:1287, 1987.

Talner LB: Does hydration prevent contrast material renal injury? *AJR* 136:1021, 1981.

VanZee BE, Hoy WE, Talley TE, Jaenike JR: Renal injury associated with intravenous pyelography in nondiabetic and diabetic patients. *Ann Intern Med* 89:51, 1978.

Treatment of Adverse Reactions to Contrast Media

Cohan RH, Dunnick NR, Bashore TM: Treatment of reactions to radiographic contrast material. *AJR* 151:263, 1988.

Freitag JJ, Miller LW (eds): *Washington Manual of Medical Therapeutics,* ed 23. Boston: Little, Brown, 1980.

Hamilton G: Severe adverse reactions to urography in patients taking beta-adrenergic blocking agents. *Can Med Assoc J* 133:122, 1985.

Siegle RL: Iodinated contrast material reactions: treatment and prevention. *Contemp Diagn Radiol* 9(16):1, 1986.

vanSonnenberg E, Neff CC, Pfister RC: Life-threatening hypotensive reactions to contrast media administration: comparison of pharmacologic and fluid therapy. *Radiology* 162:15, 1987.

CHAPTER 5

RENAL CYSTIC DISEASE

Renal cysts, cystic disease, and cystic masses are the most common abnormalities encountered in uroradiology. In some cases the renal cysts are part of a systemic process that also involves the kidneys. In most patients, however, one or several cystic masses are detected and the question is whether the lesion is benign or malignant. In the vast majority of cases, the radiographic findings are sufficiently characteristic that surgery is not required. However, use of various radiographic modalities may be necessary before a confident diagnosis can be reached.

The classification of renal cystic diseases reflects both morphologic features and pathophysiology. In 1964, Osathanondh and Potter used microdissection studies to divide renal cysts into four groups. They felt type 1 cysts were due to dilation of collecting tubules which resulted in infantile polycystic kidney disease. In type 2 cysts, inhi-

bition of the development of ampullae result in inadequate branching of the collecting tubules which terminate in cysts. This results in multicystic nephroma or multicystic dysplastic kidneys. In type 3 cysts, normal collecting tubules are interspersed among abnormal tubules that have undergone cystic enlargement. The abnormality involves the interstitial or ampullary parts of some collecting tubules. In adult polycystic kidney disease (APCD), cysts associated with systemic diseases such as tuberous sclerosis and medullary sponge kidney are included. In type 4 cysts, the cystic disease is due to urethral obstruction and resulting back-pressure on the kidney.

Other investigators including Gleason et al. and Grossman et al. have developed classification systems based on radiologic-pathologic correlation or the appearance at urography. In 1969, Elkin and Bernstein suggested a classification of renal cysts based on genetic, clinical and morphologic criteria. It is a modification of this classification that is used here.

CORTICAL CYSTS

Simple Cysts

The most common renal mass lesion is a simple cortical cyst. Cortical cysts are uncommon in children or young adults but are seen by excretory urography (IVP) in as many as 20% of men with prostatic enlargement. Many more cysts can be detected with computed tomography (CT) and ultrasound (US) than with urography. In fact, with more routine use of CT and US, renal cysts are estimated to occur in 50% of the population older than 50 years of age. Thus, they are considered acquired lesions and probably arise from obstructed ducts or tubules.

Simple cysts are composed of fibrous tissue and are lined by flattened cuboidal epithelium. They contain clear serous fluid and do not communicate with the collecting system.

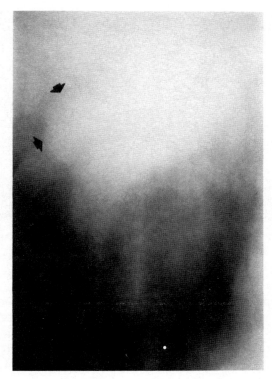

Figure 5.1.   Simple cyst. A cortical bulge (*arrows*) is seen projecting into the perinephric fat.

Most patients with a simple cyst are asymptomatic, and the cyst is detected as an incidental finding. Hematuria is occasionally attributed to a benign cyst. Rarely a large cyst may obstruct the collecting system or cause hypertension. Local pain may be due to distention of the cyst wall or spontaneous bleeding into the cyst.

Although simple cysts have been described in all age groups, they are unusual in children. A cyst in a child must be carefully examined to differentiate a benign cyst from a cystic Wilms' tumor.

Cortical cysts can occasionally be detected on plain abdominal radiographs. The water density cyst is seen as a cortical bulge projecting into the perinephric fat (Fig. 5.1). Calcification is seen in the wall of a simple cyst in only 1% of cases.

During urography, a simple cyst is seen as a lucent mass in the renal parenchyma. Radiographs taken soon after intravenous contrast injection (1 or 2 minutes) optimize visualization of cortical masses, as this is the peak parenchymal opacification (Chapter 4). A cyst is well defined and has a sharp interface with the normal renal cortex (Fig. 5.2). The cyst does not enhance but does distort the adjacent parenchyma. If the cyst extends beyond the surface of the kidney, the parenchyma is extended to produce a "beak" or "claw sign." The margin of

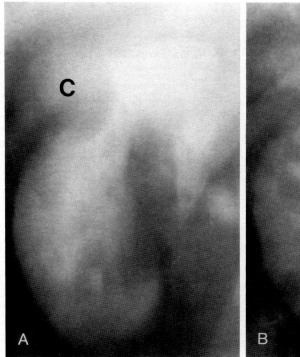
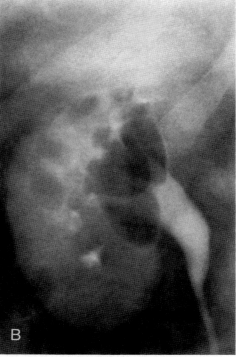

Figure 5.2.   Simple cyst. **A,** The early nephrotomogram demonstrates a rounded, peripheral mass (C) which has an imperceptibly thin wall and sharp interface with the normal renal parenchyma. **B,** The cyst is obscured by bowel gas and cannot be seen on the plain radiograph obtained 5 min after contrast injection.

the cyst with the kidney is smooth and the cyst wall is too thin to be seen during urography. If the cyst is entirely intrarenal, its wall cannot be distinguished from the adjacent renal parenchyma and its thickness can not be assessed.

These same findings are present on CT examination. Computed tomography has superior contrast resolution, allowing measurement of the density of the cyst fluid which should be near that of water (Fig. 5.3). A density greater than about 15 Hounsfield units (HU) is suspicious for a complicated cyst or even a solid mass lesion. There should be no contrast enhancement of a simple cyst. However, small increases (2–5 HU) in density are normally seen after intravenous contrast injection. Renal cysts are often detected as an incidental finding during a contrast enhanced CT examination of the abdomen, and there is no opportunity to test for contrast enhancement. However, if the density of the cyst fluid is less than 15 HU and other criteria of a simple cyst are present, the lesion will almost certainly be benign.

The wall of a benign cortical cyst is too thin to be seen on CT. However, when evaluating wall thickness with CT, it is important to look at a portion of the cyst that extends well away from the parenchyma so that a portion of adjacent renal tissue ("beak") is not included in the section. If the cyst is completely intrarenal, wall thickness cannot be assessed.

Although these same features are also seen with US, the terminology is different because sound waves are used rather than x-rays. A simple cyst is still a rounded homogeneous mass with a sharp interface with the normal renal parenchyma (Fig. 5.4). However, rather than being lucent, it is echo-free with enhanced through-transmission. Thin septations that are too fine to be detected with CT may be seen with US.

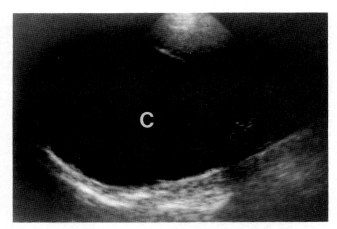

Figure 5.4.   Simple cyst. A well-defined, echo-free mass (C) is seen in the upper pole of the kidney.

Angiography is not routinely used to evaluate a suspected renal cyst. However, if performed, the cyst is seen as an avascular mass displacing adjacent blood vessels. A few tiny vessels may be seen supplying the cyst wall.

Simple cortical cysts are also readily detected with magnetic resonance imaging (MRI) (Fig. 5.5). The appearance of a homogeneous rounded mass with a thin wall and sharp interface with normal renal parenchyma is similar to that on CT. The long T_1 values result in a low signal intensity on T_1-weighted images. However, they have a very high signal intensity on T_2 weighted images, which reflects the long T_2 value of water.

The accuracy of the radiographic diagnosis of a renal cyst depends on how well it is seen with each modality. When all of the criteria of a benign simple cyst are present, it is highly unlikely to be anything else and further evaluation is not warranted. However, cysts often are not visualized well enough by IVP to make this determination. Due to cost considerations, US is the most efficient method of confirming the presence of a simple cyst that is poorly seen during urography. Ultrasound has the added advantages of not requiring ionizing radiation and avoiding the potential adverse reactions associated with intravenous contrast injection.

Computed tomography is currently the gold standard for the evaluation of renal mass lesions, but it is a more expensive examination than US and requires intravenous contrast material. It is indicated when the US examination is indeterminate or technically inadequate due to obesity or overlying gas. It is also appropriate to proceed directly to CT if the urogram indicates that the mass is complex or likely to be solid. Although there is insufficient experience with the magnetic resonance imaging of renal cystic masses, MRI should also be highly accurate in the diagnosis of these benign lesions.

Renal cysts occasionally regress in size or disappear completely. Although this phenomenon may be due to

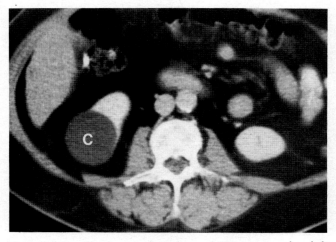

Figure 5.3.   Simple cyst. An enhanced CT scan reveals a left renal mass (C) with the same cystic characteristics seen with urography. The cyst fluid measured 4 HU.

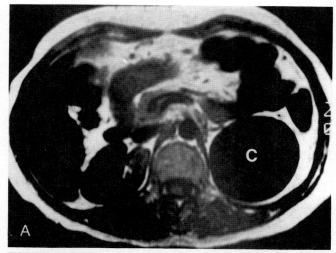

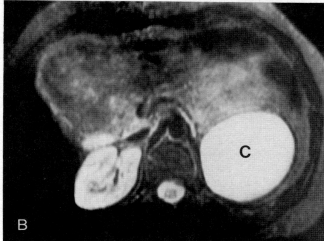

Figure 5.5. Simple cyst. **A,** T₁-weighted (TR 500, TE 15) images demonstrate a low signal intensity (C) which is much higher on **B,** T₂ weighted (TR 2000, TE 40) images.

resorption of a hematoma misdiagnosed as a cyst, most cases are probably due to spontaneous cyst rupture. An increase in pressure within the cyst relative to either the collecting system or the perinephric space may result in rupture. Such a pressure rise could be caused either by hemorrhage into the cyst or by a change in the composition of the cyst fluid.

The most common clinical manifestations of cyst rupture are hematuria and flank pain. The diagnosis can be made by either IVP or retrograde pyelography if the cyst communicates with the collecting system. The cyst cavity was opacified by urography in 88% of cases reported by Papanicolaou et al. In most cases, the communication of the cyst with the collecting system closes spontaneously. Once the diagnosis is made, management is conservative.

Complicated Cysts

Cystic masses that do not satisfy the criteria of a benign simple cyst must be further evaluated to exclude malig-

nancy. Various abnormalities are now recognized which exclude the diagnosis of a simple cyst.

Septations

Thin internal septations can be detected by US, but their presence alone does not suggest malignancy. Many of these thin septations are not seen during either urography or CT, and it is likely that they will be classified as typical simple cysts.

Other septations are thick enough to be seen during CT examination. If the septa are thin, smooth, and do not have localized areas of thickening or irregularity, a diagnosis of benign cyst can be made (Fig. 5.6). However, if there is an associated solid mass, the lesions must be considered malignant.

Calcification

The presence of calcification is also a nonspecific finding (Fig. 5.7). When evaluation of the kidney depended primarily on urography, the presence of calcification, especially central calcification, was an ominous sign. However, CT has made the presence or absence of calcification almost irrelevant, because wall thickening and soft tissue masses can easily be detected without the help of calcification. Thin calcification in the wall of a cyst or in a septation does not, in itself, warrant surgical exploration.

Thick Wall

A thick wall is incompatible with a simple cyst. It indicates either that the lesion is another cystic mass or that the cyst has become complicated by some process such as infection or hemorrhage. Inflammatory or infectious cavities may result in this appearance or the lesion may

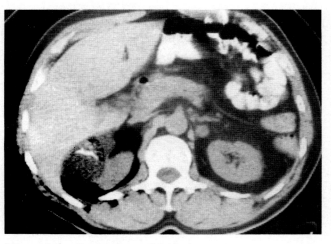

Figure 5.6. Septated cyst. Calcified septations are seen in this cystic mass which otherwise has the characteristics of a benign cyst.

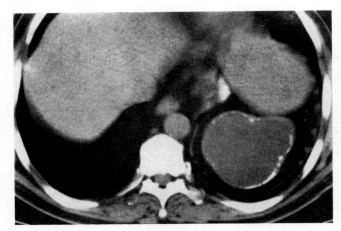

Figure 5.7. Calcified cyst. Calcification is seen in the wall of this benign cyst.

be a cystic renal adenocarcinoma (Chapter 6). These lesions must be considered indeterminate, and surgical exploration is indicated (Fig. 5.8). The presence of an associated soft tissue tumor mass is an even more ominous finding and is highly suspicious for a malignancy.

Increased Density

A cystic mass with a density above water must contain more than simple cyst fluid. On current scanners a density greater than 10–15 HU is worrisome, but this reading should be checked against the water bath phantom, as there may be considerable drift in the CT numbers. If an increased density is present, further evaluation with US, pre- and post-contrast-enhanced CT, or aspiration is warranted.

One category of atypical renal cyst that has an increased attenuation coefficient is the hyperdense cyst. These lesions look like typical simple cysts on CT examination in that they are rounded, well-defined, homogeneous masses that do not enhance with intravenous contrast injection. They are usually small, peripheral lesions, measuring less than 3 cm in diameter (Fig. 5.9). However, instead of having a density near water, they measure 60–90 HU. They are easily recognized on an unenhanced CT examination but are often masked by the enhanced renal parenchyma, because their densities are similar. Thus, it is probable that these lesions are more common than is appreciated, inasmuch as most abdominal CT scans are performed after intravenous contrast injection.

There are several possible etiologies for a hyperdense renal cyst. The most common are hemorrhage and a high protein content of the cyst fluid. However, a diffuse paste-like calcified material has also been found. The vast majority of these hyperdense cysts are benign, but they must be carefully examined for other atypical features. Computed tomography examination prior to and following intravenous contrast injection is often helpful. A cyst will not enhance while a solid tumor will increase in density.

Ultrasound examination is another useful modality in the evaluation of the hyperdense renal mass. It enables the examiners to distinguish between a cystic and solid lesion. With US, blood elements can sometimes be seen floating within the cyst. However, if the lesion cannot be clearly evaluated, surgical exploration may still be needed.

Hemorrhagic cysts can also be identified with MRI. Simple cysts have a low signal intensity on T_1-weighted images while hemorrhagic cysts have a high signal intensity on all pulse sequences. Because the blood elements tend to settle out, the more intense signal of the paramagnetic methemoglobin can be seen in the dependent portion of the cyst on T_1-weighted images. The relative intensity of the two cyst layers reverses on T_2-weighted

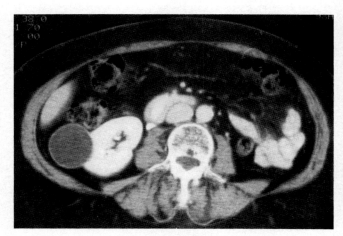

Figure 5.8. Thick-walled cyst. The thick wall in this cystic mass indicates a complicated cyst or other cystic mass. Further evaluation is warranted.

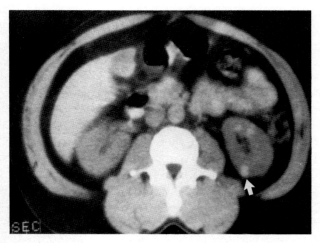

Figure 5.9. Hyperdense cyst. A small peripheral dense mass is seen (*arrow*) in the posterior aspect of the left kidney. At surgery this was a benign hemorrhagic cyst. Several similar tiny lesions in the same kidney are presumably hemorrhagic cysts as well.

sequences. A renal adenocarcinoma can usually be distinguished by its inhomogeneity, indistinct or irregular margins, and lack of a fluid-hemoglobin level.

Milk of Calcium Cyst

Milk of calcium is a collection of small calcific granules in the cyst fluid. The granules, usually calcium carbonate, are in suspension and layer out in the dependent portion of the cyst (Fig. 5.10). They are seen most frequently in calyceal diverticulae (Chapter 11) but may also be present in simple cysts or polycystic kidneys. Milk of calcium cysts have no sex predilection but are more common in the upper poles of the kidneys.

The milk of calcium nature of these calculi may not be appreciated on a supine radiograph, but the fluid-calcium layer is easily detected on upright films or CT examination. A horizontal line of calcium density can also be detected by US, regardless of the patient's position. Most of these cysts are detected as an incidental finding, and intervention is unnecessary.

MEDULLARY CYSTIC DISEASE

This disease complex includes medullary cystic disease and related diseases such as juvenile nephronophthisis and retinal-renal dysplasia. The kidneys are small to normal in size, and maintain a normal configura-

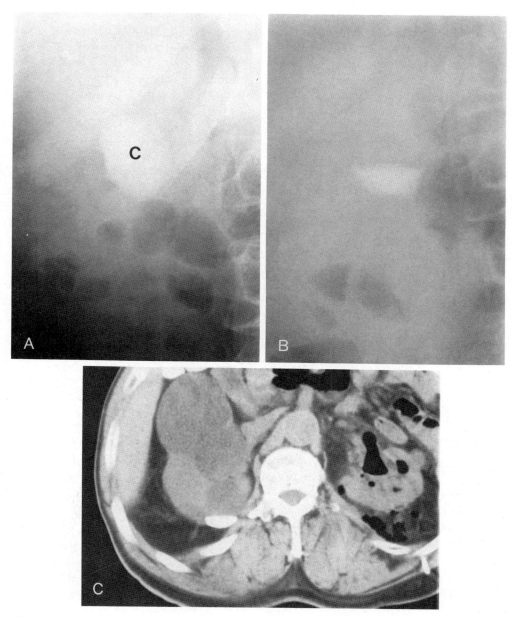

Figure 5.10. Milk of calcium cyst. **A,** A homogeneous calcific density (C) is identified on this supine abdominal radiograph. **B,** A "fluid/calcium" level is seen on an upright film. **C,** This level is also appreciated on an unenhanced CT scan.

tion and smooth contour. There are a variable number of small cysts, up to 2 cm in diameter, which are located primarily in the medulla. The cortex is thin but does not contain cysts. Biopsy shows interstitial and periglomerular fibrosis as well as tubular atrophy. However, the diagnosis cannot be made if cysts are not included in the biopsy specimen because the fibrotic changes are nonspecific.

The uremic medullary cystic diseases can be classified by the age of onset. The adult form is transmitted by autosomal-dominant inheritance. Patients usually present as young adults with anemia, which may be severe, and have progressive renal failure. They have a salt-wasting nephropathy that is not corrected with mineralocorticoids. Other than a fixed low specific gravity, the urine sediment is normal. Hypertension may develop near the end of the disease course.

Juvenile nephronophthisis typically presents at 3–5 years of age with polydipsia and polyuria. The clinical course with anemia and progressive renal failure is similar to the adult onset variety, but progression is slower with 8–10 years before terminal uremia. Juvenile nephronophthisis is transmitted by autosomal-recessive inheritance.

Abdominal radiographs may demonstrate small kidneys without calcification. High-dose nephrotomography reveals a thin renal cortex. Linear contrast collections radiating from the pyramids may be seen. However, excretory urography is not likely to be helpful, and is seldom performed because of the renal failure. Computed tomography demonstrates small smooth kidneys and may reveal the small medullary cysts.

High-resolution US may be the examination of choice in these patients. The corticomedullary differentiation is lost and the parenchyma appears isoechoic or hypoechoic with the liver or spleen. In patients with severe uremia, medullary cysts can usually be demonstrated, but they may not be detectable in milder cases.

POLYCYSTIC RENAL DISEASE

Infantile Polycystic Disease

Infantile polycystic disease (IPCD) is transmitted by autosomal-recessive inheritance and is frequently referred to as autosomal-recessive polycystic kidney disease. IPCD includes a spectrum of abnormalities ranging from newborns with grossly enlarged spongy kidneys to older children with medullary ductal ectasia. The older children also develop hepatic fibrosis that progresses to portal hypertension and esophageal varices.

Congenital hepatic fibrosis (CHF) may represent yet another disease transmitted by autosomal recessive inheritance in which the renal disease is different and milder than IPCD. Other entities associated with CHF include APCD, multicystic dysplastic kidneys, choledochal cyst, and Caroli's disease. However, medullary ductal ectasia is found in all forms of IPCD, with or without CHF.

Patients with the infantile form of IPCD have renal failure at birth and most die within the first few days of life. Patients with the juvenile form have a milder renal disease characterized by tubular ectasia and renal cysts. They often present with symptoms arising from hepatic fibrosis with portal hypertension and varices rather than renal failure.

The radiographic manifestations reflect the age of onset and the severity of renal involvement. In the neonatal form there is massive enlargement of the kidneys which maintain their reniform shape. The kidneys are enlarged but function poorly. The nephrogram is faint with blotchy opacification. Linear striations due to stasis of contrast material in the dilated renal tubules have been described. The numerous small (1- to 2-mm) cysts in both the cortex and medulla result in increased echogenicity on sonography. However, with high-resolution scanners a peripheral sonolucent rim can be seen representing compressed renal cortex (Fig. 5.11). A prominent renal pelvis and calyces may result in a sonolucent central zone.

Polycystic Disease of Childhood

Among older children, fewer than 10% of the renal tubules are affected and hepatic fibrosis dominates the clinical course. This is sometimes referred to as congenital hepatic fibrosis. The clinical presentation is usually a result of portal hypertension with splenomegaly, gastric, and esophageal varices. The kidneys are only mildly enlarged but contain variably sized cysts that are predominantly medullary in location. The appearance of tubular ectasia in these children is similar to that seen in medul-

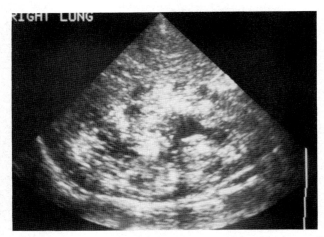

Figure 5.11. Infantile polycystic disease. Numerous small cysts create increased echogenicity. A peripheral sonolucent rim represents compressed parenchyma. (Case courtesy of Kate Feinstein, M.D.)

lary sponge kidney in adults (Chapter 11). An increased echogenicity with loss of the normal corticomedullary junction is seen with US. The sonolucent rim of compressed renal parenchyma may also be seen in the juvenile form.

Adult Polycystic Kidney Disease

APCD is the most common form of cystic kidney disease and is responsible for 10–12% of patients on chronic dialysis. It is transmitted by autosomal-dominant inheritance. However, due to variable expressivity and spontaneous mutations, as many as 50% of patients with APCD may have no family history of renal disease. Although the etiology is unknown, the cysts seem to arise from nephrons that initially were able to function normally.

The age at which patients with APCD present is most commonly the third or fourth decade. However, APCD may be seen in children or in older adults. The initial complaint is usually pain that may be lumbar, groin, or upper abdominal. The enlarged kidneys may be palpable as abdominal masses.

Hypertension, which occurs in over half of patients with APCD, is due to increased renin production by the kidneys. Hematuria may be due to rupture of one of the renal cysts into the renal pelvis or the presence of a stone.

Patients with APCD often suffer from flank pain that can be due to a variety of etiologies. Acute pain may result from swelling of one of the cysts due to hemorrhage or infection. Colicky pain may arise from ureteral obstruction by stone, blood clot, or rarely a cyst. Chronic pain is more likely due to progressive enlargement of the cysts with stretching of the renal capsule.

All patients with APCD have progressive renal failure. The rate of progression of the azotemia is related to the age of onset; those patients whose symptoms begin after age 50 years have a better prognosis. Almost half of patients with APCD have cerebral (berry) aneurysms in the circle of Willis, and stroke from rupture of a berry aneurysm is a significant cause of morbidity and mortality.

Excretory urography is seldom used to evaluate patients with known APCD. However, new cases may be diagnosed with IVP because the findings are characteristic. The plain abdominal radiograph is remarkable for the poor visualization of the renal outlines. Three-quarters of the renal outline is seen in less than 10% of patients with APCD as compared with 80% of patients with unilateral renal enlargement due to other causes. Calcification in the cyst walls is common, and nephrolithiasis may be detected. If renal function is adequate, the urogram will demonstrate enlarged kidneys with a mottled renal parenchyma due to the many cysts. The collecting system is splayed by the parenchymal cysts, which may cause infundibular obstruction. Although its appearance is typical for APCD, it may not be distinguishable from the renal involvement by multiple cysts and hamartomas in patients with tuberous sclerosis.

Sonography and CT have replaced nephrotomography as the standard method of examination of patients with APCD. Innumerable renal cysts are seen with either modality. The kidneys are markedly enlarged but maintain their basic reniform shape.

Computed tomography has the advantage of clearly demonstrating the cysts and collecting systems of both kidneys. Precontrast scans are needed to demonstrate renal stones and facilitate the diagnosis of hemorrhagic cysts (Fig. 5.12). Since the kidneys are typically riddled with innumerable cysts that abut each other, the cysts are

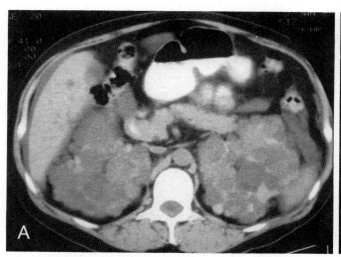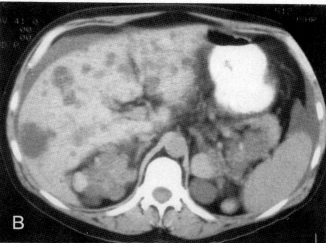

Figure 5.12. Adult polycystic disease. **A,** This unenhanced CT scan demonstrates bilateral renal enlargement by numerous cysts. Several dense cysts are presumably hemorrhagic. **B,** At a higher level hyperdense renal cysts, as well as associated hepatic cysts, are seen.

not round in shape but assume a variety of irregular contours.

Computed tomography is also useful in demonstrating hepatic cysts that are present in 57 to 74% of patients with APCD. These liver cysts develop from dilatation of aberrant bile ducts that embryologically failed to establish communication with the biliary tree. The cysts gradually accumulate fluid secreted by the lining cuboidal epithelial cells. Fewer than 5% of patients have associated cysts in other organs such as the spleen or pancreas.

Multiple renal cysts are easily identified on MRI. Uncomplicated cysts resemble simple cortical cysts with a homogeneous low signal intensity on T_1-weighted images and high intensity on T_2-weighted images. Complicated cysts reflect the presence of infection or age of the hemorrhage. Acute bleeding results in a hyperintense image regardless of the pulse sequence. However, the appearance varies with the age of the bleed. The high protein content of an infected cyst results in a signal intensity between a simple cyst and one with an acute hemorrhage.

Bleeding into renal cysts is common and may be the source of acute flank pain. If the cyst ruptures into the renal pelvis, hematuria will occur. Cyst hemorrhage may be more common in APCD because of the associated hypertension or the increased bleeding tendency of uremia or heparinization during dialysis. Hemorrhagic renal cysts may be seen in 70% of patients with APCD. Perinephric hemorrhage has been reported but is rare.

Both kidneys are affected with APCD, but involvement may be asymmetric. Rare cases of unilateral APCD are reported but these may represent manifestations too small for macroscopic imaging.

There is no treatment for APCD and patients must often be sustained by dialysis or transplantation. By informing patients of the heritability of APCD, genetic counseling can help them with family planning. Thus, it is important for the diagnosis to be made before the patients reach child-bearing age. Excretory urography with nephrotomography and sonography are both able to detect changes of APCD among children of affected families. Since ultrasound is less invasive, it is the preferred screening examination.

MULTICYSTIC DYSPLASTIC KIDNEY

A multicystic dysplastic kidney (MCDK) consists of a collection of irregularly sized cysts and fibrous tissue but no functioning renal parenchyma. The cysts do not communicate, the renal collecting system is small or absent, and there are atretic ipsilateral renal vessels. The anomaly results from occlusion of the fetal ureters usually before 8–10 weeks of gestation.

A variant, the hydronephrotic type of multicystic dysplasia, may result from incomplete ureteral obstruction

later in gestation. In such cases, the cysts communicate with the renal pelvis.

In rare cases MCDK may be confined to one segment of the kidney. Most of these cases occur in the upper-pole moiety of a duplicated collecting system.

Most renal dysplasias are detected as an abdominal mass in infancy. MCKD is the second most common cause of an abdominal mass in the neonate, trailing only hydronephrosis in frequency. Males are more commonly affected than females, and there is a predilection for the left kidney.

Malformations including bilateral MCDK, ureteropelvic junction (UPJ) obstruction, hypoplasia of the opposite kidney, and horseshoe kidney are commonly associated with MCKD. These occurred in 41% of fetuses examined sonographically by Kleiner et al. Since some of these contralateral anomalies are fatal, less severe changes are more common, and UPJ obstruction is the most common malformation seen in children or adults. If the MCDK is not detected in infancy it may remain asymptomatic and be detected as an incidental finding in an adult.

Abdominal radiographs may demonstrate a soft tissue flank mass. In adults calcification is common, usually in the cyst walls (Fig. 5.13). There is no functioning renal parenchyma on the affected side, but excretory urography demonstrates compensatory hypertrophy of the contralateral kidney.

If retrograde pyelography is performed, an atretic ureter may be demonstrated (Fig. 5.14). Extravasation is

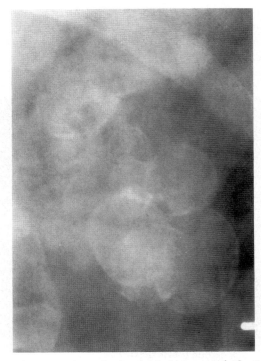

Figure 5.13. Multicystic dysplastic kidney. Calcification can be seen in cyst walls.

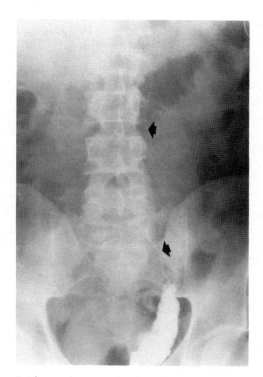

Figure 5.14. Multicystic dysplastic kidney. Retrograde pyelography demonstrates a small atretic ureter (*arrows*) which does not reach the kidney. Extravasation is present around the distal ureter.

common because cannulation of the small ureteric opening may be difficult.

The multiple cysts with thick septa are nicely demonstrated by CT (Fig. 5.15). Mural calcifications can be demonstrated in the cyst walls, but there is no evidence of contrast excretion.

Sonography is particularly valuable in assessing infants and demonstrates multiple cysts of varying sizes (Fig. 5.16). There is no connection between adjacent cysts, nor is there renal parenchyma surrounding the cysts. If angiography is performed, no ipsilateral renal artery will be seen.

Segmental multicystic renal dysplasia in an upper-pole moiety may be seen in patients with obstruction from an ectopic ureterocele. The dysplastic segment has the same features as the multicystic dysplastic kidney and causes compression of the normally functioning lower pole moiety.

Focal multicystic renal dysplasia has also been reported. This presumably results from in utero infundibular obstruction. This entity is fortunately rare as it cannot be distinguished radiographically from other renal cystic masses.

The classic multicystic dysplastic kidney must be distinguished from the "hydronephrotic type of multicystic dysplasia." This hydronephrotic form probably results from incomplete obstruction of the ureter after the tenth week of gestation. In this form, there is a renal pelvis that communicates with the multiple cysts. Function may be demonstrated by excretion of contrast material during

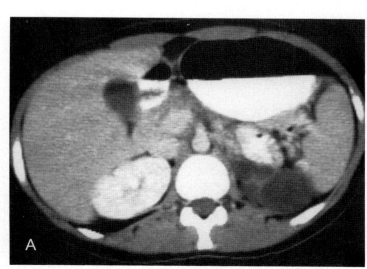

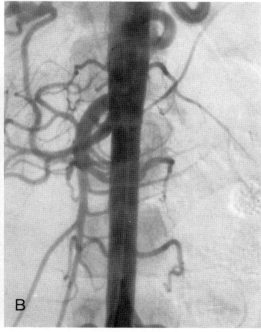

Figure 5.15. Multicystic dysplastic kidney. **A,** On CT, multiple cysts, but no functioning renal tissue, are present on the left. The right kidney is normal. **B,** An abdominal aortogram demonstrates absence of the left renal artery.

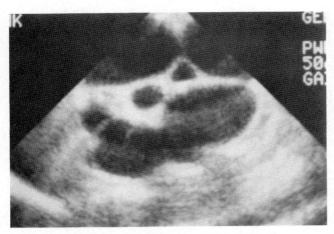

Figure 5.16.   Multicystic dysplastic kidney. Multiple cysts of varying sizes are seen in an infant. (Courtesy of Kate Feinstein, M.D.)

urography or CT, or excretion of radionuclide during nuclear medicine studies. If the diagnosis is uncertain, percutaneous aspiration with antegrade pyelography may be required. Surgery is indicated in patients with the hydronephrotic type of disease because significant renal function can often be preserved.

Treatment

Our knowledge of the natural history of MCDK is increasing with the use of in utero US. As many as 41% of fetuses with MCDK have a contralateral renal anomaly. This is much higher than the 11–15% incidence seen in neonates. This is due to the fact that many of these associated anomalies are fatal and that in some cases there is involution of MCDK to what appears in the neonate as renal agenesis.

This may also occur after birth. In a review of 30 patients with MCDK by Vinocur et al., 13.5% decreased in size or disappeared. This is presumably due to leakage or reabsorption of cyst fluid. The majority (73%) did not change in size and 13.5% increased. Surgery is needed if there is significant growth during the first year of life, the diagnosis is inconclusive or complications arise which require nephrectomy.

MULTILOCULAR CYSTIC NEPHROMA

This uncommon lesion has been described by various names including multilocular renal cyst, cystic adenoma, lymphangioma, segmental multicystic kidney, segmental polycystic kidney, cystic harmartoma, benign cystic nephroma, and Perlman's tumor. It is a congenital renal lesion which is not genetically transmitted.

Multilocular cystic nephroma (MLCN) is a well-circumscribed lesion containing many cysts of variable sizes. The cystic mass is surrounded by a thick fibrous capsule that compresses adjacent renal parenchyma and often

projects into the renal pelvis. The cysts are lined by flattened or cuboidal epithelium and contain clear fluid. Hemorrhage and necrosis are uncommon.

The presenting signs and symptoms depend on the patient's age. Males are usually younger than 4 years of age and present with a palpable abdominal mass. Females typically present between the ages of 4 and 20 years, or over 40 years. Among children presenting under 4 years of age, 73% are male; when the patient is older than 4 years at presentation, 89% are female. In the adult, MLCN may be found during examination of an unrelated complaint or during the investigation of pain, hematuria, or urinary tract infection. Hematuria may result from herniation of the tumor into the renal pelvis causing tissue necrosis of the overlying thin layer of transitional cell epithelium.

Calcification is uncommon, especially in pediatric patients. However, radiographically detected calcifications were found in 7 of 12 adult patients reported by Banner et al. It is usually in the cyst walls or intervening stroma. The pattern of calcification is nonspecific and may be central or peripheral. A large renal mass is seen with excretory urography. The cystic mass occurs with equal frequency on either side, but is more common in the lower pole. Projection of the mass into the renal pelvis can often be demonstrated (Fig. 5.17). The mass is hypovascular and mottled in appearance.

The multiple cystic spaces are best demonstrated with US. If the cysts are large, multiple locules separated by echogenic stroma suggest the diagnosis of MLCN (Fig. 5.18). If the cysts are small, they may not be defined by US and the echogenic stroma may suggest a complex or solid renal mass.

The CT appearance is usually characteristic. The masses are large, averaging about 10 cm in diameter. They are sharply delineated from the normal renal parenchyma. MLCN is hypovascular but the septations enhance

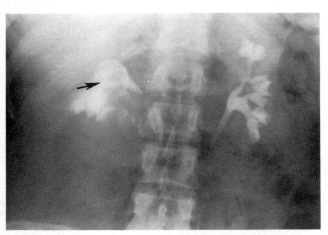

Figure 5.17.   Multilocular cystic nephroma. A large mass in the lower pole of the right kidney is projecting into the renal pelvis (*arrow*).

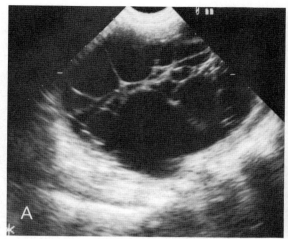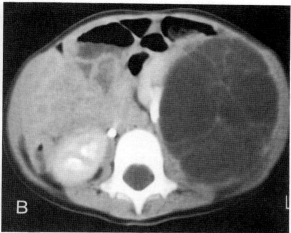

Figure 5.18. Multilocular cystic nephroma. **A,** Multiple cysts are separated by echogenic stroma on ultrasound. **B,** A large cystic mass with multiple septations is seen on CT.

after intravenous contrast injection (Fig. 5.18). When large cysts are present, the internal septations are well defined. If the cysts are small, the mass may have a pitted appearance.

Angiography demonstrates most lesions to be hypovascular, but the degree of vascularity depends on the size of the cysts and the amount of intervening stroma. Tortuous vessels and modest neovascularity can be seen, but signs of frank tumor vascularity, such as encasement, arteriovenous shunting, or vascular pooling are not present.

MLCN must be differentiated from a cystic renal adenocarcinoma. Although adenocarcinoma arising in MLCN has been reported, Madewell et al. at the Armed Forces Institute of Pathology believe these cases are multiloculated renal adenocarcinoma as the pathologic features of MLCN are not present.

Radiologic imaging studies are not adequate to exclude malignancy and further evaluation is needed. Cyst aspiration is usually inadequate because the locules do not communicate and an excessive number of punctures would be required to evaluate all portions of the lesion. Thus, surgical excision is indicated.

Since MLCN is a benign lesion and can often be suggested preoperatively. Local excision may be appropriate. Frozen sections should be obtained, however, to exclude malignancy. If malignant tissue is seen, a radical nephrectomy could be performed.

CYSTS ASSOCIATED WITH SYSTEMIC DISEASE

The phakomatoses are a group of neurologic disorders which include congenital abnormalities of the skin and other organs. Two of these, tuberous sclerosis and von Hippel-Lindau disease, are associated with renal cysts.

Tuberous Sclerosis

The complex of tuberous sclerosis (Bourneville's disease) includes small cutaneous angiofibromas on the face (adenoma sebaceum) and hamartomas in a variety of organs, such as the brain, eyes, heart, and kidneys. It is transmitted as an autosomal-dominant, but with incomplete penetrance. Sporadic cases, presumably due to spontaneous mutation, may also occur.

Patients may present with mental retardation, seizures or the characteristic skin lesions. Approximately 80% of patients have renal angiomyolipomas which may cause hematuria.

In addition to the angiomyolipomas found in patients with tuberous sclerosis (Chapter 6), there is an increased incidence of renal cysts. These cysts are small and rarely exceed 3 cm in diameter. They have a distinctive microscopic appearance with hyperplastic epithelium. Severe renal involvement can lead to renal failure. Computed tomography may demonstrate only hamartomas, hamartomas and cysts (Fig. 5.19), or only cysts.

Sonography clearly distinguishes the anechoic cysts from angiomyolipomas which are typically very echogenic. The appearance of the cysts is the same as simple cortical cysts. The appearance of an angiomyolipoma reflects the proportion of each tissue element within the tumor.

Computed tomography is often used to confirm the presence of an angiomyolipoma by demonstrating the fatty nature of the tumor. Tumors without fat will be indistinguishable from a renal adenocarcinoma.

von Hippel-Lindau Disease

This syndrome consists of cerebellar and retinal hemangioblastomas, renal carcinomas, pheochromocytomas, and a variety of visceral cysts including renal cysts. It

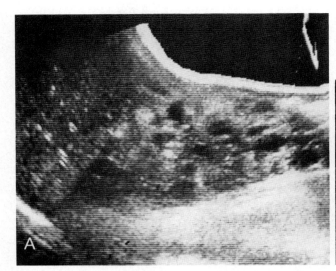

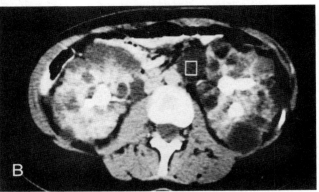

Figure 5.19. Tuberous sclerosis. Ultrasound and CT both demonstrate multiple mass lesions. **A,** On ultrasound, echogenic masses represent hamartomas while the echo-free areas are cysts. **B,** Computed tomography reveals fatty density hamartomas and water density cysts.

is transmitted by autosomal-dominant inheritance, but with only moderate penetrance.

The most common presentation is with symptoms of a cerebellar hemangioblastoma. Capillary angiomas involve the retina and may cause progressive visual loss. Renal cysts occur in approximately three-fourths of patients, and renal adenocarcinomas arise in 25–45% of patients (Chapter 6). The renal tumors are often bilateral and usually multifocal. Other urologic manifestations include adrenal pheochromocytomas and papillary cyst adenomas of the epididymis.

The renal cysts, which usually range in size from 0.5 to 3.0 cm, may be numerous and described as "simple" (Fig. 5.20). However, the hyperplastic epithelial lining may be a precursor of malignancy. Radiographic evaluation of

patients with von Hippel-Lindau disease is difficult. The numerous cysts distort the normal renal architecture. Tumors arise in the cyst wall, so careful evaluation is essential. Narrowly collimated CT is the most useful modality for this purpose. However, the tumors are often small and difficult to distinguish from cysts. Levine et al. recommend annual follow-up CT examination of any lesions that do not satisfy the criteria for either a benign cyst or a frank neoplasm.

Selective magnification renal arteriography may be useful to detect the small renal tumors (Chapter 6). Angiography is particularly valuable if surgical resection is contemplated, and precise knowledge of the vascular anatomy is needed to remove the tumor and spare as much renal parenchyma as possible.

MISCELLANEOUS RENAL CYSTS

Hydatid Disease

Hydatid disease in man is usually due to *Echinococcus granulosus,* but it may also be caused by *E. multilocularis.*

The adult worm lives in the intestine of a dog (definitive host) and discharges the egg-containing proglottid into the feces. The intermediate host is usually a sheep that ingests the eggs while grazing on contaminated ground. The protective chitinous layer is dissolved in the duodenum and the hydatid embryo passes through the intestinal wall into the portal vein. Thus, the liver is the organ most commonly involved. The embryo develops into a slowly growing cyst. The cycle is completed when the intermediate host (sheep) dies and the larva are eaten by the definitive host (dog). The human being is infected as an accidental host by eating contaminated food.

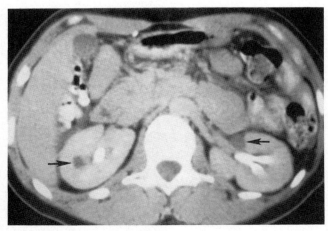

Figure 5.20. von Hippel Lindau disease. A simple renal cyst (*arrows*) is seen in each kidney.

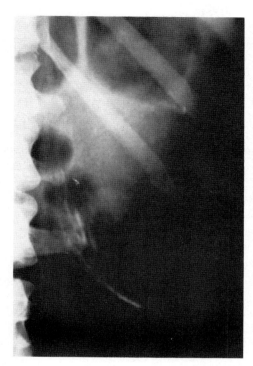

Figure 5.21. Hydatid disease. A calcified cyst wall is appreciated on the plain radiograph.

Hydatid cysts are composed of three layers: an outer protective pericyst, an easily broken middle membrane, and a thin inner germinal layer that produces the scolices. The organs most commonly involved in humans are the liver (75%) and lung (15%). Other organs, such as brain, bone, and kidney are infected in less than 10% of cases.

Although most cases are acquired in childhood, they are not usually detected until adulthood. The symptoms of renal hydatid disease are nonspecific and many patients are asymptomatic. Flank pain, hematuria, or signs of urinary tract infection may be present. A serologic test is available for patients suspected of having hydatid disease, either on the basis of contact or radiologic findings.

Curvilinear calcifications in the wall of the hydatid cyst may be detected on plain radiographs (Fig. 5.21). A hypovascular mass is detected with urography. However, the thick rim distinguishes the hydatid cyst from a simple cortical cyst.

Thick wall cysts are also well demonstrated by either CT or US. If daughter cysts are present, they can be detected by internal echoes or a high-density component next to the clear, water density cyst fluid.

Acquired Cystic Disease of Uremia

With improvements in dialysis and renal transplantation, patients with end-stage renal disease are now living much longer. As a result, examiners are beginning to detect acquired cystic disease, benign tumors, and an occasional renal adenocarcinoma in the native kidneys (Chapter 6).

Although the mechanism of cyst formation in these uremic patients is unknown, it is postulated that dialysis incompletely removes toxins and their build up may induce these changes. The cysts are thought to develop as a result of fusiform dilations of the proximal renal tubules. The involution of these cysts after successful renal transplantation supports this hypothesis.

Cysts occur in approximately 45% of patients followed for 3 years and may be seen in as many as 90% of patients on long-term dialysis. Solid tumors are also seen with increased frequency, up to 7%. These solid neoplasms include adenomas, oncocytomas, and adenocarcinomas. From pathologic examination it is not easy to determine the biologic behavior of these tumors, but the incidence of malignant adenocarcinomas is probably small. Many of these tumors which are classified as malignant histologically do not demonstrate malignant behavior. In a review of 14 long-term dialysis series, Grantham et al. found that only 2 of 601 (0.33%) patients developed metastatic cancer. This is similar to the incidence in the general population.

The US examination of native kidneys is difficult because they are often small, distorted, and surrounded by highly echogenic fat. Calcification frequently occurs, either in the cyst walls or the renal interstitium, making US evaluation even more difficult. It is easier to examine the native kidneys with CT (Fig. 5.22) than US and the sensitivity of CT in detecting small lesions is greater than with US.

Communicating Cysts

Occasionally a renal cyst communicates with the collecting system and opacifies with intravenous contrast material on IVP, CT, or retrograde pyelography. Any cys-

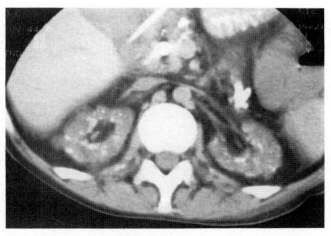

Figure 5.22. Acquired cystic disease of dialysis. Dystrophic calcification and multiple renal cysts are present on this unenhanced CT scan.

tic renal mass, such as a benign cortical cyst, inflammatory cyst, or even cystic carcinoma may rupture into the collecting system and produce this appearance. However, the most common etiology is a pyelogenic cyst or calyceal diverticulum (Chapter 11).

A pyelogenic cyst is lined with transitional epithelium and communicates with the collecting system through a narrow isthmus. The connection is usually at the fornix but can be at any portion of the calyx. Most cysts are small, usually less than 2 cm in diameter. Pyelogenic cysts are usually asymptomatic but occasionally may contain calculi or milk of calcium.

Since excreted contrast material enters the calyces from the tubules of Bellini, the calyces opacify before the calyceal diverticulum. This is a useful differentiating feature distinguishing them from papillary necrosis or focal hydronephrosis. Communicating cysts are also well demonstrated by CT where contrast accumulation can be clearly seen (Fig. 5.23).

EXTRAPARENCHYMAL CYSTS

Various investigators have used different terms to describe extraparenchymal cysts. To minimize this ambiguity, we consider cysts in two anatomic locations. The term *parapelvic cyst* is applied to those lying in the region of the renal sinus and the term *perinephric cyst* for those just beneath the renal capsule.

Amis and Cronan have suggested cysts in the renal sinus are further subdivided into etiologies. They use the term parapelvic cyst for a renal parenchymal cyst that projects into the renal sinus. Those cysts that arise in the renal sinus, probably from lymphatics, are termed peripelvic cysts. Using this terminology, parapelvic cysts are usually large but solitary while peripelvic cysts are more often small and multiple.

Parapelvic Cysts

These benign cysts lie in the region of the renal hilum and cause extrinsic compression on the collecting system. Smooth bowing or displacement of the infundibuli is seen on the IVP. The CT appearance is that of a benign cyst that is located in the hilar area (Fig. 5.24) rather than the cortex of the kidney.

Parapelvic cysts may not be renal in origin but could be lymphocysts or may arise from embryologic remnants in the renal hilum. With increased use of CT and US, they are frequently recognized and are often multiple and bilateral (Fig. 5.24). Problems arise when they are confused with other entities.

On urography the mass effect of the parapelvic cyst on the collecting system could also be caused by a renal tumor or metastases to lymph nodes in the hilar region. Ultrasound demonstrates their benign cystic nature (Fig. 5.25). However, on US the multiple echo-free areas in the central portion of the kidney may suggest hydronephrosis. Care must be taken to demonstrate that a dilated calyx is continuous with an enlarged infundibulum and pelvis before hydronephrosis is diagnosed.

Parapelvic cysts should not be confused with renal sinus fat (sinus lipomatosis). Both of these entities produce extrinsic compression on the renal collecting system and may be indistinguishable by urography. However, CT and US can easily distinguish between these processes. The low-density fat is clearly different from the water density cysts on CT examination. Fat is highly echogenic on US where it can be easily differentiated from the echo-free parapelvic cysts.

Perinephric Cysts

A perinephric cyst is renal in origin but not a true cyst. It represents a collection of fluid, presumably extrava-

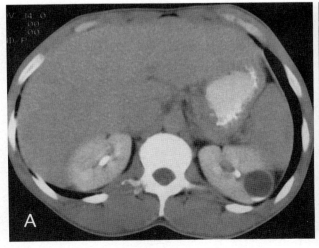
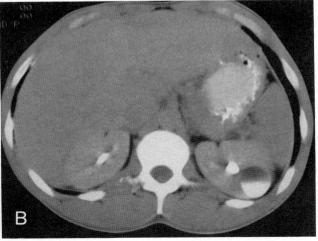

Figure 5.23.   Communicating cyst. A small amount of contrast material is seen in the left renal cyst. The thick wall suggests it is most likely a calyceal diverticulum. Later images demonstrate further contrast accumulation.

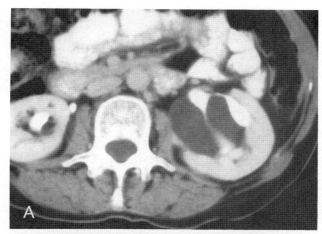

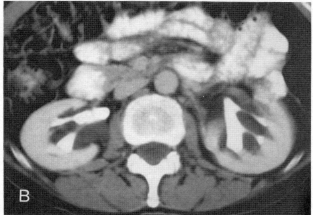

Figure 5.24. Parapelvic cyst. **A,** A large cyst in the left renal hilus is bowing the collecting system. **B,** Computed tomography demonstrates that these cysts are often multiple and bilateral.

sated urine, that is formed, often after renal trauma, but trapped beneath the renal capsule. Perinephric cysts may also be seen in infants with congenital lower urinary tract obstruction. The cyst walls are composed of fibrous tissue and do not have an epithelial lining. They are seldom of any clinical significance but, if large, could result in hypertension due to the compressive force on the renal parenchyma (Page kidney).

CYST PUNCTURE

Percutaneous aspiration of renal cysts may be performed for either diagnostic or therapeutic purposes. Therapeutic cyst aspiration is discussed in more detail in Chapter 3.

Cystic masses which do not meet the criteria for benign cysts may be aspirated to obtain material for cytologic evaluation. Fluid from a simple cyst is clear and straw colored. Occasionally, the aspiration procedure causes bleeding. However, there should be progressive clearing of the aspirate if the blood is due to the puncture.

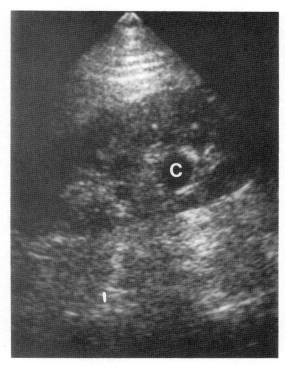

Figure 5.25. Parapelvic cyst. A cyst (C) in the region of the renal hilus is seen with ultrasound.

As CT and US provide increasingly precise information about the character of cystic renal masses, cyst aspiration is used less frequently for diagnosis. Furthermore, when a renal adenocarcinoma occurs in the wall of a cyst, the fluid may be clear and the cytology negative.

A recent survey of the membership of the Society of Uroradiology reported that CT is considered the gold standard in evaluating cystic renal masses. Cyst aspiration is indicated for lesions that are indeterminate on CT and US, or for the diagnosis of lesions suspected of being malignant in patients who are poor surgical risks. Aspiration can also be diagnostic in patients with infected renal cysts, as the organism can be identified by Gram stain and culture. Percutaneous drainage of infected renal cysts and abscesses is also discussed in Chapter 22.

Complications of renal cyst puncture are usually minor and consist of microscopic or transient hematuria or extravasation of contrast material. Major complications were reported in 1.4% of cases surveyed by Lang and included perirenal hemorrhage, pneumothorax, infection, and arteriovenous fistula formation. However, this incidence decreased to 0.75% for institutions with extensive experience with cyst puncture.

SUGGESTED READINGS

Cortical Cysts
Bosniak MA: The current radiological approach to renal cysts. *Radiology* 158:1, 1986.

Coleman BG, Arger PH, Mintz MC, et al: Hyperdense renal masses: a computed tomographic dilemma. *AJR* 143:291, 1984.

Dunnick NR, Korobkin M, Clark WM: CT Demonstration of hyperdense renal carcinoma. *J Comput Assist Tomogr* 8(5):1023, 1984.

Dunnick NR, Korobkin M, Silverman PM, et al: Computed tomography of high density renal cysts. *J Comput Assist Tomogr* 8(3):458, 1984.

Elkin M, Bernstein J: Cystic diseases of the kidney: radiological and pathological considerations. *Clin Radiol* 29:65, 1969.

Friedland GW: Shrinking and disappearing renal cysts. *Urol Radiol* 9:21, 1987.

Gleason DC, McAlister WH, Kissane J: Cystic disease of the kidneys in children. *AJR* 100:135, 1967.

Grossman H, Winchester PH, Chisari FV: Roentgenographic classification of renal cystic disease. *AJR* 104:319, 1968.

Hartman DS: Cysts and cystic neoplasms. *Urol Radiol* 12:7, 1990.

Levine E, Grantham JJ: High-Density renal cysts in autosomal dominant polycystic kidney disease demonstrated by CT. *Radiology* 154:477, 1985.

Osathanondh V, Potter EL: Pathogenesis of polycystic kidneys. *Arch Pathol* 77:459, 1964.

Papanicolaou N, Pfister RC, Yoder IC: Spontaneous and traumatic rupture of renal cysts: diagnosis and outcome. *Radiology* 160:99, 1986.

Reynolds WF, Goldstein AMB, Williams EJ, et al: Uncommon radiologic observations in renal milk-of-calcium stone. *Urology* 11(4):419, 1978.

Rosenberg ER, Korobkin M, Foster W, et al: The significance of septations in a renal cyst. *AJR* 144:593, 1985.

Sussman S, Cochran ST, Pagani JJ, et al: Hyperdense renal masses: a CT manifestation of hemorrhagic renal cysts. *Radiology* 150:207, 1984.

Extraparenchymal Cysts

Amis ES Jr, Cronan JJ: The renal sinus: an imaging review and proposed nomenclature for sinus cysts. *J Urol* 139:1151, 1988.

Cronan JJ, Yoder IC, Amis ES Jr, et al: The myth of anechoic renal sinus fat. *Radiology* 144:149, 1982.

Elkin M, Bernstein J: Cystic diseases of the kidney: radiological and pathological considerations. *Clin Radiol* 29:65, 1969.

Hidalgo H, Dunnick NR, Rosenberg ER, et al: Parapelvic cysts: appearance on CT and sonography. *AJR* 138:667, 1982.

Polycystic Renal Disease

Bosniak MA, Ambos MA: Polycystic kidney disease. *Semin Roentgenol* 10:133, 1975.

Grossman H, Rosenberg ER, Bowie JD, et al: Sonographic diagnosis of renal cystic disease. *AJR* 140:81, 1983.

Hayden CK Jr, Swischuk LE, Smith TH, et al: Renal cystic disease in childhood. *Radiographics* 6:97, 1986.

Kirks DR: *Practical Pediatric Imaging: Diagnostic Radiology of Infants and Children.* Boston, Little, Brown, 1984.

Lee JKT, McClennan BL, Kissane JM: Unilateral polycystic kidney disease, *AJR* 130:1165, 1978.

Levine E, Cook LT, Grantham JJ: Liver cysts in autosomal-dominant polycystic kidney disease: clinical and computed tomographic study. *AJR* 145:229, 1985.

Levine E, Grantham JJ: Perinephric hemorrhage in autosomal dominant polycystic kidney disease: CT and MR findings. *J Comput Assist Tomogr* 11(1):108, 1987.

McCallum RW, Gildiner M: Diminished visualization of renal outlines in adult renal polycystic disease. *J Can Assoc Radiol* 32:13, 1981.

Segal AJ, Spataro RF: Computed tomography of adult polycystic disease. *J Comput Assist Tomogr* 6(4):777, 1982.

Walker FC Jr, Loney LC, Root ER, et al: Diagnostic evaluation of adult polycystic kidney disease in childhood. *AJR* 142:1273, 1984.

Cysts Associated with Systemic Disease

Chonko AM, Weiss SM, Stein JH, et al: Renal involvement in tuberous sclerosis. *Am J Med* 56:124, 1974.

Kadir S, Kerr WS Jr, Athanasoulis CA: The role of arteriography in the management of renal cell carcinoma associated with von Hippel-Lindau disease. *J Urol* 126:316, 1981.

Levine E, Collins DL, Horton WA, et al: CT screening of the abdomen in von Hippel-Lindau disease. *AJR* 139:505, 1982.

Loughlin ER, Gittes RF: Urologic management of patients with von Hippel-Lindau's disease. *J Urol* 136:789, 1986.

Mitnick JS, Bosniak MA, Hilton S, et al: Cystic renal disease in tuberous sclerosis. *Radiology* 147:85, 1983.

Acquired Cystic Disease of Uremia

Cho C, Friedland GW, Swenson RS: Acquired renal cystic disease and renal neoplasms in hemodialysis patients. *Urol Radiol* 6:153, 1984.

Grantham JJ, Levine E, Acquired cystic disease: replacing one kidney disease with another. *Kidney Int* 28:99, 1985.

Levine E, Grantham JJ, Slusher SL, et al: CT of acquired cystic kidney disease and renal tumors in long-term dialysis patients. *AJR* 142:125, 1984.

Mindell HJ: Imaging studies for screening native kidneys in long-term dialysis patients. *AJR* 153:768, 1989.

Taylor AJ, Cohen EP, Erickson SJ, et al: Renal imaging in long-term dialysis patients: a comparison of CT and sonography. *AJR* 153:765, 1989.

Medullary Cystic Disease

Garel LA, Habib R, Pariente D, et al: Juvenile nephronophthisis: sonographic appearance in children with severe uremia. *Radiology* 151:93, 1984.

Rego JD Jr, Laing FC, Jeffrey RB: Ultrasonographic diagnosis of medullary cystic disease. *J Ultrasound Med* 2:433, 1983.

Steele B, Lirenman DS, Beattle CW: Nephronophthisis. *Am J Med* 68:521, 1980.

Multicystic Dysplastic Kidney

Kleiner B, Filly RA, Mack L, et al: Multicystic dysplastic kidney: observations of contralateral disease in the fetal population. *Radiology* 161:27, 1986.

Pedicelli G, Jequier S, Bowen A, Boisvert J: Multicystic dysplastic kidneys: spontaneous regression demonstrated with US. *Radiology* 160:23, 1986.

Sanders R, Hartman D: The sonographic distinction between neonatal multicystic kidney and hydronephrosis. *Radiology* 151:621, 1984.

Vinocur L, Slovis TL, Perlmutter AD, et al: Follow-up studies of multicystic dysplastic kidneys. *Radiology* 167:311, 1988.

Multilocular Cystic Nephroma

Banner MP, Pollack HM, Chatten J, et al: Multilocular renal cysts: radiologic-pathologic correlation. *AJR* 136:239, 1981.

de Wall JG, Schroder FH, Scholtmeijer RJ: Diagnostic workup and treatment of multilocular cystic kidney. *Urology* 28(1):73, 1986.

Madewell JE, Goldman SM, Davis CJ, et al: Multilocular cystic nephroma: a radiographic-pathologic correlation of 58 patients. *Radiology* 146:309, 1983.

Parienty RA, Pradel J, Imbert MC, et al: Computed tomography of multilocular cystic nephroma. *Radiology* 140:135, 1981.

Hydatid Disease

Beggs I: The radiology of hydatid disease. *AJR* 145:639, 1985.

Lewall DB, McCorkell SJ: Rupture of echinococcal cysts: diagnosis, classification and clinical implications. *AJR* 146:391, 1986.

Cyst Aspiration

Amis ES Jr, Cronan JJ, Pfister RC: Needle puncture of cystic renal masses: a survey of the Society of Uroradiology. *AJR* 148:297, 1987.

Lang EK: Renal cyst puncture and aspiration: a survey of complications. *Am J Roentgenol* 128:723, 1977.

Sandler CM, Houston GK, Hall JT, et al: Guided cyst puncture and aspiration. *Radiol Clin North Am* 24(4):527, 1986.

RENAL TUMORS

Since any cell type found in the kidney or renal capsule has the potential to become neoplastic, there are many renal tumors which may be seen. Unfortunately, few of these tumors have a radiographic appearance sufficiently characteristic to make a confident diagnosis. Thus, the majority of solid renal masses must be considered malignant until proven otherwise.

RENAL PARENCHYMAL TUMORS

Adenocarcinoma

Renal adenocarcinoma is a malignant neoplasm that arises from proximal convoluted tubular epithelial cells. The many synonyms that have been applied to this tumor, such as hypernephroma, Grawitz tumor, clear cell carci-noma, and malignant nephroma are either misleading or inadequate and are best ignored.

Renal carcinoma is twice as common among men than women. The tumor may occur at any age, but the inci-dence peaks in the sixth decade. No etiologic agents are recognized, but there is an increased incidence with the use of tobacco. Patients with von Hippel-Lindau disease often develop renal carcinomas which are smaller but frequently multiple and bilateral. There is also a familial renal cell carcinoma unrelated to von Hippel-Lindau dis-ease.

There is an increased incidence of renal adenocarci-noma among patients on chronic dialysis, either hemo-dialysis or peritoneal dialysis. These tumors begin to ap-pear as early as 3 years after initiation of dialysis but are very difficult to detect as the kidneys are not functioning and usually contain multiple cysts.

The classic clinical presentation with a flank mass, pain, and hematuria occurs in only a minority of patients. Often patients first complain of nonspecific symptoms such as weight loss, fatigue, or even gastrointestinal or neurologic symptoms. Less common presenting com-plaints include weight loss, fever, or a new varicocele. Fatigue may be due to a normochromic normocytic ane-mia. A variety of other hormones may be secreted by renal adenocarcinomas in sufficient quantity to cause dis-tinct clinical manifestations (Table 6.1). These hormones include renin, erythropoietin, parathormone, adrenocor-ticotropic hormone (ACTH), prolactin, and gonadotro-pin. Thus, renal adenocarcinoma has sometimes been called the "internist's tumor."

Hematuria is the most common sign, occurring in over 50% of patients. It is usually gross but is occasionally only microscopic. Flank pain, present in over one-third of patients, is probably due to distension of the renal cap-sule. A flank mass is palpable at presentation in approxi-mately one-third of patients. As abdominal computed to-mography (CT) and ultrasound examinations are being

Table 6.1.
Endocrine Manifestations of Renal Adenocarcinoma

Hormone	Manifestation
Renin	Hypertension
Erythropoietin	Erythrocytosis
Parathormone	Hypercalcemia
Prolactin	Galactorrhea
Gonadotropin	Gynecomastia
ACTH	Cushing's syndrome

performed more commonly, there has been an increase in the discovery of small, asymptomatic renal carcinomas.

It is difficult to predict the natural history of renal adenocarcinoma. Some tumors demonstrate aggressive behavior by growing rapidly and metastasizing early. On the other hand, occasional patients may live for years with an untreated primary tumor. Metastases have been reported as late as 31 years after nephrectomy and spontaneous regression of either metastases or a primary tumor may occur.

Radiology

The radiologic investigation of patients suspected of having a renal carcinoma usually begins with excretory urography. However, urography is not as sensitive as CT in the detection of renal masses. Urography detects only half the renal masses between 2 and 3 cm in diameter that are seen by CT. In a retrospective review of 65 consecutive patients with renal tumors, Demos et al. found

that excretory urography missed four (6%) tumors. Curry et al. found only three (33%) of nine small renal neoplasms (less than 3 cm) using screening urography. Thus, CT is needed in patients with a strong clinical suspicion of a renal tumor even if the IVP is unrevealing.

Calcification can be detected on the preliminary radiograph in as many as 20% of renal adenocarcinomas (Fig. 6.1). However, calcification may also be seen in other renal masses including common lesions such as benign cysts.

The character of the calcification is helpful in determining the etiology of a renal mass. Peripheral curvilinear calcification is more commonly seen in a cyst while central calcification means the lesion is more likely a renal carcinoma. However, the importance of calcification has decreased since ultrasound (US) and CT can be used to more clearly define the nature of a renal mass (Fig. 6.1). Either of these cross sectional imaging modalities can directly detect the presence of a soft tissue mass or tumor nodule within a cystic mass without relying on the presence of a central calcification. Furthermore, calcification of a central septation within a cyst may give the misleading impression of a solid mass on urography.

In all but very large tumors, renal function is preserved. The carcinoma is identified as a vascular mass with mottled density which causes a focal bulge in the renal contour. Involvement of the collecting system is seen as irregularity of the urothelial surface or complete occlusion of a calyx or infundibulum. A filling defect within the collecting system may represent blood clot or tumor invasion.

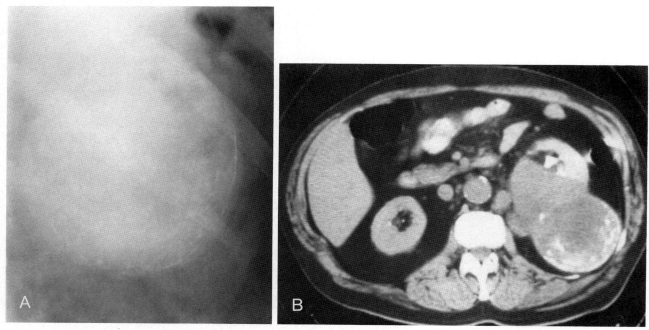

Figure 6.1. Renal carcinoma. **A,** Calcification is appreciated in a left renal mass on the preliminary radiograph. **B,** Computed tomography confirms a large calcified renal tumor.

Hypovascular or cystic renal carcinomas may be difficult to distinguish from benign cysts on IVP. Benign cortical cysts are sharply defined and have an imperceptibly thin wall (Chapter 5). If the wall of a cystic mass can be detected by either IVP or CT, the lesion is not a simple cyst and further evaluation is warranted.

Even with routine nephrotomography, it is often impossible to define a renal mass well enough by IVP to make a benign diagnosis. Further study with either US or CT is needed. Those lesions that are most likely benign cysts are most efficiently confirmed sonographically. On the other hand, if the lesion is complex or solid, CT will probably be needed and it may be more expeditious to omit US and proceed directly to CT.

Ultrasound is particularly helpful in distinguishing solid from cystic renal masses. A renal adenocarcinoma is usually seen as a solid mass, although cystic regions representing areas of hemorrhage or necrosis are common.

The echogenicity of renal carcinomas is variable. They may be more echogenic, less echogenic (Fig. 6.2), or isoechoic with the normal renal parenchyma. Highly echogenic tumors may mimic the increased echogenicity of fat-containing tumors such as an angiomyolipoma. Isoechoic tumors may be difficult to detect with US, especially if they are small and do not displace the collecting system or produce a contour deformity. Less echogenic tumors simulate more homogeneous tumors such as lymphoma or may be confused with a renal cyst. However, these solid tumors have poorly defined margins and do not have the increased sound transmission seen with cysts. A few renal adenocarcinomas are frankly cystic. However, even these tumors can usually be distinguished from simple cysts by their irregularly thick walls and the presence of some internal echoes.

Computed tomography is the single most valuable modality in assessing a renal mass. It is the most sensitive radiographic examination for the detection of renal masses. Computed tomography can also diagnose simple cysts with a high degree of accuracy. Other mass lesions that are indeterminate or clearly solid must be considered renal adenocarcinoma until proven otherwise.

Renal adenocarcinomas are readily detected by CT. The density is variable and depends on the presence of tissue necrosis, hemorrhage, or calcification. Although a contour bulge may often be appreciated, smaller masses may easily be missed on precontrast images (Fig. 6.3).

After intravenous contrast injection, renal carcinomas usually demonstrate an inhomogeneous enhancement. Portions of the tumor become as dense as the normal renal cortex while other areas show little enhancement (Fig. 6.4). Cystic carcinomas are recognized by their thick irregular wall or the presence of a tumor nodule.

The use of angiography as a method of diagnosing renal carcinoma has decreased as CT has assumed this role. However, arteriography may be employed to identify small vascular tumors when CT is equivocal. Arteriog-

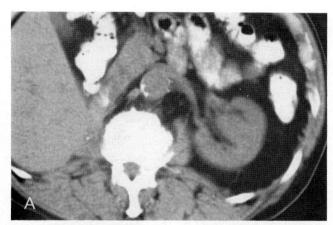

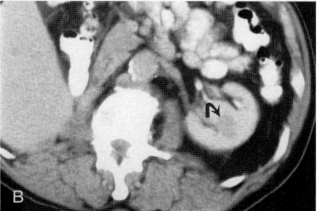

Figure 6.3.   Renal carcinoma. **A,** The precontrast image is unremarkable. **B,** After contrast injection, a small low-density mass (*arrow*) is seen.

Figure 6.2.   Renal carcinoma. Ultrasound reveals a mass (M) in the upper pole that is slightly less echogenic than the normal renal parenchyma.

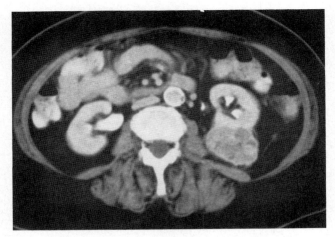

Figure 6.4. Renal carcinoma. Computed tomography reveals inhomogeneous enhancement of the tumor.

raphy is often needed when the renal parenchyma is abnormal or distorted, as when examining patients with von Hippel-Lindau disease. The definition of the tumor vascularity and identification of the number and location of the renal arteries may contribute to a safer surgical resection.

Most renal adenocarcinomas are vascular tumors and display tumor neovascularity. The most specific vascular appearance is encasement, where a vessel decreases in caliber as it is entrapped by tumor but then increases in caliber farther along its course (Fig. 6.5). This phenomenon is rarely seen in inflammatory masses. Arteriovenous shunting is common and there may be a dense tumor stain, vascular puddling, or the formation of venous lakes.

These changes may be less obvious in the minority of renal carcinomas which are hypovascular. Such tumors often have large areas of hemorrhage or tumor necrosis but still demonstrate some abnormal vessels.

Small tumors whose vascularity is similar to that of the normal renal parenchyma may also be difficult to detect with arteriography. In this setting, epinephrine injected prior to the arteriogram may demonstrate a tumor not seen on the routine films. Five to 10 μg of epinephrine is injected through the catheter into the renal artery. This constricts the normal renal arteries and diminishes blood flow to the normal renal parenchyma. However, tumor vessels do not have a muscular wall and are unable to constrict. Thus, more blood (and contrast material) go to the tumor, making it easier to identify (Fig. 6.6).

Arteriography is seldom needed to stage renal carcinoma but may be employed as a diagnostic tool or as part of a therapeutic technique with vascular occlusion. It may occasionally be used to evaluate the liver, especially to distinguish a hemangioma from a metastasis. A hepatic dysfunction syndrome associated with renal adenocarcinoma has been reported. It consists of nonspecific constitutional symptoms, hepatomegaly, and abnormal liver function tests. The liver is hypervascular with accentua-

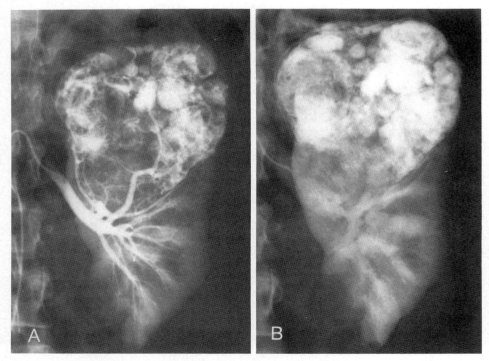

Figure 6.5. Renal carcinoma. **A** and **B,** The arteriographic findings of neovascularity, encasement, and venous laking indicate renal carcinoma.

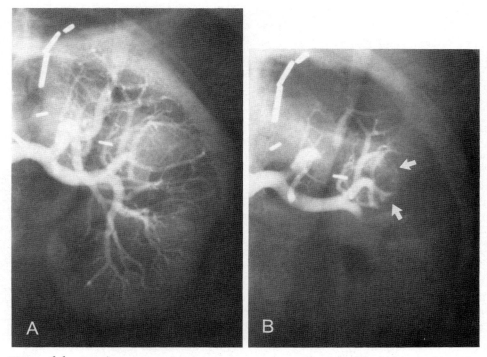

Figure 6.6. Renal carcinoma. Previous surgery makes evaluation of the kidney in this patient with von Hippel-Lindau disease difficult. **A,** A renal arteriogram is suggestive of a solid renal mass. **B,** After epinephrine, the normal renal arteries constrict, making the tumor vessels more conspicuous (*arrows*).

tion of the normal fine granular pattern. The hepatomegaly and abnormal liver function tests return to normal after nephrectomy.

Magnetic resonance imaging (MRI) has not yet been shown to be helpful in identifying renal carcinoma. Renal masses are more difficult to detect on MRI than CT, due to the poorer spatial resolution of MRI. Furthermore, the signal intensity of renal carcinoma is similar to that of the normal renal parenchyma. Small renal tumors are often isointense with normal renal parenchyma on both T_1- and T_2-weighted spin echo images. Thus, renal carcinomas must be diagnosed on the basis of contour deformity, disruption of the corticomedullary junction, or the heterogeneous signal intensities seen in large tumors that contain areas of tumor necrosis.

Contrast-enhanced studies with gadolinium (Gd-DTPA) are more promising for the detection of renal mass lesions. MRI has been shown to be useful, however, in staging renal carcinoma, particularly in detecting and defining the limits of tumor extension into the renal vein and inferior vena cava.

Staging

The two most commonly used staging systems are the classic system described by Robson et al. in 1969 and the TNM system described by the American Joint Committee for Cancer Staging. The Robson classification (Table 6.2)

is simpler, has been in use longer, and provides both anatomic and prognostic information.

In the Robson system, Stage I disease is confined to the kidney. Tumor does not extend beyond the renal capsule. The 5- and 10-year survivals for these patients are 67% and 56%, respectively.

Tumor that has grown through the renal capsule into the perinephric space is considered Stage II. The ipsilateral adrenal gland may be involved. Since the entire contents of Gerota's fascia are removed during formal nephrectomy, the distinction between Stage I and Stage II disease does not usually affect surgical treatment. The 5- and 10-year prognoses are 51% and 28%, respectively.

Table 6.2
Renal Carcinoma Staging

Stage I	Confined within renal capsule
Stage II	Penetrates beyond renal capsule but remains within Gerota's fascia
Stage IIIA	Extends into renal vein and may progress into IVC
Stage IIIB	Involves regional lymph nodes
Stage IIIC	Includes both venous extension and lymph node involvement
Stage IVA	Tumor growth through Gerota's fascia into adjacent tissues
Stage IVB	Distant metastases

Stage III is subdivided into A, B, and C categories. Tumor that involves the main renal vein is classified as Stage IIIA. The tumor may grow into the inferior vena cava (IVC) and up to the right atrium. The precise delineation of the tumor thrombus is critical to planning the surgical approach.

Involvement of regional lymph nodes indicates Stage IIIB, while Stage IIIC is used when tumor involves both the main renal vein and regional lymph nodes. The 5- and 10-year prognoses for Stage III disease are 34 and 20%, respectively.

Stage IV disease indicates disseminated tumor. Direct extension through Gerota's fascia into the adjacent organs is classified as Stage IVA. Hematogenous or lymphatic metastases to distant sites results in a Stage IVB classification. The 5- and 10-year prognoses for Stage IV disease are 14 and 3%, respectively. Interestingly, patients with solitary metastases do better than those with multiple metastatic deposits.

This presurgical staging can usually be accomplished with CT (Fig. 6.7). However, venography may be needed to better define the presence and limit of venous extension. In some centers intravenous digital angiography has also been used to identify the vascularity of the tumor and the number and location of the renal arteries.

The overall accuracy of CT in staging renal carcinoma is greater than 90%. However, some distinctions are more crucial than others. In most patients, for instance, a radical nephrectomy is performed, and it is inconsequential whether or not there is penetration of the renal capsule by tumor. Since it is difficult to make this distinction by CT, the elimination of this category raises the accuracy of CT staging to over 95%.

On the other hand, precise delineation of the venous extension is essential to plan the surgical approach and gain vascular control of the kidney (Fig. 6.8). If the CT

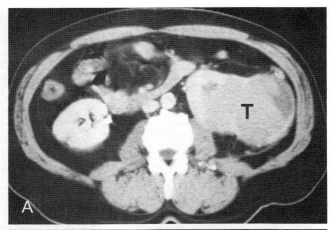

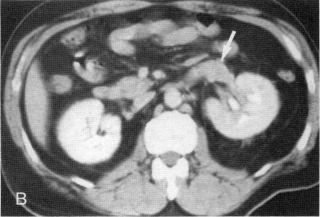

Figure 6.8. Renal carcinoma. **A,** A large tumor (T) lies in the left kidney. **B,** Enlargement and diminished enhancement of the left renal vein (*arrow*) indicate tumor extension.

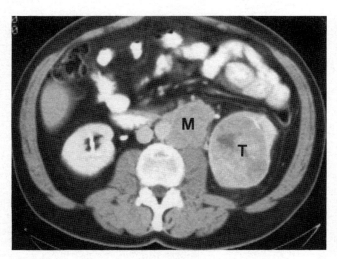

Figure 6.7. Renal carcinoma. A large tumor (T) is seen in the lower pole of the left kidney. Regional lymph node metastases (M) indicates Stage IIIB.

examination is equivocal, venography or MRI may be required.

Inferior vena cavography obtained after injection of contrast material in the iliac vein will detect tumor extension into the IVC. Selective catheterization of the renal vein is usually needed to identify tumor that has grown into the vein but not reached the cava. In some patients a large tumor thrombus completely occludes the IVC (Fig. 6.9). If surgery is contemplated, a cavogram performed "from above" via access through a vein in the right antecubital fossa and the superior vena cava may be needed to define the cephalad extent of the tumor (Fig. 6.9).

Although MRI has not been useful in diagnosing renal adenocarcinoma, it has shown utility in staging. Since flowing blood does not impart signal, a patent vein can easily be distinguished from the higher signal intensity of tumor extending into the vein. Furthermore, limited flip angle techniques such as the GRASS technique rapidly assess the status of the major veins (Fig. 6.10).

MRI may also prove accurate in assessing the small opacities seen in the perinephric space in many of these patients on CT examination. Some of these represent

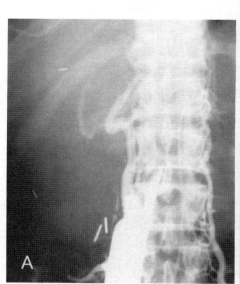
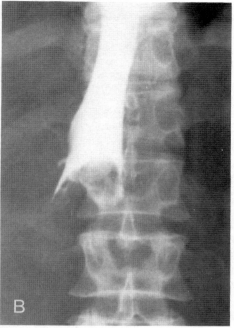

Figure 6.9.   Renal carcinoma. **A,** An inferior vena cavagram demonstrates complete occlusion. **B,** A cavagram "from above" delineates the cephalad extent of the tumor.

inflammatory changes while others may be due to involved lymph nodes or collateral vessels. MRI can clearly identify patent vessels and distinguish them from lymphadenopathy (Fig. 6.11).

Papillary Adenocarcinoma

Renal adenocarcinomas may be subdivided into papillary and nonpapillary types based on the pattern of cellu-

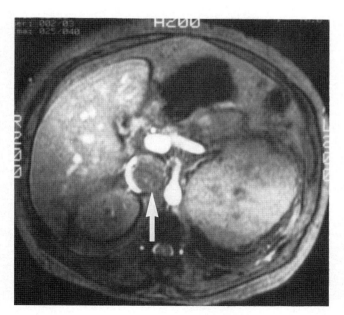

Figure 6.10.   Renal carcinoma. Limited flip angle techniques, such as GRASS, are useful in identifying tumor extension into the inferior vena cava (*arrow*).

lar architecture. Papillary carcinomas comprise only 5–15% of all renal adenocarcinomas but are characterized by a lower stage at presentation, slower growth, and a better prognosis than nonpapillary carcinomas.

Papillary tumors are less vascular than nonpapillary types as seen by either CT (Fig. 6.12) or angiography. They show less vascular enhancement and often do not have the frankly malignant hypervascular pattern seen with nonpapillary tumors. Calcification is also seen more commonly in papillary tumors, presumably reflecting slower growth.

Sarcomatoid Carcinomas

Sarcomatoid renal cell carcinomas contain elements of renal adenocarcinoma, transitional cell carcinoma, and sarcoma. They occur more frequently in elderly patients but are radiographically indistinguishable from renal adenocarcinoma.

Treatment

Surgical resection is the primary mode of therapy for patients with renal adenocarcinoma. Most patients undergo radical nephrectomy, which is why the distinction between Stage I and Stage II is seldom of value other than for assessing prognosis. In this operation the entire contents of the perirenal space are removed without opening Gerota's fascia. The regional lymph nodes, paraaortic for left-sided tumors and paracaval for tumors of the right kidney, are also resected. Tumor extending into the renal vein and IVC can often be removed, as this tumor is

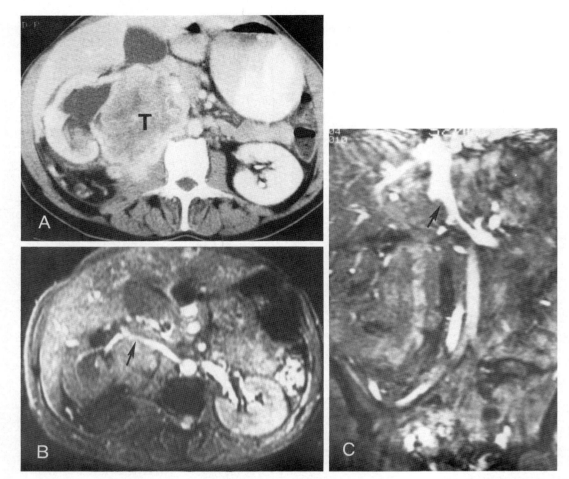

Figure 6.11.   Renal carcinoma. **A,** A large right renal tumor (T) is obstructing the upper pole collecting system and obscuring the inferior vena cava on CT. **B,** On MRI a GRASS image demonstrates encasement of the right renal artery (*arrow*) by the tumor. **C,** On a coronal image, tumor (*arrow*) extends into the inferior vena cava.

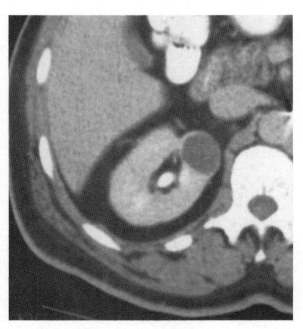

Figure 6.12.   Renal carcinoma. The homogeneous low density is typical of papillary adenocarcinoma.

usually well encapsulated and not attached to the vessel wall.

Patients with Stage IV disease may also be treated with surgical resection. This may be done as palliation or to prevent complications such as hematuria, pain, or even congestive heart failure due to large arteriovenous fistulae. Occasionally cases of regression of metastatic disease following removal of the primary tumor are reported.

Angiography may also play a valuable role in the therapy of renal adenocarcinoma. Presurgical embolization of the tumor may dramatically reduce the vascularity of the tumor making resection easier by diminishing blood loss. Work at the M.D. Anderson Hospital suggested that a delay in surgical resection after embolization would improve survival due to an enhanced immunologic response to the tumor antigen. However, these results have not been supported by long-term studies and embolization is usually performed within 24 hours of surgical resection.

Arterial embolization can also be used to treat complications in patients who are not surgical candidates. Hematuria can often be stopped with particulate embolization of materials such as Gelfoam and steel coils.

Absolute ethanol may also be used to occlude the renal artery. However, this should be done with an occlusion balloon to prevent reflux and unwanted damage to other vessels.

Adenoma

These benign tumors are often confused with and may be difficult to distinguish from renal adenocarcinoma. Both tumors arise from the proximal convoluted tubule and cannot be distinguished by histologic or histochemical means. They occur in the same age groups, and both show a marked male predominance. Many authors feel that an adenoma is a small renal carcinoma that has not yet metastasized.

Since most of these small renal adenomas are detected at autopsy, they have little clinical significance. However, when they are detected at surgery the nomenclature used to describe these cortical glandular tumors implies prognostic significance. It may be best to describe these tumors as renal adenocarcinomas, but with a low likelihood of metastasis. Search for evidence of metastases and arranging appropriate follow-up may be beneficial.

Oncocytoma

An *oncocyte* is a large transformed epithelial cell which has a finely granular eosinophilic cytoplasm. Oncocytes increase in number with age and are found in a variety of organs including salivary glands, thyroid, pancreas, and kidney. A *renal oncocytoma* is an uncommon tumor arising from the proximal tubule. The existence of these tumors as distinct from renal adenocarcinoma has been recognized relatively recently.

Oncocytomas have a male predilection and a mean age of presentation in the seventh decade. They comprise 4–7% of renal tumors. Oncocytomas are most often detected as an incidental finding and average over 7 cm in diameter. Occasional patients may complain of a flank mass, pain, or hematuria.

The gross appearance of an oncocytoma is a well-defined tan to brown tumor which often contains a prominent central stellate scar.

Although there are occasional reported cases of involvement of regional lymph nodes and tumor extension into the vein, the vast majority of oncocytomas are well differentiated and benign. In the series reported by Lieber et al., the actuarial survival curve for the 90 patients with an oncocytoma was not significantly different from an age- and sex-matched cohort.

Oncocytomas can be detected as a solid renal mass by excretory urography. They are moderately vascular tumors and cannot be distinguished from a renal adenocarcinoma.

On CT an oncocytoma is often well defined with a relatively sharp interface with the normal renal parenchyma (Fig. 6.13). The central stellate scar is best seen with CT but is not pathognomonic for an oncocytoma as it can be seen in renal adenocarcinoma.

Angiography demonstrates a vascular renal tumor with a dense tumor blush (Fig. 6.14). A "spoke wheel" pattern of vessels penetrating into the center of the tumor is common. Although this vascular configuration is often described in an oncocytoma, it is not pathognomonic as it can also be seen in renal adenocarcinoma.

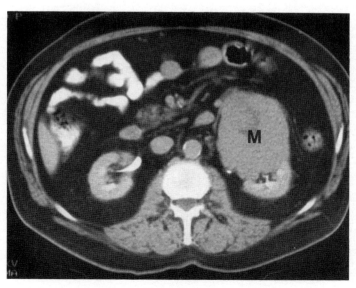

Figure 6.13.   Oncocytoma. A large left renal mass (M) is present, but has a well-defined interface with the normal renal parenchyma.

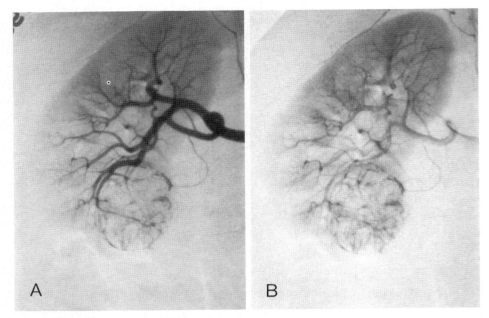

Figure 6.14.   Oncocytoma. **A** and **B,** Arteriography demonstrates circumferential vessels with penetrating central vessels, giving a "spoke wheel" configuration.

Since an oncocytoma cannot be reliably diagnosed radiographically, treatment is surgical. If typical radiographic features of an oncocytoma, such as a central stellate scar and a spoke wheel vascular pattern are present, an oncocytoma may be suggested. However, neither appearance is pathognomonic and surgery is required. Alerting the surgeon to the possible diagnosis of oncocytoma may encourage inspection and biopsy or local excision. Thus, more normal renal parenchyma may be preserved than if the more radical formal nephrectomy is performed.

Wilms' Tumor

Wilms' tumor (nephroblastoma) arises from metanephric blastema. It is a tumor of young children, with 50% of cases diagnosed in the first 2 years of life and 75% before the age of 5 years. There is no sex predilection, but there is a high association with several malformation syndromes.

Approximately one-third of children with sporadic aniridia develop Wilms' tumor. Patients with aniridia and Wilms' tumor present at an earlier age and more frequently have bilateral tumors than patients with Wilms' tumor in general. An anomaly localized to the short arm of chromosome 11 has been found in 33% of patients with aniridia and Wilms' tumor.

Patients with hemihypertrophy have an increased incidence of nephroblastomas, adrenal cortical neoplasms, and hepatoblastomas. The side of hypertrophy and the tumor are unrelated.

In 1970, Drash reported the association of male pseu-

dohermaphroditism, glomerulonephritis, and Wilms' tumor. The components of this syndrome may not occur at the same time. Thus, the development of any two should alert physicians to the possibility of the third component arising.

The Beckwith-Wiedemann syndrome is also related to Wilms' tumor. This syndrome, comprised of macroglossia, omphalocele, adrenal cytomegaly, and visceromegaly, often includes a proliferation of nephrogenic blastema (from which Wilms' tumors arise). Other anomalies including microcephaly, malformed ears, a variety of genitourinary anomalies such as horseshoe kidneys, and developmental retardation are also associated with Wilms' tumor.

Wilms' tumor is usually a mixed tumor containing epithelial, blastemal, and stromal elements. The nonepithelial elements may differentiate into striated muscle, adipose, cartilage, or bone. This may explain the rare case in which the detection of fat may cause confusion with an angiomyolipoma. There is usually a pseudocapsule that separates the tumor from the rest of the kidney.

Radiology

Most children with Wilms' tumor present with a palpable abdominal mass. Abdominal pain, anorexia, fever, and hypertension are also commonly present. Gross hematuria occurs in less than 10% of cases.

Wilms' tumors are usually large (averaging 12 cm) by the time they are detected. Since they arise from the cortex, much of the tumor growth may be exophytic. Thus, the splaying of the collecting system seen with intrarenal masses may not be present. However, the large size of these tumors makes them readily detected. The expansile tumor mass compresses the normal kidney but maintains a relatively sharp margin.

Ultrasound has become the preferred examination for these young children presenting with an abdominal mass (Fig. 6.15). The solid nature and renal origin of the tumor mass can be determined. Most tumors will be hypo- to hyperechoic solid masses, are usually well defined, and may be demarcated from the normal parenchyma by a tumor pseudocapsule or compressed renal cortex.

Hypoechoic areas within the tumor may represent regions of hemorrhage or tissue necrosis. Dystrophic calcification is uncommon, but may cause hyperechoic foci with shadowing when they occur. Ultrasound is also useful in detecting tumor extension into the renal vein or IVC and for identifying hepatic metastases.

The paucity of retroperitoneal fat in young children makes CT evaluation of Wilms' tumor more difficult than adult renal neoplasms. Furthermore, the ionizing radiation and need for intravenous contrast material makes

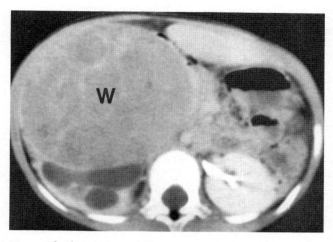

Figure 6.16. Wilms' tumor. A huge Wilms' tumor (W) is obstructing the collecting system.

this examination less desirable than ultrasound in children.

Wilms' tumor is seen as a large mass which enhances less than the normal renal parenchyma. The degree of heterogeneity depends on the presence of tissue necrosis or hemorrhage. The tumor mass is usually large, causing compression of the remainder of the kidney (Fig. 6.16).

Computed tomography is valuable, however, in contributing to the staging evaluation (Fig. 6.17) and providing precise delineation of the size of the tumor mass. It is also useful in evaluating the contralateral kidney when ipsilateral nephrectomy is contemplated.

Arteriography is seldom necessary to evaluate patients with Wilms' tumor. The tumors are moderately vascular with splaying of intrarenal branches. Neovascularity is common and areas of vascular puddling may be seen.

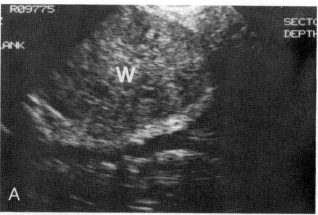

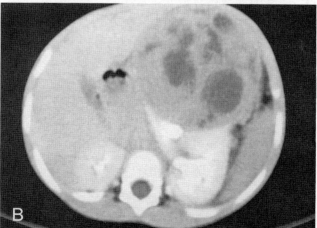

Figure 6.15. Wilms' tumor. **A,** On ultrasound a large solid tumor (W) is detected in the upper pole of the left kidney. **B,** Splaying of the renal parenchyma and distortion of the collecting system on CT confirm its renal origin.

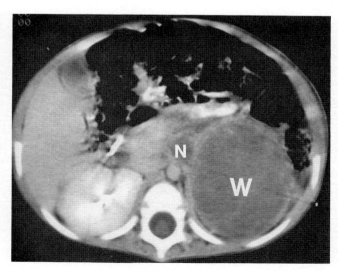

Figure 6.17. Wilms' tumor. Involvement of regional lymph nodes (N) as well as the primary tumor (W) is seen by CT.

The angiographic appearance is not specific and is not helpful in making the diagnosis, other than confirming the presence of a vascular mass.

MRI appears to be no more valuable in Wilms' tumor than in adult renal neoplasms. Although ionizing radiation is spared, the children require sedation and monitoring to undergo an MRI examination. The most promising application of MRI is in definition of the venous extent of tumor.

The most common sites for metastases are the lung and liver. Involvement of the adjacent retroperitoneum, the peritoneum, or mediastinum is not uncommon. Tumor staging is similar to renal adenocarcinoma (Table 6.3).

Nephroblastomatosis

Nephroblastomatosis is a group of pathologic entities characterized by persistent nephrogenic blastema. It results from an arrest in normal nephrogenesis with persistence of residual blastema. Although nephroblastomatosis is not malignant, it is associated with Wilms' tumor and those conditions with a high incidence of Wilms' tumor.

Nephroblastomatosis may be either diffuse, or more commonly, multinodular. The radiographic features are dependent on the size and distribution of the embryologic remnants. The lesions in the multifocal form are usually microscopic nodules and are difficult to image. In the diffuse form the kidneys are enlarged and the collecting system may be deformed by parenchymal nodules.

The lesions are often hypoechoic but may also be iso- or hyperechoic. Their subcapsular location suggests nephroblastomatosis and helps to distinguish this condition from polycystic renal disease or lymphoma. This distribution is also seen on CT. Nephroblastomatosis is clearly distinguished from normal renal tissue by the difference in contrast enhancement (Fig. 6.18).

Typical angiographic features include a normal caliber main renal artery. Peripheral nodules are hypovascular, they do not blush with contrast, and the kidney has a scalloped appearance.

Patients with nephroblastomatosis are at increased risk of developing Wilms' tumor. Many are treated with

Table 6.3
Staging Wilms' Tumor

Stage I	Limited to kidney
Stage II	Extends beyond kidney but is completely resected
Stage III	Residual nonhematogenous tumor confined to the abdomen
Stage IV	Hematogenous metastases to lung, liver, bone, or brain
Stage V	Bilateral renal involvement

antineoplastic drugs which often decreases the renal size. However, they remain at risk and should be followed to detect the subsequent development of a Wilms' tumor.

Mesoblastic Nephroma

This benign tumor is usually present at birth and has been described as a congenital Wilms' tumor or fetal mesenchymal hamartoma. It is comprised of interlacing sheets of fibromatous cells. Small bundles of these fibromatous cells are characteristically found diffusely interspersed in the adjacent renal parenchyma.

The tumor is large, averaging over 6 cm in diameter, and often replaces almost the entire renal parenchyma. The cut surface has a whorled appearance resembling leiomyoma of the uterus. It is not encapsulated, and finger-like extensions of the tumor penetrate the adjacent kidney. Although the tumor may penetrate the capsule and involve the perinephric space, it rarely extends into the renal vein or renal pelvis. Cases with a low grade of malignancy have been reported and it may be confused with Wilms' tumor.

The typical presentation is with a nontender abdominal mass. It is detected at birth or the first few months of life, and there is no sexual predilection.

If urography is performed, a large mass replacing most of the ipsilateral kidney will be seen. Calcification is uncommon.

Ultrasound is the most commonly used modality in the evaluation of these patients. The most common pattern, homogeneously echoic, reflects the smooth mass of fibromatous cells. Occasionally hyperechoic foci are seen. Although uncommon, areas of necrosis or hemorrhage are readily detected as hypoechoic regions.

A fairly uniform, solid, intrarenal mass has been reported on CT. Angiography may occasionally be needed for preoperative evaluation. Most mesoblastic nephromas are moderately vascular and demonstrate tumor vascularity.

Treatment is surgical excision and cure is usually achieved with nephrectomy. In some patients extensive tumor necrosis, extrarenal infiltration, and mesenchymal immaturity suggest more aggressive behavior. In these patients, who usually present beyond 3 months of age, adjunctive chemotherapy or radiation therapy may be given.

MESENCHYMAL TUMORS

Angiomyolipoma

These hamartomatous tumors are composed of mature adipose tissue, thick-walled blood vessels and sheets of smooth muscle. The amount of each component varies in each tumor. Some pathologists prefer to use the name reflecting the predominant tissue to describe the tumor.

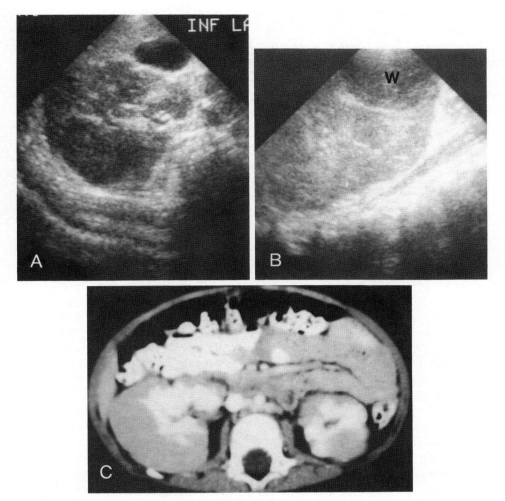

Figure 6.18. Nephroblastomatosis. **A,** A lobulated kidney with indistinct corticomedullary junction is seen on ultrasound. **B,** A Wilms' tumor (W) is seen as a hypoechoic mass in the lower pole. **C,** On CT the diffuse confluent nephroblastomatosis is clearly demarcated from the functioning renal paren-chyma. (Reprinted with permission from Fernback SK, Feinstein KA, Donaldson JS, Baum ES: Nephroblastomatosis: comparison of CT with US and Urography. *Radiology* 166:153, 1988.)

Thus, a *myoangiolipoma* is comprised primarily of smooth muscle. Other tumors may have only two of the three tissue elements and may be referred to as myolipoma, angiomyoma, etc.

Angiomyolipomas are found more often in females than in males, and the mean age at presentation is 41 years. Most patients are asymptomatic, however, intra- or perirenal hemorrhage may cause flank pain. Hematuria and hypertension are occasionally reported.

There is a strong association of angiomyolipomas and tuberous sclerosis. However, sporadic angiomyolipomas are being recognized with increasing frequency on CT and US examinations. Although 80% of patients with tuberous sclerosis have an angiomyolipoma, less than 40% of patients with an angiomyolipoma have an element of the tuberous sclerosis complex.

Tuberous sclerosis, or Bourneville's disease, is caused by an autosomal-dominant gene with variable expressiv-

ity. Only approximately 50% of patients with tuberous sclerosis have family members with one or more manifestations of the disease. The tuberous sclerosis syndrome includes epilepsy, mental retardation, and various hamartomas. In addition to renal angiomyolipomas and multiple renal cysts, patients often develop retinal phakomas and cerebral hamartomas. Adenoma sebaceum are seen in the face in the malar areas. In some patients the clinical syndrome is incompletely manifest.

Among patients with tuberous sclerosis, the angiomyolipomas are usually multiple and bilateral. In patients without tuberous sclerosis, the tumors are usually solitary. As the spatial resolution of CT and US continues to improve, tiny angiomyolipomas are being detected in asymptomatic patients as incidental findings.

Lymphangiomyomatosis is an idiopathic disease of young women consisting of smooth muscle hamartomas along the lymphatic system. It most commonly involves intrathoracic lymphatics but abdominal involvement can be extensive. It is considered by many to be a "forme fruste" of tuberous sclerosis. Renal hamartomas are found in approximately 15% of patients with lymphangiomyomatosis.

Plain abdominal radiographs may demonstrate a relatively lucent mass if there is a large fatty component to the tumor. Calcification is seldom seen, but may be due to previous hemorrhage. Urography may demonstrate a renal mass. However, the urogram is often unrevealing as the tumors frequently have an exophytic growth pattern.

The typical US finding of a highly echogenic renal mass (Fig. 6.19) depends upon the fat content of the tumor. If there is relatively little fat, the sonographic pattern will be indistinguishable from other renal masses. Even the very echogenic appearance can occasionally be mimicked by renal adenocarcinoma. If there has been hemorrhage, sonolucent areas may be seen.

The most reliable imaging modality for angiomyolipoma is CT. The detection of a renal mass of fat density virtually assures the diagnosis of angiomyolipoma (Fig. 6.20). However, the absence of demonstrable fat does not exclude the diagnosis of an angiomyolipoma. Both lipomas and liposarcomas may also be fatty density and thus indistinguishable from an angiomyolipoma by CT, but they are rare renal tumors.

Examination of a fatty renal mass by CT must be done carefully to avoid volume-averaging adjacent perinephric fat and a falsely low-density reading. In small tumors narrow collimation is essential. Small, less than 1 cm, lesions are commonly seen in the kidneys during enhanced CT examinations of the abdomen. These lesions are often cysts, but are too small for adequate analysis and are considered indeterminant. However, rescanning through these lesions with narrow collimation, such as 1.5-mm sections, may demonstrate the fatty component

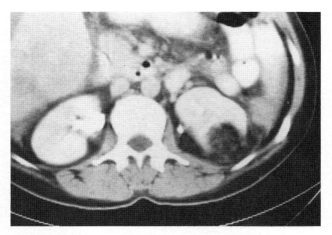

Figure 6.20.   Angiomyolipoma. An angiomyolipoma can be diagnosed by the macroscopic fat detected by CT.

and allow the diagnosis of angiomyolipoma. The presence of multiple angiomyolipomas or associated renal cysts suggests tuberous sclerosis (Fig. 6.21).

MRI can also detect fat within an angiomyolipoma. A high signal intensity is seen on both T_1- and T_2-weighted images. When clearly imaged, MRI should have the same accuracy as CT in diagnosing an angiomyolipoma. However, MRI is probably not as sensitive as CT in detecting fat in small tumors.

Arteriography can be quite helpful in diagnosing an angiomyolipoma and distinguishing it from a liposarcoma. If significant vascular components are present, tortuous almost aneurysmally dilated vessels are seen. Contrast flows slowly through these dilated vessels with continued opacification well into the venous phase. Vascular encasement found in malignant tumors is not present in angiomyolipomas. Arteriography is also valu-

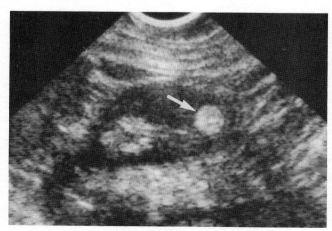

Figure 6.19.   Angiomyolipoma. The highly echogenic pattern (*arrow*) is typical of an angiomyolipoma.

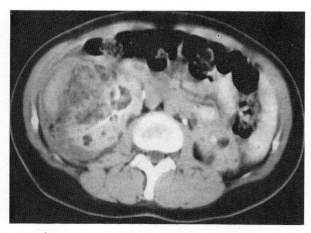

Figure 6.21.   Angiomyolipoma. Multiple fatty density renal lesions are seen in this patient with tuberous sclerosis.

able in defining the vascular supply to tumors in which local resection is planned. Growth of angiomyolipomas is usually expansile, but venous extension into the inferior vena cava has been reported.

Treatment of angiomyolipomas has traditionally been surgical. This reflects the predominance of symptomatic and large lesions detected. Since a benign diagnosis can be made with confidence, tumorectomy or partial nephrectomy is appropriate. When angiomyolipomas, especially small lesions, are detected in asymptomatic patients, no therapy is needed. Should hemorrhage occur, surgery or catheter embolization may be performed. Some investigators, however, recommend elective exploration with renal sparing surgery as there is a slightly increased incidence of renal adenocarcinoma in patients with an angiomyolipoma.

Fibrous Tumors

Fibromas are usually small tumors that occur more frequently in the medulla than the cortex. Although occasionally large enough to cause symptoms, most fibromas are detected as incidental findings at autopsy. Fibrosarcomas are rare tumors which usually arise from the renal capsule.

Osteosarcoma

This tumor is rarely a primary renal neoplasm, but may arise from a fibrosarcoma undergoing metaplasia to tumor osteocytes. It is easily diagnosed by the presence of formed bone. The main differential is a metastasis to the kidney from a primary skeletal osteosarcoma. The age of the patient helps with this distinction as patients with primary renal osteosarcoma are usually elderly while primary skeletal osteosarcomas occur in adolescents and young adults.

Lipoma

Intrarenal lipomas are rare tumors that are usually small and seldom symptomatic. All but one of the 18 cases reviewed by Dineen et al. were in middle-aged women. They should be easily detected by CT but may not be distinguishable from an angiomyolipoma.

Leiomyoma and Leiomyosarcoma

Smooth muscle tumors may arise from vessel walls or scattered muscle fibers of the renal capsule. They are the most common tumors of the renal cortex. Most leiomyomas are small and asymptomatic.

Leiomyosarcomas are usually large and locally invasive by the time they become clinically apparent. They tend to metastasize widely and the prognosis is poor. Both leiomyomas and leiomyosarcomas are more common in postmenopausal women.

Malignant Fibrous Histiocytoma

Although malignant fibrous histiocytoma (MFH) is common elsewhere in the body, it is rare as a primary renal tumor. It has been reported in patients ranging in age from 13 to 68 years. Symptoms are nonspecific, and most tumors are large by the time they are detected. Common metastatic sites include liver, lung, and bone. Local recurrence is common and the prognosis is poor.

Hemangioma

Hemangiomas are uncommon renal tumors of endothelial cells and capillary size vessels. If the vessels are dilated the tumor may be called a *cavernous hemangioma*. The tumors are usually small, ranging from several millimeters to 5 cm in diameter and are most frequently located at the apex of the renal pyramids.

The most common presenting complaint is hematuria, and some patients may experience colicky pain due to passage of blood clots. Males and females are affected equally and present most often during the third or fourth decade.

The plain radiograph and urogram are usually normal although sometimes a small defect can be appreciated in the urothelium. The lesions are usually too small to be detected by US or CT.

Selective renal angiography is the most useful modality in diagnosing these small vascular tumors. The ipsilateral renal artery is not usually enlarged. A dense tangle of vessels which may allow arteriovenous shunting is seen. Since these endothelial lined spaces lack contractile elements they do not react to vasoactive stimuli. Thus, vasoconstrictive drugs may improve the diagnostic capability by constricting normal renal arteries and shunting contrast into the hemangioma.

Treatment has traditionally been surgical for symptomatic lesions. However, transcatheter ablation should be effective therapy and may minimize loss of renal tissue.

Juxtaglomerular Tumors

Robertson first described this tumor of the juxtaglomerular (JG) apparatus in 1967. Although a rare tumor, it is a curable cause of significant hypertension. Patients with JG tumors (reninomas) are usually younger than those with essential hypertension, and there is a marked female preponderance.

The JG tumor is composed of small uniform cells with little nuclear pleomorphism or mitotic activity. The presence of renin can be confirmed with an immunofluorescence antibody test. Juxtaglomerular cells are similar to smooth muscle and it may be difficult to distinguish these tumors from hemangiopericytomas.

Juxtaglomerular tumors range from 3 to 7 cm in diameter when they are detected. The tumors are benign;

neither local invasion nor distant metastases have been reported.

Patients usually present with symptoms of hypertension that is moderate to severe. Elements of secondary aldosteronism such as hypokalemia may also be present. Rarely, acute flank pain, hypotension, or anemia may reflect hemorrhage from the tumor.

The plain abdominal radiograph is unrevealing as the tumors are not calcified. Excretory urography can demonstrate a mass in the majority of cases. The tumor is often peripheral in location and may not distort the collecting system unless it is quite large.

Sonography reveals an echogenic mass due to the abundant small vascular channels within the tumor. This is most helpful in distinguishing the tumor from a cortical cyst.

The CT findings are nonspecific since a JG tumor can not be distinguished from most other solid neoplasms. Contrast enhancement is necessary as the tumor is isodense with normal renal parenchyma.

Arteriography is often performed in patients with a JG tumor. Many patients undergo aortography to look for stenosis of the main renal artery. It is essential, however, to study both kidneys as well as the main renal arteries to detect these tumors. Despite the abundant vascular spaces, JG tumors are hypovascular (Fig. 6.22). Thus, selective renal arteriography should be performed even if aortography is normal.

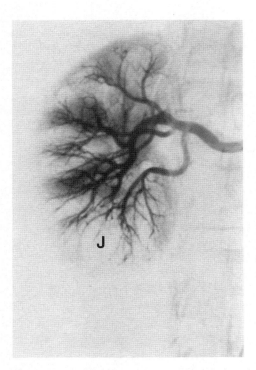

Figure 6.22.   Juxtaglomerular tumor. The hypovascular mass (J) in the lower pole of the right kidney is a JG tumor causing hypertension by excess renin secretion.

A small amount of tumor vascularity can often be appreciated, but splaying of adjacent vessels by a hypovascular mass is the most obvious finding. The nature of the tumor can be confirmed by measuring selective renal vein renin levels.

Treatment of juxtaglomerular tumors is surgical. Since the tumors are benign, local tumorectomy or partial nephrectomy are often performed to preserve as much normal renal parenchyma as possible. Arteriography is useful to define the vascularity of the tumor and the region of the arterial supply.

RENAL PELVIS TUMORS

Most of the tumors arising from the renal pelvis are malignant, with transitional cell carcinoma the most common type. Less often, squamous cell, undifferentiated, or adenocarcinomas may occur. Papillomas comprise approximately half of the benign tumors with the remainder being angiomas, fibromas, myomas, or polyps.

Transitional Cell Carcinoma

Primary tumors of the renal pelvis are relatively uncommon as they comprise less than 10% of renal tumors. The most common tumor, transitional cell carcinoma occurs twice as often in men than women and peaks in occurrence in the 7th decade.

Transitional cell carcinoma may occur anywhere along the urothelium. The incidence of carcinoma is roughly proportional to the surface area. For every 50 bladder tumors, there are three transitional cell carcinomas in the renal pelves or intrarenal collecting systems and one tumor in the ureters.

Metabolites of aminophenols may cause carcinoma of the renal pelvis, ureter, or bladder. The incidence of renal pelvic carcinoma is markedly increased in patients who consume large amounts of phenacetin, which is metabolized to aminophenol. Infection with *Schistosoma hematobium* is associated with squamous cell carcinoma of the bladder or ureter but does not usually reach the renal pelvis. An increased incidence of carcinoma of the renal pelvis is seen, however, in patients with Balkan nephropathy.

Transitional cell carcinomas may be either flat or papillary, and approximately 20% also contain metaplastic squamous changes. Papillary-type carcinomas are more common and tend to be of low-grade malignancy with a relatively benign course. Nonpapillary tumors (including squamous cell carcinoma) tend to be flat and may be more difficult to detect radiographically. These tumors are generally of a higher-grade malignancy and spread by direct extension as well as lymphatic and hematogenous metastases. Multicentric lesions are seen in approximately 30% of renal pelvic carcinomas and are even more common among transitional cell carcinomas of the bladder.

Hematuria is the most common presentation, present in about 80% of patients. Flank pain, dysuria, and abdominal mass or pyuria are infrequent. Obstruction of the collecting system may be due to the tumor mass, sloughed pieces of tumor, or blood clot.

The plain abdominal radiograph is usually unrevealing as transitional cell carcinomas are rarely calcified. It is important, however, to exclude a radiopaque renal stone which may be the etiology of a filling defect seen with urography. During excretory urography or retrograde pyelography the tumor is seen as a filling defect arising from the wall of the renal pelvis (Fig. 6.23). Transitional cell carcinomas, especially nonpapillary types, may be flat. Papillary tumors often grow in a frond-like pattern which allows contrast into the interstices of the tumor.

An intraluminal filling defect must be distinguished from the smooth extrinsic compression defect of crossing vessels. A sloughed papillae or fungus ball (mycetoma) should be detected by either radiographic evidence of papillary necrosis or the clinical findings of fungus infection. One common problem is distinguishing a renal pelvic tumor from a radiolucent stone such as a urate calculus. This can easily be accomplished with CT as even uric acid stones are much denser than soft tissue tumors.

Ultrasound is not routinely used in the evaluation of patients with renal pelvic tumors, but can distinguish them from the highly echogenic appearance of renal stones. A transitional cell carcinoma may be detected as a soft tissue mass within the lumen of the collecting system.

It may be difficult to image small renal pelvic tumors with CT, but larger lesions are well defined after intravenous contrast injection (Fig. 6.24). They are seen as soft tissue masses causing filling defects in the collecting system. The greatest contribution of CT in this setting is the identification of renal stones that are not sufficiently opaque to be seen on the plain abdominal radiograph.

Preoperative staging of transitional cell carcinoma is an important aspect of determining whether or not the tumor can be locally resected. Since the tumors tend to be multifocal, renal sparing surgery is desirable. Computed tomography is useful in detecting regional invasion and lymph node metastases if the nodes are enlarged. Metastases to normal size lymph nodes cannot be detected by CT.

Although transitional cell carcinomas can be imaged with MRI, it has little role in either the detection or staging of these neoplasms. The magnetic resonance findings of transitional cell carcinoma are similar to those of other renal tumors with an increased signal intensity on T_2-weighted images. However, small lesions may be missed, especially if there is motion artifact.

Angiography is seldom used to diagnose or evaluate renal pelvic tumors. Transitional cell carcinomas are usually hypovascular, but neovascularity and encasement may be seen.

Treatment of transitional cell carcinoma of the renal pelvis is by nephroureterectomy. Since these tumors are often multifocal, the rest of the urothelium must be closely examined for the presence of additional tumors. It is important for the entire ipsilateral ureter and a cuff

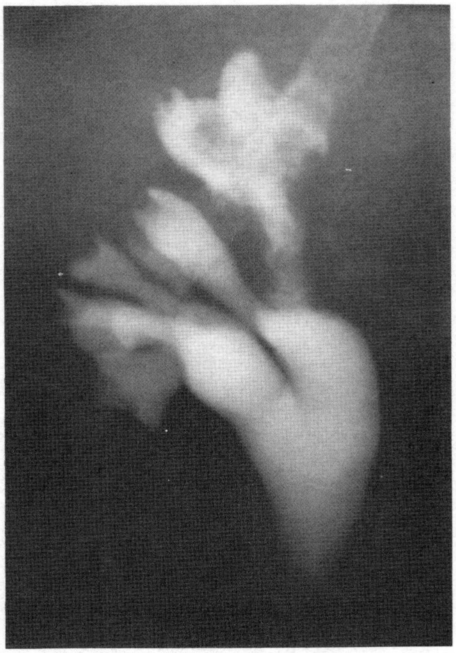

Figure 6.23. Transitional cell carcinoma. An irregular filling defect involves the upper pole infundibulum and calyces.

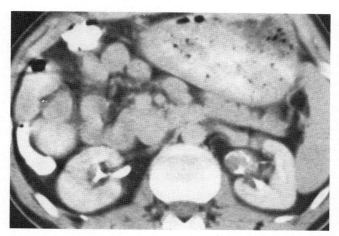

Figure 6.24. Transitional cell carcinoma. Several soft tissue masses in the renal pelvis are defined after intravenous contrast injection.

of bladder to be removed as the distal ureter is otherwise a common site for recurrent disease.

Squamous Cell Carcinoma

Squamous cell carcinomas constitute only about 7% of tumors of the renal pelvis. They are frequently associated with leukoplakia or chronic irritation from stones or urinary tract infection. They are also associated with schistosomiasis when there is involvement of the upper tracts. Most are flat and extend along the urothelium and ulcerate.

Although multifocal lesions are less common than with papillary types, squamous cell carcinomas tend to be of a higher-grade malignancy and local invasion is common. The presence of renal stones or infection makes it difficult to recognize these tumors.

Radiographically, squamous cell carcinomas are difficult to detect. A renal stone is often present and an associated mass may be indistinguishable from xanthogranulomatous pyelonephritis.

SECONDARY TUMORS OF THE KIDNEY

Lymphoma

Since the kidneys do not contain lymphoid tissue, primary renal lymphoma is rare. However, the kidneys may become involved by either hematogenous dissemination or direct extension from adjacent retroperitoneal disease. Thus, renal lymphoma is usually part of a generalized process involving multiple sites.

Renal involvement is much more common in non-Hodgkin lymphomas than in Hodgkin's disease. When present, involvement is more often bilateral than unilateral. At presentation, involvement of the kidneys by non-Hodgkin lymphoma is seen in 5.8% of cases; at autopsy the frequency of renal involvement rises to 41.6%

Renal involvement is more frequent among certain subgroups of non-Hodgkin lymphoma. Poorly differentiated lymphoma of Burkitt type is often described as an extranodal tumor and the kidneys are affected in approximately 10% of cases at presentation. AIDS-related lymphomas were found by CT to involve the kidneys in 11% of patients in one recent series.

Most patients with renal lymphoma have disease in other locations which dominates the clinical presentation. Fever, weight loss, and palpable adenopathy are common complaints. Occasionally, diffuse involvement of both kidneys or ureteral obstruction by adenopathy may compromise renal function. Renal lymphoma is usually clinically silent and occurs late in the course of the disease.

Renal lymphoma may have several different appearances. The most common is multiple lymphomatous masses which is seen in over half the cases. A solitary mass or diffuse infiltration of the kidney by lymphoma may also be seen. Although most renal lymphoma has spread by hematogenous dissemination, CT may demonstrate local extension from paraaortic disease in some cases.

The plain abdominal radiograph is seldom revealing. Lymphadenopathy or renal enlargement may occasionally be detected in patients with abundant retroperitoneal fat. Excretory urography may demonstrate either diffuse renal enlargement or one or more discrete renal masses. If there is extensive involvement, there may be delayed contrast excretion or even absent function. Lymphadenopathy may cause obstruction anywhere from the ureter to the renal pelvis. Bulky lymphadenopathy will often displace the ureters. Since the proximal ureters lie lateral to the paraaortic lymph nodes, they are displaced laterally. The distal ureters are pushed medially as the external iliac lymph nodes are lateral to the ureters.

With US lymphoma is usually hypoechoic, reflecting the homogeneous nature of the tumor (Fig. 6.25). However, a lymphomatous mass shows little sound through transmission, which helps to distinguish it from a cyst. Ultrasound is often helpful in identifying hydronephrosis and is the examination of choice in patients with renal failure or other contraindications to intravenous contrast material.

Computed tomography is routinely used to stage and monitor patients with malignant lymphoma and is an ex-

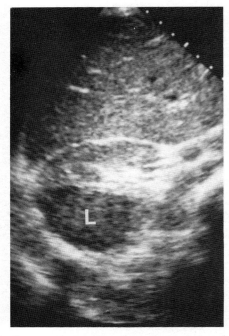

Figure 6.25. Lymphoma. On ultrasound, a hypoechoic mass (L) is seen in the posterior aspect of the right kidney.

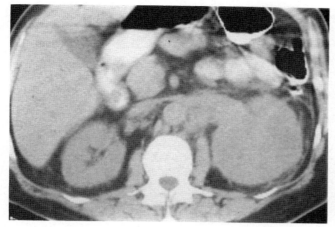

Figure 6.26. Lymphoma. Lymphomatous involvement of the left kidney is appreciated by enlargement of the kidney and replacement of the normal hilar structures.

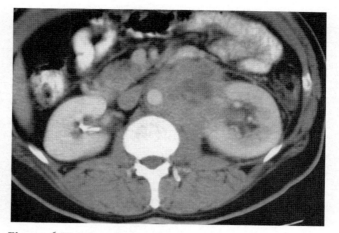

Figure 6.28. Lymphoma. Extension of paraaortic tumor invades the left kidney.

cellent method of detecting renal involvement. Lymphomatous masses are homogeneous, rounded masses. It is difficult to detect renal lymphoma on unenhanced examinations unless the masses are large (Fig. 6.26). After intravenous contrast injection, lymphoma is usually well demarcated from the normal parenchyma by its diminished enhancement (Fig. 6.27). The CT pattern reflects the pathologic involvement as a solitary mass, multiple nodules, or diffuse involvement. Adjacent lymphadenopathy and direct tumor extension to the kidney are also well depicted with CT (Fig. 6.28).

Angiography is not often needed in the evaluation of patients with renal lymphoma, but may be used if a primary renal carcinoma with regional lymph node metastases is suspected. Renal lymphoma is typically hypovascular but may show encasement and modest neovascularity. The major renal arteries are displaced by the tumor masses which also efface the nephrogram.

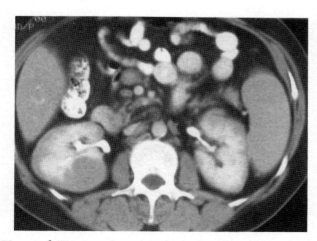

Figure 6.27. Lymphoma. Multiple lymphomatous nodules are seen after contrast enhancement.

Leukemia

Involvement of the kidneys in leukemia is usually due to diffuse infiltration by leukemic cells. It occurs more often with lymphocytic than granulocytic forms. Occasionally a discrete mass such as a chloroma may be produced. Intrarenal hemorrhage and hematuria are common.

With leukemic infiltration both kidneys are symmetrically enlarged. The collecting system is attenuated and filling defects may be seen due to blood clots. Occasionally acute urate nephropathy occurs.

Multiple Myeloma

Multiple myeloma is a disorder of older adults characterized by proliferation of plasma cells and abnormal serum and urine proteins. Renal failure results from precipitation of Bence-Jones proteins in the tubules which may cause mechanical obstruction or damage of tubular cells. Intravascular contrast media causes in vitro precipitation of these proteins and may worsen renal failure in these patients. However, many patients undergo contrast studies without difficulty and underlying renal disease is probably necessary before contrast-induced nephropathy occurs.

Hypercalcemia results from bone lesions and causes nephrocalcinosis. The kidneys are smoothly enlarged and the collecting system is attenuated. Precipitation of abnormal proteins in the tubules or uric acid nephropathy may impair contrast excretion.

Solid Tumor Metastases

Metastatic disease involving the kidneys is relatively common in autopsy series where it may be seen in as many as 20% of patients. The most common primary tumors are carcinomas of the lung, breast, colon, and malignant melanoma. About half of these patients have metastases to both kidneys and half have involvement of only one kidney.

The patient's symptoms are usually dominated by manifestations of the primary tumor, but hematuria and proteinuria are common. Tumors that are especially vascular may cause significant renal hemorrhage resulting in gross hematuria or a perinephric hematoma. Unless extensive metastases involve both kidneys, the renal function is normal. Occasionally urine cytology may be positive.

Although renal metastases are common in autopsy series, where they outnumber primary renal malignancy 4 : 1, they are not commonly seen clinically. Most patients with renal metastases have widespread metastatic disease and imaging studies are not needed to demonstrate renal involvement as well. In the series reported by Choyke et al., over half of the patients died within 3 months of the demonstration of renal metastases.

More recent use of CT to stage and monitor patients with an underlying malignancy has made detection of metastases more common. In a patient with extensive metastases, a renal mass is most likely another metastasis. However, among patients whose disease is in remission, a new renal mass is more likely to be a primary renal tumor.

Plain radiographs are seldom revealing in patients with renal metastases. A solid renal mass may be detected with excretory urography, especially if the tumor is 2 cm or more in size.

Ultrasound is often used to monitor patients with an underlying malignancy for the development of hydronephrosis. Renal metastases are seen as a solid renal mass. Echo-free areas may represent tumor necrosis or local hemorrhage.

The most common modality to detect renal metastases is CT as this is the examination most frequently used to stage and monitor oncology patients (Fig. 6.29). Unenhanced scans are seldom useful in detecting metastases, but may be helpful in excluding renal calculi. Metastases are often small and multiple but certain primary tumors such as colonic carcinomas may produce a solitary large renal metastasis. These may be indistinguishable from a primary renal adenocarcinoma. Renal biopsy may be required to make this distinction (Fig. 6.30). Tumor invasion of the renal vein and extension into the inferior vena cava is commonly seen in renal adenocarcinoma but rare in renal metastases. Although vascular lesions may enhance as much as the normal renal parenchyma during the early vascular phase, they later become hypodense. Small lesions may resemble cysts but can be differentiated by their higher density.

Renal metastases demonstrate high signal intensity on T_2-weighted images. However, MRI is seldom useful, as other entities such as primary renal malignancy or an

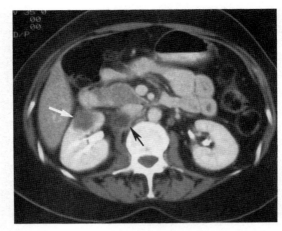

Figure 6.29. Metastasis. The low-density mass in the right kidney (*arrow*) is a metastatic tumor. Another metastasis is just posterior to the inferior vena cava (*arrow*).

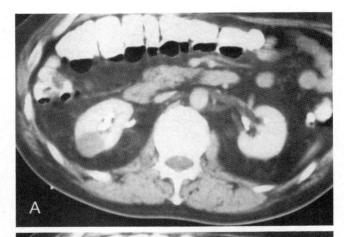

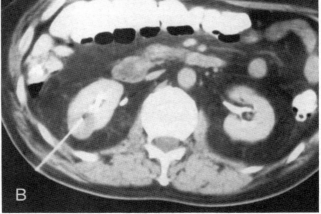

Figure 6.30. Metastasis. **A,** A solitary renal mass is detected in this man with lung carcinoma. **B,** A renal biopsy confirmed metastatic disease rather than a second primary tumor.

inflammatory process may have similar signal characteristics.

Arteriography may be used to help distinguish a metastasis from a primary renal adenocarcinoma. The vascularity of the metastasis reflects the vascularity of the primary tumor. Furthermore, selective angiography may reveal small tumors that may be missed by CT, US, or MRI. Multiple tumors makes metastatic disease more likely. A definitive diagnosis can usually be made with fine-needle biopsy.

RENAL CAPSULAR TUMORS

The renal capsule is composed not only of fibrous tissue, but also of nerves, smooth muscle, blood vessels, and perirenal fat. Any of these tissues may give rise to a tumor, benign or malignant. However, tumors of the renal capsule are rare.

Malignant capsular tumors are often quite large when diagnosed. Presenting complaints include a flank mass, abdominal pain, and weight loss. Unless the renal parenchyma is invaded, hematuria is uncommon. The prognosis is usually poor.

If the tumor is large, a soft tissue mass may be appreciated on the plain abdominal radiograph. Calcification is uncommon, but a lipoma or liposarcoma may be recognized by the fat density. Extrinsic compression or displacement of the kidney is seen with urography. If the kidney is invaded, distortion of the collecting system or poor function may be present.

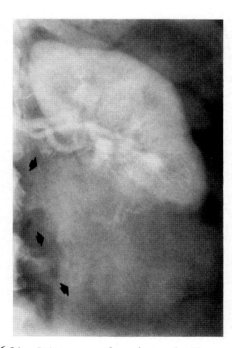

Figure 6.31. Leiomyoma of renal capsule. The capsular nature of this tumor is revealed by the feeding capsular vessels (*arrows*).

Computed tomography is helpful in identifying the mass, especially if the growth is exophytic. Preservation of the collecting system suggests an extrarenal mass, but a capsular tumor cannot be distinguished from an exophytic renal neoplasm in this manner.

Angiography is very helpful in the diagnosis of renal capsular tumors as the mass is fed by enlarged capsular arteries (Fig. 6.31). The intrarenal arteries remain intact, although they may be compressed by a large capsular tumor. The capsular vessels are often stretched and separated from the kidney while the renal parenchyma is displaced inwardly.

SUGGESTED READING

Renal Parenchymal Tumors

Ambos MA, Bosniak MA, Valensi QJ, et al: Angiographic patterns in renal oncocytomas. *Radiology* 129:615, 1978.

Beahrs OH, Myers MH: (eds) *Manual for Staging of Cancer,* 2nd ed. JB Lippincott, Philadelphia 1983, p 177.

Choyke PL: MR imaging in renal cell carcinoma. *Radiology* 169:572, 1988.

Choyke PL, Filling-Katz MR, Shawker TH, et al: Von Hippel-Lindau disease: radiologic screening for visceral manifestations. *Radiology* 174:815, 1990.

Curry NS, Schabel SI, Betsill WL Jr: Small renal neoplasms: diagnostic imaging, pathologic features, and clinical course. *Radiology* 158:113, 1986.

Demos TC, Schiffer M, Love L, et al: Normal excretory urography in patients with primary kidney neoplasms. *Urol Radiol* 7:75, 1985.

Drash A, Sherman F, Hartman WH, et al: A syndrome of pseudohermaphroditism, Wilms' tumor, hypertension and degenerative renal disease. *J Pediat* 76:585, 1970.

Ekelund L: Pharmacoangiography of the kidney: an overview. *Urol Radiol* 2:9, 1980.

Fein AB, Lee JKT, Balfe DM, et al: Diagnosis and staging of renal cell carcinoma: a comparison of MR imaging and CT. *AJR* 148:749, 1987.

Fernback SK, Feinstein KA, Donaldson JS, et al: Nephroblastomatosis: comparison of CT with US and urography. *Radiology* 166:153, 1988.

Foster WL Jr, Halvorsen RA, Jr, Dunnick NR: The clandestine renal cell carcinoma: atypical appearances and presentations. *Radiographics* 5:175, 1985.

Hartman DS: Cysts and cystic neoplasms. *Urol Radiol* 12:7, 1990.

Hartman DS, Davis CJ Jr, Madewell JE, et al: Primary malignant renal tumors in the second decade of life: Wilms' tumor versus renal cell carcinoma. *J Urol* 127:888, 1982.

Hartman DS, Lesar MSL, Madewell JE, et al: Mesoblastic nephroma: radiologic-pathologic correlation of 20 cases. *AJR* 136:69, 1981.

Johnson CD, Dunnick NR, Cohan RH, et al: Renal adenocarcinoma: CT staging of 100 tumors. *AJR* 148:59, 1987.

Kioumehr F, Cochran ST, Layfield L, et al: Wilms' tumor (nephroblastoma) in the adult patient: clinical and radiologic manifestations. *AJR* 152:299, 1989.

Levine E, Huntrakoon M, Wetzel LH: Small renal neoplasms: clinical, pathologic, and imaging features. *AJR* 153:69, 1989.

Lieber MM, Tomera KM, Farrow GM: Renal oncocytoma. *J Urol* 125:481, 1981.

Ljungberg B, Holmberg G, Sjodin JG, et al: Renal cell carcinoma in a renal cyst: a case report and review of the literature. *J Urol* 143:797, 1990.

Lowe RE, Cohen MD: Computed tomographic evaluation of Wilms' tumor and nephroblastoma. *Radiographics* 4(6):915, 1984.

Mena E, Bull FE, Bookstein JJ, et al: Angiography of the nephrogenic hepatic dysfunction syndrome. *Radiology* 111:65, 1974.

Mesrobian HGJ: Wilms' tumor: past, present, future. *J Urol* 149:231, 1988.

Press GA, McClennan BL, Melson GL, et al: Papillary renal cell carcinoma: CT and sonographic evaluation. *AJR* 143:1005, 1984.

Quinn MJ, Hartman DS, Friedman AC, et al: Renal oncocytoma: new observations. *Radiology* 153:49, 1984.

Robson CJ, Churchill BM, Anderson W: The results of radical nephrectomy for renal cell carcinoma. *J Urol* 101:297, 1969.

Shirkhoda A, Lewis E: Renal sarcoma and sarcomatoid renal cell carcinoma: CT and angiographic features. *Radiology* 162:353, 1987.

Siegel SC, Sandler MA, Alpern MB, et al: CT of renal cell carcinoma in patients on chronic hemodialysis. *AJR* 150:583, 1988.

Smith SJ, Bosniak MA, Megibow AJ, et al: Renal cell carcinoma: earlier discovery and increased detection. *Radiology* 170:699, 1989.

Stigsson L, Ekelund L, Karp W: Bilateral concurrent renal neoplasms: report of eleven cases. *AJR* 132:37, 1979.

Wallace S, Chuang VP, Swanson D, et al: Embolization of renal carcinoma. *Radiology* 138:563, 1981.

Zagoria RJ, Wolfman NT, Karstaedt N, et al: CT features of renal cell carcinoma with emphasis on relation to tumor size. *Invest Radiol* 25:261, 1990.

Mesenchymal Tumors

Blute ML, Malek RS, Segura JW: Angiomyolipoma: clinical metamorphosis and concepts for management. *J Urol* 139:20, 1988.

Bosniak M, Megibow AJ, Hulnick DH, et al: CT diagnosis of renal angiomyolipoma: the importance of detecting small amounts of fat. *AJR* 151:497, 1988.

Curry NS, Schabel SI, Garvin AJ, Fish G: Intratumoral fat in a renal oncocytoma mimicking angiomyolipoma. *AJR* 154:307, 1990.

Dineen MK, Venable DD, Misra RP: Pure intrarenal lipoma: report of a case and review of the literature. *J Urol* 132:104, 1984.

Dunnick NR, Hartman DS, Ford KK, et al: The radiology of juxtaglomerular tumors. *Radiology* 147:321, 1983.

Rofsky NM, Bosniak MA, Megibow AJ, et al: Adrenal myelolipomas: CT appearance with tiny amounts of fat and punctate calcification. *Urol Radiol* 11:148, 1989.

Rumancik WM, Bosniak MA, Rosen RJ, et al: Atypical renal and pararenal hamartomas associated with lymphangiomyomatosis. *AJR* 142:971, 1984.

Sant GR, Ayers DK, Bankoff MS, et al: Fine needle aspiration biopsy in the diagnosis of renal angiomyolipoma. *J Urol* 143:999, 1990.

Srinivas V, Sogani PC, Hajdu SI, et al: Sarcomas of the kidney. *J Urol* 132:13, 1984.

Stillwell TJ, Gomez MR, Kelalis PP: Renal lesions in tuberous sclerosis. *J Urol* 138:477, 1987.

Renal Pelvic Tumors

Baron RL, McClennan BL, Lee JKT, et al: Computed tomography of transitional cell carcinoma of the renal pelvis and ureter. *Radiology* 144:125, 1982.

Narumi Y, Sato T, Hori S, et al: Squamous cell carcinoma of the uroepithelium: CT evaluation. *Radiology* 173:853, 1989.

Pollack HM, Arger PH, Banner MP, et al: Computed tomography of renal pelvic filling defects. *Radiology* 138:645, 1981.

Yousem DM, Gatewood OMB, Goldman SM, et al: Synchronous and metachronous transitional cell carcinoma of the urinary tract: prevalence, incidence, and radiographic detection. *Radiology* 167:613, 1988.

Secondary Tumors of the Kidney

Choyke PL, White EM, Zeman RK, et al: Renal metastases: clinicopathologic and radiologic correlation. *Radiology* 162:359, 1987.

Dunnick NR, Reaman GH, Head GL, et al: Radiographic manifestations of Burkitt's lymphoma in American patients. *AJR* 132:1, 1979.

Hamper UM, Goldblum LE, Hutchins GM, et al: Renal involvement in AIDS: sonographic-pathologic correlation. *AJR* 150:1321, 1988.

Hartman DS, Davis CJ Jr, Goldman SM, et al: Renal lymphoma: radiologic-pathologic correlation of 21 cases. *Radiology* 144:759, 1982.

Pagani JJ: Solid renal mass in the cancer patient: second primary renal cell carcinoma versus renal metastasis. *J Comput Assist Tomogr* 7(3):444, 1983.

Richmond J, Sherman RS, Diamond HD, et al: Renal lesions associated with malignant lymphomas. *Am J Med* 32:184, 1962.

Renal Capsular Tumors

Mohler JL, Casale AJ: Renal capsular leiomyoma. *J Urol* 138:853, 1987.

Myerson D, Rosenfield AT, Itzchak Y: Renal capsular tumors: the angiographic features. *J Urol* 121:238, 1979.

Steiner M, Quinlan D, Goldman SM, et al: Leiomyoma of the kidney: presentation of four new cases and the role of computerized tomography. *J Urol* 143:994, 1990.

CHAPTER 7

RENAL INFLAMMATORY DISEASE

Inflammatory conditions involving the urinary tract are among the most common infectious disorders affecting humankind. In most cases, the infection is confined to the lower urinary tract and the diagnosis is established by clinical or laboratory studies; there is prompt resolution with appropriate therapy and imaging studies are not required. When, however, the kidney is involved by the inflammatory process or the precise diagnosis is not known, renal imaging studies play an important role, in both their diagnosis and management.

Pathologically, inflammatory disease involving the kidney can be divided into two broad groups: (*a*) glomerulonephritis—those that involve an immunologic injury of the glomerulus, and (*b*) interstitial nephritis—those that result from an effect of an infectious or toxic agent on the renal parenchyma. Radiologic studies play a limited role in the diagnosis and management of glomerulonephritis (Chapter 20). Interstitial nephritis is divided into two major subgroups: (*a*) noninfectious interstitial nephritis which is usually caused by the action of toxic agents on the kidney, and (*b*) infectious interstitial nephritis, the result of the action of a pathogen. Noninfectious interstitial nephritis will also be discussed in Chapter 20. In most cases, infectious interstitial nephritis is due to a bacterial organism; such cases are commonly called *acute pyelonephritis* or one of its variations.

BACTERIAL INFECTIONS

Bacteria usually reach the kidney via the ureter as a result of ascending infection from the lower urinary tract. Since women have a much higher incidence of lower urinary tract infection owing to the short length of the female urethra, bacterial infections of the kidney are, therefore, much more common in women than in men before the age of 50 years. Beyond this age, however, the incidence of urinary tract infection in men increases, as a result of urinary stasis caused by benign prostatic hypertrophy and other factors. Much less commonly, bacterial infections are spread to the kidney hematogeneously. Clinically, there are fever, flank pain, chills, and other systemic symptoms such as nausea, vomiting, and malaise. These symptoms usually help to differentiate infections involving the kidney from those that purely involve the lower urinary tract. In some cases, however, clinical differentiation may be difficult as these symptoms may be present in patients with infection solely confined to the lower urinary tract. Conditions that may predispose patients with lower urinary tract infection to renal involvement include (*a*) vesicoureteral reflux, (*b*) urinary tract obstruction, (*c*) calculi, (*d*) altered bladder function, (*e*) altered host resistance, (*f*) pregnancy, and (*g*) congenital urinary tract anomalies. Nonetheless, there is usually a prompt response to appropriate antibiotic therapy and diagnostic imaging studies are either done after the fact or are not necessary.

In those cases where response to therapy is slow, the precise diagnosis is in doubt, or the clinical picture is complicated by the presence of an underlying systemic disease such as diabetes mellitus, radiologic investigation on a more immediate basis is indicated to (*a*) look for an underlying abnormality that may have predisposed the patient to the infection; (*b*) search for an abnormality such as obstruction, calculus, or papillary necrosis that may prevent a rapid response to therapy from taking place; or (*c*) diagnose a complication of the parenchymal infection such as a renal or perinephric abscess.

The optimal imaging approach for patients with bacterial infections of the kidney depends on the acuity of the illness, the predisposing conditions that may be present, and the preference of the individual physicians involved. In general, in patients with normal or near-normal renal function, urography is the best overall screening study, as a normal examination virtually precludes the presence of significant pathology. When the urogram suggests a parenchymal abnormality or is equivocal, computed tomography (CT) more precisely defines the nature and extent of the suspected abnormality. Antegrade or retrograde pyelography is generally the next study performed if urography suggests obstruction is present. In patients with abnormal renal function, sonography is generally preferable to urography as the screening study.

Computed tomography, while more sensitive to the detection of parenchymal pathology than is urography, does not reliably demonstrate calyceal abnormalities and may not demonstrate the precise nature of an associated urinary obstruction; thus it is rarely indicated as the *initial* imaging study in patients with renal inflammatory disease.

Bacterial infections of the kidney represent a spectrum of clinical disorders that are interrelated. Most commonly Gram-negative enteric pathogens, including *Escherichia coli, Proteus mirabilis, Pseudomonas aeruginosa,* and *Klebsiella*, are found on urine culture. In the preantibiotic era, Gram-positive urine pathogens including *Staphylococcus* and *Streptococcus* were relatively common, however, today they represent only a small minority of infections.

Pathologically, acute pyelonephritis is an acute bacterial infection of the kidney manifested by infiltration of the renal interstitium with neutrophils. Grossly, the kidney exhibits swelling and the tissues appear hyperemic. Small microabscesses 1–5 mm in diameter may be present. These changes tend to occur focally within the kidney interspersed with zones of unaffected renal tissue.

When there is a heavier leukocyte infiltration of the kidney with resultant increased edema and hyperemia and focal areas of tissue necrosis, a more severe form of bacterial infection is present which has been termed *acute bacterial nephritis.* Clinically, acute bacterial nephritis presents with evidence of severe infection secondary to a Gram-negative organism. Approximately half of these patients have underlying diabetes mellitus and

there is frequently a component of frank sepsis. When this severe inflammatory process is confined to a single lobe of the kidney, the process has been termed *acute lobar nephronia* or *acute focal bacterial nephritis* (AFBN).

If there is coalescence of the small microabscesses present in acute pyelonephritis with underlying tissue liquefication, an *acute renal abscess* is formed. An acute renal abscess may complicate acute pyelonephritis, AFBN, or acute bacterial nephritis. Some investigators have felt that AFBN actually represents an intermediate form of renal inflammatory disease between acute pyelonephritis and acute renal abscess. Following formation of the abscess, fibroblasts migrate into the area of inflammation to build a wall between the normal parenchyma and necrotic tissue. This walling-off process is characteristic of more mature abscesses. A *chronic renal abscess,* therefore, represents a walled-off abscess and the remainder of the renal parenchyma returns to normal. If the walling-off process is incomplete and the renal abscess breaks through the renal capsule, a *perinephric abscess* is formed.

If the infection is confined to the collecting system and the patient also has ureteral obstruction, the process is termed *pyonephrosis.* In patients with pyonephrosis, inflammatory changes may be present throughout the renal parenchyma, but the collecting system itself is filled with pus as a result of inadequate drainage. If pylosinus extravasation should occur in such patients, a perinephric abscess may be formed by this mechanism as well.

Acute Pyelonephritis

Acute uncomplicated pyelonephritis presents the most common and most benign bacterial infection involving the kidney. The infection responds quickly (within 48–72 hours) to antibiotic therapy and unlike acute pyelonephritis in children, does not lead to any permanent morphological change in the kidney. It is not surprising, therefore, that the results of urography and ultrasonography are normal in three-quarters of the cases. In the remainder, abnormal urographic findings include (Fig. 7.1): (*a*) diffuse renal enlargement, generally attributed to the edema that accompanies the infection; (*b*) a delay in the appearance of the contrast material in the renal collecting system; (*c*) attenuation of the calyces, also the result of parenchymal edema; and (*d*) a decrease in the density of the nephrogram in the affected portion of the kidney. In general, the degree of radiographic abnormality and the degree of impairment of contrast excretion that is present reflect the severity of the interstitial inflammatory disease.

Rarely, caliectasis that is not attributable to concomitant obstruction may be present as the result of pyelonephritis. In such cases, this finding is attributed to

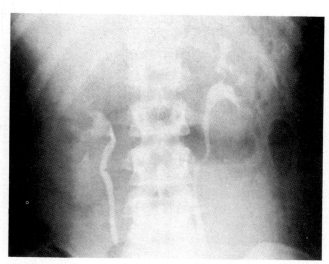

Figure 7.1. Urographic appearance of acute pyelonephritis. The right kidney is enlarged and there is decreased filling of the collecting system.

the presence of an endotoxin elaborated by some Gram-negative bacteria that is said to have an effect on ureteral peristalsis. In the vast majority of cases, however, the finding of caliectasis in association with acute pyelonephritis implies the presence of either past or present underlying urinary tract obstruction.

Mucosal striations, sometimes referred to as "ridging" of the mucosa, are an uncommon manifestation of acute pyelonephritis in the renal collecting system. These striations are thought to be a manifestation of mucosal edema but are not specific for acute pyelonephritis; they are found in a variety of other conditions including vesicoureteral reflux.

Sonographic findings in patients with acute uncomplicated pyelonephritis are either normal or show renal enlargement and diffusely hypoechogenic renal parenchyma. Dinkle et al. has demonstrated an increase in renal size of as much as two standard deviations over normal as determined by sonography to be present in children with acute renal inflammatory disease. The authors reported, however, that the finding of renal enlargement appears to be somewhat age dependent with the youngest children showing the greatest degree of change.

Radionuclide imaging in patients with acute pyelonephritis has been reported using both renal cortical imaging agents such as ^{99m}Tc DMSA and inflammatory imaging agents such as ^{67}gallium (^{67}Ga) citrate. Handmaker reported that the nuclear imaging studies assisted in confirming the diagnosis of acute pyelonephritis in 10 of 60 patients studied for this reason. Renal cortical imaging studies may show an inhomogeneous distribution of the radionuclide within the affected kidney or polar defects with asymmetric tracer uptake. In some cases, a pattern

that was specific for the diagnosis of pyelonephritis, termed the "flare" pattern, representing a striate distribution of decreased radioactivity was present. ^{67}Gallium will localize in any area of inflammation and is reported to have an accuracy of 86% in distinguishing upper-tract from lower-tract infection at 48 hours. Difficulties with gallium imaging for patients with pyelonephritis include the fact that within the first 24 hours there is normal excretion of the radiotracer by the kidneys and the study cannot differentiate infection within the kidney from that in the surrounding perinephric tissues. In addition, gallium uptake in the kidneys is relatively nonspecific and may be present in a variety of other renal diseases including acute tubular necrosis and vasculitis. Other investigators have reported utilizing ^{111}indium (^{111}In)-labeled autologous leukocytes in imaging renal inflammatory disease. Indium leukocyte studies have the advantage in comparison to ^{67}Ga in that the radiopharmaceutical is not normally excreted by the kidneys and that delayed images are not generally required. However, the sensitivity of such studies for the diagnosis of acute pyelonephritis has never been confirmed in large clinical studies.

As a rule, CT of the kidney should not be performed as the initial study on patients with uncomplicated acute pyelonephritis. Computed tomography is indicated when there is a discrepancy between the clinical picture and the result of urography or sonography; in other cases, the findings of renal inflammatory disease may be discovered in a search for another source of the patient's symptomatology. Noncontrast enhanced scans are normal. Following contrast administration, however, narrow striate areas of decreased contrast enhancement are seen either focally or generally in the kidney depending on the degree of involvement that is present (Fig. 7.2). Because of CT's superior contrast resolution, as compared to urography, CT scans may show these changes even in patients in whom urography is considered normal. These striate areas of decreased contrast enhancement most probably represent decreased areas of excretion of the contrast material secondary to the inflammatory disease. Gold has postulated that they represent areas of slow urine flow within the tubular lumen secondary to elevated interstitial pressure. In the absence of a discrete mass, they should not be interpreted as evidence of a more severe form of renal inflammatory disease, that is, AFBN.

Acute Focal Bacterial Nephritis

The characteristic feature of acute focal bacterial nephritis (AFBN) is that the inflammatory process produces a mass effect which thereby simulates the presence of a frank renal abscess. AFBN is a more severe form of renal inflammatory disease than is acute uncomplicated pyelonephritis. The entity is also known as acute focal pyelonephritis and because the inflammatory process is

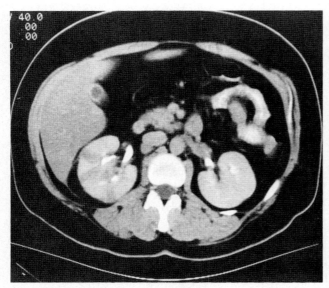

Figure 7.2. Computed tomography appearance of acute pyelonephritis. Relatively narrow striate zones of decreased contrast enhancement are present in the right renal parenchyma.

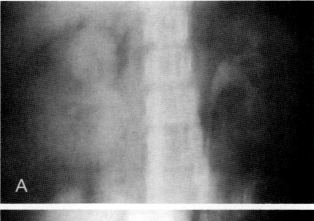

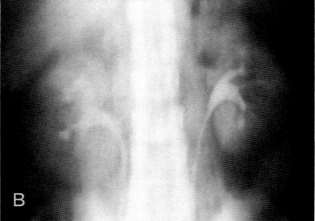

Figure 7.3. Acute focal bacterial nephritis. **A,** Initial urogram demonstrates bulbous enlargement of the lower pole of the right kidney suggesting the presence of a mass. There is poor opacification of the renal collecting system, as well. **B,** Follow-up study after 10 days of antibiotic therapy shows marked improvement. (From McDonough WD, Sandler CM, Benson GS: Acute focal bacterial nephritis: Focal pyelonephritis that may simulate renal abscess. *J Urol* 126:670, 1981.)

generally confined to a single renal lobe, it is also sometimes referred to as acute lobar nephronia. Some authorities feel, however, that this latter term should be reserved for the inflammatory lesion that accompanies intrarenal reflux in association with reflux nephropathy.

On urography, the involved segment of the kidney appears enlarged and there is evidence of mass effect (Fig. 7.3) with diminution of the nephrogram, and either compression of the calyces in the involved segment or complete nonvisualization of the calyces in the affected segment. The mass is typically intrarenal in location. In some cases a combination of focal and diffuse abnormalities may be present in the kidney. The findings on urography, however, may be indistinguishable from that produced by an acute renal abscess or other forms of renal inflammatory disease.

On sonography, the mass is typically sonolucent, poorly marginated, and may contain low-level echoes that may disrupt the corticomedullary junction. In some patients, areas of involvement have been described as being slightly hyperechoic, but this appearance is uncommon. Differentiating these phlegmatous areas of involvement from true liquefaction may be difficult even using high-resolution equipment.

Acute focal bacterial nephritis demonstrates a relatively characteristic appearance on CT (Figs. 7.2 and 7.4). On noncontrast scans, some swelling of the affected region of the kidney may be appreciated; however, this area will have the same or only slightly less density as the adjacent unaffected renal parenchyma. After contrast administration, however, the affected area of the kidney is

clearly demonstrated as a large wedge-shaped mass-like lesion secondary to diminished contrast enhancement. This wedge-shaped area is thought to represent the lobar architecture of the kidney. This appearance is in contrast to a frank abscess which will be present both before and after contrast administration.

The appearance of AFBN may be modified by antibiotic therapy. Partially treated patients may demonstrate a rounded or ovoid area of decreased enhancement with poorly defined margins (Fig. 7.5); this appearance may be a source of confusion as it is less characteristic of AFBN.

Acute Bacterial Nephritis

Acute bacterial nephritis represents the most severe form of renal inflammatory disease short of frank abscess.

Urography typically demonstrates marked swelling of the kidney (Fig. 7.6) and there is usually severe impair-

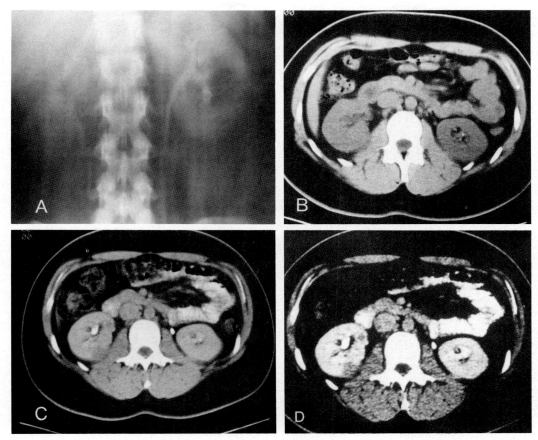

Figure 7.4. Acute focal bacterial nephritis. **A,** IVP demonstrates poor definition of the renal outline with decreased calyceal filling. These findings are difficult to distinguish from those produced by uncomplicated acute pyelonephritis. **B,** Noncontrast CT scan demonstrates slight swelling of the inferomedial portion of the right kidney, but the renal parenchyma appears homogeneous. **C,** After contrast, a poorly defined wedge-shaped area of decreased contrast enhancement is present which is better appreciated at a narrow window setting **(D).**

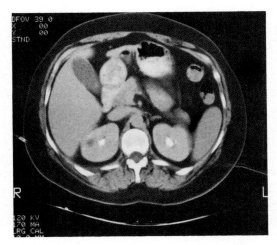

Figure 7.5. Atypical appearance produced by partially treated AFBN. Computed tomography shows a rounded area of decreased enhancement in the right kidney without significant mass effect.

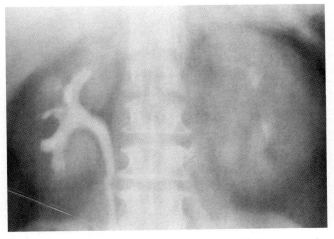

Figure 7.6. Acute bacterial nephritis. The left kidney is markedly swollen and demonstrates poor excretion of the contrast material. The calyces, while poorly opacified, are seen well enough to exclude concomitant ureteral obstruction.

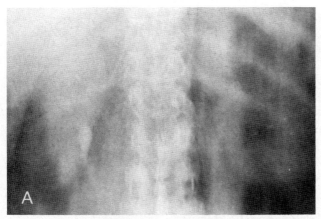

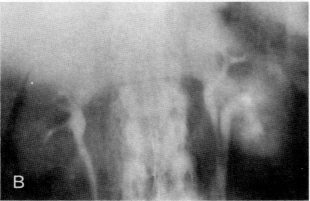

Figure 7.7. Acute bacterial nephritis. **A,** Initial study demonstrates swelling of the left kidney with virtually no excretion of contrast into the renal collecting system. **B,** Follow-up study after 2 weeks of parenteral antibiotics shows marked improvement. A bifid renal pelvis is now evident.

ment of contrast material excretion (Fig. 7.7). The nephrogram is typically of normal or increased intensity and persists for several hours after the administration of the contrast material. This appearance is similar to the nephrogram which has been described in association with acute tubular necrosis and must be differentiated from the nephrogram of acute extrarenal obstruction. In the later instance, the nephrogram becomes progressively more intense during the course of the study. The pyelogram typically is markedly delayed in appearance or may be entirely absent. The urographic changes, while generally more pronounced, may be difficult to distinguish from other forms of renal inflammatory disease.

Angiographic findings in acute bacterial nephritis include a slowing of arterial flow, splaying of the intrarenal vascular tree, a decrease in the caliber of the intrarenal arteries, and a striate or mottled nephrogram, similar to that found in acute renal vein thrombosis.

Sonography reveals diffuse renal enlargement and large zones of hypoechogenic parenchyma (Fig. 7.8) similar in appearance to those present in a more limited fashion in patients with acute focal bacterial nephritis.

Computed tomography is the imaging study of choice for the demonstration of acute bacterial nephritis. The kidney is diffusely enlarged and nearly homogeneous in density on noncontrast studies. Following contrast administration, however, there are multiple wedge-shaped zones of diminished enhancement that radiate from the collecting system to the renal capsule (Fig. 7.8). When compared with the attenuation of the kidney prior to contrast enhancement, these zones demonstrate a modest increase in density, but less than that present in the unaffected areas of the kidney.

As in patients with AFBN, the appearance of these wedge-shaped areas may be modified following antibiotic therapy, although not as rapidly as in patients with the focal form of involvement.

Davidson and Talner have shown that long-term follow-up studies in patients with acute bacterial nephritis may demonstrate generalized wasting of the kidney and focal calyceal clubbing, suggestive of papillary necrosis. The appearance of such structural changes as a sequela of acute bacterial nephritis must be contrasted with acute uncomplicated pyelonephritis in which no long-term structural changes occur in adults. The etiology of these morphologic changes has been postulated to involve ischemic insult to the kidney as a result of the inflammatory process.

Acute Renal Abscess

Prior to the availability of broad-spectrum antibiotics, the majority of renal abscesses formed as a result of hematogeneous dissemination of *Staphylococcus aureus* from a site usually in the skin or bone. With the widespread availability of antibiotics, most renal abscesses form as a result of the coalescence of small microabscesses that are present as a part of acute pyelonephritis or one of its variations. The predominate organisms responsible for abscesses today are Gram-negative enteric species and occur in the setting of diabetes mellitus, drug abuse, vesicoureteral reflux, and renal calculus disease. Acute abscesses may be solitary or form in multiple locations in the kidney simultaneously. The appearance of multiple lesions is less common and suggests hematogenous dissemination (Fig. 7.9).

The signs and symptoms of an acute renal abscess are difficult to distinguish from less virulent forms of bacterial infection of the kidney. There is usually a low-grade fever, leukocytosis, and flank pain; urinalysis may demonstrate pyuria, but may also be normal, especially if some walling-off of the process has occurred. There is frequently a history of prior antibiotic therapy with recrudesence on cessation.

Urography may demonstrate decreased opacification of all or part of the kidney and there is typically decreased calyceal opacification with either compression or

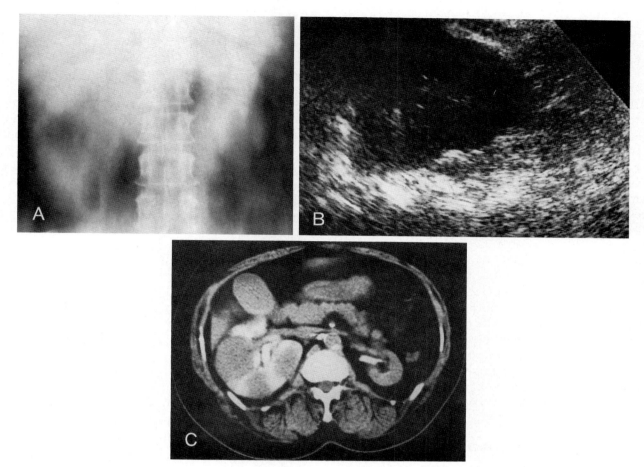

Figure 7.8. Acute bacterial nephritis. **A,** Excretory urogram shows a swollen kidney with impaired contrast excretion on the right. An incidental adrenal calcification is present. **B,** Sonogram shows a diffuse decrease in echogenicity throughout the renal parenchyma. **C,** computed tomography shows multiple wedge-shaped areas of decreased contrast enhancement. (B and C from Corriere JN Jr, Sandler CM: The diagnosis and immediate therapy of acute renal and perirenal infections. *Urol Clin North Am* 9(2):219, 1982.)

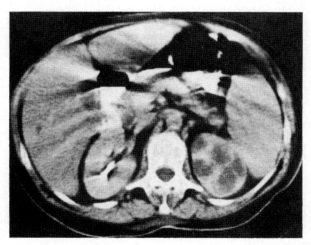

Figure 7.9. Multiple acute renal abscesses. On CT, multiple rounded areas of decreased attenuation are present which were also present before contrast administration. Needle aspiration revealed *Staphylococcus aureus.*

amputation of the calyces in the affected segment. Tomography may demonstrate an ill-defined lucency within the renal parenchyma associated with mass effect. The findings on urography are rarely specific and it may be difficult to distinguish abscess from other forms of inflammatory disease.

Angiography is no longer utilized as a first-line imaging study to diagnose renal abscesses, but may be performed in an attempt to differentiate an atypical CT appearance of an abscess from that of tumor. The study typically demonstrates generalized pruning of the vascular tree and, in addition, there may be draping of vessels around a poorly defined mass, usually best appreciated on the capillary phase.

On sonography, abscesses appear as sonolucent lesions that contain low-amplitude echoes reflecting the necrotic nature of the mass. There is typically poor through-transmission of the ultrasound beam; the findings are usually best characterized as representing a complex mass.

Computed tomography is the imaging study of choice for the diagnosis of an acute renal abscess. The lesion is a low attenuation, rounded or ovoid mass (typically between 10 and 20 HU) which, in contrast to other nonnecrotic inflammatory masses, is present both before and after contrast enhancement. The attenuation of the mass may increase slightly after the administration of the contrast, but not to the extent that is present with renal tumors. Depending on the degree of the surrounding inflammatory process, the borders of the mass may be relatively sharply defined or indistinct. In some cases, gas may be present within the abscess; this finding, when present, is virtually pathognomonic. There is usually thickening of Gerota's fascia, and increased density may be found in the adjacent perinephric and mesenteric fat. This later finding has been termed "dirty fat" by some investigators but is not specific for a renal inflammatory process.

Radionuclide studies performed with either ^{67}Ga citrate or ^{111}In-labeled leukocytes will localize in an acute renal abscess. Neither study, however, permits differentiation of a frank abscess from a phlegmon or a focal area of pyelonephritis, nor do they permit separation of those inflammatory masses that are confined to the kidney from those that have extended into the perinephric space.

Chronic Renal Abscess

When fibroblasts migrate into the area of an acute renal abscess and form a barrier between the abscess and the remainder of the kidney, a chronic renal abscess is formed. Extension of the abscess into the perinephric space may or may not be present.

On imaging studies, a chronic renal abscess presents as an intrarenal mass. Angiographically, while the interior of the mass is avascular, there is frequently a prominent hypervascular rim surrounding the avascular center, representing the granulation tissue at the lesion's periphery. This same finding may be seen on CT where the rim of the lesion enhances after contrast administration to a greater extent than does the surrounding normal renal parenchyma. It is the finding of this hypervascular rim that helps to identify the lesion as a chronic renal abscess. The presence of a rim, however, is not pathognomonic of a chronic renal abscess; such a pattern of enhancement may be found in some necrotic or cystic renal neoplasms. On sonography, chronic renal abscesses appear as complex intrarenal masses. In some instances, the rim of granulation tissue may be identified by its echogenic nature; however, sonography has not proven to be as reliable as CT in identifying the nature of the lesion. Hoddick et al. reported a significant number of false-negative sonograms among 12 patients with renal or perirenal abscesses in whom both modalities were obtained; there were no false-negative CT studies in this group.

Perinephric Abscess

A *primary* perinephric abscess forms when an intrarenal abscess breaks through the renal capsule into the perinephric space. On discovery, the intrarenal component may be large or may have healed and the extrarenal component is all that can be identified. Primary perinephric abscesses may also form as a result of pyelosinus extravasation of infected urine. *Secondary* perinephric abscesses may form when infection is spread to the perinephric space hematogeneously from an external source. A third mechanism by which perinephric abscesses occur is direct extension into the perinephric space of an infection in an adjacent organ, i.e., a ruptured appendix or diverticulitis.

The signs and symptoms of a perinephric abscess are nonspecific in that clinical differentiation of this process from less advanced forms of renal inflammatory disease is usually not possible. In some patients, however, referred pain to the thorax, the groin, thigh, or hip may be a clue that the disease has spread beyond the kidney. In most cases, symptoms of urinary infection are present for periods longer than 2 weeks. Fever is usually present but tends to be intermittent and low-grade. As many as 25% are said to have normal urinalysis. The development of a perinephric abscess as a complication of renal inflammatory disease is more common in patients with large staghorn calculi (Fig. 7.10), pyonephrosis, diabetes, and in patients with neurogenic bladder disease.

On plain films a large perinephric abscess may be identified as a soft tissue mass in the perinephric space (Fig. 7.11). A scoliosis of the lumbar spine convex to the opposite side may also be present. The psoas margin may be obscured on the involved side; however, such a find-

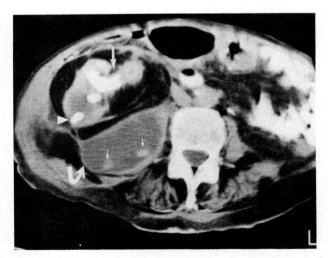

Figure 7.10. A small right kidney containing multiple calculi (*arrow*) is present. An abscess containing an extruded calculus is present in the inferior portion of the kidney (*arrowhead*). A chronic perinephric abscess with an enhancing rim (*curved arrow*) also contains extruded calculi (*small white arrows*).

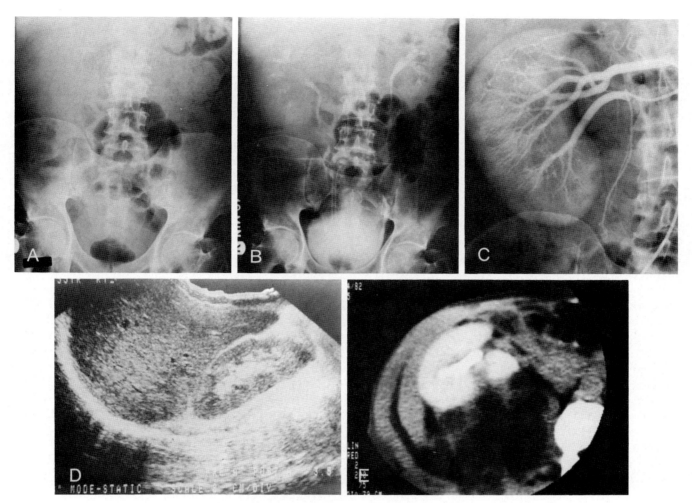

Figure 7.11. Perinephric abscess. **A,** Plain film shows a large soft tissue mass in the right flank with obliteration of the psoas margin. **B,** IVP shows extrinsic compression of the renal collecting system, with generalized renal enlargement. **C,** Selective right renal angiogram shows no evidence of an intrarenal mass, but there is displacement of the capsular vessels from the renal margin, suggesting fluid in the perinephric space. Two renal arteries which have been injected simultaneously are present. **D,** Sonogram shows anterior displacement of the lower pole of the kidney, but a definite abscess is not seen. **E,** Computed tomography shows a large posterior perinephric abscess with multiple loculation. The abscess displaces the right kidney almost to the anterior abdominal wall.

ing may be present in up to 10% of normal patients. Air within the abscess is found in a number of large perinephric abscesses secondary to gas-forming organisms; extensive gas collection, however, may be confused with gas normally present within the colon.

Urography generally demonstrates changes in the renal parenchyma previously described with less severe forms of renal inflammatory disease. With a large abscess, a soft tissue density outside the confines of the kidney may be appreciated. Tomography demonstrates thickening and displacement of Gerota's fascia (Fig. 7.12). In addition, it may demonstrate that the two kidneys do not appear in focus on the same tomographic section; the affected kidney may be displaced anteriorly due to fluid behind it. In some cases, however, the findings on urography will be subtle with compression of the kidney by the surrounding soft tissue mass being present (Fig.

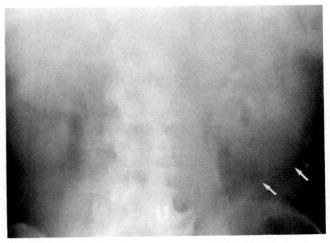

Figure 7.12. Tomogram demonstrates thickening and displacement of Gerota's fascia (*arrows*) secondary to a perinephric abscess.

7.11**B**). Loss of the normal mobility of the kidney (Mathe's sign) may be present; in such cases the position of the affected kidney appears fixed on upright radiographs and the respiratory excursion of the kidney is reduced. Maneuvers described in the older literature specifically designed to demonstrate this phenomenon on urography are no longer necessary as the diagnosis will be established on cross-sectional imaging.

On sonography, perinephric abscesses appear as masses of variable echogenicity adjacent to the kidney. Gas within the abscess will demonstrate acoustic shadowing, but the presence of gas within the abscess may be a source of confusion, especially when it is relatively anterior to the kidney, since it may be confused with shadowing from intestinal gas. Depending on its sonographic characteristics, US may underestimate the size of or even fail to detect the perinephric fluid collection entirely because its borders may blend into the normally echogenic perinephric fat (Fig. 7.11**D**).

There is consensus that CT is the imaging study of choice for the detection of perinephric abscess. Such abscesses are best detected when contrast-enhanced scans are obtained, but the abnormality is usually readily detected even when only unenhanced studies are possible. The strength of CT is its ability to define precisely the boundaries of the process so that extension into the psoas muscle, the posterior pararenal space, and into the true pelvis may all be accurately detected. As in intrarenal abscess, chronic perinephric abscess may demonstrate an enhancing rim (Fig. 7.10).

Percutaneous Drainage of Renal and Perinephric Abscesses

It is now well established that percutaneous drainage of renal and perinephric abscesses utilizing radiologic guidance is the preferred method of therapy, at least initially. Percutaneous drainage provides satisfactory clinical results utilizing local anesthesia and obviates the need for open surgical drainage.

Either fluoroscopic, ultrasonic, or CT guidance may be utilized. The method used largely depends on the experience and preference of the radiologist and the size and location of the cavity to be drained. When possible, we prefer the fluoroscopic method as it generally allows the drainage to be performed most quickly. Appropriate antibiotic coverage should be started. A variety of catheters and techniques may be utilized including the placement of a guidewire and catheter using the Seldinger technique and direct placement of the drainage catheter using a trocar catheter combination. Catheters ranging in size from 8 to 16 French may be used depending on the technique that is utilized for placement and the characteristics of the material to be drained. Self-retaining pigtail, sump, or malecot catheters may be utilized with equal degrees of success.

With large perinephric collections, it is preferable to place the drainage catheter in the most dependent portion of the abscess cavity. Loculated collections may require the placement of more than one catheter. When both renal and perinephric abscesses coexist, placement of separate drainage catheters in each collection provides the most efficient method of drainage (Fig. 7.13).

In most of the reported series, renal and perinephric abscesses are grouped in larger series of abdominal and pelvic abscesses. Sacks et al., however, have reported a series of renal and perirenal abscesses, separately, totaling 18 patients. Percutaneous drainage, as the sole therapy, was successful in management in 61% of the cases; in 39% successful temporization of the abscess was achieved by percutaneous methods. In these cases, surgery to correct the underlying condition that was associated with the development of the renal or perirenal abscess was performed. The period of drainage varied and ranged from a few days to 2 months. The drainage catheter may be removed when there is radiologic demonstration that the abscess cavity has resolved, there is absence of continued drainage, and the patient's clinical condition has improved.

Complications of renal abscess drainage include the exacerbation of urosepsis and hemorrhage. Migration of the drainage catheter into the GI tract also has been described.

Pyonephrosis

Pyonephrosis represents an obstructed, infected renal collecting system. Most authorities consider it to represent one of the few true urologic emergencies in that untreated pyonephrosis leads to sepsis and death. Until the advent of cross-sectional imaging studies and interventional uroradiologic techniques, the diagnosis of pyonephrosis was established by clinical or urologic methods. Radiologic techniques now provide a method for the diagnosis of pyonephrosis as well as its therapy.

Most patients with pyonephrosis have clinical evidence of urinary tract infection. In one series, however, the aspiration of infected urine under fluoroscopic guidance was the first evidence of urinary tract infection in approximately 10% of the cases. Calculi are the cause of the associated urinary tract obstruction in a majority of cases; metastatic disease, postoperative ureteral strictures, and such processes as retroperitoneal fibrosis account for the remainder.

The role of imaging studies in the diagnosis of pyonephrosis has been reported by Yoder et al. in a series of 70 patients. Plain abdominal radiographs demonstrated obvious urinary calculi in approximately one-half of the cases. Urography demonstrates findings typical of acute urinary tract obstruction in those cases where sufficient renal function permitted excretion of the contrast material; in approximately one-third of Yoder's

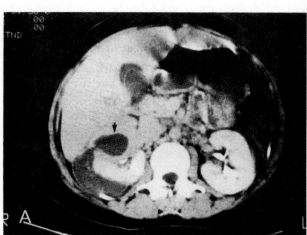

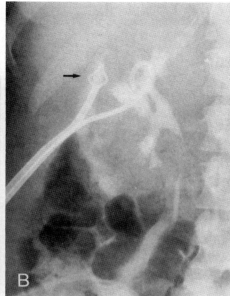

Figure 7.13. **A,** Computed tomography scan demonstrates an acute intrarenal abscess (*arrow*) with a large perinephric component inferior to the kidney. **B,** Two catheters were used for drainage; a pigtail catheter was placed in the intrarenal component, while a malecot catheter (*arrow*) was placed in the perinephric space.

cases, the involved kidney demonstrated no discernible contrast material excretion. In patients with ileal conduits, loopograms may be helpful by demonstrating partial or complete obstruction of the affected ureter. Radionuclide studies generally demonstrate diminished excretion of ^{99m}Tc-DTPA, but a dilated renal collecting system may be found on delayed images. Computed tomography usually shows evidence of hydronephrosis and generally demonstrates the cause and level of the associated obstruction. Rarely, layering of contrast material above purulent material in the collecting system is present, which allows a specific diagnosis of pyonephrosis to be entertained.

Sonography is the most reliable method by which pyonephrosis can be distinguished from uninfected hydronephrosis on imaging studies. The findings on US include: (*a*) persistent dependent echoes within the collecting system, (*b*) shifting urine-debris levels, (*c*) dense peripheral echoes with shadowing secondary to gas in the collecting system, and (*d*) low-level echoes within the dilated collecting system with poor through-transmission (Fig. 7.14). Subramanyam has reported sonography to have a sensitivity of 90% and an overall accuracy of 96% for this diagnosis among a group of 73 patients. Jeffrey, however, has reported that while the findings of medium- to coarse-intensity echoes within the collecting system had a specificity of 100% for pyonephrosis, the sensitivity of the study was only 62%. In this series, 10% of the patients with proven pyonephrosis had sonographic findings indistinguishable from uninfected hydronephrosis.

Percutaneous aspiration of infected urine utilizing radiologic guidance is the definitive diagnostic study in suspected pyonephrosis and is usually performed in association with percutaneous nephrostomy. Yoder has reported that percutaneous nephrostomy and antibiotics were successful as the only therapy for pyonephrosis in 33% of their cases; in 40% the procedure permitted successful temporization prior to a surgical procedure to remove the cause of obstruction. Nephrectomy was ultimately required in 20% while 5% of the patients died, commonly from sepsis. Twenty-eight percent of the pa-

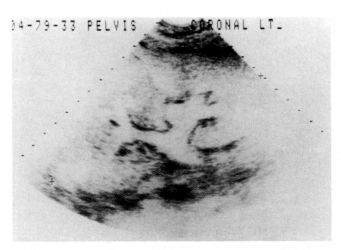

Figure 7.14. Multiple echoes representing pyonephrosis are present within a dilated renal collecting system. (Courtesy of Patricia Athey, M.D.)

tients in this series, however, suffered serious complications from the procedure including the development of temporally related frank sepsis, fever, shaking chills, and hemorrhagic shock.

Gas-forming Renal Infections

Gas may be present in the kidney from a variety of etiologies including the iatrogenic introduction of air during a surgical or radiologic procedure, as a result of a surgical procedure (i.e., the construction of an ileal conduit), or as the result of a renoalimentary fistula, external penetrating trauma, or urinary infection. In the later instance, the presence of gas usually indicates infection with a Gram-negative pathogen (*Escherichia coli* in 70%, followed by *Klebsiella, Aerobacter,* and *Proteus*) and is most common in diabetics in whom the presence of glycosuria is said to promote its production via the fermentation of glucose into carbon dioxide and hydrogen. Diabetes, however, is not a necessary precondition for the development of a gas-forming infection and its rare occurrence, even in diabetics, suggests that other factors such as altered host resistance play a role in its pathogenesis. As described earlier, gas may be present in acute or chronic renal abscesses or perinephric abscesses.

A variety of confusing terminology is used to describe other gas-forming infections. Most authorities agree that the term *emphysematous pyelonephritis* be reserved for those cases in which gas is found diffusely infiltrating the renal parenchyma (Fig. 7.15). More than 90% of the reported cases of this condition have been in diabetics. When the gas is confined to the kidney alone, a mortality rate of 60% has been reported in patients treated with antibiotics with or without surgical drainage. When there is extension of the gas into the perirenal space, the mortality rate on medical therapy alone is said to exceed 80%, however, with nephrectomy, there is a reduction in mortality to the 30–50% range. Gas within the lumen of the renal pelvis or calyces, termed an *air pyelogram* (Fig. 7.16), or gas within the walls of the renal pelvis with or without an air pyelogram, termed *emphysematous pyelitis* (Fig. 7.17), has a less grave implication than does true emphysematous pyelonephritis. Diabetes is present in approximately one-half of this group of patients and the condition has a considerably lower mortality, in the range of 15–20%.

Radiologic studies including plain films, excretory urography, and CT aid in the diagnosis of these conditions and especially in distinguishing gas-containing renal abscesses from gas either in the collecting system or in the renal parenchyma (Fig. 7.18). Emphysematous pyelonephritis has three sequential stages. Initially, a mottled lucency may be present extending radially along the renal pyramids. In more extensive renal emphysema, air may be found in a bubbled pattern within the paren-

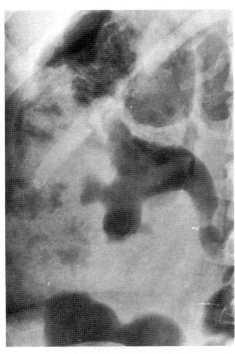

Figure 7.15. Emphysematous pyelonephritis. Coned view of the right kidney showing a bubbled appearance within the renal parenchyma secondary to diffuse infiltration of the kidney by gas. An air pyelogram and ureterogram are also present. (Courtesy of Davis S. Hartman, M.D., and the Armed Forces Institute of Pathology.)

chyma and there is associated air within the confines of Gerota's fascia. As the process ensues, air diffusely infiltrates the renal parenchyma and extends beyond the confines of Gerota's fascia within the retroperitoneum. These changes are well demonstrated by CT. Intramural gas or gas within the collecting system is usually also well

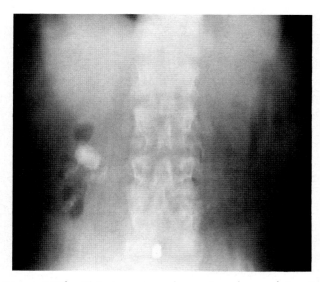

Figure 7.16. Plain tomogram shows air and several struvite calculi to be present within the right renal collecting system.

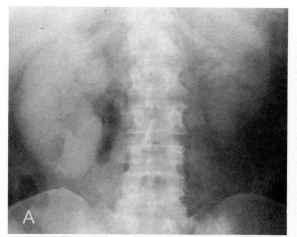

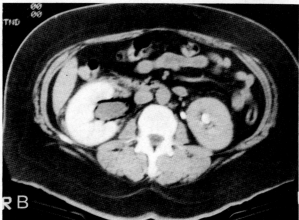

Figure 7.17.   A, Twelve-hour delayed film from an IVP demonstrates a persistent nephrogram in the right kidney with air in the walls of the renal pelvis and proximal ureter. **B,** Computed tomography clearly demonstrates the mural location of the air.

shown on CT where it can be distinguished from parenchymal air even in kidneys that fail to excrete contrast material.

Renal Fistula

The development of a renoalimentary fistula may result from Crohn's disease, tumors in either the kidney or the gastrointestinal tract, or severe renal trauma. Most commonly, however, they occur as a result of renal inflammatory disease. Usually fistulas develop between the kidney and the colon (Fig. 7.19), but the duodenum (Fig. 7.20), the stomach, and the distal small bowel may also be involved. The site of fistulization is principally determined by the anatomic proximity of the organ to the kidney. Renocutaneous fistulae and fistulae to the pleura or lung have also been described.

Renal fistulae occur in the setting of renal or perinephric abscesses or pyonephrosis, usually complicated by the presence of calculi. In the older literature, renal tubercu-

losis was described as the causative factor in 25% of the cases.

The diagnosis of renal fistulae will almost always require either retrograde or antegrade pyelography as the severe inflammatory disease requisite for the development of the fistula will preclude sufficient contrast material excretion for visualization on urography. A single case of a renal colic fistula in association with xanthogranulomatous pyelonephritis diagnosed by CT has been reported.

Xanthogranulomatous Pyelonephritis

Xanthogranulomatous pyelonephritis (XGP) is a relatively uncommon form of renal inflammatory disease characterized histologically by the presence of lipid-laden macrophages (xanthoma cells), as well as other inflammatory cells including plasma cells, leukocytes, and histiocytes. The classically described triad of findings include: (*a*) a staghorn calculus, (*b*) absent or diminished excretion of contrast material on urography, and (*c*) a poorly defined renal mass. The signs and symptoms of the disease are nonspecific with fever, malaise, flank pain or tenderness, weight loss and leukocytosis being the most common presenting complaints. Lower urinary tract symptoms (frequency, dysuria) are present in only one-half of the patients. Anemia is present in 70%, approximately 25% of the patients demonstrate abnormalities in liver function tests, and about 10% have underlying diabetes mellitus. Some series report as much as a 4 : 1 female preponderance. While most patients range in age from 45 to 65 years, patients as young as 5 years of age have been reported. Active urinary tract infection with *E. coli, Proteus mirabilis, Klebsiella,* or *Pseudomonas aeruginosa* either alone or in combination is present in virtually every case. Before the advent of cross-sectional imaging, the diagnosis of XGP was rarely established preoperatively.

XGP probably represents an uncommon reaction by the kidney to urinary tract obstruction in the presence of urinary tract infection. The obstruction is usually secondary to a calculus (75%), but less commonly may be secondary to ureteropelvic junction obstruction or a ureteral tumor. Symptoms of XGP are generally of long duration, being present in 40% of the cases for periods of greater than 6 months, from 1 to 6 months in another 40%, and less than 1 month in only 20%. Rarely, XGP may present as a fulminant illness and may be accompanied by an acute renal abscess. Either total or partial nephrectomy is the usual treatment.

Two forms of XGP have been described. The most common (85%) results in diffuse involvement of the affected kidney. Diffuse XGP may be staged as follows: Stage I, involvement is limited to the kidney; Stage II, involvement extends to the renal pelvis or the perirenal

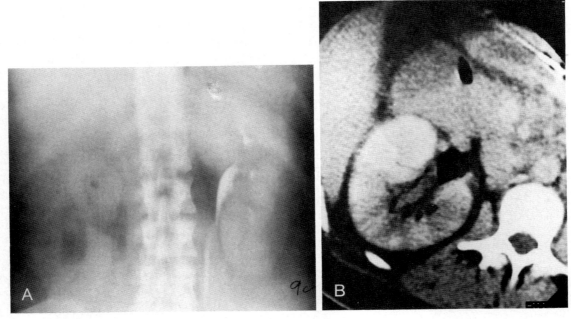

Figure 7.18. **A,** IVP shows a small amount of gas to be present within the poorly functioning right kidney, but it is not possible to distinguish whether this air collection is in the renal parenchyma or in the collecting system. **B,** Computed tomography scan clearly shows the gas is present within the renal collecting system.

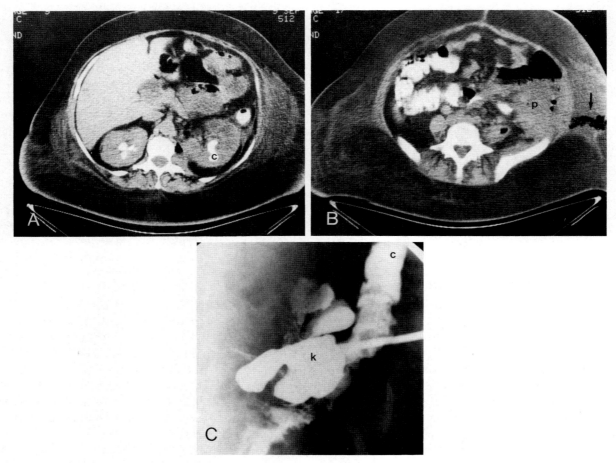

Figure 7.19. **A,** Computed tomography scan in an obese diabetic patient shows inflammatory changes involving the left kidney. A renal calculus (c) is also present. **B,** A more inferior section reveals a large amount of pus (p) in the perinephric space with an air-fluid level. Gas also extends into the soft tissues of the flank (*arrow*). **C,** A percutaneous drainage catheter was placed. Contrast injection reveals a fistula between the renal collecting system (k) and the descending colon (c).

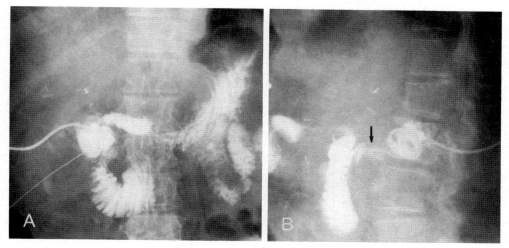

Figure 7.20. Anteroposterior **(A)** and lateral **(B)** radiographs after nephrostomy tube placement demonstrate a pyeloduodenal fistula (*arrow*).

fat within the confines of Gerota's fascia; Stage III, involvement extends beyond Gerota's fascia into the retroperitoneum, other organs, or both. A renoalimentary fistula may also rarely be present. The localized form of XGP (15%) is much less common; in such cases the inflammatory process is limited to a portion of the kidney. This form is sometimes referred to as the "tumefactive" form of XGP as the findings are more easily confused with those produced by a frank renal tumor. The majority of cases of both forms of XGP demonstrate extensive perinephric extension.

Plain abdominal radiography demonstrates the staghorn calculus and there is usually a poorly defined mass in the perinephric space. Loss of the psoas margin may be present but, as in perinephric abscess, is not a reliable sign. Urography demonstrates absent or reduced excretion of the contrast material in 85% of the cases (Fig. 7.21); where excretion sufficient for visualization is present, hydronephrosis is generally evident. Retrograde pyelography may be performed to demonstrate the point of obstruction. The calyces may be grossly irregular with evidence of superimposed papillary necrosis. Angiogra-

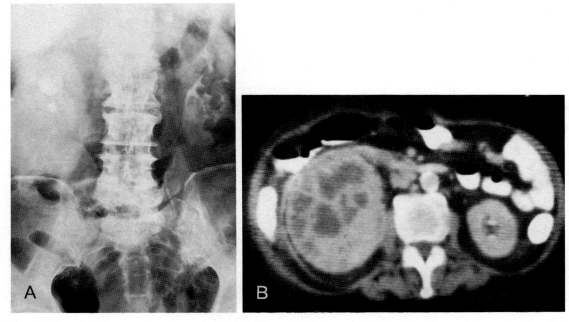

Figure 7.21. Diffuse xanthogranulomatous pyelonephritis. **A,** IVP shows a swollen poorly functioning right kidney containing multiple calculi. **B,** Computed tomography scan demonstrates multiple low-attenuation abscesses; however, the process is confined to the renal capsule.

phy, which is no longer routinely employed, shows marked splaying of the intrarenal branch vessels around avascular zones of tissue. In some cases neovascularity, reminiscent of a renal adenocarcinoma, may be found. Enlargement of the capsular branches, reflecting perinephric extension of the inflammatory process, may be present.

Sonography demonstrates diffuse renal enlargement with a central echogenic focus representing the staghorn calculus (Fig. 7.22). The renal parenchyma demonstrates a diffuse anechoic pattern which corresponds to the areas of inflammatory reaction or abscess. In some cases, however, the infected parenchyma may produce an echo pattern similar to that produced by normal renal parenchyma and is a source of potential confusion. The calyces may be shown as multiple fluid-filled masses with echo-producing debris.

While the CT findings in XGP are not specific for the disease, they usually strongly suggest the correct diagnosis. The kidney is diffusely enlarged but retains its reniform shape. The renal pelvis is characteristically poorly defined or normal in size, unless there is concomitant ureteropelvic junction obstruction. One or more calculi are generally present and there may be small flecks of parenchymal calcification as well. There are high-density areas at the periphery of the kidney representing atrophic parenchyma with inflamed columns of Bertin rimming low-attenuation central areas representing dilated calyces filled with pus and necrotic material. Subramanyam has suggested that the pus in patients with XGP will demonstrate an attenuation which ranges from −15 and +10 Hounsefield units, with the negative values being a reflection of the lipid-laden macrophages which characterize the disease process. Other investigators have found that the attenuation of the pus in XGP is indistinguishable from that found in conventional renal or peri-

nephric abscesses. Contrast-enhanced scans demonstrate hyperemia at the periphery of the kidney, around the calyces, and in the renal fascia. The degree of the extension to the perinephric space, the posterior pararenal space, the psoas, or the muscles of the back, is well demonstrated (Fig. 7.23). In the tumefactive form of XGP, CT may demonstrate a localized water-density mass which contains a calculus. In other cases, the findings are identical to that produced by diffuse XGP, albeit localized to one portion of the kidney.

Malacoplakia

Malacoplakia is an uncommon form of granulomatous renal inflammatory disease characterized histologically by the presence of distinctive histiocytes (von Hansemann cells) which contain basophilic staining inclusions called Michaelis-Gutmann bodies. These inclusions are thought to represent phagocytized fragments of bacteria. It has been postulated that malacoplakia represents an enzymatic defect within the histiocytes such that intracellular digestion of the phagocytized bacteria is incomplete. Malacoplakia may occur throughout the urinary tract as well as in a variety of other organs including the gastrointestinal tract, the uterus, the vagina, the adrenal gland, the breast, skeleton, and brain. Renal parenchymal malacoplakia (RPM) accounts for 16% of the reported cases in the urinary tract.

RPM occurs in women 4 times as frequently as in men. Patients ranging in age from as young as 6 weeks to 85 years have been reported. The peak incidence is in patients over 50 years of age. Fever, flank pain, and a palpable flank mass are the most common presenting complaints. Most patients have active urinary tract infection

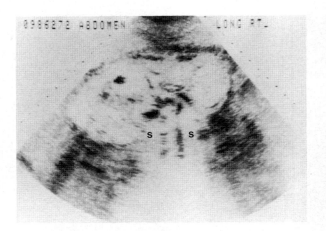

Figure 7.22. Xanthogranulomatous pyelonephritis. A longitudinal sonogram demonstrates a diffusely enlarged kidney. Multiple acoustic shadows (s) are produced by a staghorn calculus. (Courtesy of Patricia Athey, M.D.)

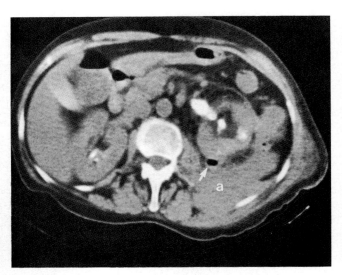

Figure 7.23. Computed tomography scan in a patient with xanthogranulomatous pyelonephritis showing extension of the inflammatory process into the perinephric space (a). A gas-containing intrarenal abscess is also present (*arrow*).

(*E. coli* in 90%). There is often a history of altered host resistance including autoimmune disease, alcoholism, carcinoma, or rheumatoid arthritis.

Two forms of RPM have been described. Multifocal involvement occurs in 75% of the cases and is reported to be bilateral in half of these. The kidney is enlarged and contains multiple yellow-brown masses which range in size from a few millimeters to a few centimeters. Unifocal RPM (25% of the cases) presents as a solitary mass ranging in size from 2 to 8 cm which is sharply demarcated from the remainder of the kidney.

The radiologic findings depend on the pattern of involvement that is present. With multifocal RPM there is frequently diffuse enlargement of the kidney. Excretion of contrast is diminished in more than half of the cases, presumably secondary to extensive renal parenchymal replacement. In some cases, the urogram may demonstrate a mass impressing the calyces. Sonography may demonstrate multiple ill-defined masses of varying echo intensity. Computed tomography demonstrates multiple soft tissue masses within the kidney that enhance less than normal renal parenchyma. Extension of the inflammatory process into the retroperitoneum may also be demonstrated (Fig. 7.24**A**). Angiography demonstrates stretching of intrarenal branch vessels with an inhomogeneous angiographic nephrogram (Fig. 7.24**B**). Neovascularity of the parenchymal masses may be present making differentiation from renal tumors difficult. Renal vein thrombosis complicating multifocal RPM has also been described.

With unifocal RPM, the dominant radiographic findings are that of a mass. On urography, the mass is indistinguishable from those produced by frank renal tumors or other inflammatory conditions. The sonographic features are that of a complex mass.

Because the radiographic findings in malacoplakia are not specific, the diagnosis is only rarely established preoperatively. Major organ involvement is reported to have a 50% mortality. Nephrectomy is the usual treatment for unilateral disease. With bilateral disease, renal failure is the rule.

Chronic Pyelonephritis

The term *chronic pyelonephritis* is used to denote a set of morphologic changes in the adult kidney that result from a previous episode of acute renal infection. As such, the term chronic pyelonephritis is a source of confusion in that the term implies an indolent or recurrent state of infection. Since this is not the case, many authorities feel that the term *chronic atrophic pyelonephritis* or the etiologic appellation, *reflux nephropathy,* is better suited to describe the morphologic changes that occur.

Much of the current understanding of the pathology of chronic pyelonephritis derives from the work of the

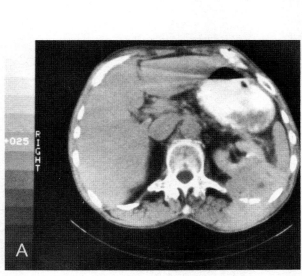
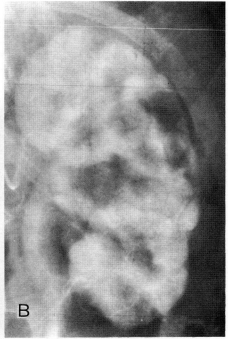

Figure 7.24.   Renal parenchymal malacoplakia. **A,** Computed tomography scan shows a large, inhomogeneous, poorly marginated mass arising from the posterior aspect of the left kidney. There is extension into the perinephric space and left flank. **B,** Nephrogram phase from a selective renal angiogram shows a diffusely inhomogeneous nephrogram consistent with the multifocal form of involvement. (Courtesy of Davis S. Hartman, M.D., and the Armed Forces Institute of Pathology.)

late C. J. Hodson who extensively investigated the relationship between renal parenchymal scarring, vesicoureteral reflux, and renal infection. Hodson proposed that the parenchymal scarring that characterizes chronic pyelonephritis is actually the result of vesicoureteral reflux and the subsequent reflux of urine back into the renal tubules, a process known as *intrarenal reflux*. He demonstrated experimentally in pigs that intrarenal reflux of infected urine produced pathologic changes in the kidney identical to those found in chronic pyelonephritis. Thus, chronic atrophic pyelonephritis may be thought of as the residua of a previous episode of acute pyelonephritis.

Ransley and Risdon, expanding on the work of Hodson, discovered that the anatomy of the papilla was the determining factor governing its propensity for intrarenal reflux. In a simple papilla, the openings of the papillary ducts are slit-like; when there is elevated pressure in the collecting system as a result of vesicoureteral reflux, these slit-like orifices close and no intrarenal reflux occurs. However, in the compound calyces found in the polar regions of the kidney, the orifices of the ducts of Bellini tend to be circular; when intrapelvic pressure rises these circular openings allow intrarenal reflux to occur. Further observations have shown that the shape of the opening of the papillary ducts in all compound calyces is not uniform; some are more prone to reflux than others.

The effect of the intrarenal reflux of infected urine is to cause an acute inflammatory reaction in the renal parenchyma that overlies that papilla; this ultimately results in parenchymal scarring which extends throughout the thickness of the renal cortex and causes retraction of the overlying calyx. Hodson referred to this inflammatory reaction as "acute lobar nephronia," as its distribution reflects the lobar architecture of the kidney. Thus, scarring associated with this intrarenal reflux has a characteristic appearance; it must extend through the entire thickness of the renal parenchyma and must be associated with deformity of the calyx adjacent to the scar. *It is important to note that the scarring associated with reflux nephropathy occurs only in early childhood, usually before the age of 4 years.* Older children and adults appear to recover from an episode of intrarenal reflux without permanent structural damage to the kidney. Thus, the radiologic picture in the adult reflects disease in early childhood.

The question as to whether changes of reflux nephropathy can also develop as a result of reflux of *uninfected* urine is unsettled. Although most authorities believe that the presence of urinary infection is an essential component of this process, there is experimental evidence that scarring from high pressure intrarenal reflux can occur with sterile urine. Indeed, reflux of sterile urine in utero has been postulated as being the etiology

of Ask-Upmark kidney, a segmental hypoplastic renal anomaly.

A small number of adults with characteristic changes of reflux nephropathy present with a clinical picture of renin-mediated hypertension. If the process is bilateral, renal failure may also occur. Thus the importance of detecting significant vesicoureteral reflux in children with urinary tract infections is underscored.

The radiologic findings in chronic pyelonephritis on urography include the demonstration of one or more parenchymal scars typically in the polar regions of the kidney overlying a deformed calyx (Fig. 7.25). There may be focal areas of compensatory hypertrophy adjacent to the areas of cortical scarring. The intervening areas of the kidney appear normal. In less severe cases, only an area of parenchymal thickening will be present and there may be no adjoining calyceal abnormality. It is not possible, in such cases, to be certain of the etiology of the parenchymal abnormality as other causes of parenchymal scarring (i.e., renal infarction) may produce an identical appearance. Only when the characteristic radiologic picture is present can a definitive diagnosis be established.

Ultrasound changes in patients with chronic atrophic pyelonephritis include a focal loss of parenchyma which can be appreciated on longitudinal or cross-sectional images. Increased echogenicity in the area of the scar may also be demonstrated. The central renal sinus echoes may be extended to the periphery of the kidney in the area of abnormality. Once again the process appears focal in contrast to other causes of generalized increased cortical echogenicity. Similarly, anatomic abnormalities may

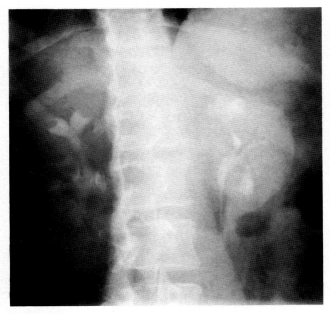

Figure 7.25.   Oblique film from an IVP shows scarring in the polar regions of the kidney associated with calyceal clubbing as a result of reflux nephropathy.

also be demonstrated on CT, but the degree to which the calyceal deformity is present may not be appreciated on this study.

RENAL TUBERCULOSIS

Renal tuberculosis results from hematogenous dissemination of mycobacterium tuberculosis from a distant site, usually in the lungs or bones. Bacilli lodge in the corticomedullary junction of the kidney where most heal without sequela. Since the initial lesions occur as a result of hematogenous dissemination, multiple bilateral lesions are initially produced; in approximately three-quarters of the cases, however, active tuberculomas form in only one kidney. The lesions then progress along the nephron to rupture into the pelvocalyceal system.

While there has been a decline in the incidence of pulmonary tuberculosis, the incidence of extra-pulmonary tuberculosis has largely remained unchanged. New cases continue to be diagnosed in the United States, particularly among the immigrant population. A history of tuberculosis in another site is present in virtually all cases, however, that site may be inactive at the time of presentation of the renal involvement. Kollins et al. report that evidence of pulmonary tuberculosis is found on chest radiography in only about 50% of the patients with active urinary tract infection. In only 10% of the patients is active pulmonary disease present in coexistence with the renal lesions.

Within the urinary tract the renal lesions progress in an indolent fashion, often producing little clinical symptomatology until the entire urinary tract is affected. As such, lower urinary tract symptoms including frequency, dysuria, and nocturia are the most common presenting complaints. About one-quarter of the patients have gross hematuria. Approximately 10% of the patients will be completely asymptomatic, but will be found on examination to have the classical laboratory findings of sterile pyuria—the presence of white blood cells in the urine with subsequently sterile cultures on conventional culture media. Generalized constitutional symptoms are unusual; in one series they were present in less than 10% of the cases.

The radiologic findings in renal tuberculosis depend upon the extent of the disease process. In one-third of the patients in Kollins' series, plain film examination provided evidence of extraurinary tract tuberculosis that alerted the radiologist to the presence of the disease. Such findings include evidence of skeletal tuberculosis in the hip or sacroiliac joints, or in the spine, with or without a paraspinous abscess, and calcification in abdominal or retroperitoneal lymph nodes.

Radiologic abnormalities are demonstrated in the majority of cases of renal tuberculosis. In approximately 10% of the cases in Kollins' series, however, urography

was considered normal even when active infection was demonstrated with positive urinary cultures. Urographic abnormalities include the following:

Papillary Abnormalities

In the earliest stages of renal tuberculosis, the tips of the papilla demonstrate a moth-eaten, irregular appearance. As the disease progresses, extensive papillary necrosis may be present with the formation of frank cavities which may communicate with each other as a result of caseous necrosis within the renal parenchyma.

Parenchymal Calcification

Calcification occurs throughout the renal parenchyma in approximately one-third to one half of the cases (Fig. 7.26). Two types of calcification are described: (*a*) an amorphous granular opacity associated with granulomatous masses, and (*b*) dense, punctate calcifications which likely represent healed tuberculomas. In addition, approximately 20% of the patients demonstrate frank renal calculi.

Parenchymal Scarring

Parenchymal scarring may be present in 20% of the cases and may be either localized to a single area of the kidney or may involve the entire kidney. The scars are generally associated with underlying calyceal abnormalities and parenchymal calcifications.

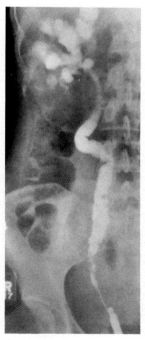

Figure 7.26. Renal tuberculosis. Retrograde pyelogram shows multiple ureteral strictures and infundibular stenoses characteristic of tuberculosis.

Calyceal Abnormalities

The hallmark of renal tuberculosis is the development of multiple irregular infundibular stenoses or strictures with subsequent hydrocalycosis (Figs. 7.26 and 7.27). When the strictures are complete, the entire calyx may be excluded from the remainder of the collecting system. The renal pelvis is typically small and contracted. These stenoses are the result of fibrosis that accompanies the healing process.

The degree to which these changes will be shown on urography depends on the degree to which renal function is compromised. In more than 50% of the cases, renal function is sufficiently compromised at the time of presentation so that either antegrade or retrograde pyelography is necessary. As a majority of cases are associated with inflammatory changes in the urinary bladder as well, retrograde catheterization of the ureteral orifices may be either difficult or impossible. Advanced renal tuberculosis presents with a completely nonfunctioning kidney—the so-called autonephrectomy (Fig. 7.28). Extensive parenchymal calcification is typically present in such cases. In other cases where poor excretion of contrast is demonstrated, a tuberculous pyonephrosis (Fig. 7.27) will be present as a result of obstruction from extensive ureteral stricture formation.

Since demonstration of the typical calyceal and ureteral abnormalities is critical to establishing the diagnosis of renal tuberculosis, conventional radiologic contrast studies remain the procedures of choice. While calyceal clubbing may be demonstrated by CT, the delineation of infundibular stenoses may be difficult on cross-sectional imaging. Sonography will also rarely demonstrate specific features of renal tuberculosis. The parenchyma may demonstrate intrarenal masses of varying echogenicity which represent liquefying tuberculous cavities. A sonographic clue to the diagnosis is the demonstration of dilated calyces without commensurate dilatation of the renal pelvis.

UNCOMMON RENAL INFECTIONS

Fungal Infections

Fungal diseases of the kidney develop as opportunistic infections occurring principally in the setting of altered host resistance from such diverse entities as diabetes mellitus, the use of systemic antibiotics, immunosuppressive and chemotherapeutic agents, the use of indwelling intravenous or urinary catheters, acquired immunodeficiency, and renal transplantation. Renal involvement most commonly occurs with infections secondary to *Candida albicans* or other candida species, but has been reported in association with *Coccidiomycosis immitis, Cryptococcus neoformans, Torulopsis glabrata,* and *Aspergillus fumigatus.* Fungal infections may also complicate conventional Gram-negative urinary tract infections.

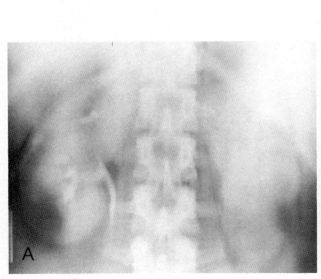 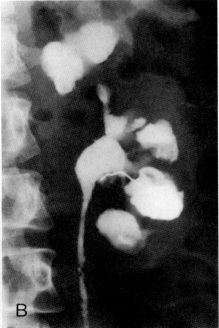

Figure 7.27.   Renal tuberculosis. **A,** IVP demonstrates multiple lucencies in the left kidney which represent dilated, but unopacified calyces (negative pyelogram). **B,** Antegrade pyelogram shows characteristic infundibular stenoses, calyceal dilatation, and a contracted renal pelvis. Strictures are also present in the proximal ureter.

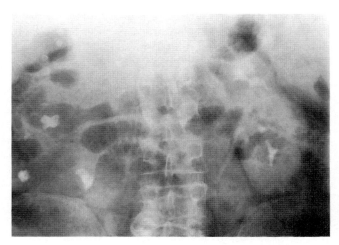

Figure 7.28.   There is a nonfunctioning right kidney containing multiple course calcifications representing a tuberculous autonephrectomy.

Candidiasis

Candida is a ubiquitous organism normally found in the pharynx, the gastrointestinal tract, or vagina. Two patterns of renal involvement with *Candida* have been described. In systemic candidiasis, infection is spread to the kidneys as a result of hematogenous dissemination of the organisms with involvement of the kidneys and multiple other organs including the brain and lungs. The patient is desperately ill with fever, leukocytosis, splenomegaly, and azotemia. Disseminated candidiasis is invariably fatal if not treated.

Primary renal candidiasis occurs without associated hematogenous or major organ involvement. It is a less fulminant illness than renal involvement associated with systemic candidiasis. Most of the reported patients have been women and there is a strong association with diabetes mellitus. The pathogenesis of primary renal candidiasis is also thought to be a result of hematogenous dissemination of the organism, but in a mild form. Ascending spread from the lower urinary tract has also been implicated. In many of the reported cases, however, asymmetric involvement of the kidneys is present with demonstrable lesions in only one kidney. The fungi are filtered by the glomerulus and lodge in the distal tubules. Proliferation of the fungi results in multiple medullary and cortical abscesses producing an acute fungal pyelonephritis. There is a diffuse fungal infiltration of the tips of the renal papilla, producing papillary necrosis. The fungi are then extruded into the renal collecting system with subsequent formation of fungus balls (mycetoma), which may then obstruct the renal pelvis or ureter producing hydronephrosis or renal colic. With severe infection, renal failure may ensue. The diagnosis is established by the demonstration of the fungal hyphae on direct examination of the urine.

Radiologic findings include diminished excretion of the contrast material on urography, papillary necrosis, and hydronephrosis. The characteristic finding of candidiasis is the demonstration of multiple filling defects ranging in size from 1 to 4 cm within the collecting system representing fungus balls (Fig. 7.29). Scalloping of the ureters related to submucosal edema, analogous to the changes in the esophagus produced by oral thrush, has also been reported. With diminished renal function, antegrade or retrograde pyelography may be necessary for demonstration of the changes in the renal collecting system. On sonography, the fungus balls may be recognized as hyperechogenic masses within the collecting system with no acoustic shadowing. On CT, low-attenuation lesions, representing microabscesses that are best demonstrated following contrast enhancement, may be found.

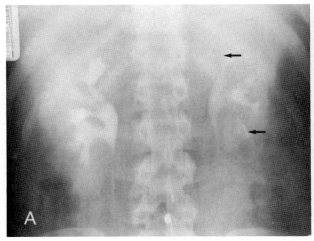
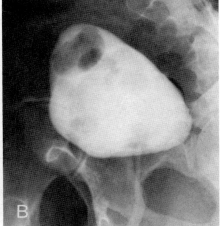

Figure 7.29.   Renal candidiasis. **A,** IVP demonstrates papillary necrosis in the left kidney with multiple small filling defects (*arrows*) representing fungus balls. **B,** Cystogram in the same patient shows multiple large fungus balls.

Percutaneous nephrostomy with percutaneous removal of the fungus balls has been reported as an adjunctive therapy.

Other Fungal Infections

Infection with coccidiomycosis occurs as a result of an active focus of infection elsewhere, usually in the lungs. Renal manifestations including papillary necrosis, cavitation, and parenchymal calcification have all been reported. Cryptococcus infection may produce cavitation, papillary necrosis, and multiple parenchymal abscesses.

Brucellosis

Brucellosis of the kidney occurs primarily in meat packers or from the ingestion of unpasteurized milk. The renal infection occurs as a result of hematogenous dissemination of the organism. The renal involvement is radiologically similar to that produced by tuberculosis with extensive calcification, cavitation, and the production of infundibular strictures.

Actinomycosis

Actinomycosis of the kidney usually occurs as a result of infection of the gastrointestinal tract with spread to the kidney via a renoalimentary fistula or by fistulization through the diaphragm from the lung. The causative organism, *Actinomycosis israelii,* while producing mycelial colonies similar to fungi, is actually a bacterium usually sensitive to penicillin. Infection may result in a picture of acute pyelonephritis, a pyonephrosis, or a granulomatous renal abscess.

Hydatid Disease

Renal hydatid disease is caused by infestation of a tapeworm, usually *Echinococcus granulosis.* Dogs or other canines constitute the primary host for the disease. The eggs of the worm are swallowed, hatch in the gastrointestinal tract, and then enter the portal circulation where the oncospheres lodge in multiple organs, mainly the liver and lungs. Renal hydatid disease occurs in approximately 2–3% of the patients. The renal involvement may be primary or secondary. In primary hydatid disease, the worms reach the kidney via the arterial circulation; in secondary renal infestation, the worms spread to the urinary tract as a result of involvement of an adjacent organ, such as the liver.

Within the kidney, the worms form a characteristic three-layered hydatid cyst which may grow rapidly and destroy the kidney or may progress very slowly, producing minimal clinical symptoms. One or more daughter cysts may form from the mother cyst. Symptoms of renal involvement are nonspecific, but include flank pain, renal colic, and eosinophilia. At the time of presentation, the average hydatid cyst is approximately 8 cm in diameter.

Radiologic manifestations include the presence of a well-defined soft tissue mass in the renal fossa on plain films. Curvilinear calcification is present in the wall of the cyst in about one-third of the cases. On urography, distortion of the renal pelvis or calyces may be evident (the "crescent sign"). Communication between the cyst and the collecting system results in a characteristic appearance, especially when there is also filling of the daughter cysts. This finding has been called the "bunch of grapes" sign. Extensive renal destruction may result in a nonfunctioning kidney.

On sonography, hydatid cysts appear as round, homogeneous, echo-free masses. The presence of daughter cysts may be readily identified. Dependent echoes within the cyst secondary to hydatid sand (hooks, scolices, and brood capsules of the worms) may be present. When the patient is moved or changes position, movement of these echoes produces the "falling snowflake" sign, said to be pathognomonic of the disease.

The advisability of diagnostic cyst puncture in hydatid disease has been debated for many years. While such a procedure is diagnostic, concern that the puncture will cause spread of the disease to uninfected areas has been raised. In addition, venous intravasation of the cyst fluid has been reported to cause acute anaphylaxis.

SUGGESTED READINGS

General References

Benson M, Li Puma JP, Resnick MI: The role of imaging studies in urinary tract infection. *Urol Clin North Am* 13(4):605, 1986.

Corriere JN, Jr, Sandler CM: The diagnosis and immediate therapy of acute renal and perirenal infections. *Urol Clin North Am* 9(2):219, 1982.

Gold RP, McClennan BL, Rottenberg RR: CT appearance of acute inflammatory disease of the renal interstitium. *AJR* 141:343, 1983.

Hoddick W, Jeffrey RB, Goldberg HI, et al: CT and sonography of severe renal and perirenal infections. *AJR* 140:517, 1983.

Morehouse HT, Weiner SN, Hoffman JC: Imaging in inflammatory disease of the kidney. *AJR* 143:135, 1984.

Rauschkolb EN, Sandler CM, Patel S, et al: Computed tomography of renal inflammatory disease. *J Comput Assist Tomogr* 6(3):502, 1982.

Soulen MC, Fishman EK, Goldman SM, Gatewood OMB: Bacterial renal infection: role of CT. *Radiology* 171:703, 1989.

Wicks JD, Thornbury JR: Acute renal infections in adults. *Radiol Clin North Am* 115(2):245, 1979.

Acute Pyelonephritis

Dinkle E, Orth S, Dittrich M, et al: Renal sonography in the differentiation of upper from lower urinary tract infection. *AJR* 146:775, 1986.

Edell SL, Bonavita JA: The sonographic appearance of acute pyelonephritis. *Radiology* 132:683, 1979.

Handmaker H: Nuclear renal imaging in acute pyelonephritis. *Semin Nucl Med* 12(3):246, 1982.

Harrison RB, Shaffer HA: The roentgenographic findings in acute pyelonephritis. *JAMA* 241(16):1718, 1979.

Mendez G, Jr, Morilo G, Alonso M, et al: Gallium-67 radionuclide imaging in acute pyelonephritis. *AJR* 134:17, 1980.

Senn E, Zaunbauer W, Bandhauer K, et al: Computed tomography in acute pyelonephritis. *Br J Urol* 59:118, 1987.

Silver TM, Kass EJ, Thornbury JR, et al: The radiological spectrum of acute pyelonephritis in adults and adolescents. *Radiology* 118:65, 1976.

Acute Focal Bacterial Nephritis

McDonough WD, Sandler CM, Benson GS: Acute focal bacterial nephritis: focal pyelonephritis that may simulate renal abscess. *J Urol* 126:670, 1981.

Rosenfield AT, Glickman MG, Taylor KJW, et al: Acute focal bacterial nephritis (acute lobar nephronia). *Radiology* 132:553, 1979.

Zaontz MR, Pahira JJ, Wolfman M, et al: Acute focal bacterial nephritis: a systematic approach to diagnosis and treatment. *J Urol* 133:752, 1985.

Acute Bacterial Nephritis

Davidson AJ, Talner LB: Late sequelae of adult-onset acute bacterial nephritis. *Radiology* 127:367, 1978.

Ishikawa I, Saito Y, Onouchi Z, et al: Delayed contrast enhancement in acute focal bacterial nephritis: CT features. *J Comput Assist Tomogr* 9(5):894, 1985.

Lillienfeld RM, Lande A: Acute adult onset bacterial nephritis: long term urographic and angiographic followup. *J Urol* 114:14, 1975.

Renal and Perirenal Abscesses

Gerzof SH, Gale ME: Computed tomography and ultrasonography for diagnosis and treatment of renal and retroperitoneal abscesses. *Urol Clin North Am* 9:185, 1982.

Morgan WR, Nyberg LM, Jr: Perinephric and intrarenal abscesses. *Urology* 26(6):529, 1985.

Percutaneous Drainage of Renal and Perinephric Abscesses

Bernardino ME, Baumgartner BR: Percutaneous abscess drainage in the genitourinary tract. *Radiol Clin North Am* 24:539, 1986.

Gobien RP, Stanley JH, Schabel SI, et al: The effect of drainage tube size on adequacy of percutaneous abscess drainage. *Cardiovasc Intervent Radiol* 8:100, 1985.

Sacks D, Banner MP, Meranze SG, et al: Renal and related retroperitoneal abscesses: Percutaneous drainage. *Radiology* 167:447, 1988.

Pyonephrosis

Jeffrey RB, Laing FC, Wing VW, et al: Sensitivity of sonography in pyonephrosis: a reevaluation. *AJR* 144:71, 1985.

Subramanyam BR, Raghavendra BN, Bosniak MA, et al: Sonography of pyonephrosis: a prospective study. *AJR* 140:991, 1983.

Yoder IC, Pfister RC, Lindfors KK, et al: Pyonephrosis: imaging and intervention. *AJR* 141:735, 1983.

Gas-forming Renal Infections

Evanoff GV, Thompson CS, Foley R, et al: Spectrum of gas within the kidney. Emphysematous pyelonephritis and emphysematous pyelitis. *Am J Med* 83:149, 1987.

Lautin EM, Gordon PM, Friedman AC, et al: Emphysematous pyelonephritis: optimal diagnosis and treatment. *Urol Radiol* 1:93, 1979.

Zweig GJ, Li YP, Srinantaswarny S, Chandramouli S, et al: Gas-forming infections of the abdomen: plain film findings. *Appl Radiol* 19:37, 1990.

Xanthogranulomatous Pyelonephritis

Goldman SM, Hartman DS, Fishman EK, et al: CT of xanthogranulomatous pyelonephritis: radiologic-pathologic correlation. *AJR* 141:963, 1984.

Parker MD, Clark RL: Evolving concepts in the diagnosis of xanthogranulomatous pyelonephritis. *Urol Radiol* 11:7, 1989.

Sandler CM, Foucar E, Toombs BD: Xanthogranulomatous pyelonephritis with air containing intrarenal abscesses. *Urol Radiol* 2:113, 1980.

Subramanyam BR, Megibow AJ, Raghavendra BN, et al: Diffuse xanthogranulomatous pyelonephritis: Analysis by computed tomography and sonography. *Urol Radiol* 4:5, 1982.

Van Kirk OC, Go RT, Wedel VJ: Sonographic features of xanthogranulomatous pyelonephritis. *AJR* 134:1035, 1980.

Zafaranloo S, Gerard PS, Bryk D: Xanthogranulomatous pyelonephritis in children: analysis by diagnostic modalities. *Urolog Radiol* 12:18, 1990.

Malacoplakia

Arap S, Denes, FT, Silva J, et al: Malakoplakia of the urinary tract. *Eur Urol* 12:113, 1986.

Hartman DS, Davis DJ Jr, Lichtenstein JE, et al: Renal parenchymal malacoplakia. *Radiology* 136:33, 1980.

Long JP Jr, Althausen AF: Malacoplakia: A 25-year experience with a review of the literature. *J Urol* 141:1328, 1989.

Miller OS, Finck FM: Malacoplakia of the kidney: the great impersonator. *J Urol* 103:712, 1970.

Chronic Pyelonephritis

Hodson CJ: Reflux nephropathy: a personal historical review. *AJR* 137:451, 1981.

Kay CJ, Rosenfield AT, Taylor KJW, et al: Ultrasonic characteristics of chronic atrophic pyelonephritis. *AJR* 132:47, 1979.

Ransley PG, Risdon RA: Reflux and renal scarring. *Br J Radiol* (Suppl 14):1, 1978.

Renal Tuberculosis

Cohen MC: Granulomatous nephritis. *Urol Clin North Am* 13(4):647, 1986.

Kollins SA, Hartman GW, Carr DT, et al: Roentgenographic findings in urinary tract tuberculosis. A 10 year review. *AJR* 121(3):487, 1974.

Roylance J, Penry JB, Davies ER, et al: The radiology of tuberculosis of the urinary tract. *Clin Radiol* 21:163, 1970.

Fungal Infections

Clark RE, Minagi H, Palubinskas AJ: Renal candidiasis. *Radiology* 101:567, 1971.

Dembner AG, Pfister RC: Fungal infection of the urinary tract: demonstration by antegrade pyelography and drainage by percutaneous nephrostomy. *AJR* 129:415, 1977.

Fisher J, Mayhall G, Duma R, et al: Fungus balls of the urinary tract. *South Med J* 72(10):1281, 1979.

Gerle RD: Roentgenographic features of primary renal candidiasis. *AJR* 119:731, 1973.

Irby PB, Stoller ML, McAninch JW: Fungal bezoars of the upper urinary tract. *J Urol* 143:447, 1990.

Michigan S: Genitourinary fungal infections. *J Urol* 116:390, 1976.

Shirkhoda A: CT findings in hepatosplenic and renal candidiasis. *J Comput Assist Tomogr* 11(5):795, 1987.

Stuck KJ, Silver TM, Jaffe MH, et al: Sonographic demonstration of renal fungus balls. *Radiology* 142:473, 1981.

Zirinsky K, Auh YH, Hartman BJ, et al: Computed tomography of renal aspergillosis. *J Comput Assist Tomogr* 11:177, 1987.

Hydatid Disease

Aragona F, DiCandio G, Serretta V, et al: Renal hydatid disease: report of 9 cases and discussion of urologic diagnostic procedures. *Urol Radiol* 6:182, 1984.

Saint Martin G, Chiesa JC: "Falling snowflakes", an ultrasound sign of hydatid sand. *J Ultrasound Med* 3:257, 1984.

CHAPTER 8

VASCULAR DISEASES

ANATOMY

Arterial

The renal arteries arise from the aorta near the level of the L1-L2 interspace. The right renal artery usually arises from the lateral or anterolateral aspect of the aorta and slightly lower than the left renal artery, which arises from the lateral or posterolateral aspect of the aorta. Thus, aortography should be performed in the anteroposterior or slight right posterior oblique projections to demonstrate the origin of the renal arteries to best advantage.

In as many as 40% of patients, one or both kidneys are supplied by more than one renal artery. Accessory renal arteries arise from the aorta and are usually distal to the main renal artery (Fig. 8.1). Occasionally an accessory renal artery supplies the upper pole of the kidney, and rarely an accessory renal artery may arise from the celiac, hepatic, or mesenteric arteries. Anomalous kidneys, such as a horseshoe or pelvic kidney, almost always have multiple accessory renal arteries.

The inferior adrenal artery and arteries supplying the renal capsule, renal pelvis, and ureter arise from the main renal artery. Occasionally, the gonadal, middle adrenal, or inferior phrenic arteries may also arise from the renal artery.

The main renal artery divides into dorsal and ventral rami that run posterior and anterior to the renal pelvis. The larger ventral division supplies the anterior and superior aspects of the kidney while the dorsal division supplies the posterior and inferior portions.

Segmental branches arise from the dorsal and ventral rami and run along the infundibulae before dividing into interlobar arteries. These interlobar arteries course between the pyramid and the cortical column before branching into arcuate arteries which run along the bases of the medullary pyramids.

Collateral pathways which provide arterial supply to the kidney when the main renal artery is compromised include the inferior adrenal, capsular, ureteric, gonadal, intercostal, lumbar, and pelvic arteries. The upper three lumbar arteries allow blood from the aorta to communicate with pelvic, ureteral, or capsular arteries which anastomose with renal branch arteries. When the ureteral artery serves as a major collateral, the dilation and tortuosity resulting from increased blood flow may impinge on the ureter, causing notching (Fig. 8.2).

Although the intrarenal arteries have been considered end arteries, some intrarenal collateral pathways exist. Trueta described small coiled arteries which lie near the calyces. They arise from the interlobar arteries and communicate with vessels in the pelvic mucosa, as well as adjacent interlobar arteries. Perforating arteries also provide communication between renal arcuate or interlobular arteries and capsular vessels. These intrarenal collateral arteries are not sufficient to prevent renal infarction but may minimize the effects of ischemia by helping to preserve renal parenchyma.

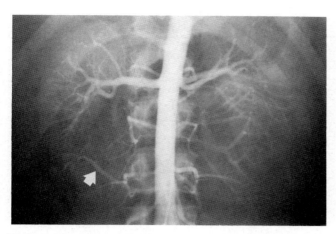

Figure 8.1.   Accessory renal artery. An abdominal aortogram demonstrates an accessory renal artery (*arrow*) supplying the lower pole of the right kidney.

Venous

In general, the venous anatomy parallels the arterial circulation. Accessory renal veins are less frequent than accessory arteries, and when they occur they are more common on the right. However, the left renal vein may bifurcate to encircle the aorta and become a circumaortic renal vein. This is due to persistence of the posteriorly located left supracardinal vein and a midline supracardinal anastomosis between right and left vessels. It is a relatively common anomaly, reported in 2–16% of pa-

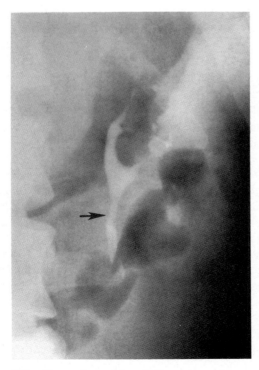

Figure 8.2.   Ureteral notching. Collateral arteries create extrinsic compression (*arrow*) on the proximal ureter in this patient with renal artery stenosis.

tients, according to anatomic and angiographic studies. Using CT, Reed et al. found a circumaortic left renal vein in 19 (4.4%) of 433 cases (Fig. 8.3). The posterior portion of this venous collar typically runs inferiorly before crossing behind the aorta to reach the inferior vena cava.

Patients with a circumaortic left renal vein are asymptomatic, although one case with hematuria and proteinuria has been reported. Knowledge of this anomaly is important when surgery is contemplated or during collection of renal or adrenal vein samples. The ventral vein usually drains the ventral and inferior portions of the kidney while the dorsal component drains the dorsal and superior segments.

A circumaortic left renal vein can also be seen during angiography. Late films from a selective left renal arteriogram may demonstrate both ventral and dorsal components. During venography care must be taken not to overlook the more inferior entrance of the dorsal vein into the inferior vena cava (IVC). Both left renal veins may also be seen during inferior vena cavography.

Another common anomaly, the retroaortic left renal vein, is seen less frequently. In the same series of CT examinations reported by Reed et al., 8 (1.8%) of 433 patients had a single retroaortic renal vein (Fig. 8.4). Both of these anomalies can be recognized by CT, and venography is seldom necessary for confirmation. Patients are asymptomatic but recognition is important if surgery involving this region is planned.

The left renal vein receives the inferior phrenic, capsular, ureteric, adrenal and gonadal veins. In addition, there are usually rich collateral vessels that anastomose with branches of the hemiazygos and ascending lumbar veins. These vessels are particularly important as they may preserve the kidney should venous thrombosis occur.

The right renal vein is shorter than the left, and has a more oblique course to the inferior vena cava. It receives capsular and ureteric veins as well as some retroperitoneal collaterals, but the right inferior phrenic and gonadal veins enter directly into the vena cava.

Valves may occur in the renal veins. There is a marked variation in the reported incidence of renal vein valves in anatomic studies, ranging from 28 to 70% on the right and from 4 to 36% on the left. Not surprisingly, they are demonstrated less frequently at venography. Their significance lies in surgical planning but they can also cause difficulty to the angiographer by inhibiting reflux of contrast material or passage of a catheter during venography or venous sampling (Fig. 8.5).

Renal vein varices may be idiopathic or the result of renal vein thrombosis or portal hypertension. Varices are felt to cause hematuria in some patients although this causal relationship is difficult to prove.

Renal vein varices, like varicoceles, are more common on the left than on the right. Thus, an anatomic etiology is

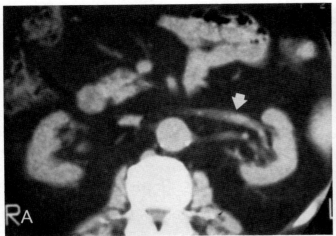

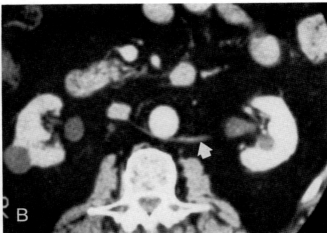

Figure 8.3. Circumaortic left renal vein. **A,** The anterior portion (*arrow*) of a circumaortic left renal vein is in its normal location. **B,** The posterior portion (*arrow*) runs behind the aorta.

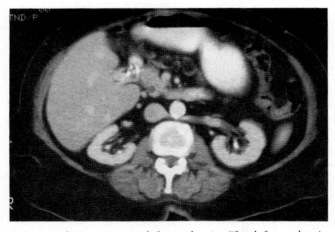

Figure 8.4. Retroaortic left renal vein. The left renal vein passes behind the aorta to enter the inferior vena cava.

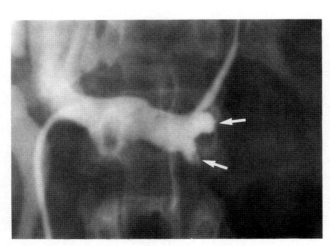

Figure 8.5. Renal vein valves. Contrast is prevented from reaching the intrarenal veins by valves (*arrows*).

postulated. Compression of the left renal vein between the superior mesenteric artery and the aorta ("nutcracker" phenomenon) may result in left renal vein hypertension hematuria and varix formation.

Collateral pathways exist for venous drainage of blood from the kidney in case of occlusion of the main renal vein. Inferior phrenic or adrenal, gonadal, and ureteric veins commonly enter the left renal vein while only the ureteric vein enters the right renal vein. Any of these vessels as well as a variety of small retroperitoneal veins that enter the renal veins may function as collateral vessels. The right adrenal, inferior phrenic, and gonadal veins enter directly into the inferior vena cava.

In renal vein thrombosis the clot usually propagates along the entire renal vein and these collateral vessels are also occluded. A local occlusion, such as surgical ligation, however, may allow these collaterals to take over drainage of the kidney. This occurs much more readily with occlusion of the left renal vein as it receives more potential collateral vessels than the right renal vein.

Circumcaval (Retrocaval) Ureter

Venous anomalies may affect the ureter. Persistence of the right subcardinal vein traps the ureter behind the inferior vena cava. The ureter crosses posterior to the IVC and then passes around the medial border anteriorly to partially encircle the cava. This anomaly, which occurs in approximately one in 1100 patients, has been termed a *retrocaval* or *circumcaval ureter*. The term circumcaval ureter is preferred as it is possible for the ureter to lie behind the vena cava without encircling it. A circumcaval ureter is more common in men than women.

A retrocaval ureter is usually found as an incidental finding. Most patients are asymptomatic, although right flank pain may be sufficient to bring this anomaly to attention.

The most common complication is obstruction, caused by constriction of the retrocaval segment of the ureter by the IVC. In a few cases, fibrous bands or adhesions of this segment of the ureter have been reported. The hydronephrosis and stasis predispose to stone formation and infection.

Two radiographic patterns of circumcaval ureter have been recognized by Bateson and Atkinson. The more common form has an **S**-shaped deformity of the mid-ureter as it courses around the IVC. The narrowing of the ureter occurs at the lateral border of the psoas muscle suggesting that the obstruction is not caused by compression by the vena cava. The second type has less severe hydronephrosis, but the point of obstruction is at the lateral wall of the IVC. However, ureteral obstruction is not necessarily present in a circumcaval ureter.

When the classic (Type I) appearance is seen in urography, the diagnosis of circumcaval ureter can be suggested (Fig. 8.6). However, an inferior vena cavagram or CT is needed for confirmation. In the less severe form (Type II), medial deviation must be distinguished from other etiologies such as retroperitoneal fibrosis or a retroperitoneal mass.

Circumcaval ureter can be recognized on CT by following the opacified ureter around the IVC. Computed tomography also demonstrates the more lateral location of the cava which usually lies lateral to the right pedicle of the L3 lumbar vertebral body.

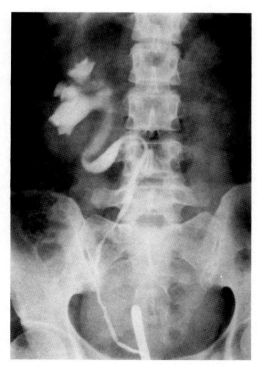

Figure 8.6. Circumcaval ureter. Failure of regression of the postcardinal vein traps the ureter behind the inferior vena cava.

Lymphatic

There is an extensive lymphatic system within the kidney which provides an accessory drainage route for excess fluid. In normal states approximately one-fourth of lymphatic flow from the kidney is via small lymphatic vessels which permeate the capsule and communicate with lymph vessels in the perinephric space. The remainder of the renal lymph fluid is drained into large lymph vessels in the renal hilum. The renal lymphatics are not directly imaged but enlarged vessels may be detected by CT.

DISEASES OF INTRARENAL ARTERIES

A variety of entities affect intrarenal arteries. Although the etiology and clinical course may be different, the radiographic manifestations are similar. Since the disease process is usually generalized, both kidneys are affected and are reduced in size. Small infarcts result in a slightly irregular contour. Renal function may be markedly impaired, but if imaged by either urography or retrograde pyelography the renal collecting system will be normal. The most characteristic findings are the multiple microaneurysms seen with renal arteriography.

Collagen Vascular Diseases

The vasculitides affect the glomeruli and other small renal vessels. They may be classified as primarily involving either medium and large renal arteries or small vessels and capillaries. Although any of the systemic vasculitides may involve the kidneys, this discussion will concentrate on those that do so commonly.

Polyarteritis Nodosa

Renal involvement occurs in 90% of patients with polyarteritis nodosa (PAN). The clinical presentation is often with hematuria, and other abnormalities such as proteinuria are detected on urinalysis. Renal ischemia occurs as a result of involvement of medium-sized vessels, and renin mediated hypertension is common. The small aneurysms seen in PAN may occasionally rupture and produce an intraparenchymal or perinephric hematoma.

With the exception of arteriography, radiographic imaging studies demonstrate nonspecific findings. Parenchymal scarring may be seen with urography, US, or CT. Areas of hemorrhage, due to aneurysm rupture are best defined by CT (Fig. 8.7), but if large, can also be detected by urography or sonography. The most definitive radiographic examination is arteriography, where small aneurysms occur at the bifurcation of interlobular or arcuate arteries (Fig. 8.7). These aneurysms are not limited to the kidneys, as arteries in the liver, spleen, pancreas, muscle, and gastrointestinal tract are often involved.

Although these small aneurysms are typical of PAN, they are not pathognomonic. Similar aneurysms may be

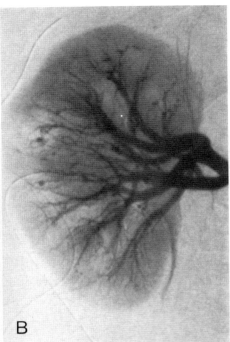

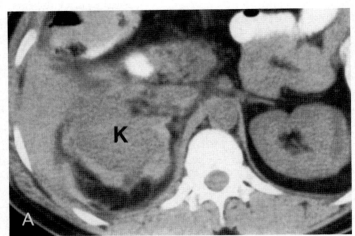

Figure 8.7.   Polyarteritis nodosa. **A,** A CT scan demonstrates high-density fluid surrounding the right kidney (K), indicating an acute perinephric and subcapsular hematoma. **B,** An arterio-gram reveals multiple small aneurysms of the small intrarenal arteries.

seen in patients with systemic lupus erythematosus, Wegener's granulomatosis, intravenous drug abuse, and have even been reported with renal metastases.

Wegener's Granulomatosis

Patients with Wegener's granulomatosis have necrotizing granulomas of the respiratory tract, a focal necrotizing angiitis involving small arteries and veins, and a focal necrotizing glomerulitis which leads to fibrin thrombi and local necrosis of individual glomerular tufts. It occurs most commonly in the fourth and fifth decades and has a slight male preponderance.

Symptoms of upper airway involvement, including sinusitis, otitis media, pharyngitis, and epistaxis, dominate the clinical presentation. Although nodular, infiltrative, or cavitary lung lesions are commonly seen, the pulmonary involvement is generally asymptomatic.

Renal disease may be absent in the limited form of Wegener's granulomatosis, but a rapidly progressive glomerulonephritis is life-threatening in the full syndrome. The most common manifestations of renal disease are hematuria and proteinuria. Hypertension is uncommon.

The radiographic manifestations in the kidneys are nonspecific and reflect the degree of renal failure. Microaneurysms, parenchymal scarring, and areas of hemorrhage may be seen. The findings are indistinguishable from those of PAN.

Systemic Lupus Erythematosus

Most patients with systemic lupus erythematosus have renal involvement, and many die of renal failure. The larger renal vessels are usually unaffected but interlobular arteries may be affected by inflammatory changes and may be narrowed. The predominant renal changes consist of a focal glomerulonephritis with thickening of the basement membrane resulting in the "wire loop" appearance on histologic preparations.

The radiographic appearance depends on the stage of involvement. Before the onset of renal failure, the kidneys appear normal. Microaneurysms, similar to those seen in PAN, may occasionally be seen on angiography. Although renal infarcts are common (Fig. 8.8), they are usually too small to be seen without selective magnification arteriography.

Scleroderma

Progressive systemic sclerosis is a generalized disorder manifested by vascular and connective tissue fibrosis. There is narrowing of the interlobular arteries due to intimal thickening, and there may be fibrinoid necrosis of the afferent arterioles.

Scleroderma is most common in the fourth and fifth decades, and shows a significant female preponderance. The incidence of renal involvement is variously reported,

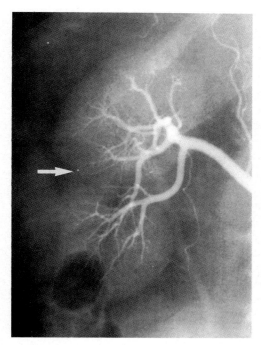

Figure 8.8. Systemic lupus erythematosus. A renal infarct can be appreciated by the cortical scar (*arrow*).

but the kidneys may be affected in up to 80% of cases. Renal failure is often the cause of death.

The radiographic manifestations are nonspecific. Before the onset of renal failure the kidneys may appear normal. Hypertension is common, such that the vascular changes seen on angiography may be due to either nephrosclerosis or scleroderma. However, the microaneurysms seen with the vasculitides are not seen with scleroderma.

Radiation Nephritis

Radiation nephritis may be either acute or chronic, may cause hypertension, or may result merely in proteinuria. It is a degenerative process that affects the tubules and glomeruli. The vascular changes that consist of fibrinoid necrosis occur late in the course and involve primarily arcuate and interlobar arteries. As little as 1000 rads may induce radiation nephritis, and microscopic changes can be seen with lower doses. Typically, however, doses of at least 2000–2500 rads within a 5-week period are needed to cause significant renal damage.

Acute radiation nephritis is manifested by proteinuria and hypertension following a latent period of 6–13 months. Uremia, malignant hypertension, and congestive heart failure follow. The prognosis is poor, with a mortality of approximately 50%.

Patients who develop chronic radiation nephritis may or may not have been affected by acute radiation nephri-

tis. Chronic radiation nephritis has an insidious onset of mild proteinuria, anemia, and azotemia, beginning 18 months to several years after radiation exposure. Although the clinical course is more protracted, the mortality of 50% is similar to acute radiation nephritis.

Arteriolar Nephrosclerosis

Systemic hypertension affects the vascular tree of the kidney more consistently and more extensively than any other region of the body. The degree of change is largely a function of the severity and duration of the hypertension.

Benign Nephrosclerosis

The vascular sclerotic process is accelerated by hypertension. There is arteriolar vasospasm with intramural edema followed by muscular hypertrophy and later intramural arteriolar fibrosis and hyaline degeneration. Glomerular and tubular changes are the result of ischemia. The kidneys are small due to irregular cortical thinning.

The clinical symptoms of patients with benign nephrosclerosis are usually limited to those of hypertension, and the physical examination reveals primarily cardiac and retinal changes. Mild proteinuria may be present.

Malignant Nephrosclerosis

The walls of the arterioles are markedly thickened by an eosinophilic granular material. An endothelial proliferation with concentric layers of collagen occurs in the afferent arterioles and intralobular arteries.

Males develop malignant hypertension more often then females, and most patients have a long history of benign hypertension. Patients with malignant hypertension have a diastolic blood pressure greater than 130 mm Hg and have papilledema. Neurologic symptoms and renal failure are common.

Laboratory tests reveal proteinuria in almost all patients. Elevated plasma renin and aldosterone along with hypokalemia are manifestations of secondary aldosteronism. Untreated malignant hypertension has a poor prognosis, with renal failure the most common cause of death.

The radiographic findings reflect the degree of involvement of the kidneys. Unless there is a renal artery stenosis to protect one of the kidneys, involvement is systemic.

On excretory urography the kidneys are normal to small in size. The calyces remain normal, even in areas of marked cortical thinning.

Increased tortuosity and more rapid tapering of intrarenal arteries is seen with angiography (Fig. 8.9). More severe changes include filling defects and loss of cortical vessels.

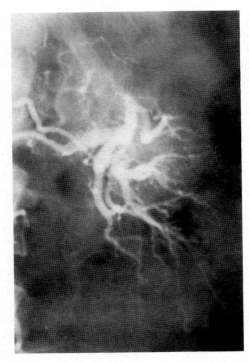

Figure 8.9. Arteriolar nephrosclerosis. A selective left renal arteriogram demonstrates tortuosity and rapid tapering of intrarenal arteries in this man with long-standing hypertension.

EMBOLISM AND INFARCTION

The most common source of renal artery emboli is a diseased heart. Patients with atrial enlargement secondary to valvular heart disease or a dyskinetic left ventricle after myocardial infarction provide the source of mural thrombi that may dislodge and become renal artery emboli. Smaller emboli may arise from an ectatic or aneurysmal aorta or even from cholesterol plaques in a patient with severe atherosclerosis.

Unlike arterial stenoses that are slowly progressive and may cause atrophy or collateralization, emboli produce acute ischemia that may result in infarction. The typical clinical features include the sudden onset of flank pain, hematuria, fever, and leukocytosis. However, the presentation is variable, and the diagnosis is often missed. Despite documented unilateral involvement, a decrease in renal function is seen in many patients.

The radiographic appearance of renal embolism depends on the size of the embolus and location of the arterial occlusion. Excretory urography demonstrates an absence of enhancement of the affected segment of the kidney, reflecting lack of vascular perfusion. If the main renal artery is occluded, there is no renal function in the affected kidney. A swollen, edematous kidney is seen on US as an enlarged kidney with decreased echogenicity.

Retrograde pyelography reveals a normal collecting system with sharply cupped calyces. If there is much swelling, there may be attenuation of the intrarenal collecting system.

The absence of contrast enhancement in the affected renal tissue is best demonstrated by CT. Smaller infarcts are seen as wedge shaped, low density areas within an otherwise normal appearing kidney (Fig. 8.10). If the entire kidney is affected, the increase in size due to edema can be identified by the large size and more rounded configuration. Even if the entire renal artery is occluded, capsular branches remain patent and enhance the outer rim of the kidney. The preservation of this outer 2–4 mm of cortex has been described on excretory urography, but it is best seen on CT (Fig. 8.10).

Radionuclide renography may suggest the diagnosis by demonstrating an area devoid of radionuclide activity. However, arteriography is needed for a definitive diagnosis. Sharp vessel cut off will be seen if the embolus completely occludes arterial flow. Incompletely occluding emboli appear as a filling defect within a contrast-filled artery (Fig. 8.11).

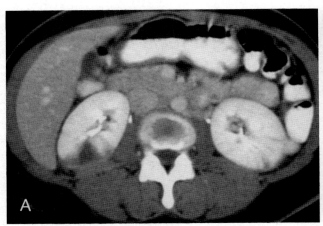
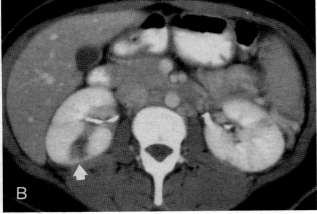

Figure 8.10. Renal infarction. **A,** Several wedge-shaped unenhancing areas indicate infarction due to emboli from subacute bacterial endocarditis. **B,** Capsular vessels preserve a thin peripheral rim (*arrow*).

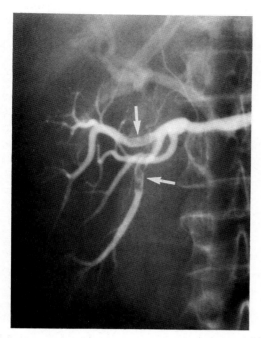

Figure 8.11. Renal embolus. Emboli are seen (*arrows*) as filling defects within the contrast-filled arteries.

After the acute phase of renal infarction, atrophy begins. The infarcted tissue contracts leaving a cortical scar (Fig. 8.12). The parenchymal loss reflects the distribution of the affected artery. If the main renal artery is occluded, the entire kidney will be affected. The kidney atrophies uniformly. There is no appreciable renal function, but renin may be elaborated and cause hypertension.

Treatment of renal artery embolism depends on the patients' underlying medical condition and the status of the contralateral kidney. Attempts at revascularization can be made with lytic therapy delivered directly into the renal artery via an arterial catheter. However, this is not rewarding nearly as often as lysis of clot that forms behind an arterial stenosis. Many patients are treated with anticoagulant therapy although surgical revascularization may be attempted in selected cases.

ARTERIAL THROMBOSIS

Thrombosis of the renal artery occurs most commonly as a complication of severe atherosclerosis. In such cases atherosclerosis usually involves a variety of other arteries, including coronary and carotid arteries, which dominate the clinical picture. This gradual occlusion of the renal artery which finally results in thrombosis is usually clinically silent and results in ipsilateral renal atrophy.

Acute thrombosis of the renal artery may occur after trauma. It usually follows blunt abdominal trauma in which the forces of acceleration or deceleration produce intimal tears with resulting disection of the renal artery and thrombosis. Renal artery thrombosis may also result from subintimal dissection of the renal artery during arteriography. This is more likely to occur during an attempted transluminal angioplasty than a diagnostic renal arteriogram.

With acute renal artery thrombosis, the kidney remains normal in size. Unless extensive renal artery collaterals have developed, there is no renal function, and intravascular contrast material will not be excreted. Retrograde pyelography demonstrates a normal collecting system.

Computed tomography reveals lack of enhancement, although a thin peripheral rim often remains viable due to collateral circulation through capsular arteries. Arteriography may be used to confirm the diagnosis of an occluded main renal artery.

With gradual occlusion, the kidney has usually diminished in size over time and a small kidney remains (Fig. 8.13). If collateral vessels are present, there may be a

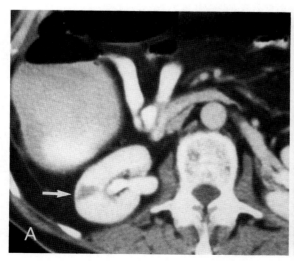

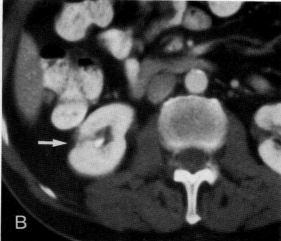

Figure 8.12. Chronic infarction. **A,** An acute infarction is seen as a wedge-shaped unenhanced area with preservation of the periphery by capsular vessels (*arrow*). **B,** Six months later a cortical scar is present (*arrow*).

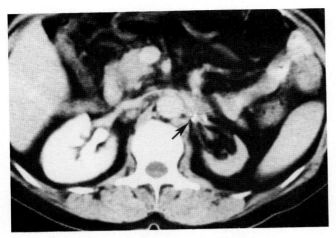

Figure 8.13. Chronic infarction. The left renal artery was sacrificed during retroperitoneal tumor resection. Surgical clips (*arrow*) are seen on the renal artery. The kidney is atrophic and does not enhance.

small amount of renal function preserved. The renal contour is smooth unless small infarcts have already occurred. The calyces remain normal if visualized by retrograde pyelography or if there is sufficient function remaining to image the collecting system during urography.

ANEURYSM

Aneurysms of the renal arteries are uncommon. They are rare in autopsy series, but may be seen during angi-

ography. The most common etiology is atherosclerosis but a dissecting aneurysm may also involve the renal artery. Mycotic aneurysms usually involve the aorta but may occasionally affect the renal artery.

Most patients are asymptomatic and the aneurysm is discovered incidentally during abdominal arteriography. Since hypertensive patients often undergo angiography looking for a renovascular etiology, it is not surprising that many patients found to have a renal artery aneurysm are hypertensive. In some patients, surgical resection of the aneurysm results in cure of the hypertension. However, these are usually patients with an associated renal artery stenosis and lateralizing renal vein renin levels.

Renal artery aneurysms often contain clot and may give rise to renal emboli with or without infarction. The risk of rupture is small but is more likely in hypertensive or pregnant patients. Calcified aneurysms rarely, if ever, rupture.

If calcified, a renal artery aneurysm can be recognized on the plain abdominal radiograph (Fig. 8.14). However, the appearance of a curvilinear calcification could be due to a tortuous or wandering splenic artery or even a nonvascular etiology.

Arteriography is required for a definitive diagnosis (Fig. 8.15), and even small, noncalcified aneurysms are easily identified unless thrombosed. The aneurysm may be partially or completely filled with thrombus, which prevents its opacification. Thus, thrombosed uncalcified aneurysms may be missed by arteriography.

Surgical treatment for a renal artery aneurysm is usu-

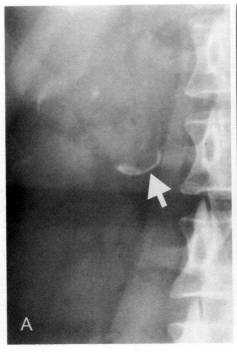

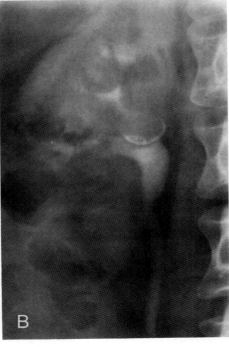

Figure 8.14. Renal artery aneurysm. **A,** Curvilinear calcification (*arrow*) in the region of the renal hilum indicates a renal artery aneurysm. **B,** Excretory urography confirms that it is extrinsic to the collecting system.

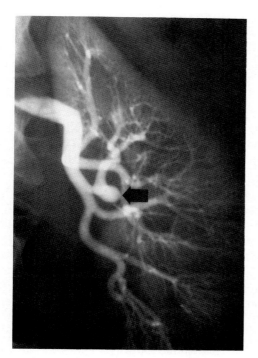

Figure 8.15. Renal artery aneurysm. A selective left renal arteriogram reveals a renal artery aneurysm (*arrow*).

ally not necessary. If renin-dependent hypertension can be demonstrated, resection is indicated. However, the presence of symptoms including flank pain or hematuria may be coincidental with but not caused by the aneurysm and surgery should be undertaken with caution.

Mycotic Aneurysm

A mycotic aneurysm is one that arises as a result of an infectious process in the arterial wall. They may occur as a result of septic emboli, often from bacterial endocarditis, but are also seen in intravenous drug abusers. Septic emboli tend to lodge at a branch point, a site of rapid vessel tapering, or a sharp bend in the artery. Mycotic aneurysms may also result from direct spread from a contiguous infection or from bacteria lodging in the vasa vasora or in the diseased intima.

Once established, the infection weakens the arterial wall and has a high incidence of rupture. Identification of a mycotic aneurysm may also be the first clue to an underlying bacterial endocarditis. Since the aneurysm may harbor bacteria despite antibiotic therapy, surgery may be needed to eradicate the site of infection.

ARTERIOVENOUS FISTULA

An *arteriovenous fistula* is an abnormal communication between the arterial and venous circulation that bypasses the capillary bed. Congenital fistulae or arteriovenous malformations, also known as angiomas or angiodysplasias, are uncommon.

Congenital

Congenital arteriovenous malformations (AVMs) are often asymptomatic and may not be detected until well into adult life. They are found more often in women than men, and hematuria is the most common presenting complaint. If large enough, an AVM may decrease perfusion to the renal parenchyma resulting in renal ischemia and renin mediated hypertension.

The findings on excretory urography are dependent on the size and location of the lesion. Large AVMs located near the collecting system may create extrinsic compression on the renal pelvis. If there is hematuria, blood clots may be seen.

Arteriography is needed for a definite diagnosis, and many small AVMs can only be detected with selective magnification renal arteriography. They are often classified as either cirsoid or aneurysmal. Cirsoid AVMs have multiple small arteriovenous communications (Fig. 8.16) while the aneurysmal type has only a solitary communication. The cirsoid variety tends to be located adjacent to the collecting system and often causes hematuria. The aneurysmal AVM is more likely to cause an abdominal bruit and hypertension.

Acquired

Acquired AV fistulae do not have the female preponderance seen with congenital AVMs. Since trauma due to a penetrating injury or biopsy is the most common etiology, they are often seen in males.

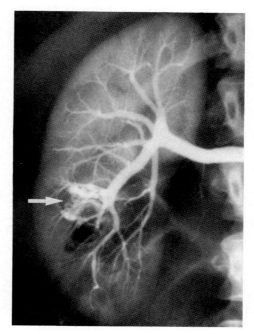

Figure 8.16. Congenital arteriovenous malformation. A tangle of vessels is seen in the right kidney (*arrow*).

The physiologic effect of an AV fistula depends on the size of the fistula and its specific location. The artery supplying the fistula enlarges and collateral vessels may develop if the fistula is larger than the artery feeding it. In some cases retrograde flow may occur in the artery distal to the fistula. The draining veins are dilated and their walls thickened. This venous arterialization may even be associated with the development of atherosclerotic plaques.

The most common clinical manifestation of renal arteriovenous fistulae is an abdominal bruit. Approximately half of symptomatic patients have cardiomegaly and congestive heart failure. Hematuria is also common.

Hypertension, which is usually diastolic, is renin mediated. The renal artery blood pressure and flow distal to the shunt are diminished. This relative renal ischemia stimulates renin secretion.

With increased use of renal biopsy, this has become the most frequent etiology of an acquired AV fistula (Fig. 8.17). It is probable that many more occur than are diagnosed, as angiography is performed only in those patients symptomatic enough to suggest a large fistula. Arteriovenous fistulae may also be seen as a complication of selective renal arteriography, especially during percutaneous transluminal angioplasty. In such cases, a stiff guidewire is often needed to lead the angioplasty catheter through the site of the renal artery stenosis. If the guidewire is passed out too far into the kidney, it will penetrate the renal artery and may enter an adjacent vein.

Small AV fistulae may heal spontaneously. Thus, many patients who develop a fistula after renal biopsy or angiography may be followed for the development of symptoms. Some of these fistulae may enlarge and require treatment.

Significant AV fistulae may be treated with transcatheter occlusion. It is critical to assess the size of the communication and be sure that any embolic material will be captured in the fistula and not pass through to become a pulmonary embolus. The most common indications for treatment are persistent hematuria or hypertension that can be localized to the kidney containing the fistula. If all the communicating branches can be occluded, percutaneous therapy should be successful. If transcatheter occlusion cannot be performed surgery may be needed.

Postnephrectomy

Although uncommon, a fistula may develop between the stump of the renal artery and the stump of the renal vein or vena cava after nephrectomy. Postoperative infection or excessive bleeding requiring packing during surgery contribute to their development. These fistulae tend to be large and may be hemodynamically significant.

RENAL VEIN THROMBOSIS

Thrombosis of the renal vein is usually due to an underlying abnormality of hydration, the clotting system, or the kidney. Occasionally extrinsic compression may occlude either the IVC or the renal vein and cause clot

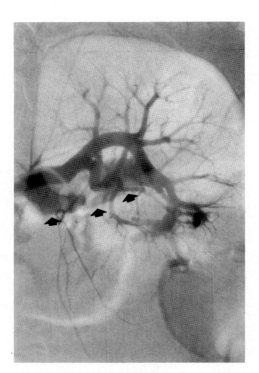

Figure 8.17.   Acquired arteriovenous fistula. An arteriogram demonstrates rapid filling of the renal vein (*arrows*) after renal biopsy. Both the supplying artery and draining vein are enlarged.

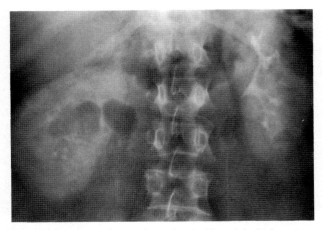

Figure 8.18.   Renal vein thrombosis. The right kidney is enlarged and functions poorly. A small amount of contrast material opacifies the intrarenal collecting system which is attenuated but shows no evidence of obstruction.

formation due to absent or slow flow. Renal or left adrenal tumors may grow along the veins resulting in tumor thrombus in the renal vein. Renal vein thrombosis is more common on the left side, presumably reflecting the longer left renal vein as compared to the right.

The clinical manifestations of renal vein thrombosis depend on the age of the patient, the specific disease process, and the speed with which it occurs. In infants, renal vein thrombosis is often an acute event incited by dehydration due to a volume depleting illness such as severe diarrhea. The kidney swells and renal function deteriorates. If the venous occlusion is not relieved, the kidney will infarct and atrophy.

In adults, the most common underlying abnormality is membranous glomerulonephritis. Approximately 50% of patients with membranous glomerulonephritis have renal vein thrombosis. Thrombosis occurs less frequently in lipoid nephrosis, immunoglobulin A (IgA) nephropathy or minimal change disease. Although patients with renal vein thrombosis often present with the nephrotic syndrome, the protein loss is due to the underlying renal disease rather than the venous thrombosis. In patients with no renal disease and renal vein thrombosis, there is little or no proteinuria.

Masses that produce extrinsic compression on the renal vein may also induce renal vein thrombosis. Retro-

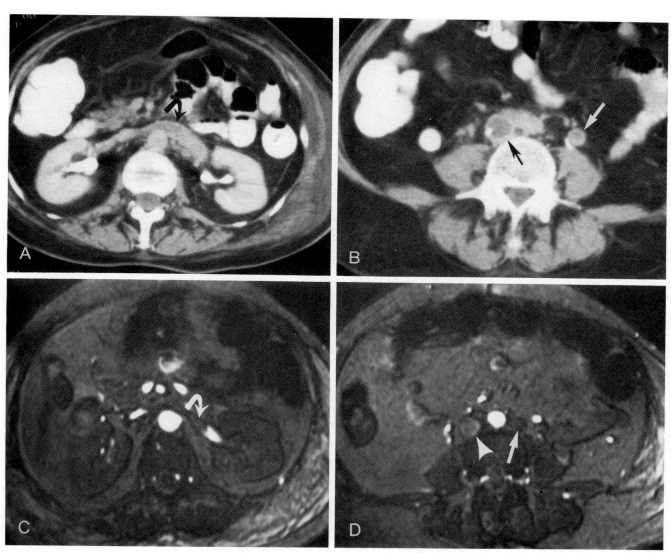

Figure 8.19.   Renal vein thrombosis. **A,** A CT scan through the level of the left renal vein demonstrates thrombosis (*arrow*) by the absence of enhancement. **B,** Below the kidneys, there is thrombosis of the inferior vena cava (*black arrow*) and left gonadal vein (*white arrow*). **C,** A magnetic resonance image using limited flip angle technique (GRASS) confirms the renal vein thrombosis by the absence of signal (*arrow*). **D,** At a lower level, thrombosis of the inferior vena cava (*arrowhead*) and left gonadal vein (*arrow*) are also seen.

peritoneal fibrosis, a tumor mass, acute pancreatitis, trauma, and retroperitoneal surgery may each incite renal vein thrombosis. Thrombocytosis, elevated clotting factors, or dehydration are other processes that may induce renal vein thrombosis. When thrombosis is gradual in onset, symptoms may be mild. If sufficient collateral vessels exist, renal function may be unaffected. If thrombosis occurs more acutely, collateral vessels are less likely to develop and clinical symptoms such as back pain are common. Laboratory abnormalities are nonspecific; the marked proteinuria seen in these patients is due to the underlying nephrotic syndrome rather than the renal vein thrombosis. Pulmonary embolism is a common associated problem.

The radiographic findings also depend on the underlying disease process and extent of collateral venous flow. If collateral veins are unable to drain the kidney adequately, the kidney will be enlarged. A persistent nephrogram is seen on excretory urography and the collecting system is attenuated. However, since renal function is impaired, retrograde pyelography may be required to exclude obstruction. However, sharp calyces are usually seen well enough on an excretory urogram to exclude obstruction.

Sonography is often used to exclude ureteral obstruction but can also demonstrate an enlarged, relatively hypoechoic kidney. In some cases, the renal vein thrombosis can also be imaged.

Computed tomography may be used to exclude a renal mass such as a carcinoma growing into the renal vein. Renal enlargement with diminished opacification reflecting impaired function is seen. Intravenous contrast should opacify the renal veins; absence of enhancement of a kidney that has arterial flow implies venous thrombosis (Fig. 8.18).

The most definitive test is renal venography. The normal renal vein should be visualized during the venous phase of a renal arteriogram. Absence of venous opacification implies obstruction. Direct renal venography may also be used to demonstrate venous thrombosis, but it is seldom necessary.

MRI is rapidly gaining use in vascular imaging. It is often used to evaluate renal vessels in patients with renal adenocarcinoma, but can also be applied to renal vein or caval thrombosis. Rapidly acquired images using a program such as gradient refocused acquisition in the steady state (GRASS) are especially useful for this purpose (Fig. 8.18).

Anticoagulation is the standard therapy for renal vein thrombosis. This prevents clot propagation while endemic enzyme systems lyse or recanalize the thrombosed vessel. Pulmonary embolism is a common complication of renal vein thrombosis. Lytic therapy may be used in patients in whom the thrombosis is more acute and the clinical manifestations more severe.

SUGGESTED READINGS

Anatomy

Bateson EM, Atkinson D: Circumcaval ureter: a new classification. *Clin Radiol* 20:173, 1969.

Beckmann CF, Abrams HL: Renal vein valves: incidence and significance. *Radiology* 127:351, 1978.

Beckmann CF, Abrams HL: Circumaortic venous ring: incidence and significance. *AJR* 132:561, 1979.

Beckmann CF, Abrams HL: Idiopathic renal vein varices: incidence and significance. *Radiology* 143:649, 1982.

Beinart C, Sniderman KW, Weiner M, et al: Left renal vein hypertension: a cause of occult hematuria. *Radiology* 145:647, 1982.

Crosse JEW, Soderdahl DW, Teplick SK, Clark RE: Nonobstructive circumcaval (retrocaval) ureter. *Radiology* 116:69, 1975.

Hoeltl W, Hruby W, Aharinejad S: Renal vein anatomy and its implications for retroperitoneal surgery. *J Urol* 143:1108, 1990.

Lautin EM, Haramati N, Frager D, et al: CT diagnosis of circumcaval ureter. *AJR* 150:591, 1988.

Nielsen PB: Retrocaval ureter: report of a case. *Acta Radiol* 51:179, 1959.

Reed MD, Friedman AC, Nealy P: Anomalies of the left renal vein: analysis of 433 CT scans. *J Comput Assist Tomogr* 6(6):1124, 1982.

Sampaio FJB, Aragao AHM: Anatomical relationship between the intrarenal arteries and the kidney collecting system. *J Urol* 143:679, 1990.

Trueta, J: *Studies of the Renal Circulation.* Springfield, Illinois, Charles C Thomas, 1947.

Collagen Vascular Diseases

Anderson R: Arteriography in polyarteritis nodosa. *Br J Urol* 40(5):556, 1968.

Easterbrook JS: Renal and hepatic microaneurysms: report of a new entity simulating polyarteritis nodosa. *Radiology* 137:629, 1980.

Fauci AS, Haynes BF, Katz P, Wolff SM: Wegener's granulomatosis: prospective clinical and therapeutic experience with 85 patients for 21 years. *Ann Intern Med* 98:76, 1983.

Litvak AS, Lucas BA, McRoberts JW: Urologic manifestations of polyarteritis nodosa. *J Urol* 115:572, 1976.

Longmaid HE, Rider E, Tymmkiw J: Lupus nephritis—new sonographic findings. *J Ultrasound Med* 6:75, 1987.

Radiation Nephritis

Jongejan HTM, van der Kogel AJ, Provoost AP, Molenaar JC: Radiation nephropathy in young and adult rats. *Int J Radiat Oncol Biol Phys* 13:225, 1987.

Willett CG, Tepper JE, Orlow EL, Shipley WU: Renal complications secondary to radiation treatment of upper abdominal malignancies. *Int J Radiat Oncol Biol Phys* 12:1601, 1986.

Renal Embolism and Infarction

Hann L, Plister RC: Renal subcapsular rim sign: new etiologies and pathogenesis. *AJR* 138:51, 1982.

Lessman RK, Johnson SF, Coburn JW: Renal artery embolism—clinical features and long-term follow-up of 17 cases. *Ann Intern Med* 89(4):477, 1978.

Renal Artery Aneurysm

DuBrow RA, Patel SK: Mycotic aneurysm of the renal artery. *Radiology* 138:577, 1981.

Tham G, Ekelund L, Herrlin K, et al: Renal artery aneurysms—natural history and prognosis. *Ann Surg* 197(3):348, 1983.

Arteriovenous Fistulae

Chew QT, Madayag MA: Post-nephrectomy arteriovenous fistula. *J Urol* 109:546, 1973.

Ekelund L, Gothlin J: Renal hemangiomas—an analysis of 13 cases diagnosed by angiography. *AJR* 125:788, 1975.

Takaha M, Matsumoto A, Ochi K, et al: Intrarenal arteriovenous malformation. *J Urol* 124:315, 1980.

Renal Vein Thrombosis

Bradley WG, Jacobs RP, Trew PA, et al: Renal vein thrombosis: occurrence in membranous glomerulonephropathy and lupus nephritis. *Radiology* 139:571, 1981.

Brennan RE, Curtis JA, Koolpe HA, et al: Left renal vein obstruction associated with nonrenal malignancy. *Urology* 19(3):329, 1982.

Clark RA, Wyatt GM, Colley DP: Renal vein thrombosis: an underdiagnosed complication of multiple renal abnormalities. *Radiology* 132:43, 1979.

Gatewood OMB, Fishman EK, Burrow CR, et al: Renal vein thrombosis in patients with nephrotic syndrome: CT diagnosis. *Radiology* 159:117, 1986.

Keating MA, Althausen AF: The clinical spectrum of renal vein thrombosis. *J Urol* 133:938, 1985.

O'Dea MJ, Malek RS, Tucker RM, Fulton RE: Renal vein thrombosis. *J Urol* 116:410, 1976.

Winfield AC, Gerlock AJ, Shaff MI: Perirenal cobwebs: a CT sign of renal vein thrombosis. *J Comput Assist Tomogr* 5(5):705, 1981.

RENAL HYPERTENSION

Hypertension is a common medical problem that affects as many as one-third of the population at some time in their life. It is defined as a diastolic pressure of 90 mm Hg or more and is graded as mild, moderate, severe, or malignant. Unfortunately, most hypertension is idiopathic. No etiology can be found, and the patient must be treated with antihypertensive medication. There is a minority of patients, however, in whom a specific etiology can be identified. In many of these patients appropriate therapy results in cure.

The major etiologic categories of hypertension are renovascular, renal, endocrine, and neurologic. This chapter discusses renal parenchymal and renovascular hypertension. Adrenal etiologies are addressed in Chapter 13.

ETIOLOGIES

Renal Parenchymal

A large number of parenchymal abnormalities have been associated with hypertension including pyelonephritis, glomerulopathies, ureteral obstruction, and renal mass lesions. Although many of these entities are common, they are seldom causally related to hypertension. However, documentation of a causal role has been shown in some cases, with relief of hypertension when the parenchymal abnormality has been alleviated.

Hydronephrosis

Unilateral ureteral obstruction may cause hypertension by activating the renin-angiotensin system. It has been shown experimentally in dogs that acute ureteral occlusion results in unilateral renin secretion and the development of hypertension. Human data confirm this increased renin secretion in acute but not chronic ureteral obstruction. Surgical intervention should cure those patients with lateralizing renin levels.

Renal Cyst

Renal cysts, as well as other masses, may cause renin-mediated hypertension. This may be due to compression of either the main renal artery or a branch renal artery causing ischemia. The resultant increased renin secretion leads to hypertension. Decompression of the cyst relieves the pressure on the renal artery and cures the hypertension. Cyst drainage can be done percutaneously, but sclerosis may be needed to prevent recurrence. If this cannot be done, surgery may be required.

Chronic Pyelonephritis

Chronic pyelonephritis is another curable etiology of hypertension, although the hypertension in most patients with chronic pyelonephritis is idiopathic. Patients more likely to become normotensive after nephrectomy for chronic pyelonephritis are younger, have a more recent onset of hypertension, a more severely involved ipsilateral kidney, and a nearly normal contralateral kidney. Lateralizing renal vein renins may be used to predict patients likely to respond to surgery.

Renal Carcinoma

Both renal adenocarcinoma and Wilms' tumor may cause hypertension in several different ways. The mass may cause extrinsic compression on the renal artery resulting in ischemia and increased renin secretion. Other, very vascular tumors may cause hypertension due to arteriovenous shunting. Rarely, a renal carcinoma or Wilms' tumor may produce renin. In some cases the hypertension may be the presenting finding with the renal tumor detected during the hypertension workup. Arteriography performed in these patients must include both main renal arteries in order to exclude a significant renal artery stenosis and possible renovascular hypertension in the contralateral kidney.

Juxtaglomerular Tumors

Renin secreting tumors of the juxtaglomerular cells (JG tumor) are a rare cause of hypertension. Patients with a JG tumor, or reninoma, tend to be young and are often less than 20 years old. The most frequent symptoms are related to the hypertension and include headache, polydipsia, polyuria, and neuromuscular complaints resulting from hypokalemia. The hypertension is usually moderate to severe.

The tumor is usually small and confined to the kidney, although a large (6.5 cm) tumor and a reninoma arising in the perinephric space have been reported. Juxtaglomerular tumors are usually sharply marginated and may be separated from the normal renal parenchyma by a pseudocapsule.

Detection of a renal mass by excretory urography depends on the size and location of the tumor. Calcification is not seen. Ultrasound is most frequently useful in demonstrating that the mass seen at urography is solid rather than cystic. The JG tumor is relatively echogenic due to the numerous interfaces caused by the small vascular channels in the tumor.

Although CT is quite sensitive in detecting these tumors, the appearance is nonspecific. Contrast enhancement is needed as the tumor may be isodense with normal renal parenchyma on unenhanced scans.

Reninomas are often detected at arteriography during an evaluation for possible renovascular hypertension. The tumor is typically hypovascular, even on selective renal arteriography. It is detected by displacement of small intrarenal arteries (Fig. 9.1).

Renal vein renin sampling will demonstrate elevated levels arising from the tumor. However, selective sampling from branch renal veins may be needed to confirm the abnormal renin secretion.

Although few JG tumors have been reported, they appear to be benign. Thus, simple tumorectomy or partial nephrectomy is curative.

Ask-Upmark Kidney

Segmental hypoplasia has been recognized as a cause of hypertension since the report of six patients by Ask-Upmark in 1929. The affected kidney is small and has few pyramids and a deep cortical groove overlying an abnormal calyx or recess extending from the renal pelvis. Hyperplasia of JG cells has been reported and excess renin

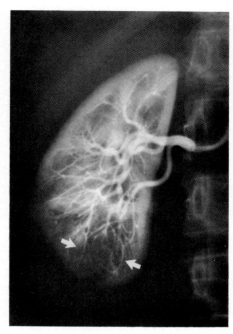

Figure 9.1. Juxtaglomerular tumor. A small hypovascular mass (*arrows*) is seen in the lower pole.

secretion documented in some cases. The process may be unilateral or bilateral.

An Ask-Upmark kidney may be seen in both children and adults. Most children are hypertensive and often the hypertension is severe. The condition is more common in females and there is a high association with vesicoureteral reflux and urinary tract infection.

Since many patients have vesicoureteral reflux, there is some controversy over the etiology. The renal abnormalities are similar and it may be impossible to distinguish the changes due to vesicoureteral reflux from an Ask-Upmark kidney radiographically.

On excretory urography the affected kidney is small and contains one or more deep cortical scars. The contralateral kidney often demonstrates compensatory hypertrophy. The calyx underlying the cortical scar is dilated and clubbed. Hypertrophy of adjacent renal tissue may splay the infundibulum creating a mass effect.

Arteriography demonstrates a normal renal artery. The size of the renal artery is proportional to the size of the kidney, which is often small. The size of the orifice of the renal artery is also proportional to the size of the vessel, indicating its congenital etiology (Fig. 9.2).

Trauma

Trauma may cause hypertension by causing injury to the renal artery or it may be due to the compressive effect of a subcapsular hematoma. Traumatic injury may create an intimal hematoma or partial tear of the renal artery which results in renal ischemia. Selective renal arteriography is needed to detect the arterial lesion which may

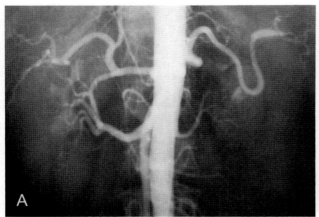

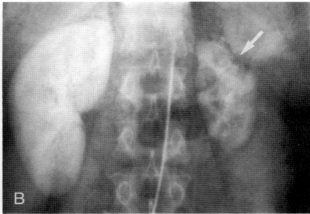

Figure 9.2. Ask-Upmark kidney. **A,** Aortography demonstrates a small left renal artery but no focal stenosis. **B,** A focal parenchymal scar (*arrow*) is seen on later-phase films. Elevated renins were measured from the left renal vein.

affect the main renal artery or a branch vessel. Those patients with partial renal damage may be treated medically, as the hypertension may resolve spontaneously. If the kidney is threatened, however, urgent repair is needed.

Another mechanism of trauma-induced hypertension is the development of a subcapsular hematoma which compresses the renal parenchyma creating local ischemia resulting in increased renin secretion. This phenomenon was first demonstrated by Page in 1939 when he produced arterial hypertension in laboratory animals by wrapping one kidney in cellophane. This induced a proliferative reaction which formed a fibrocollagenous shell compressing the renal parenchyma. The hypertension results from excess renin secretion due to ischemia caused by the mass effect of the hematoma compressed against the kidney by the renal capsule. The development of hypertension is not acute but may take months or even years after the trauma.

A subcapsular hematoma is easily seen on CT (Fig. 9.3). If hypertension develops subsequently, renal vein renin levels should be measured. These will usually lateralize to the affected kidney. Arteriography shows no arterial injury, but the renal distortion by the subcapsular mass is seen. Evacuation of the hematoma should result in cure.

Renovascular Hypertension

Only a small minority of hypertensive patients have a renovascular etiology; the vast majority of patients have essential hypertension. Estimates vary, but the prevalence of renovascular hypertension among all hypertensive patients is approximately 1 to 4%. It is difficult to predict on a clinical basis which patients have renovascular hypertension, but some characteristics make it more likely.

Renovascular hypertension is more common among patients at either age extreme. Patients under 20 or over 50 years of age are more likely to have a renovascular etiology while those with essential hypertension are usu-

ally between 30 and 50 years old at onset. However, fibromuscular dysplasia, the second most common cause of renovascular hypertension, typically affects women between the ages of 30 and 55 years. Rapid acceleration or severe hypertension is another indication of a renovascular etiology as is a severe hypertensive retinopathy. A flank bruit is the other finding on physical examination that suggests a renovascular etiology; it is especially common in patients with fibromuscular dysplasia. A family history of hypertension, on the other hand, is found more often in patients with essential hypertension.

Renovascular hypertension is renin mediated and occurs as a response to renal ischemia. Renin is an enzyme produced in the JG apparatus of the kidney. It acts on the circulating serum protein angiotensinogen to produce angiotensin I, which in turn is converted to angiotensin II. Angiotensin II has several properties that increase blood pressure. It stimulates aldosterone secretion, causes arteriolar constriction, and exerts antidiuretic and antinatriuretic effects on the kidney.

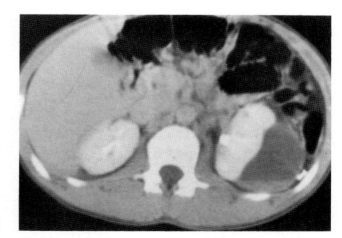

Figure 9.3. Subcapsular hematoma. Compression of the renal parenchyma indicates the subcapsular location. The compression creates local ischemia resulting in increased renin secretion.

The most important factor governing renin release is the afferent arteriole which acts as a baroreceptor. The transmural pressure across this arteriole may decrease as a result of a reduction in perfusion pressure or decreased compliance of the arteriole.

In patients with renovascular hypertension, the hypertension is dependent on the high circulating levels of angiotensin II. Thus, either saralasin, an angiotensin II antagonist, or the converting enzyme inhibitor captopril may be used to control the hypertension.

Although many different processes may cause stenosis of the main renal artery, the most common are atherosclerosis and fibromuscular dysplasia. Rarely, renal artery stenoses may be congenital, due to Takayasu's aortitis, the middle aortic syndrome, irradiation, or may be associated with neurofibromatosis.

Atherosclerosis

Atherosclerosis accounts for approximately two-thirds of cases of significant narrowing of the main renal artery. The lesions usually occur at the origin of the renal artery or within the first 2 cm (Fig. 9.4). They are often circumferential but may be eccentric. Since atherosclerosis is a generalized process, both renal arteries are frequently affected. If atherosclerosis is present at the renal ostia, it may not be possible to determine whether the plaque is renal or aortic in location.

Atherosclerosis begins as a proliferation of smooth muscle cells in the intima and creates a mound that protrudes into the lumen. Lipid deposition follows with inflammation, necrosis, and formation of atherosclerotic plaque.

Atherosclerosis is more common in men than women, and is accelerated by smoking. The age at which patients present with hypertension is considerably older than in those with fibromuscular dysplasia.

Fibromuscular Dysplasia

Fibromuscular dysplasia (FMD) has only been recognized for the past 30 years, but it accounts for almost one-third of cases of renovascular hypertension. It may involve any layer of the renal artery and is classified as intimal, medial, or adventitial. The medial variety can be subdivided into several more categories.

Intimal fibroplasia consists of a concentric accumulation of collagen beneath the internal elastic membrane. This creates a smooth stenosis, usually in the midportion of the renal artery. It is more common among children and is progressive.

Medial dysplasia is the most common type and accounts for approximately 95% of cases. The subcategories reflect involvement of the inner or outer media and the presence of collagenous infiltration, smooth muscle hypertrophy, or medial dissection.

Medial fibroplasia is the most common subtype of dysplasia. There is replacement of smooth muscle by collagen that forms thick ridges. These alternate with areas of small aneurysm formation and result in the classic "string of beads" appearance seen with arteriography (Fig. 9.5). This type of medial dysplasia is most commonly seen in women from 20 to 50 years of age. Although it is progressive, it is usually responsive to percutaneous transluminal angioplasty.

Collagen infiltrates the outer layer of the media in perimedial fibroplasia. A similar beaded appearance is present in the renal arteries but is less dramatic as true aneurysms do not develop.

True medial hyperplasia is an uncommon form of medial dysplasia and consists of hyperplastic smooth muscle and fibrous tissue. Focal stenoses are seen but aneurysm formation is not present (Fig. 9.6).

Medial dissection is also uncommon and may be histologically indistinguishable from other forms of medial

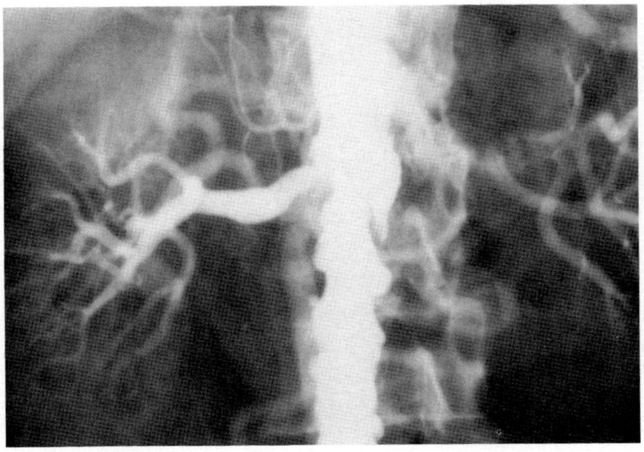

Figure 9.4. Atherosclerosis. Diffuse atherosclerotic changes are seen in the abdominal aorta as well as the right renal artery.

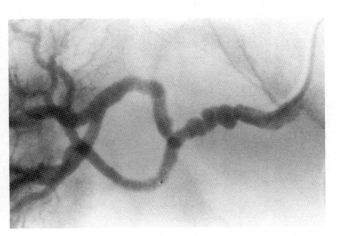

Figure 9.5. Fibromuscular dysplasia. Thick ridges of collagen alternate with aneurysms to create a "string of beads" appearance typical of medial fibroplasia.

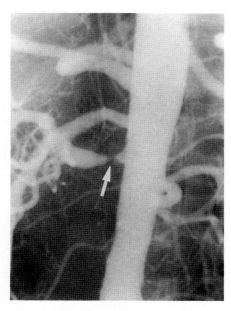

Figure 9.6. Fibromuscular dysplasia. The focal stenosis (*arrow*) suggests medial hyperplasia.

dysplasia. In this form a new channel is formed in the outer third of the media.

In adventitial dysplasia a collagenous infiltrate surrounds the adventitia. Either discrete focal or longer tubular stenoses may be produced.

Fibromuscular dysplasia is not limited to the renal arteries but is also seen in cephalic, visceral, and peripheral arteries. FMD involves the carotid and vertebral arteries but tends to spare the intracranial vessels. Transient ischemia attacks may be due to involvement of cephalic vessels by FMD.

Most patients are asymptomatic when the visceral arteries are affected by FMD. Symptoms of intestinal angina have been reported due to lesions in the superior mesenteric artery. The hepatic artery may also be involved but is seldom symptomatic.

Peripheral arteries are seldom affected but reports have confirmed involvement of most medium and large muscular arteries. Claudication may result if arterial flow is compromised.

Takayasu's Aortitis

Takayasu's disease is a granulomatous arteritis that commonly involves the aorta and its major branches. It has a marked female preponderance and is usually seen in patients under 35 years of age. Although primarily seen in Orientals, cases are being reported with increasing frequency in western civilizations. Temporal arteritis is histologically similar but is confined to small vessels and is typically found in older patients.

Since major branches of the abdominal aorta are often affected, hypertension is a common complication of Ta-

kayasu's disease. The hypertension may be due to either coarctation of the aorta or main renal artery stenosis.

Symptoms of Takayasu's disease are nonspecific and it is often not recognized until well advanced. Takayasu's disease is classified into four types.

Arteriography demonstrates vascular narrowing of the aortic arch or great vessels arising from the arch (Type 1); descending thoracic and upper abdominal aorta (Type 2); aortic arch vessels, abdominal aorta, and major branches (Type 3); or pulmonary arteries (Type 4). Typically, there is a smooth tapered narrowing of the affected artery. Skip areas may occur and multiple vessels are commonly involved. The disease may progress to complete occlusion. Treatment is usually surgical, but successful transluminal angioplasty has been reported.

Middle Aortic Syndrome

This rare syndrome of diffuse narrowing of the abdominal aorta often affects the visceral and renal arteries. It occurs in young patients, most often in the second decade of life. Hypertension is typically severe. An abdominal bruit and diminished femoral pulses in a young patient may suggest the diagnosis. The prognosis is poor with patients dying from cerebral hemorrhage, hypertensive encephalopathy, stroke, and congestive heart failure.

The middle aortic syndrome is distinct from aortic coarctation, which is a congenital lesion. Multiple etiologies are responsible for the middle aortic syndrome including a chronic inflammatory aortitis, atherosclerosis, and cystic medial necrosis. The disease is progressive and does not respond well to transluminal angioplasty. Thus, treatment consists of surgical revascularization. Although surgery is best performed after the patient is fully grown, the severity of disease may mandate an earlier aggressive surgical approach.

The radiographic manifestations depend on the specific vessels involved. Stenosis of a renal artery may result in a small kidney with delayed excretion of contrast material on urography.

Arteriography is required to define the vascular involvement. A smooth tapering of the distal thoracic or abdominal aorta is seen. Narrowing is often severe and is usually most marked in the infrarenal aorta. The renal arteries are commonly affected with long stenoses (Fig. 9.7). Lateral views may demonstrate narrowing of the celiac or superior mesenteric arteries in as many as 90% of patients.

The middle aortic syndrome must be distinguished from Takayasu's disease. Patients with Takayasu's disease are usually slightly older and have other manifestations of arteritis, such as fever and an elevated sedimentation rate. The great vessels of the chest are often involved in Takayasu's disease but not in the middle aortic syndrome.

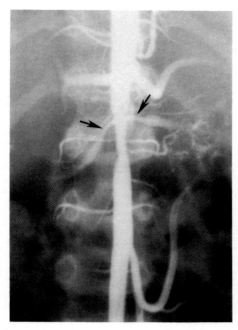

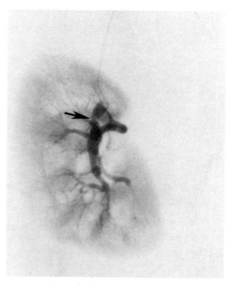

Figure 9.8.   Renal transplant. A focal transplant renal artery stenosis (*arrow*) is seen on this selective arteriogram.

Figure 9.7.   Middle aortic syndrome. Tubular narrowing of the mid-aorta has resulted in bilateral right renal artery stenoses (*arrows*).

Renal Transplantation

Approximately 50% of patients develop hypertension after receiving a renal allograft. In the early period after transplantation, acute rejection is the most common cause of hypertension. High-dose glucocorticoid therapy contributes to hypertension, but this can be reduced by using an alternate-day regimen for long-term therapy. Stenosis of the transplant renal artery is another possible cause of hypertension (Fig. 9.8). This may be due to acute angulation or extrinsic compression of the artery, ischemic injury during vascular clamping, or intimal fibrosis due to rejection.

The incidence of hypertension is higher if the native kidneys are left in place than if they are removed. This is most likely due to activation of the renin-angiotensin system as elevated renin levels can be measured in the native renal veins.

Renal Artery Aneurysm

There is an association between renal artery aneurysms and hypertension. However, it is not clear how often the hypertension is caused by the aneurysm. Renin-mediated hypertension may be produced by extrinsic compression of the main renal artery or an intrarenal branch artery by the aneurysm, or by thrombus formation and occlusion of a branch artery.

Vaughn et al. reported 41 hypertensive patients with renal artery aneurysms but without associated renal or renal artery lesions. Narrowed vessels with delayed flow of contrast and a segmental decreased nephrogram distal

to the aneurysm was interpreted as evidence of ischemia. Seven of eight (88%) patients followed for at least 1 year who underwent ipsilateral nephrectomy were cured. Other investigators, however, have found additional renal artery stenoses that were likely responsible for the hypertension.

SCREENING

Since it is extremely difficult to predict on a clinical basis which patients have renovascular hypertension, a radiographic screening test is needed. However, the prevalence of renovascular hypertension is less than 5% of all hypertensive patients, so that it is impractical to apply these tests to all hypertensive patients. Thus a group of patients at increased risk for renovascular hypertension is selected to undergo radiographic screening for renovascular hypertension. The following criteria are often used to select patients for radiographic screening:

1. Age extreme, usually under 20 or over 50 years
2. Recent onset of hypertension (less than 1 year)
3. Rapid acceleration of hypertension.
4. Malignant hypertension
5. A flank bruit

A variety of radiographic screening tests have been used, and there is no consensus as to which is the best. The choices may reflect local institutional bias, equipment available, physician interest or expertise, and the characteristics of the patient population.

Hypertensive Urography

One of the most common radiographic screening tests for renovascular hypertension has been hypertensive urography. This is performed by rapidly injecting a bolus of contrast material into a peripheral arm vein and obtaining sequential radiographs of the kidneys at 1-minute intervals for five minutes. Additional films are also obtained to examine the kidneys and the remainder of the urinary tract for other pathology.

Findings that suggest renovascular hypertension include a small kidney with delayed excretion (Fig. 9.9) and a delayed intense pyelogram. Extrinsic impression from collateral vessels may also be seen on the ureter or renal pelvis. The most reliable findings are delayed contrast excretion and a small kidney.

Earlier reports on hypertensive urography including the 1972 publication of a multiinstitutional cooperative study by Bookstein et al. recommended the use of hypertensive urography to screen patients suspected of renovascular hypertension. Those patients with a positive urogram were recommended for arteriography. However, further analysis has not supported this approach, and the false-negative (22%) and false-positive (13%) rates were too high for use as a screening test. Improvements in competing modalities combined with the insensitivity of the hypertensive urogram have resulted in its abandonment for this purpose.

Radionuclide Renography

Radionuclide renography has been used to detect renovascular hypertension, but results with ^{131}I-orthoiodohippurate have suffered from disappointingly high false-positive and false-negative rates. However, the development of quantitative gamma camera renography and the use of technetium-99m-DTPA has improved the radionuclide results (Fig. 9.10). Grunewald and Collins, for instance, reported the results of 141 patients with severe hypertension. Quantitative renography predicted renal artery stenosis in 15 patients. Thirteen of these patients underwent arteriography where a significant renal

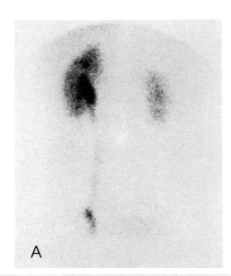

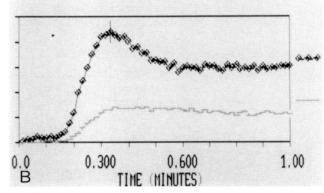

Figure 9.10. Radionuclide renogram. **A,** Posterior image of ^{99m}Tc DTPA renogram demonstrates a small right kidney with impaired function. **B,** Time-activity curves during bolus injection. The left kidney is normal but perfusion to the right kidney is markedly reduced.

artery stenosis was confirmed. Using computer acquired dynamic renal perfusion imaging, Chiarini et al. were able to generate a renal perfusion index and determine the contribution from each kidney. This radionuclide study agreed with angiography in 91% of the 200 cases. There were only 10% false-positive and 9% false-negative examinations.

The addition of captopril has further improved the results that can be obtained with radionuclide renography. Captopril is an angiotensin converting inhibitor that blocks the conversion of angiotensin I to angiotensin II. It has a peak effect within 90 minutes of oral ingestion of 25–50 mg. Several small studies have shown that there is an alteration in the pattern of radionuclide accumulation and excretion by the affected kidney with unilateral renal artery stenosis when captopril and noncaptopril studies are compared, and that the addition of captopril significantly enhances the detection of renovascular hypertension. However, in some patients both a captopril and noncaptopril study may be needed.

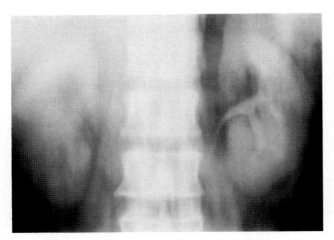

Figure 9.9. Hypertensive urogram. Delayed excretion from the right kidney indicates right renal artery stenosis.

Digital Subtraction Angiography

Digital subtraction angiography (DSA) refers to manipulation of angiographic images by a digital computer. These techniques have slightly decreased spatial resolution but much better contrast sensitivity than conventional film screen angiography. When performed with arterial contrast injections, much less contrast material is required than with conventional arteriography. However, because of the excellent contrast sensitivity, diagnostic arterial images can be obtained after intravenous contrast injections (Fig. 9.11).

Intravenous digital subtraction renal arteriography is readily applied to screening patients for renovascular hypertension, as it does not require an arterial puncture and is thus easily performed on outpatients. Either a peripheral or central vein may be used as the injection site. Diagnostic studies may be routinely obtained after injection of 40 ml of a 60% contrast material at 10 ml/sec through an 18-gauge intracath placed in a vein in the antecubital fossa. However, more consistent examinations are seen when contrast is injected through a catheter directly into the vena cava or right atrium. This may be done either through the right arm with a catheter in the superior vena cava or via the groin with the catheter in the inferior vena cava.

The arm approach is more convenient for outpatients as it avoids inadvertent puncture of the femoral artery. This approach also precludes a catheter overlying the right renal artery which is unavoidable with the groin approach. However, the groin approach is more convenient if renal vein renins are obtained at the same time.

Dunnick et al. have demonstrated improved results of intravenous digital subtraction arteriography compared to hypertensive urography for detecting patients with renovascular hypertension. Not only does intravenous digital subtraction arteriography detect more patients with renal artery stenosis than urography, but intravenous digital subtraction arteriography can also be used to detect patients with bilateral disease or patients with renal artery stenosis in a solitary kidney.

However, not all intravenous digital subtraction arteriography studies result in technically adequate examinations. Since a tight bolus of contrast material is needed to allow subtraction without changes in vessel position, patients with poor cardiac function will often have an inadequate study. Patients must also be cooperative and suspend respiration during image acquisition. Since it is a nonselective technique, overlying vessels such as the celiac and mesenteric arteries are opacified. Thus, oblique projections are usually required in addition to the standard posteroanterior view to examine the entire main renal arteries.

More recently the value of intravenous digital subtraction arteriography was demonstrated in a prospective study of 94 patients with suspected renovascular hypertension. Since technically inadequate intravenous digital subtraction arteriography studies require conventional arteriography to exclude a significant renal artery stenosis, they were considered a positive study. The positive predictive value of an abnormal intravenous digital subtraction arteriogram in this group of hypertensive patients, selected on clinical grounds to be more likely to have a renovascular etiology, was 83% and the negative predictive value 100%.

Intraarterial digital subtraction arteriography may also be used to evaluate the renal arteries. Since intraarterial digital subtraction arteriography requires an arterial puncture, it is not as suitable for screening patients as intravenous digital subtraction arteriography. However, much less contrast material is used with intraarterial digital subtraction arteriography so it is useful in patients with azotemia where a much smaller contrast volume is needed to minimize contrast nephropathy (Fig. 9.12).

Conventional Arteriography

Conventional arteriography remains the gold standard for the detection of renal artery stenosis. The spatial resolution of radiographic film is superior to digital systems,

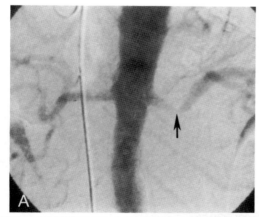
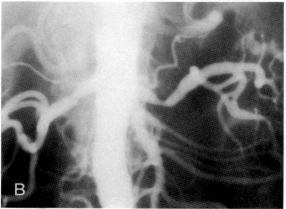

Figure 9.11. Intravenous digital subtraction angiography. **A,** A left renal artery stenosis (*arrow*) is identified. **B,** The lesion is confirmed on a conventional aortogram.

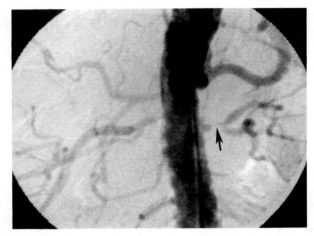

Figure 9.12. Intraarterial digital subtraction angiography. The intraarterial digital technique was used because of azotemia. Generalized atherosclerosis and stenosis of the left renal artery (*arrow*) are present.

and a variety of oblique patient positions or tube angulations may be used to optimally delineate the renal arteries. Furthermore, stenoses in accessory renal arteries that may be missed with a digital examination can be detected with conventional film arteriography (Fig. 9.13). Thus, all of the previously described diagnostic procedures are compared with conventional angiography to determine their accuracy in detecting renal artery stenosis.

Once a lesion is detected, conventional arteriography is used to further characterize the stenosis. The etiology of the vascular lesion can often be predicted by its angiographic appearance. Furthermore, the most appropriate treatment may often be determined by the nature of the stenosis. A focal stenosis of the main renal artery often responds to percutaneous transluminal angioplasty (PTA), whereas long stenoses, orifice lesions, or bilateral

disease do not do as well. In most centers, percutaneous transluminal angioplasty is the treatment of choice for a renal artery stenosis. However, surgery may be selected for lesions that will be technically difficult for PTA, or for lesions at the renal orifice, which may be due to atherosclerosis of the aorta, rather than the renal arteries.

Renin Measurement

Since renovascular hypertension is renin mediated, serum renin levels should be elevated. Indeed, peripheral renin levels are more often elevated in patients with renovascular hypertension than essential hypertension. Sodium depletion has been used to reduce renal blood flow and further stimulate renin secretion. However, measurement of peripheral renin activity is still too insensitive to be used as a screening test for renovascular hypertension.

Selective renal vein sampling provides a method of measuring the renin level being secreted by each kidney. Samples from the main renal veins and inferior vena cava are usually sufficient. If a renin-producing tumor or branch renal artery stenosis is suspected, more selective samples may be needed. The position of the catheter should be monitored fluoroscopically to make sure the catheter is correctly positioned before samples are obtained. Retroperitoneal collateral vessels and the gonadal veins must be avoided (Fig. 9.14). An ipsilateral/contralateral renal vein renin ratio of 1.5 or greater is generally considered lateralizing and predictive of renovascular hypertension. Such patients are likely to be cured by correction of the renal artery stenosis.

Multiple studies support the use of this renal vein renin ratio. A lateralizing ratio predicts a favorable response to correction of the renal artery lesion in over 90% of patients. However, not all series report such high accuracy. A nonlateralizing result is not nearly as specific,

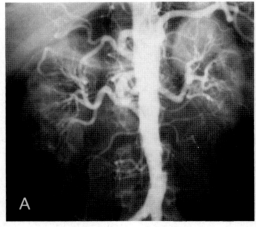
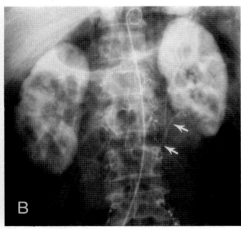

Figure 9.13. Accessory renal artery stenosis. **A,** The main renal arteries are normal. **B,** Late-phase films demonstrate incomplete opacification of the lower pole of the left kidney. An accessory renal artery (*arrows*) is now apparent. Its opacification is delayed by a stenosis.

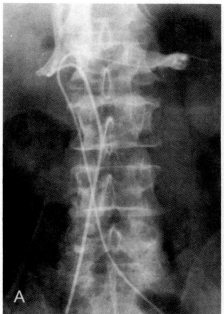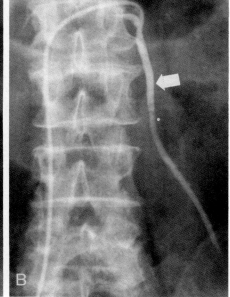

Figure 9.14. Renal vein renin collection. **A,** A catheter lies in each renal artery. **B,** Care must be taken not to draw samples from retroperitoneal or gonadal veins (*arrow*).

as false-negative rates of greater than 50% are commonly reported. Thus, many physicians prefer to correct the renal artery lesion regardless of the renin measurements.

TREATMENT

Percutaneous Transluminal Angioplasty

Percutaneous transluminal angioplasty (PTA) was first performed in 1963 and reported in 1964 by Dotter, who inadvertently cannulated an occluded iliac artery. Since then major advances by Porstmann, Zeitler, and van Andel have contributed to the increasing use and success of the procedure. In 1976, Gruntzig introduced a sophisticated balloon catheter that allowed PTA to be performed on renal and coronary arteries. Since the first report of renal artery PTA in 1978, it has rapidly become accepted as the treatment of choice for most patients with renovascular hypertension.

Mechanism

Transluminal angioplasty procedures are designed to enlarge the lumen of a stenotic artery. Since atheromatous material is not compressible, it must be fractured and pushed out into the wall of the artery. This requires a dehiscence of the intima of the renal artery. The arterial media is also split and the adventitia is stretched beyond its elastic recoil. The atheromatous plaque is forced into the medial portion of the artery. The adventitia remains intact, the media heals by fibrosis, and there is reendothelialization over the tears in the intima.

A similar process of controlled injury also occurs with nonatherosclerotic stenoses. The intima is disrupted and the lesions are split or stretched beyond their point of elastic recoil.

Technique

Details of the many techniques and technical maneuvers that may be needed to perform percutaneous transluminal renal angioplasty are beyond the scope of this text; however, some basic principles are reviewed here to facilitate understanding the results and possible complications of the procedure.

The first step in PTA is to cross the stenosis. This is sometimes difficult, especially if the stenosis is tight or if the renal artery makes an acute angle as it arises from the aorta. In some patients a brachial artery access facilitates crossing the lesion as it results in an obtuse angle of the renal artery rather than the acute angle if approached from below.

An angiographic guide wire with a floppy tip, such as a Bentson wire, is sufficient for most cases. However, steerable guidewires are now available that may be used in difficult cases with very tight stenoses. A platinum-tipped steerable guidewire that is available in 0.014- to 0.038-inch diameter may be used by itself or in coaxial fashion through a catheter.

A difficult stenosis may also be crossed without using a guidewire. A diagnostic catheter, usually 5 French, may be advanced through the stenosis while contrast is injected through the catheter. The contrast not only demonstrates the path of the catheter but also tends to keep the tip of the catheter away from the vessel wall.

Once the lesion has been crossed, access should not be surrendered until the procedure is completed. Each time the guidewire is advanced it has the potential to raise an intimal flap that may lead to further vessel damage and even arterial thrombosis. Thus, the guidewire is left across the lesion and the balloon catheter passed over the wire until it is centered at the stenosis and ready for inflation.

One of the common problems during catheter and guidewire manipulation is vascular spasm. Arterial vasospasm can be severe enough to cause local ischemia and infarction. Thus, antispasmodic and anticoagulant medications are injected, either after the diagnostic catheter has been inserted or after the stenosis has been crossed. Nifedipine (10 mg orally) is a calcium channel blocker that may be given 30 minutes before the procedure to prevent spasm. Other calcium channel blockers, such as verapamil hydrochloride may be injected intraarterially to prevent or reverse arterial spasm. Nitroglycerine (100 μg, intraarterially) is also effective at reversing arterial spasm, especially after a calcium channel blocker has been given.

The choice of the appropriate balloon angioplasty catheter is critical to the success of the procedure. The original size of the artery is judged by measuring the size of the vessel both proximal and distal to the stenosis. Magnification contributes only a small amount to the perceived vessel size if conventional angiographic films are used. However, magnification may be much greater if digital angiograms are measured. Some catheters now have centimeter markings on them to facilitate measurement. The diameter of the inflated balloon should be the size of the normal arterial lumen or 1–2 mm larger. Slight overdilation is preferable to underdilation. One commonly used method of selecting the appropriate size balloon is to use an angioplasty balloon equal to the size of the renal artery measured on a conventional arteriogram. Since there is slight magnification on the arteriogram, the fully inflated balloon will slightly overdilate the renal artery. In general, a balloon length of 2 cm is sufficient to dilate the renal artery stenosis without causing unnecessary damage to the normal renal artery.

The angioplasty balloon should be inflated with a mixture of contrast and saline. This provides sufficient opacity for easy visualization during fluoroscopy and yet is a less viscous fluid that will drain easily from the balloon once the dilation is accomplished. Most angiographers dilute the 60% contrast material used for catheter guidance with an equal amount of saline, resulting in a 30% contrast solution.

Inflation of the balloon should be monitored with a pressure gauge. Currently used polyethylene or Mylar catheters do not expand beyond their predetermined di-

ameter and too much pressure on injection could lead to balloon rupture. The balloon inflation should also be monitored fluoroscopically as the stenosis can usually be seen as an indentation on the balloon, and the elimination of this "waist" indicates dilation of the stenosis (Fig. 9.15).

In an alert and cooperative patient, pain may also help monitor the balloon dilation. Some discomfort during dilation is expected. Lack of pain is a sign of underdilation while severe pain may herald arterial rupture.

The balloon should be left inflated for 30–60 seconds, but care must be taken not to move the balloon while inflated. If a fully inflated balloon is moved, it converts the radial force into a shearing force that may completely disrupt the intima.

Results

The overall technical success rate for percutaneous transluminal angioplasty is generally reported as 80–95%. Obviously, the number, type, and location of the lesions contribute significantly to the success or failure of the procedure. Better results can be expected with increased experience and future reports should demonstrate improvement. Martin et al. reported a statistically significant rise in the technical success rate from 93 to 97% when results of the first 100 PTA cases were compared with the second 100 PTA cases. They also noted a concomitant decrease in the total complications from 20 to 13%. A variety of technical innovations also contribute to this improved success. Better guide wires, catheters, and vascular sheaths as well as the use of less contrast material, more patient hydration and digital imaging to speed the entire procedure all contribute to these improved results.

Recurrent stenoses occur in 10–20% of patients but are most commonly seen when there is incomplete dila-

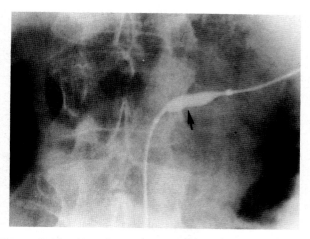

Figure 9.15. Transluminal angioplasty. Fluoroscopic monitoring confirms proper placement of the angioplasty balloon by demonstration of balloon "waisting" (*arrow*) at the site of stenosis.

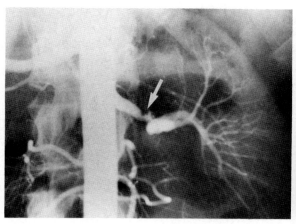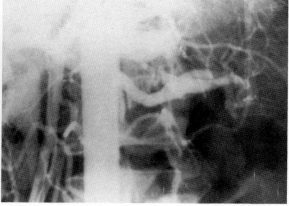

Figure 9.16. Transluminal angioplasty. **A,** A significant left renal artery stenosis (*arrow*) and poststenotic dilatation are identified. **B,** After angioplasty, an excellent result is obtained.

tion of the lesion. Thus, it is most important to get a good initial result. A restenosis can be approached as a new lesion and attempts at redilating a recurrent stenosis are generally good, but with a slightly decreased success rate.

The results of angioplasty vary with the type of lesion responsible for the renal artery stenosis. Thus, the major categories are considered separately.

ATHEROSCLEROSIS.   The best results are obtained with short, isolated stenoses in the mid-portion of the renal artery (Figs. 9.16 and 9.17). If the lesion is at the origin of the renal artery, it may not be clear whether this is due to atherosclerosis of the renal artery or plaque within the aorta, which merely overhangs the origin of the renal artery. Dilation of atherosclerotic plaque in the proximal portion of the renal artery can be performed with excellent results, however, plaque that arises from the aorta is only displaced during the dilation procedure and a large residual stenosis often persists.

When patients with atherosclerosis are analyzed, patients with occluded vessels, ostial lesions, or bilateral stenoses do not do as well as patients with unilateral nonostial lesions. Sos et al. found that two-thirds of patients with a unilateral stenosis could be successfully dilated, but only 20% of patients with bilateral stenoses had

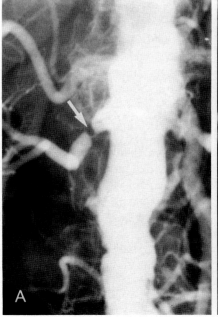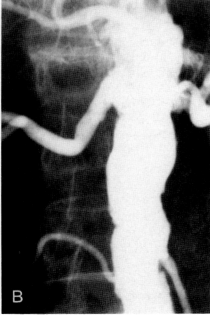

Figure 9.17. Transluminal angioplasty. **A,** Preliminary arteriogram demonstrates generalized atherosclerotic changes as well as a tight renal artery stenosis (*arrow*). **B,** The lumen is widely patent after PTA.

technical success on both sides. Most patients with a technically successful dilation experience cure or improvement in hypertension. The clinical response in patients with bilateral disease reflects the technical difficulties in obtaining technically successful dilation. If the renal arteries are adequately dilated, a good clinical response is often achieved. However, since there is a high failure rate of one or the other artery, the overall chances of a good clinical response to attempted bilateral renal artery angioplasty are relatively poor.

The clinical response to PTA cannot be measured immediately or even at discharge from the hospital as it is not uncommon for hypertension to recur during the first few months after angioplasty. Thus, at least 3–6 months of follow-up are usually required to assess the durability of the clinical response. It is uncommon for a lesion to recur after 6 months, although a new lesion may form as the underlying process of plaque formation continues.

When all patients with atherosclerotic plaques are included, approximately 75% have a good clinical response to angioplasty. Approximately 25% of patients are cured, i.e., they become normotensive off medication. Approximately 50% will be improved in that blood pressure is easier to control on fewer medications. Only approximately 25% fail due to inability to dilate the renal artery stenosis or lack of blood pressure response.

FIBROMUSCULAR DYSPLASIA. Patients with fibromuscular dysplasia almost uniformly respond to PTA with good results. Since FMD typically occurs in young or middle-aged women, the access vessels are usually free of atherosclerotic plaque and tortuosity. Thus, the lesions are easier to approach. Although tight, web-like stenoses may be present, they seldom prevent guidewire and catheter access. Tegtmeyer, Kellum, and Ayers reported technical success in each of 27 patients with FMD; 10 (37%) were cured and 17 (63%) showed improvement in hypertension. In 1985, Martin reported similarly excellent results with 25% of patients cured and 60% improved.

TAKAYASU'S DISEASE. Although experience with PTA of renal artery stenosis secondary to aortoarteritis is not as extensive as with atherosclerosis or FMD, the results have been very good. Scattered reports in the American literature have shown a high rate of technical success and frequently good clinical response. Dong et al. performed PTA on 32 patients with Takayasu's arteritis in Beijing, People's Republic of China. A 6-month follow-up was available on 22 patients, 19 of whom benefited from the procedure. Thirteen patients were cured by PTA, 6 showed improvement, while only 3 failed to respond. All patients with unilateral disease had a good clinical response to PTA, while only 62% of patients with bilateral involvement were cured or improved.

RENAL TRANSPLANTATION. PTA of a renal artery stenosis in a transplanted kidney is often technically difficult. The renal artery may be placed as either an end-to-end anastomosis with the internal iliac artery, or an end-to-side

anastomosis with the external iliac artery. Raynaud et al. performed PTA on 43 hypertensive renal transplant recipients who had stenosis of the transplant renal artery. In patients with end-to-side anastomoses, an ipsilateral femoral approach was used. In patients with an end-to-end anastomosis, a contralateral femoral approach was used most often, but an axillary approach was occasionally required. The procedure was technically successful in 35 (81%) patients, and 26 (74%) of these achieved clinical success. Most of the technical failures occurred in patients with end-to-end anastomoses.

NEUROFIBROMATOSIS. Renal artery stenosis is a common cause of hypertension in young patients with neurofibromatosis. The renal artery is surrounded by ganglioneuromatous or neurofibromatous tissue. Intimal proliferation, thinning of the media, and fragmentation of the elastic tissue lead to arterial stenosis. PTA of these lesions is extremely difficult and rarely successful. Baxi et al. reported successful PTA of a renal artery stenosis in a 19-year-old woman with neurofibromatosis. They suggested that the lesion in that patient was more likely due to dysplasia, which may also be seen in neurofibromatosis but more frequently involves small intrarenal arteries.

Complications

Complications of renal artery PTA may be considered as general complications such as adverse contrast reactions or problems at the puncture site, or specific to renal artery PTA, such as a rupture, dissection, embolus, or thrombosis of the renal artery. Idiosyncratic reactions to contrast material are rare but should be treated as a reaction to intravenous contrast injection. Contrast-induced renal failure is a frequent problem, as many of these patients have preexisting azotemia, which is the primary risk factor for contrast nephropathy. Good hydration and judicious use of contrast material will help to decrease the incidence of contrast induced renal failure. Intraarterial digital subtraction techniques are particularly helpful in avoiding this problem as much less contrast material is required. Problems related to the puncture site at either the groin or axilla include bleeding, hematoma (Fig. 9.18), or false aneurysm formation. The use of a sheath helps to reduce trauma to the vessel at the puncture site and may decrease the incidence of these complications.

Major complications involving the renal artery occur in approximately 5% of patients. Renal artery dissection may result from a subintimal position of the guidewire or may result from the dilation of the renal artery by the angioplasty balloon. The location of the catheter after crossing the stenosis should be tested with a small contrast injection. Even when the PTA proceeds without problem, a renal artery dissection may occur. Gardiner et al. reported three such cases, each of which resolved without surgical intervention.

Thrombosis of the renal artery may be incited by disruption of the arterial intima, the presence of foreign

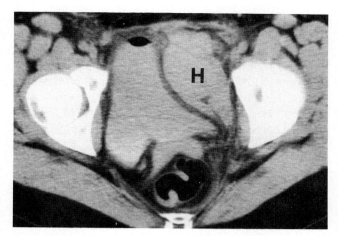

Figure 9.18. Groin hematoma. A large pelvic hematoma (H) is detected by CT after PTA.

material, or decreased flow due to occlusion of the renal artery by the angioplasty catheter. Vasospasm may also contribute to thrombosis by decreasing arterial flow (Fig. 9.19). Systemic anticoagulation is essential to prevent this problem. Prevention of arterial spasm by premedication supplemented with intraarterial nitroglycerin is also useful.

Renal artery rupture is an acute emergency that must be treated surgically. The rapid blood loss through the renal artery is life threatening. (Fig. 9.20). If rupture occurs, the catheter should be left in the renal artery and the balloon inflated in an attempt to occlude the bleeding vessel. This can be attempted while the patient is in the angiography suite but does not alleviate the need for immediate surgery.

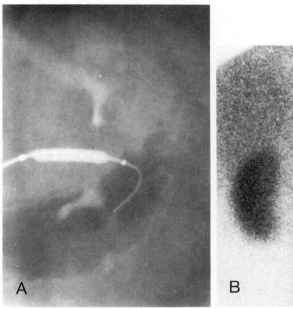

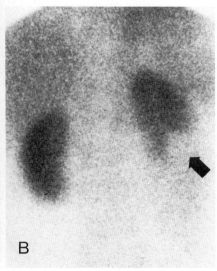

Figure 9.19. Renal infarct. **A,** During angioplasty the guide-wire was passed into a lower-pole vessel, inducing spasm. **B,** A radionuclide scan demonstrates absent perfusion to a portion of the lower pole of the left kidney (*arrow*).

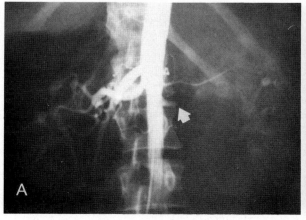

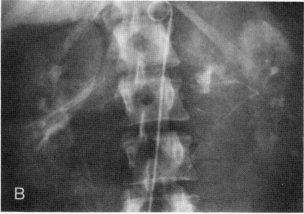

Figure 9.20. Renal artery rupture. **A,** A sharp cutoff of the left main renal artery is seen (*arrow*). **B,** Contrast extravasation is appreciated on later films. The left kidney is displaced laterally by the retroperitoneal hematoma.

Embolization

Percutaneous transcatheter renal artery embolization may be used in a variety of clinical situations in which renal ablation is desired without surgery.

Patients with end-stage renal disease may have hypertension that is difficult to control. The native kidneys of renal transplant recipients are not routinely removed, as these kidneys may help to excrete water and secrete two important hormones, vitamin D_3 and erythropoetin. These patients are poor surgical risks and mortality from bilateral nephrectomy ranges from 5 to 10%. The morbidity and mortality of transcatheter renal ablation (as judged by small series and case reports) is lower than surgical nephrectomy.

Renovascular hypertension is occasionally due to a branch renal artery stenosis that cannot be crossed for PTA. If the feeding branch artery can be cannulated, that segment of the kidney can be infarcted in an attempt to cure the hypertension.

A variety of materials may be used to occlude the main renal artery or branch vessels to infarct renal tissue. Gelatin particles have been used but recanalization may occur and an additional occluding material, such as a Gianturco coil, is needed. Cyanoacrylate, sodium tetradecol sulfate, and absolute ethanol have also been used successfully. As with embolization procedures for renal malignancy, these agents must be used with care to minimize complications.

RENOVASCULAR HYPERTENSION IN CHILDREN

The incidence of hypertension in children is 1–2%, much lower than the incidence in the adult population. The majority of these hypertensive children have a secondary cause.

Acquired renal parenchymal disease is the most common cause of hypertension among children. Other causes include the hemolytic uremic syndrome, renal trauma, nephrotic syndrome, and chronic pyelonephritis. Both acute glomerulonephritis and congenital malformation account for about 20% of cases of renal hypertension. In approximately 10%, it is renovascular hypertension. Children with renovascular hypertension tend to be younger and have higher levels of blood pressure than children with essential hypertension. Creatinine and urinalysis are usually normal in both groups.

The most common etiology of renovascular hypertension among children is FMD. Surprisingly, FMD is seen more commonly among males than females in children. As in adults, the proximal portion of the renal artery is seldom involved, but unlike the adult population, the classic "string of beads" appearance is seldom seen in children.

Renal artery stenosis due to neurofibromatosis is the next most common etiology for renovascular hyperten-

sion in children. The proximal renal artery is involved and there may be an associated hypoplasia of the abdominal aorta.

The middle aortic syndrome due to nonspecific aortitis was responsible for 4 of the 30 cases of renovascular hypertension reported by Stanley et al. (1978). An irregular narrowing of the aorta with stenosis of the proximal renal artery is seen in these patients and bilateral involvement is usual.

Hypertensive urography is even less sensitive in children than adults. Radionuclide tests are more promising, but in view of the high incidence of a secondary cause of hypertension, most children with suspected renovascular hypertension undergo conventional arteriography. Digital techniques may be used, as less contrast material is needed and the examination may be performed more quickly than with conventional angiographic filming. However, intraarterial injections are often needed to maintain a good contrast bolus and obtain optimal images.

Renal vein renin sampling is as useful in children as adults. A lateralizing result correlates with a good response to intervention. Subselective samples may be required if segmental disease is present. Thus, venous samples are best obtained after angiography.

The treatment of renal artery stenosis causing renovascular hypertension in children has traditionally been surgical. However, PTA has become the treatment of choice in adults, and is being used with increasing frequency in children.

The success rate for PTA is lower than in adults for two reasons. The smaller size of the vessel and more frequent arterial vasospasm makes children more difficult to angiogram and dilate. The most common etiologies of renal artery stenosis in adults, atherosclerosis and FMD, respond well to PTA while many children have a more fibrotic process that cannot be adequately dilated.

Mali et al. reported the use of PTA in 12 children and adolescents with renovascular hypertension. They subdivided their patients on the basis of the length and location of the renal artery stenosis. Those patients with a short stenosis in the mid- or distal portion of the renal artery responded well to PTA. The patients with a short stenosis near the origin of the renal artery were dilated but had a poor clinical response. PTA was technically unsuccessful in patients with a long stenosis at or near the origin of the renal artery.

SUGGESTED READINGS

Renal Parenchymal Hypertension

Amparo EG, Fagan CJ: Page kidney. *J Comp Assist Tomogr* 6(4):839, 1982.

Bonsib SM, Meng RL, Johnson FP Jr: Ask-Upmark kidney with contralateral renal artery fibromuscular dysplasia. *Am J Nephrol* 5:450, 1985.

Dunnick NR, Hartman DS, Ford KK, et al: The radiology of juxtaglomerular tumors. *Radiology* 147:321, 1983.

Hattery RR, Hartman GW, Williamson B: Computerized tomography of nonvascular causes of renal hypertension. *Urol Radiol* 3:261, 1982.

Himmelfarb E, Rabinowitz JG, Parvey L, et al: The Ask-Upmark kidney: roentgenographic and pathological features. *Am J Dis Child* 129:1440, 1975.

Kala R, Fyhrquist F, Halttunen P, et al: Solitary renal cyst, hypertension and renin. *J Urol* 116:710, 1976.

Messina LM, Reilly LM, Goldstone J, et al: Middle aortic syndrome: effectiveness and durability of complex arterial revascularization techniques. *Ann Surg* 204:331, 1986.

Pak K, Kawamura J, Yoshida O: Hypertension with elevated renal vein renin secondary to unilateral hydronephrosis. *Urology* 16:499, 1980.

Sonda LP, Konmnak JW, Diokno AC: Clinical aspects of nonvascular renal causes of hypertension. *Urol Radiol* 3:257, 1982.

Von Knorring J, Fyhrquist F, Ahonen J: Varying course of hypertension following renal trauma. *J Urol* 126:798, 1981.

Renovascular Hypertension

Berland LL, Koslin DB, Routh WD, Keller FS: Renal artery stenosis: prospective evaluation of diagnosis with color duplex US compared with angiography. *Radiology* 174:421, 1990.

Dunnick NR, Sfakianakis GN: Screening for renovascular hypertension. *Radiol Clin North Am* (In Press).

Ferris TF: The kidney and hypertension. *Arch Intern Med* 142:1889, 1982.

Fraley EE, Feldman BH: Renal hypertension. *N Engl J Med* 287:550, 1972.

Lagneau P, Michel JB: Renovascular hypertension and Takayasu's disease. *J Urol* 134:876, 1985.

Lewis VD, Meranze SG, McLean GK, et al: The midaortic syndrome: diagnosis and treatment. *Radiology* 167:111, 1988.

Perry MO: Fibromuscular dysplasia. *Surg Gynecol Obstet* 139:98, 1974.

Simon N, Franklin SS, Bleifer KH, et al: Clinical characteristics of renovascular hypertension. *JAMA* 220:1209, 1972.

Spies JB, LeQuite MH, Robison JG, et al: Renovascular hypertension caused by compression of the renal artery by the diaphragmatic crus. *AJR* 149:1195, 1987.

Wise KL, McCann EL, Dunnick NR, et al: Renovascular hypertension. *J Urol* 140:911, 1988.

Wylie EJ, Binkley FM, Palubinskas AJ: Extrarenal fibromuscular hyperplasia. *Am J Surg* 112:149, 1966.

Aneurysm

Cummings KR, Lecky JW, Kaufman JJ: Renal artery aneurysms and hypertension. *J Urol* 109:144, 1973.

Vaughan TJ, Barry WF, Jeffords DL, et al: Renal artery aneurysms and hypertension. *Radiology* 99:287, 1971.

Hypertensive Urography

Bookstein JJ, Abrams HL, Buenger RE, et al: Radiologic aspects of renovascular hypertension. *JAMA* 220:1225, 1972.

Kaufman JJ: Renovascular hypertension: the UCLA experience. *J Urol* 121:139, 1979.

Lalli AF: Is the hypertensive urogram a necessary examination? *J Can Assoc Radiol* 32:11, 1981.

Thornbury JR, Stanley JC, Fryback DG: Hypertensive urogram: a nondiscriminatory test for renovascular hypertension. *AJR* 138:43, 1982.

Radionuclide Renography

Chiarini C, Esposti ED, Losinno F, et al: Renal scintigraphy versus renal vein renin activity for identifying and treating renovascular hypertension. *Nephron* 32:8, 1982.

Grunewald SM, Collins LT: Renovascular hypertension: quantitative renography as a screening test. *Radiology* 149:287, 1983.

Sfakianakis GN: Renal scintigraphy following angiotensin converting enzyme inhibition in the diagnosis of renovascular hypertension (captopril scintigraphy). *J Nucl Med Technol* 17(3):160, 1989.

Sfakianakis GN, Bourgoignie JJ, Jaffe D, et al: Single-dose captopril scintigraphy in the diagnosis of renovascular hypertension. *J Nucl Med* 28:1383, 1987.

Digital Subtraction Angiography

Buonocore E, Meaney TF, Borkowski GP, et al: Digital subtraction angiography of the abdominal aorta and renal arteries. *Radiology* 139:281, 1981.

Clark RA, Alexander ES: Digital subtraction angiography of the renal arteries—prospective comparison and conventional arteriography. *Invest Radiol* 18:6, 1983.

Dunnick NR, Ford KK, Johnson GA, et al: Digital intravenous subtraction angiography for investigating renovascular hypertension: comparison with hypertensive urography. *South Med J* 78:690, 1985.

Dunnick NR, Svetkey LP, Cohan RH, et al: Intravenous digital subtraction renal angiography: use in screening for renovascular hypertension. *Radiology* 172:219, 1989.

Gomes AS, Paid SO, Barbaric ZL: Digital subtraction angiography in the evaluation of hypertension. *AJR* 140:779, 1983.

Hillman BJ, Ovitt TW, Capp MP, et al: Renal digital subtraction angiography: 100 cases. *Radiology* 145:643, 1982.

Hillman BJ, Ovitt TW, Capp MP, et al: The potential impact of digital video subtraction angiography on screening for renovascular hypertension. *Radiology* 142:577, 1982.

Kaufman SL, Chang R, Kadir S, et al: Intraarterial digital subtraction angiography: a comparative view. *Cardiovasc Intervent Radiol* 6:271, 1983.

Popsky GL, Saluk PH, Griska LB, et al: Comparison of superior vena cava and antecubital vein as DSA injection site. *AJR* 143:317, 1984.

Smith CW, Winfield AC, Price RR, et al: Evaluation of digital venous angiography for the diagnosis of renovascular hypertension. *Radiology* 144:51, 1982.

Svetkey LP, Himmelstein SI, Dunnick NR, et al: Prospective analysis of strategies for diagnosing renovascular hypertension. *Hypertension* 14:247, 1989.

Tifft CP: Renal digital subtraction angiography—a nephrologist's view. *Cardiovasc Intervent Radiol* 6:231, 1983.

Tonkin IL, Stapleton FB, Roy S, III: Digital subtraction angiography in the evaluation of renal vascular hypertension in children. *Pediatrics* 81:150, 1988.

Wilms GE, Baert AL, Staessen JA, et al: Renal artery stenosis: evaluation with intravenous digital subtraction angiography. *Radiology* 160:713, 1986.

Renal Vein Renin

Harrington DP, Whelton PK, Mackenzie EJ, et al: Renal venous renin sampling—prospective study of techniques and methods. *Radiology* 138:571, 1981.

Hietala SO, Zelenak JJ, Beachley MC, et al: Influence of contrast material on renal venous renin activity. *AJR* 132:429, 1979.

Sos TA, Vaughan ED, Pickering TG, et al: Diagnosis of renovascular hypertension and evaluation of "surgical" curability. *Urol Radiol* 3:199, 1982.

Thibonnier M, Joseph A, Sassano P, et al: Improved diagnosis of unilateral renal artery lesions after captopril administration. *JAMA* 251:56, 1984.

Thind GS: Role of renal venous renins in the diagnosis and management of renovascular hypertension. *J Urol* 134:2, 1985.

Yune HY, Rabe FE, Klatte EC, et al: Measurement of renin in segmental renal veins of hypertensives. *Radiology* 146:29, 1983.

Percutaneous Transluminal Angioplasty

Baxi R, Epstein HY, Abitbol C: Percutaneous transluminal renal artery angioplasty in hypertension associated with neurofibromatosis. *Radiology* 139:583, 1981.

Becker GJ, Katzen BT, Dake MD: Noncoronary angioplasty. *Radiology* 170:921, 1989.

Castaneda-Zuniga WR, Formanek A, Tadavarthy M, et al: The mechanism of balloon angioplasty. *Radiology* 135:565, 1980.

Clements R, Evans C, Salaman JR: Percutaneous transluminal angioplasty of renal transplant artery stenosis. *Clin Radiol* 38:235, 1987.

Dong ZJ, Li S, Lu X: Percutaneous transluminal angioplasty for renovascular hypertension in arteritis: experience in China. *Radiology* 162:477, 1987.

Dotter CT, Judkins MP: Transluminal treatment of arteriosclerotic obstruction—description of a new technique and a preliminary report of its application. *Circulation* 30:654, 1964.

Freiman DB: Transluminal angioplasty of the renal arteries. *Radiol Clin North Am* 24(4):665, 1986.

Gardiner GA, Meyerovitz MF, Harrington DP, et al: Dissection complicating angioplasty. *AJR* 145:627, 1985.

Gardiner GA, Meyerovitz MF, Stokes KR, et al: Complications of transluminal angioplasty. *Radiology* 159:201, 1986.

Gruntzig A, Kumpe GA: Technique of percutaneous transluminal angioplasty with the Gruntzig balloon catheter. *AJR* 132:547, 1979.

Gruntzig A, Vetter W, Meier B, et al: Treatment of renovascular hypertension with percutaneous transluminal dilatation of a renal-artery stenosis. *Lancet* 1:801, 1978.

Hayes JM, Risius B, Novick AC, et al: Experience with percutaneous transluminal angioplasty for renal artery stenosis at the Cleveland Clinic. *J Urol* 139:488, 1988.

Kim PK, Spriggs DW, Rutecki GW, et al: Transluminal angioplasty in patients with bilateral renal artery stenosis or renal artery stenosis in a solitary functioning kidney. *AJR* 153:1305, 1989.

Klinge J, Mali WPTM, Puijlaert CBAJ, et al: Percutaneous transluminal renal angioplasty: initial and long-term results. *Radiology* 171:501, 1989.

Martin LG, Casarella WJ, Alspaugh JP, et al: Renal artery angioplasty: increased technical success and decreased complications in the second 100 patients. *Radiology* 159:631, 1986.

Martin LG, Casarella WJ, Gaylord GM: Azotemia caused by renal artery stenosis: treatment by percutaneous angioplasty. *AJR* 150:844, 1988.

Martin LG, Price TB, Casarella WJ, et al: Percutaneous angioplasty in clinical management of renovascular hypertension: initial and long-term results. *Radiology* 155:629, 1985.

Miller GA, Ford KK, Braun SD, et al: Percutaneous transluminal angioplasty vs. surgery for renovascular hypertension. *AJR* 144:447, 1985.

Park JH, Han MC, Kim SH, et al: Takayasu arteritis: angiographic findings and results of angioplasty. *AJR* 153:1069, 1989.

Porstmann W, Wierny L: Intravasale rekanalisation inoperabler arterieller obliterationen. *Zentralbl Chir* 92:1586, 1967.

Raynaud A, Bedrossian J, Remy P, et al. Percutaneous transluminal angioplasty of renal transplant arterial stenoses. *AJR* 146:853, 1986.

Sniderman KW, Sos TA: Percutaneous transluminal recanalization and dilatation of totally occluded renal arteries. *Radiology* 142:607, 1982.

Sos TA, Pickering TG, Sniderman K, et al: Percutaneous transluminal renal angioplasty in renovascular hypertension due to atheroma or fibromuscular dysplasia. *N Engl J Med* 309:274, 1983.

Tegtmeyer CJ, Ayers CA, Wellons HA: The axillary approach to percutaneous renal artery dilatation. *Radiology* 135:775, 1980.

Tegtmeyer CJ, Kellum CD, Ayers C: Percutaneous transluminal angioplasty of the renal artery—results and long-term follow-up. *Radiology* 153:77, 1984.

Tegtmeyer CJ, Kofler TJ, Ayers C: Renal angioplasty: current status. *AJR* 142:17, 1984.

Tegtmeyer CJ, Sos TA: Techniques of renal angioplasty. *Radiology* 161:577, 1986.

Tegtmeyer CJ, Teates CD, Crigler N, et al: Percutaneous transluminal angioplasty in patients with renal artery stenosis. *Radiology* 150:323, 1981.

Van Andel GJ: *Percutaneous Transluminal Angioplasty—The Dotter Procedure.* Amsterdam, Excerpta Medica, 1976.

Zeitler E, Schoop W, Zahnow, W: The treatment of occlusive arterial disease by transluminal catheter angioplasty. *Radiology* 99:19, 1971.

Embolization

Bachman DM, Casarella WJ, Spiegel R, et al: Selective renal artery embolization—treatment of acute renovascular hypertension. *JAMA* 238:1534, 1977.

Keller FS, Coyle M, Rosch J, et al: Percutaneous renal ablation in patients with end-stage renal disease: alternative to surgical nephrectomy. *Radiology* 159:447, 1986.

Nanni GS, Hawkins IF, Orak JK: Control of hypertension by ethanol renal ablation. *Radiology* 148:51, 1983.

Reuter SR, Pomeroy PR, Chuang VP, et al: Embolic control of hypertension caused by segmental renal artery stenosis. *AJR* 127:389, 1976.

Hypertension in Children

Chevalier RL, Tegtmeyer CJ, Gomez RA: Percutaneous transluminal angioplasty for renovascular hypertension in children. *Pediatr Nephrol* 1:89, 1987.

Mali WPTM, Puijlaert CBAJ, Kouwenberg HJ, et al: Percutaneous transluminal renal angioplasty in children and adolescents. *Radiology* 165:391, 1987.

Olson DL, Lieberman E: Renal hypertension in children. *Pediatr Clin North Am* 23(4):795, 1976.

Siegel MJ, St. Amour TE, Siegel BA: Imaging techniques in the evaluation of pediatric hypertension. *Pediatr Nephrol* 1:76, 1987.

Stanley P, Gyepes MT, Olson DL, et al: Renovascular hypertension in children and adolescents. *Radiology* 129:123, 1978.

Stanley P, Hieshima G, Mehringer M: Percutaneous transluminal angioplastic for pediatric renovascular hypertension. *Radiology* 153:101, 1984.

NEPHROCALCINOSIS AND NEPHROLITHIASIS

Intrarenal calcifications may lie either in the renal parenchyma (nephrocalcinosis) or in the collecting system (nephrolithiasis). Dystrophic calcification is calcification of abnormal tissue such as tumors, cyst walls, inflammatory masses, or vessels. Since dystrophic calcification is due to the underlying parenchymal abnormality it is not usually considered nephrocalcinosis.

Nephrolithiasis is stone formation, within the collecting system. Most stones are formed in the pelvocaliceal system and may be passed distally. Occasionally they may form in a cavity that communicates with the collecting system such as a calyceal diverticulum, bladder, or urethral diverticulum. Those conditions that result in nephrocalcinosis often lead to nephrolithiasis.

Since calcification is readily detected on an abdominal radiograph, nephrocalcinosis and nephrolithiasis are routinely evaluated with conventional urography. When supplemented with computed tomography (CT), even relatively lucent stones are easily detected. The density of the stones determined by CT can be used to predict its chemical composition. Furthermore, a variety of interventional techniques are now commonly employed in the treatment of nephrolithiasis and its complications.

NEPHROCALCINOSIS

Dystrophic

Calcification of abnormal tissue is usually dystrophic. Dystrophic calcification may occur when the solubility product of calcium and phosphate is exceeded due to a change in pH or may be part of a reparative process. This may occur in a huge variety of lesions but the most common are tumor, hematoma, an inflammatory mass, or vascular abnormalities. Dystrophic calcifications will be considered in the discussion of the specific entities.

Metastatic

Calcification of normal renal tissue due to abnormally high levels of calcium is termed *metastatic*. Metastatic calcification occurs when the solubility product of calcium and phosphate or oxalate in the extracellular fluid is exceeded. Certain diseases have a predilection to calcify specific anatomic areas. Thus, metastatic nephrocalcinosis may be further subdivided by predominant location.

Cortical Nephrocalcinosis

Cortical nephrocalcinosis is peripheral in location but does include the central extension along the septa of Bertin. The medullary pyramids are spared. It may be seen on abdominal radiographs as thin peripheral lines of calcification ("tram lines") or as diffuse punctate calcifications representing necrotic cortical tubules.

The most common entities to produce cortical nephrocalcinosis are chronic glomerulonephritis and acute cortical necrosis. It may also be seen in Alport's syndrome (hereditary nephropathy and deafness), oxalosis, and in some patients with a rejected renal transplant.

Acute cortical necrosis may be due to ingestion of toxins such as ethylene glycol, exposure to methoxyflurane anesthesia, or an acute vascular insult. Both ethylene glycol and methoxyflurane exposure result in oxalate deposition which causes interstitial fibrosis. Acute hypotension may cause focal tubular necrosis which later calcifies.

Hereditary nephritis, or Alport's syndrome, is characterized by glomerulonephritis and interstitial fibrosis and is frequently associated with nerve deafness. It is inherited as an autosomal dominant trait with variable penetrance. The disease is transmitted to both sons and daughters but it is incompletely expressed in females. Hematuria often begins in childhood and mild proteinuria may be present. Progression to renal failure is slow with death by the third to fifth decade.

Medullary Nephrocalcinosis

Medullary nephrocalcinosis is central in location but with peripheral extensions along the medullary pyramids. It is usually a bilateral process with multiple stippled calcifications in the characteristic distribution.

The most common etiologies to produce medullary nephrocalcinosis are hyperparathyroidism (Fig. 10.1) and renal tubular acidosis. Other relatively common causes include tubular ectasia (medullary sponge kidney), the milk-alkali syndrome, and a variety of nephrotoxic drugs such as amphotericin B.

Hyperparathyroidism may be due to a parathyroid adenoma, carcinoma, or hyperplasia of the chief cells. It is most commonly due to a single adenoma. Typically the serum calcium is high and the phosphate is low. This helps distinguish primary hyperparathyroidism from secondary hyperparathyroidism resulting from chronic renal disease in which the serum phosphate is elevated.

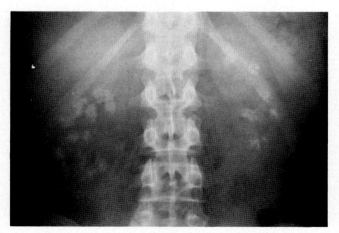

Figure 10.1. Medullary nephrocalcinosis. Multiple stippled calcifications are appreciated in the renal pyramids of both kidneys.

Patients with renal tubular acidosis (RTA) have a defect in the tubules that prevents the kidney from excreting an acid urine. Thus, the risk of stone formation is increased, as calcium salts are less soluble in alkaline urine than in an acid urine. In adults, primary RTA is due to an inherited enzymatic defect. The manifestations of urolithiasis, osteomalacia, and hypokalemia can be treated with alkalinizing salts.

A nonhereditary form of primary RTA has been described in children (Lightwood syndrome). This is a transient disorder which affects infants and lasts several years. However, if treated during the acute period, spontaneous improvement in distal tubular function occurs.

Renal tubular acidosis is also divided into proximal and distal forms. The proximal variety is a result of decreased bicarbonate reabsorption by the proximal tubule. When reabsorption of other substances is also impaired it is known as the Fanconi syndrome. Although biochemically interesting, this proximal form does not have radiographic manifestations.

In the distal form the distal renal tubule can no longer secrete hydrogen ions. This results in bicarbonate loss, reduced acid excretion, secondary aldosteronism, and hypokalemia. Nephrocalcinosis occurs in almost three-quarters of these patients and commonly appears as clusters of calcifications in the medullary pyramids.

Nephrocalcinosis may occur in patients who consume large quantities of antacids and milk for the treatment of peptic ulcer disease. This has been termed the "milk alkali syndrome." Alkaline urine facilitates precipitation of calcium containing calculi.

The stones found in medullary sponge kidney are calcium phosphate or calcium oxalate. They are usually small and many more are present than can be detected radiographically. These tiny stones are asymptomatic but may cause colic if they migrate into the collecting system, enlarge, and begin to pass down the ureter.

NEPHROLITHIASIS

Nephrolithiasis is a common problem among people from temperate climates. Smith estimates that at least 5% of the female and 12% of the male population will have at least one episode of renal colic due to stone disease by the age of 70 years. It is stimulating to note that a low urinary output is felt to aid in urinary tract stone formation, yet people from areas with hot climates such as Africa have a low incidence of stone disease. It is possible that those peoples have genetically selected individuals less likely to form stones.

In the United States, the southeastern states have the highest incidence of stone disease. Hospital admissions for stone-related problems are twice as common in the Southeast as the rest of the nation.

There are many etiologies for the production of

nephrolithiasis including genetic predisposition, diet, occupation, and lifestyle. A high water intake resulting in an increased urinary output significantly reduces the incidence of stones in patients predisposed to stone formation.

The urine must be supersaturated at least part of the time for stone formation. In addition to solute load, ionic strength complexation, and urine pH affect stone formation. Ionic strength increases the ability of urine to hold ions in solution. Anionic substances such as citrate phosphate or sulfate may complex calcium which reduces the free ionic concentration of the crystal components. The urine pH affects complexation and also has a direct effect on the solubility of organic compounds such as uric acid or cystine. Uric acid, for instance, is much more soluble as the pH increases.

Nephrolithiasis is seen three times as often in males as females. The peak age for the onset of renal stone disease is 20–30 years but the tendency for stone formation is often lifelong. The most common ages for patients treated for nephrolithiasis is 30–60 years.

The most common presenting symptom is renal colic, which is usually due to a ureteral stone. Controversy remains whether or not calyceal stones cause pain. Most calyceal stones are asymptomatic, but occasionally their removal is associated with relief of pain.

Renal colic is abrupt in onset, most frequently begins in the flank, and radiates to the groin. Men may complain of testicular pain while women feel discomfort radiating to the labia majora. Typically, patients suffering renal colic cannot find a comfortable position and continue to move around. Patients with stones in the distal ureter may present with symptoms of bladder irritability.

Hematuria is present in the vast majority of patients with urolithiasis, but may be absent in 15% of patients, particularly if the stone is completely obstructing. Pyuria is common, but a culture should be obtained to detect a urinary tract infection.

Specific Types of Urolithiasis

Calcium Stones

Calcium oxalate and calcium phosphate stones crystallize when the product of the two ions exceeds the solubility product. Thus, both the amount of calcium and the amount of oxalate are important in determining stone formation. A discussion of these factors is beyond the scope of this book, but factors affecting hypercalciuria are presented (Table 10.1).

Hypercalcemia is a common cause of hypercalciuria, although it is present in a minority of patients, and may result from a variety of metabolic processes. An abnormally large amount of calcium may be absorbed from the digestive tract. This occurs with hypervitaminosis D, sarcoidosis, and the milk alkali syndrome. Too much cal-

Table 10.1.
Causes of Hypercalciuria

Increased absorption
  Hypervitaminosis D
  Milk-alkali syndrome
  Sarcoidosis
  Beryllium poisoning
  Idiopathic hypercalciuria

Increased mobilization from bone
  Hyperparathyroidism
  Immobilization
  Bone metastases
  Multiple myeloma
  Hyperthyroidism
  Cushing's syndrome

Decreased tubular reabsorption
  Renal tubular acidosis
  Fanconi's syndrome
  Wilson's disease
  Amphotericin B toxicity

cium may be mobilized from the bony skeleton. This may result from immobilization, extensive bone metastases, or hyperparathyroidism.

Ionized calcium is filtered by the glomerulus, but most of this free calcium is reabsorbed by tubules. There is, however, a maximum reabsorption that can occur. If this is exceeded by a high calcium load in patients with hypercalcemia, hypercalciuria will result.

Hypercalciuria may also occur if there is distal renal tubular damage which interferes with hydrogen ion excretion creating RTA. Patients with primary RTA commonly develop nephrocalcinosis which characteristically involves the medullary pyramids. Secondary RTA may be due to a variety of diseases including Fanconi's syndrome, Wilson's disease, and amphotericin B toxicity, which also affects the distal renal tubule.

Calcium stones are relatively dense and usually easily seen on abdominal radiographs. Small stones may be obscured by overlying bowel gas or fecal material and nephrotomography is often needed for identification and quantification (Fig. 10.2).

Cystine Stones

Patients with cystinuria have a defect in renal tubular reabsorption of the amino acids cystine, ornithine, lysine, and arginine. A positive nitroprusside test is diagnostic and exchange column chromatography can identify the amino acids in the urine. The defect is inherited as an autosomal-recessive trait and is present in the intestinal mucosa as well as the renal tubular cells. Although in some patients a short stature is attributed to lysine deficiency, the only manifestation in most patients is nephrolithiasis. Excess cystine excreted in the urine exceeds its solubility and cystine stones are produced.

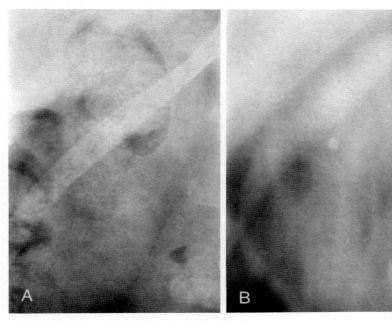

Figure 10.2. Calcium stone. **A,** Overlying bowel gas obscures a right renal stone. **B,** Nephrotomography clearly reveals a 5-mm calcium oxalate stone.

The opacity of cystine stones depends on how much contamination with calcium is present. However, many stones are pure cystine and are still easily seen on abdominal radiographs, although they are not as dense as calcium stones (Fig. 10.3).

Struvite Stones

Magnesium ammonium phosphate (struvite) stones form when the urine pH is above 7.2. They commonly occur in the setting of a urinary tract infection with a urea-splitting Gram-negative enteric organism, often *P. mirabilis.* Thus, struvite calculi are also commonly referred to as "infection stones." Struvite stones are relatively low density but are often found laminated with calcium salts forming more dense triple phosphate stones. They account for approximately 70% of staghorn calculi (Fig. 10.4).

Uric Acid Stones

Unlike other mammals, humans lack the enzyme uricase which converts uric acid into allantoin. In urine, uric acid exists either free or as the much more soluble salt, sodium urate. Acid urine (pH below 5.75) contributes to an increased concentration of the less soluble free uric acid.

Patients with uric acid calculi have hyperuricosuria but do not necessarily have hyperuricemia. Idiopathic uric acid lithiasis (see Table 10.2) occurs in patients with normal serum urate levels, but with a persistently low urine pH. This is seen in patients who take medications to acidify their urine, but it may also be present in patients with chronic diarrhea or an ileostomy.

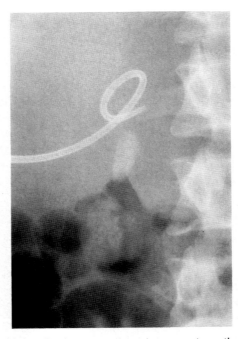

Figure 10.3. Cystine stone. A cystine stone is easily detected on an abdominal radiograph. A percutaneous nephrostomy catheter lies in the renal pelvis.

Inborn errors of metabolism may result in hyperuricemia and uric acid lithiasis. Patients with gout or the Lesch-Nyhan syndrome are prone to form uric acid stones. Similarly, an overindulgence in foods high in purine and proteins which are metabolized to uric acid may lead to hyperuricemia, hyperuricosuria, and uric acid stones. The ingestion of uricosuric drugs such as salicylates and

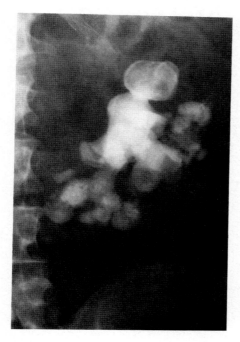

Figure 10.4. Staghorn calculus. A large staghorn calculus is easily seen in the left kidney. The alignment suggests a horseshoe kidney.

thiazides may increase the urine uric acid concentration sufficiently to allow uric acid stone formation.

In the United States uric acid stones account for 5–10% of renal stones. The reported incidence varies by country; in Israel approximately 75% of stones are uric acid.

Uric acid stones are poorly radiopaque and cannot be seen on an abdominal radiograph (Fig. 10.5). They account for the majority of "lucent" stones. However, they are still sufficiently dense to be easily seen on CT.

Xanthine Stones

These very rare stones may be seen in patients with hereditary xanthinuria but may also be present in patients treated with allopurinol, which blocks the conversion of xanthine to uric acid. Xanthine stones are relatively radiolucent, as their density is similar to uric acid stones.

Table 10.2.
Incidence of Urinary Lithiasis[a,b]

Calcium oxalate and phosphate, mixed	34
Calcium oxalate, pure	33
Calcium phosphate, pure	6
Magnesium ammonium phosphate (struvite)	15
Uric acid	8
Cystine	3

[a] From *Urol Clin North Am* 1:229, 1974.
[b] Percentage of stones analyzed.

Matrix Stones

Matrix stones are comprised primarily of coagulated mucoids with very little crystalline component. They are found most commonly in patients with urease-producing infections such as Proteus species. Matrix stones are also relatively radiolucent (Fig. 10.6) and may be confused with uric acid calculi. However, matrix stones occur in the presence of an alkaline urine while the urine is acidic in patients with uric acid calculi.

Oxalate Stones

Increased excretion of oxalate may be due to an inborn error of metabolism (primary) or may be secondary to other disorders. Hyperoxaluria may cause nephrocalcinosis and may result in calcium oxalate stones. The term *oxalosis* is used to indicate precipitation of oxalate crystals in extrarenal tissues such as the myocardium, lung, spleen, or arterial walls.

The most common cause of secondary oxalosis is small bowel disease, especially intestinal bypass operations for morbid obesity, but it may also be seen if the distal small bowel is involved with celiac disease or Crohn's disease. These patients have increased absorption of oxalate by the colon due to increased permeability of the colon or increased solubility of oxalate. Other causes of secondary hyperoxaluria include pyridoxine deficiency, methoxyflurane anesthesia, or increased consumption of leafy green vegetables which are high in oxalate.

Primary oxaluria is a rare inborn error of metabolism. There are two biochemical forms, but both result in increased urinary excretion of oxalate salts. Primary oxaluria is inherited as an autosomal recessive trait and shows no sex predilection. (Fig. 10.7) Patients present with manifestations of renal stones early in life.

Calcium oxalate crystals may precipitate out in the renal tubules which become obstructed and lead to tubular necrosis and atrophy. The crystals may stimulate an immune response in the kidney causing an interstitial nephritis. This results in progressive atrophy and renal failure.

Patients with hyperoxaluria may present with calcium oxalate stones (Fig. 10.8). However, most patients with such stones have neither a detectable abnormality of oxalate metabolism nor increased levels of oxalate excretion.

Stone Disease in Children

In developing countries, bladder calculi are common in children. They are most often uric acid and are unrelated to obstruction or infection. In industrialized countries, urinary tract calculi are found much more frequently in the upper urinary tract, just as in adults.

The male preponderance of stones seen in adults does not occur in children where males and females are

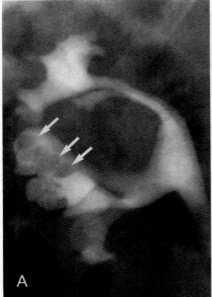
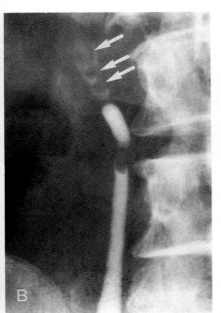

Figure 10.5. Uric acid stones. No stones could be seen on the preliminary radiograph. However, multiple filling defects (*arrows*) representing uric acid stones are identified on **A,** an excretory urogram and **B,** a retrograde pyelogram.

equally affected. Blacks are affected much less commonly than white children. Hematuria is the most common presenting symptom. Rather than the severe pain of ureteral colic seen in adults, children often complain of a more diffuse abdominal pain. The vast majority of pediatric patients have an underlying predisposing factor. Thus, children must be carefully evaluated for metabolic, anatomic, or infectious causes.

Urinary tract infection, hypercalciuria, urinary diversion procedures, congenital anomalies, and less frequently cystinuria or oxalosis may cause renal stones in children. However, the etiology remains unknown in approximately one-third of cases.

Nephrolithiasis is rare in very young children but has been reported in premature babies after furosemide therapy. Since urinary calcium excretion varies directly with urinary sodium excretion, furosemide, which increases sodium excretion, also results in hypercalciuria. This is especially marked in preterm babies as the

Figure 10.6. Matrix stones. These stones could not be seen on the abdominal radiograph. An air pyelogram demonstrated two large matrix stones (*arrows*).

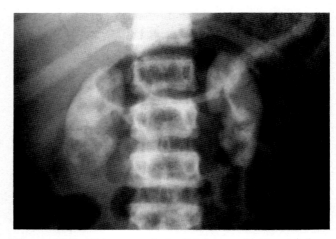

Figure 10.7. Primary oxaluria. Calcium oxalate crystals have precipitated out in the renal parenchyma.

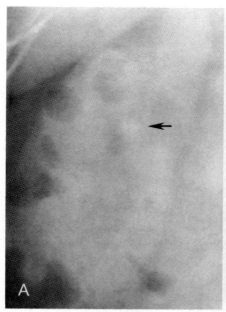
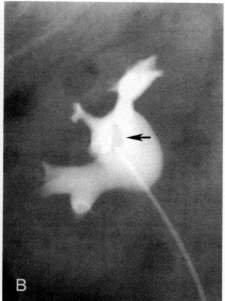

Figure 10.8. Oxalate stone. **A,** A faintly opaque oxalate stone (*arrow*) is appreciated on the preliminary film. **B,** It is seen as a filling defect (*arrow*) in the retrograde pyelogram.

marked increase in volume of amniotic fluid during the last trimester of pregnancy results from an increased excretion of sodium and water by the fetal kidney. Thus, premature babies have a higher urinary calcium at birth and are more prone to nephrolithiasis than full-term children.

Radiology

Plain Radiograph

Since approximately 90% of urinary tract calculi are radiopaque, the plain abdominal radiograph is the most useful examination in evaluating patients suspected of urolithiasis. Large stones are readily detected on a single film, but small calculi may be obscured by bowel gas or fecal material within the colon. If there are confusing overlying shadows, oblique films or nephrotomograms may be needed. With stones less than approximately 5 mm in diameter, nephrotomograms are usually more effective than oblique films, as the small opacity may be difficult to find on both the AP and oblique projection. Routine plain nephrotomography is also valuable in following patients with nephrolithiasis as tomography provides more precise delineation of the extent of the stone burden, especially when small calculi are present.

In addition to overlying bowel contents, the ribs, transverse processes, and sacrum may obscure urinary tract calculi. The lateral edge of the transverse process can be especially confusing as the cortical margin may mimic a ureteral stone.

There are many common calcifications in the abdomen that must be distinguished from urinary tract stones. Hepatic or splenic calcifications are seldom a problem, as they do not often overlie the kidneys. However, gallstones may lie over the right renal collecting system. In most cases, gallstones are larger with a characteristic ovoid shape and are easily distinguished from renal stones. However, renal calculi in an obstructed portion of the collecting system or within a calyceal diverticulum (Fig. 10.9) may precisely mimic gallstones. On an oblique radiograph, gallstones should rotate anteriorly while renal stones remain in a more posterior location.

Pancreatic calcification is most frequently seen in chronic pancreatitis. The involvement of the entire gland helps to distinguish these calcifications from renal stones.

Calcification of the costal cartilage of the lower thoracic ribs and arterial calcifications are usually linear, which helps to separate them from renal stones. Furthermore, arterial and rib calcifications lie in predictable locations.

The calcifications that are most often confused with urinary tract calculi are phleboliths (Fig. 10.10) and calcified mesenteric lymph nodes. Typically phleboliths are rounded, have a central lucency, and are seen in the true pelvis, often below the distal ureter. However, phleboliths are extremely common and are occasionally impossible to distinguish from ureteral stones without opacification of the ureter. Mesenteric lymph nodes typically have a mottled calcification, and oblique films may show them anterior to the retroperitoneum.

In these or other confusing cases, the most valuable

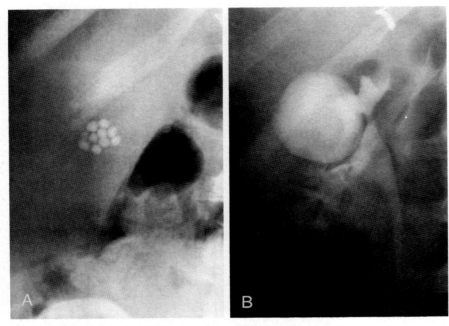

Figure 10.9. Stones in a calyceal diverticulum. **A,** Multiple stones in a spherical configuration in the right upper quadrant suggest gallstones. **B,** An excretory urogram demonstrates their location in a calyceal diverticulum.

maneuver is often comparison with old radiographs. The presence of a pelvic phlebolith that predates renal colic may be sufficient to identify a confusing calcification. In other cases, however, opacification of the collecting system is needed to separate a urinary tract calculus from an adjacent calcified structure. However, once contrast has been introduced, radiopaque stones become much more difficult to locate. Thus, care must be taken to obtain all preliminary films that are needed before proceeding to contrast injection.

Urography

Excretory urography serves two important functions in the evaluation of the patient with suspected stone disease: (*a*) It delineates the relationship of the collecting system to the calcification on the preliminary film, and (*b*) it demonstrates the degree of obstruction.

Calcifications overlying or within the kidney are seen to be renal stones when their location within the collecting system is demonstrated. Many calcium stones have a density similar to excreted contrast material, and a careful comparison with the preliminary radiograph is necessary to confirm their location. More lucent stones such as uric acid calculi are not seen on the scout film but are identified as filling defects after the collecting system has been opacified.

The anatomy of the collecting system affects the likelihood of a renal stone to be passed, and the spot where it is likely to stop if it does not pass. Patients with an abnormal collecting system may have focal dilatation due to

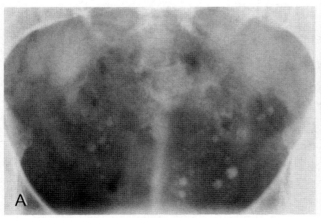
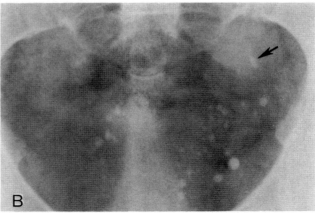

Figure 10.10. Distal ureteral stone. **A,** Multiple pelvic phleboliths are present. **B,** One week later a distal left ureteral stone (*arrow*) can be detected by comparison with the previous film.

infundibular stenosis or a calyceal diverticulum, either of which may harbor a stone that is unlikely to pass spontaneously. A ureteropelvic junction (UPJ) obstruction, or even high insertion of the ureter, is likely to keep a stone in the renal pelvis and prevent it from entering the ureter. A ureteral stricture will prevent a stone from passing further.

In patients with a normal collecting system a renal stone is most likely to be held up in the renal pelvis, the point where the ureter crosses over the pelvic brim or at the ureterovesical junction (UVJ) (Fig. 10.11). However, stones may hang up at any point along the course of the ureter, and the entire route must be carefully studied in patients with renal colic.

Stones are especially difficult to identify when they overlie the sacrum or ilium. Comparison with old radiographs, if available, is helpful (Fig. 10.10), but in many cases, urography is needed to identify the stone (Fig. 10.12) and site of obstruction.

The anatomy of the collecting system is also pertinent if interventional techniques are planned. Extracorporeal shock wave lithotripsy (ESWL) is best applied to stones in the renal pelvis, but can be used if the stone lies in the ureter above the iliac crest. If a percutaneous approach will be used, the location of the stone within the collecting system and the relationship of the collecting system to adjacent structures, such as liver, spleen, ribs and diaphragm is critical.

Stones may cause obstruction in a calyx, infundibulum, or at any point along the ureter. There is greater urgency to intervene in obstructing stones as they are more likely to create complications. If the obstruction is left unrelieved, renal function will eventually begin to deteriorate.

The most obvious sign of obstruction is delayed excretion of contrast material. The nephrogram is also delayed as compared with the normal contralateral side, but has increased intensity with time as contrast is not being excreted from the tubules (Fig. 10.13). The degree of dilation of the collecting system depends on the degree and duration of obstruction. In general, patients with ureteral obstruction, either partial or complete, have renal colic severe enough to seek medical attention. Thus, the urogram demonstrates only mild calyceal blunting and mild dilation of the ureter to the point of obstruction. Occasionally a persistent stone or recurrent stone passage may cause greater degrees of dilation of the collecting system (Fig. 10.14). Although these changes are usually quite evident, uncertainty may arise if there has been previous ureteral obstruction in which the collecting system has not returned to normal.

A more subtle change of ureteral obstruction is a persistent full column of contrast material in the ureter which ends at the stone. Upright films or a film obtained after voiding frequently exaggerates this difference in the mildly obstructed side from the normal side and helps to facilitate the diagnosis.

Stones that become impacted usually cause edema that may appear as a filling defect within the collecting system. This may have a particularly ominous appearance if a stone impacts at the UVJ. The halo appearance may suggest a ureterocele or even bladder carcinoma.

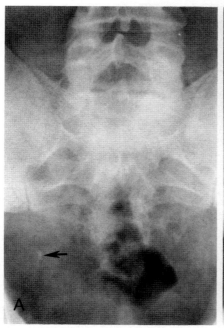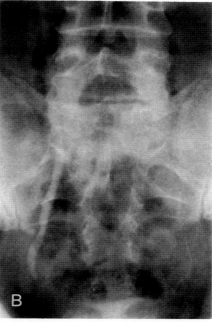

Figure 10.11. Distal ureteral stone. **A,** Preliminary radiograph demonstrates a 3 × 6 mm stone (*arrow*). **B,** A persistent column of contrast demonstrates the location of the stone at the ureterovesical junction.

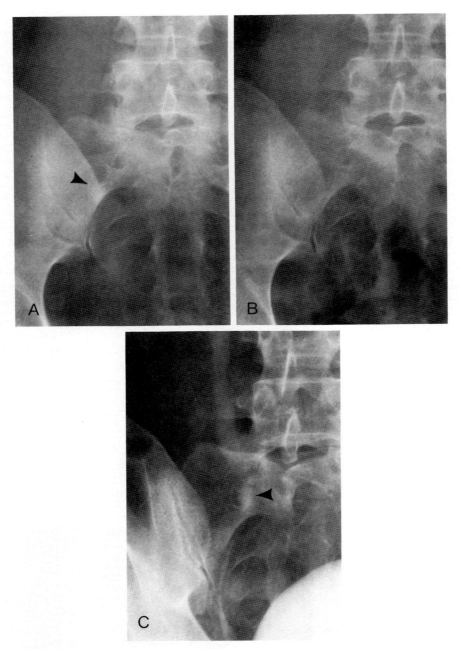

Figure 10.12. Stone obscured by sacrum. **A,** An increased density (*arrowhead*) blends with the sacrum and ilium. **B,** By comparison with a previous film, it is seen to be recently ac- quired. **C,** An excretory urogram demonstrates that this density (*arrowhead*) is a partially obstructing ureteral stone.

Retrograde Pyelography

Retrograde pyelography is indicated if an excretory urogram is contraindicated, or if there is inadequate excretion of contrast material into the affected collecting system. Patients with a severe contrast allergy or who are at increased risk for contrast-induced renal failure may be studied with retrograde pyelography. However, it should be remembered that there may be slight contrast absorption across the urothelium, and if extravasation occurs, contrast will enter the venous system. Nevertheless, retrograde pyelography is commonly employed in patients with a contraindication to an intravenous contrast injection.

Retrograde pyelography can be particularly useful prior to interventional techniques. Placing an indwelling ureteral stent catheter allows repeat contrast injection into the ureter which maximally opacifies the collecting system without the necessity of a large load of intravenous contrast material. In selected patients, such as those

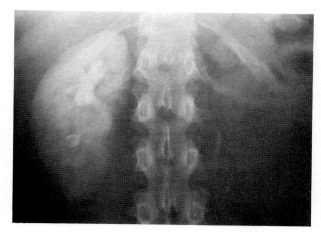

Figure 10.13. Ureteral obstruction. A persistent nephrogram of increased density is seen in this patient with an obstructing right ureteral stone.

with a severe contrast allergy or a small dense stone, another contrast agent such as air or carbon dioxide may be used (Fig. 10.15).

Antegrade Pyelography

Antegrade pyelography may be used to directly opacify the collecting system if retrograde pyelography is technically unsuccessful. It is also commonly performed in conjunction with pressure flow studies (Whitaker test) or as a prelude to a variety of interventional techniques.

Ultrasound

Both nephrocalcinosis (Fig. 10.16) and urinary tract calculi (Fig. 10.17) can be identified on ultrasound (US) by the highly echogenic focus and acoustic shadowing of the stone. This can be useful in distinguishing lucent renal stones from other etiologies of a filling defect such as blood clot or tumor. When the kidney is well seen, stones as small as 0.5 mm may be detected sonographically. In the series of 100 patients reported by Middleton et al., US was 96% sensitive in detecting renal stones as compared to abdominal radiography with renal tomography and more sensitive than an abdominal radiograph alone.

Ultrasound can also be useful in the operating room in detecting small intrarenal calculi. During an open operation, a balance must be maintained between complete stone removal and minimizing renal damage. Intraoperative radiography, US, nephroscopy, and plasma coagulum have all been used for this purpose. Ultrasonography is easily applied to the intact kidney and may be used to better define the location of a stone prior to the initial incision or to look for additional small stones or fragments after the stone is extracted. It can be especially helpful if the stone is mobile within the collecting system. However, once the collecting system has been opened, US is more difficult to interpret as small amounts of gas create confusing shadows which may mimic or hide a stone.

Ultrasound is also helpful in demonstrating obstruction of the collecting system (Fig. 10.18). Although the degree of ureteropelvocaliectasis from an acute ureteral

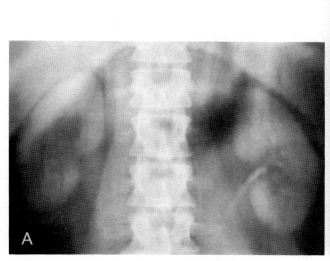

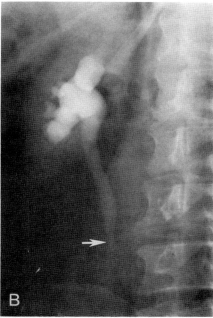

Figure 10.14. Ureteral stone. **A,** Delayed excretion from the right kidney is appreciated on an early nephrotomogram. **B,** On later films ureteropelvocaliectasis ending in the mid ureter demonstrates the stone location (*arrow*).

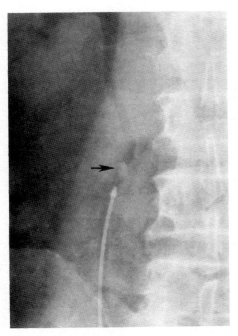

Figure 10.15.   Air pyelography. Air was used as the contrast material to better demonstrate a ureteral stone (*arrow*) during retrograde pyelography.

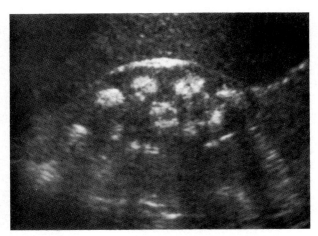

Figure 10.16.   Nephrocalcinosis. Multiple highly echogenic foci in the region of the renal pyramids with shadowing are detected with ultrasound.

Computed Tomography

obstruction due to a stone is mild, it can usually be distinguished from the normal collecting system in patients who may present with flank pain due to acute bacterial pyelonephritis or a renal infarction. Furthermore, the dilated ureter can often be followed to the point of obstruction and the stone identified (Fig. 10.19).

Computed tomography is most valuable in identifying a lucent stone as the etiology of a filling defect within the collecting system. If the defect is small, narrow collimation may be needed to avoid partial volume artifact. Even lucent stones such as uric acid calculi are easily detected on CT because their density is far greater than that of normal renal parenchyma, blood clot, or a urothelial tumor (Fig. 10.20). In vitro studies have shown the ability of CT to differentiate among renal stones on the basis of their density. Calcium oxalate stones are the densest and are usually 500–800 HU. The least dense common stones

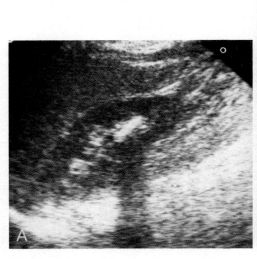

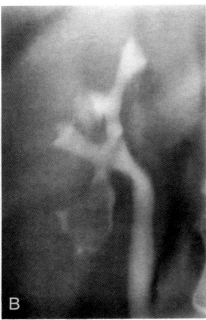

Figure 10.17.   Renal stone. **A,** Ultrasound demonstrates a highly echogenic mass with shadowing in the lower pole col-lecting system. **B,** The stone is confirmed on urography.

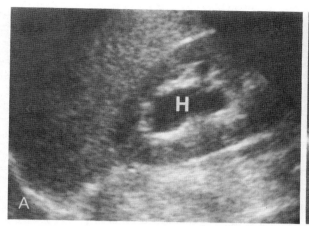

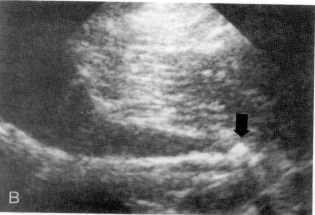

Figure 10.18.   Proximal ureteral stone. **A,** Moderate hydrone-phrosis (H) is seen with ultrasound. **B,** The ureteral dilatation ends at an obstructing ureteral stone (*arrow*).

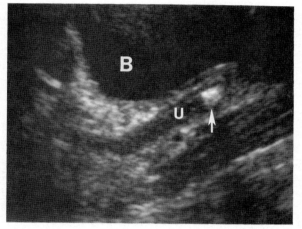

Figure 10.19.   Distal ureteral stone. A dilated ureter (U) is seen behind the bladder (B). The echogenic focus (*arrow*) is an obstructing distal ureteral stone.

are uric acid, which range from 125 to 300 HU. There is a greater variation in the density of struvite stones, which range from 300 to 700 HU, because of their greater range in mineralization. This technique is more easily applied to the intrarenal collecting system, which is easier to localize than the ureter, but can be applied to any portion of the urinary tract (Fig. 10.21).

NONSURGICAL TREATMENT OF URINARY TRACT CALCULI

Dramatic changes in the treatment of urinary tract calculi have occurred in the last 10 years. Dilation of a percutaneous nephrostomy tract to a size large enough to accommodate an endoscope has provided access to the urinary tract. A variety of catheters, stone baskets, and ultrasonic and electrohydraulic lithotriptors have been

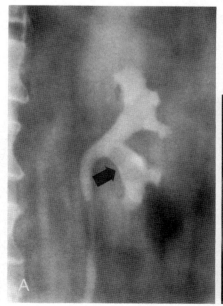

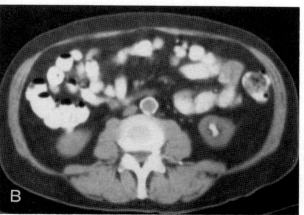

Figure 10.20.   Renal stone. **A,** A filling defect (*arrow*) is present on the excretory urogram. **B,** The high density on an unenhanced CT scan demonstrates that the filling defect is due to the presence of a stone.

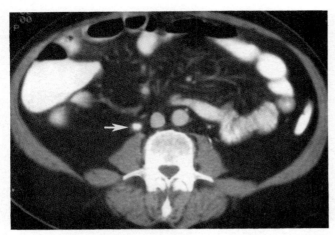

Figure 10.21. Ureteral stone. A stone (*arrow*) is readily identified in the right ureter by CT.

used to remove renal and ureteral stones. The success of these techniques has been so great that rarely are open surgical procedures needed.

The development of ESWL further advanced these nonoperative techniques. ESWL removes urinary tract calculi by fragmentation and spontaneous passage. This has eliminated the need for a percutaneous nephrostomy in most patients and has become the primary treatment for symptomatic nephrolithiasis. However, many patients still require percutaneous treatment to supplement ESWL or to treat complications arising from incomplete stone passage.

Expectant Therapy

Since approximately 80% of all urinary tract stones pass spontaneously, intervention may not be needed. Over 90% of stones less than 4 mm in diameter and 50% of stones 4–7 mm in diameter pass spontaneously. Rarely can stones 8 mm or larger be passed down the ureter into the bladder. Anatomic abnormalities and the location of the stone affect these rates.

The decision of if and when to intervene depends on the size of the stone, the anatomy of the urinary tract, the condition of the patient, and the presence or absence of other mitigating factors such as urinary tract infection or preexisting renal disease.

Percutaneous Nephrostolithotomy

Percutaneous Nephrostomy

The cornerstone of percutaneous stone removal is percutaneous nephrostomy. This determines the tract through which various instruments will be passed to remove the calculi. An ideally placed nephrostomy will avoid violating extrarenal organs (Fig. 10.22), traverse the least vascular plane of the kidney, and yet provide access to all portions of the collecting system that contain stones. The nephrostomy catheter should be sufficiently lateral so that it is not kinked or uncomfortable when the patient is lying supine. The tract should also be straight so that it can accommodate a rigid nephroscope.

The procedure is often more difficult when it is performed to remove stones as the collecting system is often not dilated and frequently a specific entry site is required to reach all of the stones. Furthermore, these access demands may necessitate entry into an upper-pole calyx, which increases the likelihood of puncturing the pleural space. The technique of percutaneous nephrostomy is discussed in Chapter 22.

In many patients, the renal stone provides an adequate target for placement of the percutaneous nephrostomy. This is usually true if a solitary calcified stone is to be removed. Multiple stones or poorly seen calculi may require opacification of the collecting system prior to nephrostomy placement.

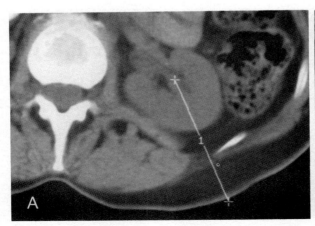

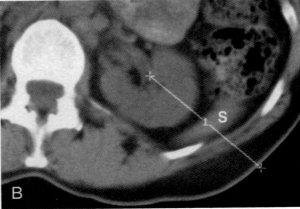

Figure 10.22. PCN route. **A,** A percutaneous nephrostomy should be placed through the least vascular plane of the kidney. **B,** A high or laterally placed nephrostomy increases the risk of injury to the spleen (S) or pneumothorax.

The collecting system can be opacified from three routes. First, if there is good renal function, intravenous contrast injection will provide adequate visualization. Furthermore, the resultant diuresis provides mild distention of the collecting system. However, optimal opacification is for only a short period of time and the patient is subjected to the hazards of intravascular contrast media.

Secondly, retrograde injection of contrast material via an indwelling catheter provides excellent opacification of the collecting system. Since the contrast is not injected intravenously, there is no limit to the volume that can be used. Furthermore, contrast can be injected during the puncture which slightly dilates the collecting system and enlarges the target for the puncture. However, this does require placement of a ureteral catheter by the urologist.

Thirdly, an antegrade pyelogram can be performed with a 22-gauge needle or via a 3 French catheter (Fig. 10.23). This method also avoids intravenous contrast injection and does provide slight dilation of the collecting system. Although ureteral catheterization is not required, an additional puncture of the renal pelvis is needed.

The definitive nephrostomy should be placed at an angle of 30–45°. This will allow the tract to pass through the least vascular plane (Brödel's line) of the kidney (Fig. 10.22) unless the kidney is malrotated. The tract should enter the calyx or infundibulum containing the stone. If more than one stone is targeted for removal, the nephrostomy tract should provide access to the locations of the other stones as well.

Tract Dilation

There are three basic methods of dilating the nephrostomy tract. Initially, coaxial stainless steel dilators were used to enlarge the tract from 8 to 24 French (Wolf) or 26 French (Storz). A bead at the end of the 8 French cannula limits the forward extent of the subsequent larger dilators (Fig. 10.24). These dilators are particularly useful when the nephrostomy tract passes through resistant fibrotic tissue.

Fascial polyurethane dilators tapered to insert over an 8F Teflon catheter can also be used to dilate the tract from 8 to 34 French (Fig. 10.25). Teflon working sheaths are available in 28 to 34 French sizes to fit over the fascial dilators. They are left in place after the dilator is removed to protect the kidney while the stones are being manipulated and removed. The Teflon sheaths are sufficiently radiopaque to be easily seen during fluoroscopy yet are translucent enough to allow visualization during manipulation.

Most interventionalists now prefer to use a modified angioplasty balloon catheter to dilate the nephrostomy tract (Fig. 10.26). A balloon that inflates to at least 8 mm in diameter and 8–15 cm in length is used. Balloon dilation is less painful to the patient and accomplishes dilation with less bleeding, and presumably less damage to the kidney and other retroperitoneal tissues.

Before catheter manipulation is started, a second or "safety" guidewire should be passed (Fig. 10.27). This second wire can be placed via a larger untapered catheter such as a Ford catheter. Two guidewires provide an extra margin of safety. If the working wire is accidentally dislodged or withdrawn, access can be regained with the safety wire. The most secure position of the working wire is down the ureter. If the tip is in the distal ureter or bladder, it usually provides sufficient stability to permit tract dilation or catheter manipulation.

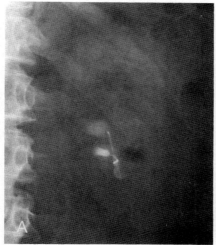 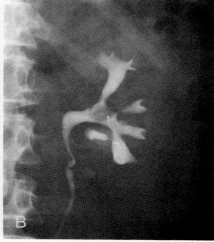

Figure 10.23. Opacification of collecting system. **A,** Faint opacification of the collecting system is seen after intravenous injection of 50 ml of contrast material. A 3 French dilator has been passed into the renal pelvis. **B,** Injection of contrast through the 3 French dilator densely opacifies and mildly distends the collecting system. (From Dunnick NR: Percutaneous approach to urinary tract calculi. In Lang EK (ed): *Percutaneous and Interventional Urology and Radiology.* Berlin, Springer-Verlag, 1986.)

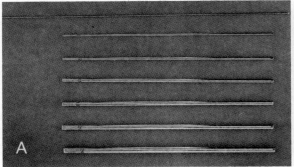

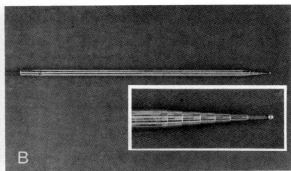

Figure 10.24.   Wolf coaxial dilator set. **A,** There are seven dilators, ranging in size from 6 to 24 French. Note the olive-tipped 6 French dilator which is longer than the others, and is passed over a 0.038-inch (0.97 mm) wire and used like a solid wire to pass progressively larger dilators through the soft tis- sues of the flank to the kidney. **B,** The seven dilators are assem- bled coaxially. The 6 French olive-tipped dilator prevents me- dial migration of the dilators where there is potential damage to the renal pedicle. (From Carson CC, Dunnick NR: *Endourol- ogy.* New York, Churchill Livingstone, 1985.)

Stone Extraction

Once access has been gained and the tract has been dilated to a working size, the stones can be directly ex- tracted, fragmented and removed in pieces or frag- mented and allowed to pass spontaneously. If possible, it is preferable to remove the stone intact as no fragments are left behind to act as a nidus for new stone formation. Furthermore, it avoids renal colic or hematuria during passage of the fragments.

A large variety of stone baskets are available. Many baskets consist of three, four, six, or eight wires in a helicoid pattern that will fit through a catheter and ex- pand after exiting the catheter tip (Fig. 10.28). This design usually includes a filiform tip of varying length and is the preferred design for ureteral stones.

Other designs such as the Hawkins stone basket use a series of two to four wires along the shaft of the catheter. They have a blunt end and can be pushed up against the

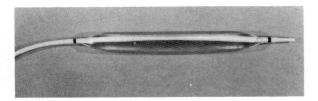

Figure 10.26.   Balloon dilating catheter. This polyurethane reinforced catheter can be inflated with pressures as high as 12 atm. (From Carson CC, Dunnick NR: *Endourology.* New York, Churchill Livingstone, 1985.)

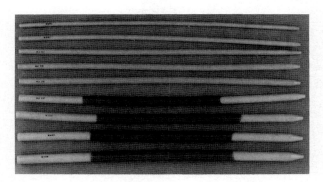

Figure 10.25.   Amplatz sequential dilators. These dilators are passed over 8F catheters. The 24- to 30-French dilators have sheaths which can be used to create a solid access for passage of baskets. (From Carson CC, Dunnick NR: *Endourology.* New York, Churchill Livingstone, 1985.)

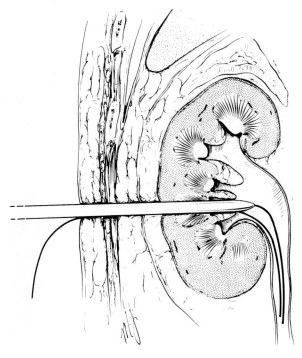

Figure 10.27.   Safety wire. A second (safety) guidewire has been passed before dilation with the fascial polyurethane dila- tors. (From Carson CC, Dunnick NR: *Endourology.* New York, Churchill Livingstone, 1985.)

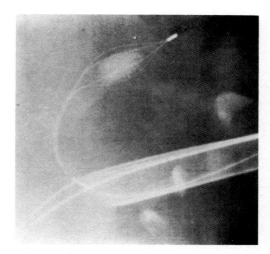

Figure 10.28. Four-wire basket. A helicoid basket has been passed through a Teflon sheath to capture the stone.

urothelium to capture a stone. This variety is especially useful in removing calyceal stones.

Forceps may also be used to grasp and extract a renal stone. Flexible forceps with an alligator grasping tip may be introduced through a catheter. Another type of flexible forceps is the three- or four-prong forceps. They may be passed through a catheter and expanded when they exit the distal end within the renal pelvis (Fig. 10.29). These are not widely used, however, as they can exert only a limited pulling force on the stone before losing their grip. Furthermore, the hooks on the grasping end

can easily dig into the urothelium and damage the collecting system.

Rigid forceps must be introduced through a straight tract. A Teflon sheath helps to prevent tissue damage during the introduction, manipulation, and withdrawal of the forceps. Three-prong rigid forceps originally designed to be used through a nephroscope are useful in removing renal pelvic or calyceal stones. Randall's forceps open with a scissors-like action (Fig. 10.30). This requires either a very short or wide tract to allow the forceps to open sufficiently to engage the stone (Fig. 10.31). The Mazzariello-Caprini forceps open by rotating along the axis (Fig. 10.30). This allows them to be used in a narrower tract. However, they are attached less securely and the two portions of the forceps may become separated during manipulation. If this occurs, the forceps are simply withdrawn and refastened. Both Randall and Mazzariello-Caprini forceps should have a groove in the tip so they can be introduced over a guidewire. Rigid forceps must be used carefully as they may damage the collecting system. Biplane or C arm fluoroscopy is helpful to direct the forceps onto the stone.

The forceps are made with several degrees of curvature. Straight forceps are too limiting once within the collecting system. They do not allow the grasping end to be directed anywhere but along the course of the nephrostomy tract. By rotating curved forceps, the grasping tip can be moved 360° around the central axis. However, if the curvature is too great, they cannot be passed through the nephrostomy tract. Thus, a slight curve is the best configuration for the rigid forceps.

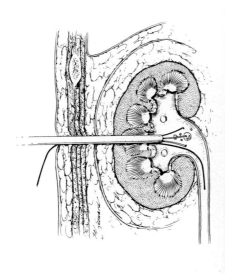

A

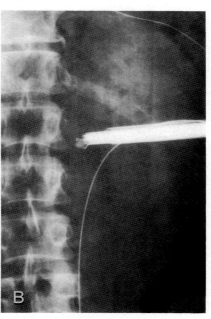

B

Figure 10.29. Three-prong forceps. The forceps are passed through the nephroscope to remove calculi. **A,** Schematic. **B,** Radiograph. (From Carson CC, Dunnick NR: *Endourology.* New York, Churchill Livingstone, 1985.)

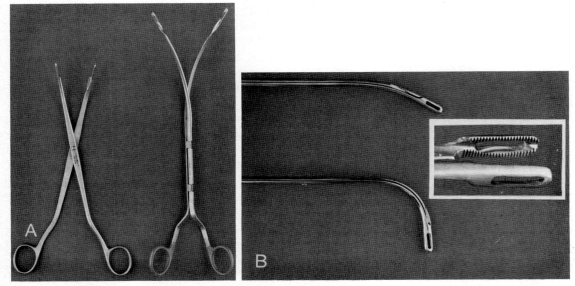

Figure 10.30. Rigid forceps. **A,** The Randall forceps (*left*) open with a conventional scissors action. The Mazzariello-Caprini forceps have a long central fulcrum, which allows better opening when used through a long tract. **B,** A variety of curves are available with either type of forceps. Insert shows the 0.97-mm hole drilled into the grasping end of the forceps, which facilitates its passage over a guide wire. (From Carson CC, Dunnick NR: *Endourology.* New York, Churchill Livingstone, 1985.)

Ultrasonic Lithotripsy

One of the most effective methods of fragmenting a renal calculus is ultrasonic lithotripsy. The transducer contains a piezoceramic crystal that will resonate at a specific frequency when it is stimulated by electrical energy (Fig. 10.32). Sound waves of 23,000–27,000 Hz are produced and transmitted via an acoustic horn down the hollow steel rod to the stone. The lithotrite probe acts as a drill as it strikes the stone several thousand times per second and gradually fragments the stone to which it is brought into contact. Unfortunately, the lithotrite probe must be a rigid rod as any articulations would result in significant energy loss.

A suction line is attached to the transducer, which aspirates stone fragments and irrigating fluid up the hollow probe. Not only does this help to minimize retained stone fragments but it also helps to keep the stone in apposition to the probe.

Saline is the preferred irrigating solution. If the irrigant does not extravasate outside the collecting system, other solutions such as water or glycine could be used. However, there is a risk of penetrating the peritoneum during ultrasonic lithotripsy, either from perforation of

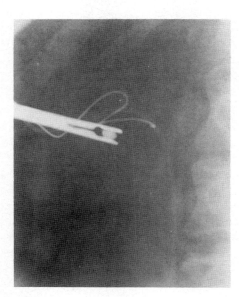

Figure 10.31. Forceps extraction. A renal pelvic stone is grasped by the rigid forceps.

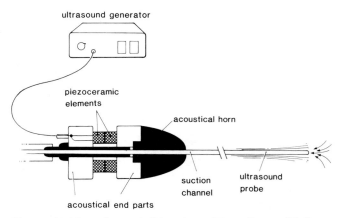

Figure 10.32. Ultrasonic lithotripter. (From Carson CC, Dunnick NR: *Endourology.* New York, Churchill Livingstone, 1985.)

the renal pelvis or because an unusually posterior peritoneal reflection is traversed by the nephrostomy tract. Extravasation of significant amounts of water or glycine may result in life-threatening electrolyte shifts and severe hyponatremia.

Electrohydraulic Lithotripsy

Another useful modality for fragmenting renal stones is electrohydraulic lithotripsy. In this technique a short spark discharge is produced at the tip of the probe. This produces intense heat that vaporizes water and creates a cavitation bubble. The resulting shock wave radiates in all directions. Both this initial shock wave and a second wave that occurs with the collapse of the bubble have an impact on the stone causing fragmentation.

The probe for electrohydraulic lithotripsy consists of a central wire core surrounded by insulation. There is a second cylindrical wire around this and then an additional layer of insulation. The probes are flexible and may be as small as 5 French.

Electrohydraulic lithotripsy is most effective in a one-sixth to one-seventh normal saline solution and is ineffective in normal saline. The heat created at the tip of the probe is easily dispersed in this fluid, but the stone must be free within the collecting system to minimize damage to the urothelium. There is no suction apparatus to remove small stones so it is desirable to break the stone into pieces just small enough to be removed through the nephrostomy tract.

Chemolysis

Chemolysis can be used either as a primary or adjunctive method of removing urinary tract calculi. It is most effective on uric acid, struvite, and cystine stones, but it is of little value on calcium oxalate or calcium phosphate stones.

The optimal chemolytic solution depends on the composition of the stone. Struvite stones contain a mixture of magnesium ammonium phosphate and calcium phosphate. They form in the presence of a urinary tract infection with urease-producing bacteria. Urease splits urea, which results in a large amount of ammonium ion in an alkaline urine. Thus, struvite stones can be dissolved with acidifying solutions such as hemiacidrin or Suby's G solution.

Acidifying solutions are used to create soluble calcium citrate complexes and dissolve calcium oxalate and calcium phosphate stones. The chelating agent ethylene-diaminetetraacetate (EDTA) may also be used for calcium stones.

Uric acid and cystine stones can be dissolved with an alkaline solution such as sodium bicarbonate or tromethamine (THAM). Uric acid stones are the easiest to dissolve and can sometimes be treated with allopurinol, hydration, and oral urinary alkalinization. Raising the urinary pH to 6.8 keeps most of the uric acid in the highly soluble monosodium urate form.

To accomplish stone dissolution effectively, a nephrostomy is needed to bathe the stone directly in a high concentration of the dissolving solution. A large nephrostomy catheter (8–10 French) is needed to provide good perfusion and the catheter tip should be placed in close proximity to the stone.

In an unobstructed system, a single catheter is sufficient. The solution is introduced through the catheter; it bathes the stone and is passed down the ureter. The tip of the nephrostomy catheter should be behind the stone so that the solution introduced through the catheter must wash over the stone before passing down the ureter. If there is ureteral obstruction, a second nephrostomy catheter is required to drain the collecting system. The two catheters should be placed on opposite sides of the stone so solvent has maximal contact with the stone during irrigation. As an alternative, a double-pigtail ureteral catheter may be used to provide drainage. Infusion rates of 75–120 ml/hr are usually sufficient.

Although chemolysis is successful in completely dissolving renal stones in approximately 70% of cases, it is a slow process, often requiring a month or more. Furthermore, most stones are not homogeneous and many contain several layers, each with different solubility characteristics. Thus, a sample of the stone should be obtained, if possible, to determine its chemical composition before beginning dissolution therapy.

Chemolysis is best suited for patients who are poor surgical risks and whose stones are particularly amenable to dissolution such as uric acid, struvite and cystine stones. It is contraindicated in patients with a urinary tract infection as infected urine may be extravasated if the irrigating pressure is excessive. This technique may also be used to eliminate tiny fragments too small to be grasped with a stone basket or forceps after ultrasonic or electrohydraulic lithotripsy.

Results

In many patients a variety of percutaneous techniques are used to remove the targeted stones. Thus, the results are reported for percutaneous nephrostolithotomy with the understanding that any or all of these methods may have been employed. For most patients, direct extraction is the technique of choice if the stone is small enough (less than 1 cm) to be removed through the nephrostomy tract. Larger stones must be fragmented, usually with ultrasonic lithotripsy, and the fragments either removed with a basket or forceps, or allowed to pass spontaneously. Chemolysis may be used as the primary therapy in selected patients or as an adjuvant method of eliminating residual fragments. Using various combinations of these techniques, excellent results have been reported.

In 1985, Segura et al. reviewed their experience in the percutaneous removal of renal or ureteral stones from 1000 consecutive patients. The targeted stone was successfully removed in 791 of 805 patients (98.3%) with renal stones. The most common reason for failure was inability to provide adequate access to the stone. A similar report by Reddy et al. described their results on 400 consecutive patients after the experience gained from the first 100 patients. As judged by plain abdominal radiographs, they were able to remove all stones from 328 of 332 patients (99%) with renal stones. Two of the four failures were due to access problems. Lee et al. echoed the importance of experience in the analysis of their first 500 patients. Their success rate for the removal of simple pelvicalyceal stones was 98% overall, but only 89% in the first 100 patients. Furthermore, 14 of the 17 patients requiring open operation after percutaneous nephrostolithotomy failed were among the first 100 patients.

Complications

Percutaneous nephrostolithotomy is a relatively safe and efficacious procedure that has largely replaced open surgical procedures for stone removal. However, it is an invasive technique and major complications do occur. In 1985, Dunnick et al. reported a 10% complication rate, with hemorrhage (Fig. 10.33) and catheter dislodgement the most common events. They noted that complications decreased with increasing experience, even though more difficult cases were accepted in the latter period. In 1987, Lee et al. found only a 4% complication rate, with fever and bleeding encountered most commonly. Two deaths

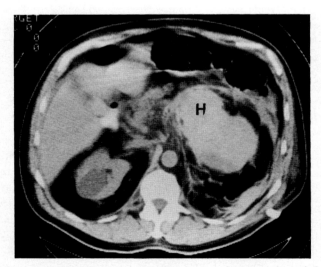

Figure 10.33. Hematoma. A CT scan demonstrates a large left hematoma (H) after percutaneous nephrostolithotomy. (From Dunnick NR, Carson CC, Braun SD, et al: Complications of percutaneous nephrostolithotomy. *Radiology* 157:51, 1985.)

were reported in this latter series of 582 patients, both in patients with serious underlying medical diseases.

A mail survey tabulating the results of 8595 percutaneous nephrostolithotomy procedures from 62 institutions was reported by Lang. Serious complications declined from a rate of 15% during the first 20 cases to 1.5% afterward. The most common serious complications reported were perirenal abscess (84), hemorrhage requiring transfusion (37), pneumo- or hydrothorax (32), arteriovenous fistula requiring intervention (26) (Fig. 10.34), perforation of the colon (16), and rupture of the renal pelvis or ureteropelvic junction (13). A total of four deaths (0.046%) were reported in this survey. Small perforations of a calyx or the renal pelvis occur frequently, but heal with nephrostomy drainage and should not be considered a significant complication.

Percutaneous stone extraction procedures require frequent radiographic monitoring to access a portion of the collecting system that will allow removal of all the targeted stones. Fluoroscopy is also used to guide tract dilation and stone removal. Since these procedures are frequently difficult and time consuming, relatively high radiation doses may be absorbed by the radiologist and other members of the interventional team. Bush et al. examined this problem during 102 procedures for percutaneous removal of renal calculi from the upper collecting system. Fluoroscopy averaged 25 minutes per case and the average radiation dose to the radiologist at the collar level was 10 mrem per case.

To minimize this radiation exposure, members of the interventional team should wear not only a lead apron, but also a thyroid shield and protective leaded glasses. A 0.5-mm lead-equivalent apron allows less than 1% of the x-rays to penetrate while a 0.25-mm lead equivalent apron allows 10% transmission. The glasses should have a side shield as the radiologist will often be facing 90° away from the x-ray beam as he/she looks at the television monitor.

The radiation exposure rate of the fluoroscope should be reduced to the lowest kVp and mA that gives a satisfactory image. Less radiation will reach the operators if the x-ray tube is below the patient rather than overhead. The field of view should be tightly collimated to only the area that must be imaged, and unnecessary fluoroscopy should be eliminated.

Another risk to the interventional team is hearing loss from the high-pitched sound produced by ultrasonic lithotriptors. On the basis of sound level measurements in an acoustic laboratory, Teigland et al. estimated that permanent hearing loss could result from 2 hours of continual operation of commercial ultrasonic lithotripsy units if performed on a daily basis. However, ultrasonic lithotripsy is intermittent and is unlikely to exceed 1 hour per patient. Thus, this is not likely to be a problem for most workers. However, those individuals who already

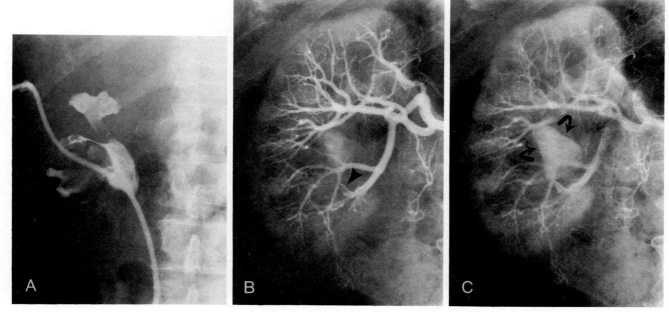

Figure 10.34. False aneurysm. **A,** Filling defect that conforms to the collecting system after nephrostomy tract placement represents a blood clot. **B, C,** Arteriogram obtained after recurrent hematuria from accidental dislodgement of the drainage catheter reveals a false aneurysm (*arrows*) arising from a lower pole branch artery (*arrowhead*). (From Dunnick NR, Carson CC, Braun SD, Miller GA, Cohan R, Illescas FF, Newman GE, Weinerth JL: Complications of percutaneous nephrostolithotomy. *Radiology* 157:51, 1985.)

have a hearing deficit or who are unusually sensitive may prefer to be more cautious and wear ear plugs during these procedures.

Extracorporeal Shock Wave Lithotripsy

ESWL has had as dramatic an impact on the treatment of urinary tract calculi as the development of percutaneous techniques. It has proven to be not only safe and efficacious but is also even less invasive than percutaneous nephrostolithotomy. Thus, it has become the primary modality for the treatment of renal and many ureteral stones.

Technique

Shock waves are produced by an underwater high voltage shock discharge of 1 microsecond duration. This is similar to electrohydraulic lithotripsy as the discharge causes water vaporization that initiates the shock wave in both techniques. The spark electrodes are located in the focus (F1) of an ellipsoid reflector such that the energy generated is concentrated at a second focal point (F2) outside the ellipsoid (Fig. 10.35). The stone to be fragmented must coincide with this point of highest energy concentration. Biplane fluoroscopy units are used to locate the stone and position the patient over the ellipsoid so that the F2 and the stone coincide.

Since shock waves are much more efficiently propagated through water than air, a path of water is needed between the ellipsoid and the stone. The initial commercial unit (Dornier) used a water bath into which the patient was immersed by a hydraulically controlled sling. Subsequent units, however, have substituted a water bag, eliminating the need for the large cumbersome bath.

Patients are prepared for the treatment with laxatives to reduce bowel gas and fecal material. This helps the fluoroscopic localization of the stones. Either general or epidural anesthesia is administered, and the patient is strapped into the sling and lowered into the water bath. Guided with biplane fluoroscopy, the stone is positioned at the F2 focus of the shock generating ellipsoid. Approximately 500–2000 shock waves are needed to fragment a renal pelvic stone into pieces small enough to be passed down the ureter.

Ureteral obstruction is a contraindication to ESWL as the stone fragments cannot pass. However, a percutaneous nephrostomy can be placed and used as the route for stone removal. Similarly, a urinary tract infection is a relative contraindication. Even when the urine clears of infection, a nidus of infection may remain in the calculus material, which can become active when the stone is fragmented. These patients must be treated cautiously and a nephrostomy catheter may be helpful in preventing obstruction by infected material.

If the stones are poorly calcified, they may be difficult to localize with fluoroscopy. In these patients a ureteral catheter can be passed and contrast injected into the col-

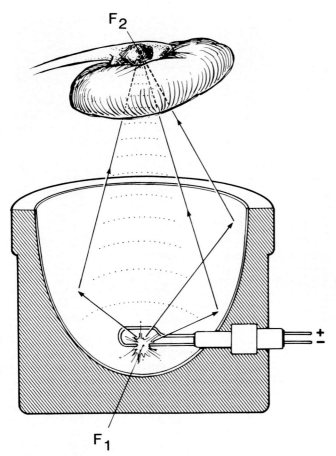

Figure 10.35. Extracorporeal shock wave lithotripsy. Spark gap electrode and semiellipsoid for focusing shock waves. Electrode is placed at first focus inside ellipsoid with stone placed at second focus. (From Carson CC, Dunnick NR: *Endourology.* New York, Churchill Livingstone, 1985.)

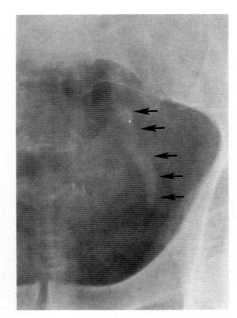

Figure 10.36. Stone fragments. After ESWL, multiple stone fragments are seen in the distal ureter (*arrows*).

lecting system to visualize the stone as a negative filling defect.

Results

The widespread acceptance of ESWL as the primary therapy for urolithiasis attests to its success. However, these shock waves merely disintegrate the stone and the many fragments must still pass through the ureter or a nephrostomy catheter. Thus, it may take days to months to achieve a stone-free status. Radiographs taken within the first few days of ESWL show only fragmentation and partial passage of the stone fragments. If the stone burden was moderate to large, many fragments may accumulate in the distal ureter as "steinstrasse" (Fig. 10.36). A ureteral catheter inserted prior to ESWL and left in place 3–5 days after treatment has been found to facilitate the passage of fragments.

Radiographs 1 to 3 months after ESWL give a more accurate appraisal of the treatment result. Riehle et al. found that 224 of 300 patients (75%) were stone-free as determined by a single abdominal radiograph 3 months after ESWL. Fragments were still present in 70 (23%) patients and in 6 (2%) patients showed no appreciable effect. Not surprisingly, patients with solitary stones less than 2 cm in diameter were more often stone free (87%) than those patients with large or multiple stones (65%).

Graff et al. were able to evaluate over 1000 patients a mean of 19.1 months after ESWL. They found that 72% of these patients remained stone free. Patients with a stone in the renal pelvis or upper ureter had the best success—85% and 89%, respectively, were stone free after follow-up. Patients with multiple stones did not do as well as only 64% were stone free. Of note, the worst group were those patients with a stone in a lower-pole calyx. Only 58% of these patients were stone free on follow up examinations.

The success of ESWL also depends on the composition of the stone. The best results in the Graff series were obtained in patients with calcium oxalate or uric acid calculi. Patients with apatite and cystine stones had the lowest stone-free rates after follow-up.

In a comparison of ESWL with percutaneous nephrostolithotomy, Lingeman et al. found similar success rates. Percutaneous nephrostolithotomy was slightly more efficacious in removing the targeted stone (98%) as compared with ESWL (95%), and was significantly better in leaving fewer fragments (7% vs. 24% for ESWL). However, patient morbidity as defined by pain, blood loss, fever, and length of hospital stay was much less in patients treated with ESWL. The significance of these retained stone fragments is unclear, however, as long-term studies have not yet shown whether or not these fragments act as a nidus for new stone formation and increase the recurrence rate.

Complications

The major advantage of ESWL is that open surgery and percutaneous nephrostomy are avoided. Thus, complications related to these invasive procedures are precluded. The stones are pulverized by shock waves focused on the stone. However, the kidney and adjacent soft tissues are also subject to some of this trauma. Intrarenal, subcapsular, and perinephric hematomas have all been seen and the incidence depends on the imaging modality used for detection.

A decrease in effective renal plasma flow (ERPF) to the kidney treated with ESWL has been demonstrated in some patients. These patients also had rises in both systolic and diastolic blood pressure. Although the mechanism of the development of hypertension after ESWL is not clear, it may be due to the compressive effect of an intrarenal or subcapsular hematoma causing decreased perfusion and compensatory renin release (Page kidney).

Staghorn Calculi

Staghorn calculi represent a special treatment problem. Not only is the stone burden great, but the collecting system is effectively obstructed. Many of these patients have an underlying urinary tract infection that may not be completely eradicated, and there is more likely to be renal damage than in patients with a smaller stone burden.

Anatrophic nephrolithotomy has been the standard surgical procedure for the removal of staghorn calculi. Although the operation is designed to minimize parenchymal damage, a decrease in renal function may be seen, and the convalescent time is long. Since many of these stones recur, repeat operations, which become increasingly difficult, may be required.

Percutaneous nephrostolithotomy may also be a difficult procedure on patients with a staghorn calculus. The stone must be fragmented prior to removal and long, often repeated sessions with ultrasonic lithotripsy are required (Fig. 10.37). The complication rate is higher than with patients with a smaller stone burden, and more than one percutaneous access is frequently needed. Furthermore, it is difficult to render these patients completely stone free, and these residual fragments may act as a nidus for more stone formation.

Snyder and Smith compared percutaneous nephrostolithotomy with anatrophic nephrolithotomy in a series of 100 patients with staghorn calculi. They found that both techniques were effective in removing the calculus. However, the shorter procedure time and decreased need for blood transfusions and narcotics favored the percutaneous technique. Furthermore, the far more rapid return to work (14.3 vs. 54.5 days after discharge from the hospital) was a very strong argument for percutaneous therapy. Although fewer retained stone fragments were seen with open surgery, percutaneous nephrostolithotomy was more amenable to a repeat procedure than anatrophic surgery.

A series of 120 patients with staghorn calculi who underwent percutaneous removal was reported by Lee et al. Most patients (73%) required two or more access routes and many (24%) had multistage procedures. Bleeding was sufficient to require transfusion in 57% of patients and 27% of patients developed a urinary tract infection. Nevertheless, symptomatic staghorn calculi were successfully removed from 85% of the patients, and the average convalescence time after discharge was only 15 days. A combination of percutaneous nephrostolithotomy and ESWL is probably the best approach to removal of staghorn calculi.

Radiology

The development and success of ESWL have had a marked impact on radiology. The number of patients undergoing percutaneous nephrostolithotomy has dropped precipitously, and it is now used for difficult or special problem cases. Bush et al. found that over 90% of patients with symptomatic stone disease are now treated with ESWL alone. Percutaneous techniques are used if there is a large stone burden (2%). They also may be applied after ESWL if obstruction occurs or to assist in removal of stone fragments. Others have reported more frequent use of percutaneous nephrostomy (PCN) after ESWL. Cochran et al. found that 9% of 1456 patients required PCN, with the most common indications being fever and obstruction. Tegtmeyer et al. performed 178 interventional procedures (12%) on 1500 patients treated with ESWL. This trend places even greater demands on the interventional uroradiologist who is expected to have a high level of technical expertise available for these complicated cases without the benefit of routine cases for training and maintenance of technical skills.

Since ESWL units are large, complex, and expensive pieces of equipment, they have become the central focus of stone treatment centers. They generate a large number of radiographic examinations essential to the treatment of these patients. Cochran et al. reviewed their experience with radiographic procedures for a single year in which 925 patients underwent ESWL. In all, 8478, radiologic studies and procedures were performed pertaining to ESWL. This is approximately 35 radiographic examinations per day. The vast majority of these were abdominal radiographs to follow the progress of stone fragmentation and passage, however, US, excretory urography, and percutaneous nephrostomies were frequently performed.

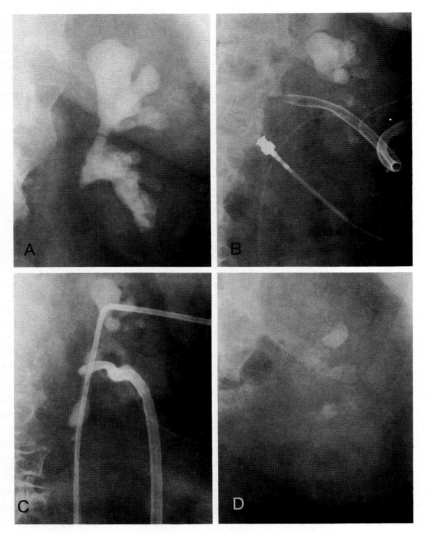

Figure 10.37. Staghorn calculi. **A,** Coned view of preoperative abdominal radiograph. Large staghorn calculus in left kidney. **B,** Retained fragments after first lithotripsy. Council catheter in renal pelvis; Gensini catheter stenting ureter. **C,** Second nephrostomy (Ford straight catheter) placed into upper pole before second lithotripsy. Contrast material in renal pelvis and ureter. **D,** Follow-up radiograph. Multiple retained fragments lodged in peripheral calyces. (From Adams GW, Oke EJ, Dunnick NR, Carson CC: Percutaneous lithotripsy of staghorn calculi. *AJR* 145:803, 1985.)

Ureteral Stones

Ureteral calculi present several problems for removal. They are often small and difficult to identify under fluoroscopy. They cannot be reached with a rigid instrument, the spine and bony pelvis limit the application of ESWL, and they may become embedded in the ureteral mucosa. Nevertheless, the variety of instruments that can be used on these stones results in successful removal for most patients.

Since approximately 80% of stones that enter the ureter pass spontaneously, it is reasonable to treat patients expectantly with analgesia and hydration while awaiting stone passage. The ureterovesical junction is the narrowest portion of the urinary tract so that stones that pass into the bladder can usually be evacuated completely with the urinary stream. Patients with bladder outlet obstruction or stasis due to bladder or urethral diverticulae may be exceptions.

The likelihood of a ureteral stone passing can be predicted by its size. Stones 4 mm or less in diameter are usually passed spontaneously and stones greater than 8 mm are unlikely to be passed. Stones that range from 4 to 7 mm in diameter lie in a gray zone where a trial of expectant therapy is often appropriate.

Percutaneous extraction techniques may be applied to ureteral as well as intrarenal stones. This is often done if a nephrostomy has already been established. Access to the ureter is usually easier if a middle or upper-pole calyx has been entered as the angle down the ureter will be less acute than if a lower pole calyx was entered with the nephrostomy. The four-wire basket with a filiform tip is

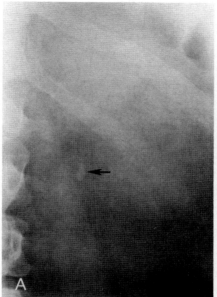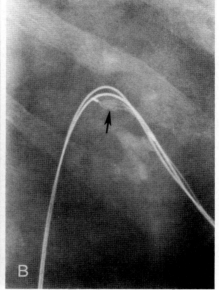

Figure 10.38. Ureteral stone. **A,** A proximal ureteral stone (*arrow*) is identified. **B,** A four-wire basket is used to extract the stone (*arrow*).

most useful in the ureter (Fig. 10.38). It is passed through the catheter beyond the stone and then opened. The stone is engaged as the basket is pulled back into the renal pelvis and then out the nephrostomy tract.

If the stone is imbedded in the ureteral mucosa, it may not be possible to capture it in the stone basket. Modifications of the four-wire basket such as the Johnson basket may be more successful by forcing the edematous mucosa to retract from the stone (Fig. 10.39). Balloon catheters passed distal to the stone and then inflated have also been used to pull the stone back into the renal pelvis where it can be removed with either a stone basket or forceps.

Ureteroscopy has been shown to be effective in reaching and removing stones from a retrograde approach. The ureter must be dilated to accommodate the ureteroscope. If a large stone is encountered, ultrasonic lithotripsy can be employed to fragment it before extraction.

In general, an antegrade approach via a percutaneous nephrostomy is used for stones in the proximal ureter, whereas a retrograde approach via the bladder is selected when the stone lies in the distal ureter. Dilation of the collecting system above the stone also favors the antegrade approach. Furthermore, if large stones are pulled into the bladder, they may damage the ureterovesical junction. Thus, stones greater than 8 mm in diameter are approached in an antegrade fashion or fragmented before being extracted.

Using a combination of these techniques as well as chemolysis for known soluble stones, Kahn was able to remove 114 of 120 (95%) ureteral stones. Two patients required surgery for ureteral avulsion and seven patients

had ureteral perforation treated with a double-J ureteral stent.

ESWL can be used on ureteral stones if they lie above the iliac crest. However, the results have not been as good as when the stone lies in the renal pelvis. However, if the ureteral stone is pushed back into the renal pelvis, the results of ESWL are excellent.

Coptcoat et al. reviewed their experience with 100 consecutive patients who required treatment for ureteral

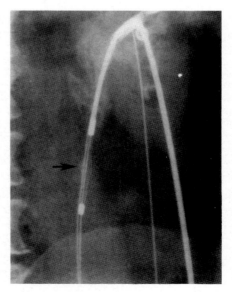

Figure 10.39. Ureteral stone. The four-wire basket was not successful in engaging this stone. The stiff wires of the Johnson basket displaced the edematous mucosa so the stone (*arrow*) could be captured.

stones. Most patients (63) had their stones removed by ESWL following retrograde manipulation. Ureteroscopic techniques were used to remove stones from 29 patients, 26 of whom had distal ureteral stones. Other techniques included percutaneous nephrostolithotomy and cystoscopic removal. Only two patients had open ureterolithotomy, although four patients required surgery either for complications of ureteroscopy or stricture.

SUGGESTED READINGS

Nephrocalcinosis and Nephrolithiasis

Drach GW: Surgical overview of urolithiasis. *J Urol* 141(Pt II):711, 1989.

Gilsanz V, Fernal W, Reid BS, et al: Nephrolithiasis in premature infants. *Radiology* 154:107, 1985.

Goldwasser B, Cohan RH, Dunnick NR, et al: Role of linear tomography in evaluation of patients with nephrolithiasis. *Urology* 33(3):253, 1989.

Hewitt MJ, Older RA: Calyceal calculi simulating gallstones. *AJR* 134:507, 1980.

Hillman BJ, Drach DW, Tracey P, et al: Computed tomographic analysis of renal calculi. *AJR* 142:549, 1984.

Lalli AF: Renal parenchyma calcifications. *Semin Roentgenol* 17:101, 1982.

Margolin EG, Cohen LH: Genitourinary calcification: an overview. *Semin Roentgenol* 17:95, 1982.

Middleton WD, Dodds WJ, Lawson TL, et al: Renal calculi: sensitivity for detection with US. *Radiology* 167:239, 1988.

Parienty RA, Ducellier R, Pradel J, et al: Diagnostic value of CT numbers in pelvocalyceal filling defects. *Radiology* 145:743, 1982.

Prien EL: The analysis of urinary calculi. *Urol Clin North Am* 1:229, 1974.

Smith LH: The medical aspects of urolithiasis: an overview. *J Urol* 141:707, 1981.

Percutaneous Nephrostolithotomy

Bush WH, Jones D, Brannen GE: Radiation doses to personnel during percutaneous renal calculus removal. *AJR* 145:1261, 1985.

Carson CC, Dunnick NR: *Endourology.* New York, Churchill Livingstone, 1985.

Dunnick NR: Percutaneous approach to urinary tract calculi. In Lang EK (ed): *Percutaneous and Interventional Urology and Radiology.* Berlin, Springer-Verlag. 1986.

Dunnick NR, Carson CC, Braun SD, et al: Complications of percutaneous nephrostolithotomy. *Radiology* 157:51, 1985.

Lang EK: Percutaneous nephrostolithotomy and lithotripsy: a multiinstitutional survey of complications. *Radiology* 162:25, 1987.

Lee WJ, Smith AD, Cubelli V, et al: Complications of percutaneous nephrolithotomy. *AJR* 148:177, 1987.

Lee WJ, Smith AD, Cubell V, et al: Percutaneous nephrolithotomy: analysis of 500 consecutive cases. *Urol Radiol* 8:61, 1986.

Pfister RC, Dretler SP: Percutaneous chemolysis of renal calculi. *Urol Radiol* 6:138, 1984.

Reddy PK, Hulbert JC, Lange PH, et al: Percutaneous removal of renal and ureteral calculi: experience with 400 cases. *Urology* 134:662, 1985.

Rodman JS, Williams JJ, Peterson CM: State of the art dissolution of uric acid calculi. *Urology* 131:1039, 1984.

Segura JW, Patterson DE, LeRoy AJ, et al: Percutaneous removal of kidney stones: review of 1,000 cases. *Urology* 134:1077, 1985.

Teigland CM, Clayman RV, Winfield HN, et al: Ultrasonic lithotripsy: the risk of hearing loss. *Urology* 135:728, 1986.

Extracorporeal Shock Wave Lithotripsy

Barloon TJ, Brown RC, Berbaum KS: Current status of adult uroradiology: a survey of members of the Society of Uroradiology. *AJR* 154:301, 1990.

Baumgartner BR, Dickey KW, Ambrose SS, et al: Kidney changes after extracorporeal shock-wave lithotripsy: appearance on MR imaging. *Radiology* 163:531, 1987.

Bush WH, Gibbons RP, Lewis GP, et al: Impact of extracorporeal shock-wave lithotripsy on percutaneous stone procedures. *AJR* 147:89, 1986.

Chaussy C, Schmiedt E, Jocham D, et al: First clinical experience with extracorporeally induced destruction of kidney stones by shock-waves. *Urology* 127:417, 1982.

Cochran ST, Barbaric ZL, Mindell HJ, et al: Extracorporeal shock-wave lithotripsy: impact on the radiology department of a stone treatment center. *Radiology* 163:655, 1987.

Cochran ST, Liu E, Barbaric ZL: Percutaneous nephrostomy in conjunction with ESWL in treatment of nephrolithiasis. *AJR* 151:103, 1988.

Graff J, Diederichs W, Schulze H: Long-term followup in 1,003 extracorporeal shock-wave lithotripsy patients. *Urology* 140:479, 1988.

Lingeman E, Coury TA, Newman DM, et al: Comparison of results and morbidity of percutaneous nephrostolithotomy and extracorporeal shock-wave lithotripsy. *Urology* 138:485, 1987.

Riehle RA, Naslund EB, Fair W, et al: Impact of shock-wave lithotripsy on upper urinary tract calculi. *Urology* 28:261, 1986.

Tegtmeyer CJ, Kellum CD, Jenkins A, et al: Extracorporeal shock-wave lithotripsy: interventional radiologic solutions to associated problems. *Radiology* 161:587, 1986.

Williams CM, Kaude JV, Newman RC, et al: Extracorporeal shock-wave lithotripsy: long-term complications. *AJR* 150:311, 1988.

Staghorn Calculi

Adams GW, Oke EJ, Dunnick NR, et al: Percutaneous lithotripsy of staghorn calculi. *AJR* 145:803, 1985.

Lee WJ, Snyder JA, Smith AD: Staghorn calculi: endourologic management in 120 patients. *Radiology* 165:85, 1987.

Snyder JA, Smith AD: Staghorn calculi: percutaneous extraction versus anatrophic nephrolithotomy. *J Urol* 136:351, 1986.

Ureteral Calculi

Banner MP, VanArsdalen KN, Pollack HM: Extracorporeal shock wave lithotripsy of ureteral calculi. *Radiology* 174:12, 1990.

Barr JD, Tegtmeyer CJ, Jenkins AD: In situ lithotripsy of ureteral calculi: review of 261 cases. *Radiology* 174:103, 1990.

Coptcoat MJ, Webb DR, Kellett MJ, et al: The treatment of 100 consecutive patients with ureteral calculi in a British stone center. *J Urol* 137:1122, 1987.

Kahn I: Endourological treatment of ureteral calculi. *J Urol* 135:239, 1986.

LeRoy AJ, Williams HJ Jr, Bender CE, et al: Percutaneous removal of small ureteral calculi. *AJR* 145:109, 1985.

CHAPTER 11

THE PELVICALYCEAL SYSTEM

PAPILLARY NECROSIS (NECROTIZING PAPILLITIS)

Papillary necrosis is due to ischemic changes in the papilla resulting in partial or complete necrosis. It is found in analgesic nephropathy, sickle cell disease, diabetes mellitus, tuberculosis, acute pyelonephritis, and long-standing chronic obstruction. Each of these conditions may result in collections of contrast medium in the papillary region outside the interpapillary line. Although the etiologies differ, each condition may result in necrotic papillae.

Analgesic Nephropathy

Analgesic nephropathy was first described in 1953 in Switzerland. A high incidence (30%) of watchmakers with interstitial nephritis were found to consume combination analgesics over a long period for eye strain and headache. The most common combination was aspirin and phenacetin. Within a few years of the Swiss report, experience from Scandinavia and Australia emphasized interstitial nephritis, papillary necrosis, and renal impairment resulting from a variety of combination drugs, all of which included phenacetin.

Phenacetin (acetophenetidin) metabolites include N-acetylparaminophenol (NAPA), which is excreted in the urine, and P-phenetidin. A recent prospective study over a period of 11 years screened over 7000 females for phenacetin intake by urine examination for NAPA. High urine concentration of NAPA was found in females who consumed 1.25 g of phenacetin per day. Those with this consumption of phenacetin and high NAPA values in the urine had higher serum creatinine levels and an increased incidence of abnormal renal function. It has also been shown that NAPA concentrates in the renal cortex and medulla, resulting in an oxidative cytotoxic effect due to production of free radicals. The second metabolite of phenacetin, P-phenetidin, produces methemoglobinemia which predisposes to vascular occlusion.

Aspirin and phenacetin together as a combination analgesic are synergistic. In the kidney, salicylates have three main deleterious actions. First, they interfere with oxidative phosphorylation, which is a protective mechanism against oxidant toxic injury. Second, they inhibit the prostaglandin peroxidase synthesis system. Inhibition of prostaglandin synthesis affects the blood vessels resulting in potential renal ischemia. Third, they reduce normal glutathione levels. Glutathione is essential in oxidative phosphorylation. Reduction in glutathione results in the production of oxidative cytotoxic agents. The concentration of aspirin and phenacetin in the papilla is at least 5 times the concentration in the cortex. Consequently, continued ingestion of this combination of drugs over a long period leads to direct toxic effects on the collecting tubules, generalized microangiopathy in the peritubular vessels, endothelial necrosis in the interstitial cells, and platelet aggregation in the vasa recta, resulting in necrosis of the whole or part of the renal papilla.

The focus of attention on phenacetin as a cause of papillary necrosis caused its removal from over-the-counter drug combinations in Europe and North America between 1961 and 1975. The United States finally removed phenacetin from the prescription drug list in 1986. Phenacetin in combination drugs has been gradually replaced by acetaminophen (paracetamol). Statistics on analgesic consumption in the Federal Republic of Germany are of interest and likely reflect the analgesic consumption statistics elsewhere including North America. In the Federal Republic of Germany the per capita ingestion of phenacetin dropped from 3.4 g in 1976 to 1.7 g in 1983. During this period acetaminophen consumption increased from 2.2 g to approximately 4.5 g per capita. Although epidemiology reports from Scandinavia and Canada suggest a reduction in the incidence of papillary necrosis from analgesic abuse since phenacetin was restricted, analgesic nephropathy continues to be implicated in a significant percentage of patients with endstage renal disease. It has been demonstrated that both aspirin and acetaminophen produce renal papillary necrosis in uninephrectomized rats. Aspirin produced severe collecting duct cellular swelling with desquamated epithelial cells of the tubules extending into the ductal lumen. In addition, periductal interstitial cells become edematous and aggregates of flocculent material accumulate in the interstitial space. These changes occur prior to any vascular changes, suggesting a direct toxic effect of aspirin on the papilla. Platelet and fibrin thrombi develop, later resulting in ischemia. Acetaminophen produces similar findings that are less severe in the interstitium and more severe in the papillary tubular epithelium. It is postulated that each substance has a significant nephrotoxic effect but that the synergistic nephrotoxic effect of both substances combined is greater than either drug alone.

In recent years numerous reports have emphasized the development of analgesic nephropathy due to nonsteroidal antiinflammatory drugs (NSAIDS) such as indomethacin (Indocid) sulindac (Clinoril), and tolmetin (Tolectin). These drugs may produce renal insufficiency by inhibition of prostaglandin synthesis leading to the development of interstitial nephritis. Nephrotoxic syndromes associated with these drugs include acute renal insufficiency, interstitial nephritis, hyperkalemia, sodium and water retention, and acute anaphylaxis. Many of these conditions are reversible on steroid therapy and removal of the offending drug. There is a marked geographic distribution of analgesic nephropathy leading to papillary necrosis. In Belgium in the area around the city of Antwerp, analgesic abuse results in 100 cases of renal insufficiency per million population, and papillary necrosis is the cause in 36% of all patients with end-stage renal disease (ESRD). The Antwerp area is unlike the remainder of Belgium where renal insufficiency is found in 19 per million population and causes only 14% of all cases of ESRD. With the exception of Antwerp in Belgium, Australia is said to have the highest incidence of analgesic nephropathy at 40 per million population and 20% of cases of ESRD. Analgesic consumption in the northern Federal Republic of Germany, Scandinavia, and Switzerland remains high but less than Australia, whereas Britain and the United States have a low incidence of analgesic nephropathy at approximately 3 per million population and 1% of patients with ESRD is due to papillary necrosis.

Recently, papillary necrosis and renal impairment has been reported in children with chronic arthritis treated with nonsteroidal antiinflammatory drugs (NSAIDS). Indomethacin, acetaminophen, aspirin, and tolmetin have been implicated as the cause of renal impairment in these children. Prostoglandin synthesis inhibition has been attributed to these antiinflammatory drugs.

Clinically the vast majority of cases of renal papillary necrosis is the result of self-administration of analgesic combination drugs and over-the-counter sales. Over 70% of patients are women approximately 50 years of age who ingest analgesics on a long-term basis for various aches and pains without medical consultation, or because medical consultation has not helped their complaints. Gastrointestinal symptoms, anemia, and eventual renal impairment result. Symptoms of renal problems present with renal colic due to sloughing of a papilla include loin pain, dysuria, and occasionally frank hematuria. Urinalysis reveals sterile pyuria, microhematuria, and mild proteinuria. Albuminuria is usually not found. Salicylate and acetaminophen derivatives are found in the urine. At this stage the disease is irreversible. Patients with renal insufficiency due to analgesic abuse also have a marked increase in the incidence of transitional cell carcinoma (Fig. 11.1), particularly affecting the infundibulae, renal pelvis, and proximal ureter.

Before the development of analgesic nephropathy, it is said that a cumulative dose of between 2 and 3 kg is required.

Sickle Cell Disease

Sickle cell disease is the result of the homozygous hemoglobin S gene and is present in approximately 10% of North American blacks and in approximately 30% of black Africans. The hemoglobin S gene alters the solubility of hemoglobulin resulting in the classic sickle cell

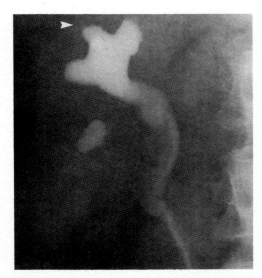

Figure 11.1. Papillary necrosis. Retrograde urogram showing faint calcification in papilla (*arrowhead*) outside the interpapillary line. The filling defect in the renal pelvis is transitional cell carcinoma.

shape of the red blood cells. Normal red cells are alleable and alter shape readily in their passage through small vessels. Sickle cells are less malleable and consequently produce aggregations of cells in small capillaries resulting in capillary occlusion and tissue anoxia. This therefore is the basis for ischemia and infarction. Up to 50% of sickle cell disease patients develop renal papillary necrosis. Unlike papillary necrosis resulting from analgesic nephropathy where the disease is due to a direct toxic effect of the drug followed by ischemia, papillary necrosis in sickle cell disease is purely ischemia, resulting in death of part or the whole papilla. Papillary necrosis may also occur in sickle cell trait (heterozygous sickle cell disease), which is recognized in India, the Middle East, and Mediterranean countries.

Diabetes Mellitus

Diabetes mellitus affects small vessels in the kidney. As in sickle cell disease, it can cause ischemia due to vascular occlusion and nephrosclerosis, leading to renal papillary necrosis.

Chronic Obstruction

Long-standing obstruction producing calyceal dilatation causes vascular insufficiency in the papilla due to vascular compression by the dilated calyx. The resulting ischemia causes papillary necrosis.

Radiology

Analgesic nephropathy, sickle cell disease, diabetes mellitus, and chronic obstruction all lead to papillary necrosis. All four conditions produce a similar radiologic appearance.

The plain film is commonly normal. Rarely the necrotic papilla develops a ring of calcification. If the whole papilla is necrotic the ring calcifications may be 5–6 mm in diameter. More commonly only part of the papilla is necrotic and when calcified is seen as a ring calcification 2–3 mm in size and of irregular shape. Rarely the plain film shows small renal outlines with several small punctate calcifications.

The plain film may also provide clues to the diagnosis. Advanced osteoarthritic change in the hips or apophyseal joints of the spine, or advanced degenerative disc disease, may be clues to excess analgesic ingestion. Vascular calcification in a young or middle-aged patient or calcification in the vas deferens and ampulla, may indicate diabetes mellitus. Bone infarction in the femoral head or neck may be due to sickle cell disease.

The classic radiologic features of renal papillary necrosis are best shown by excretory urography and retrograde pyelography. The kidneys are commonly smaller. Contrast medium outlining the collecting system generally shows cupped calyces with well-defined fornices. Small collections of contrast medium are seen in the papillary region. These may be round, elongated, or irregular in shape (Fig. 11.2). These collections extend outside the interpapillary line and indicate a space in the papilla filled with contrast medium. The space is left by a part of the papilla (medullary type) sloughing and pass-

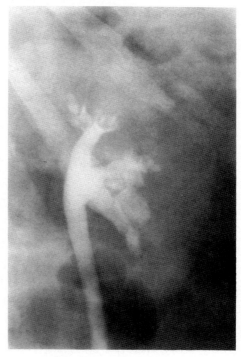

Figure 11.2. Papillary necrosis. Collections of contrast material of varying sizes are present in the papillary region adjacent to normal calyces.

ing down the ureter. These sloughed fragments are commonly not large enough to cause ureteric colic or obstruction. Follow-up serial urography may show a progressive loss of renal mass and often shows progression of these collections of contrast medium that enlarge and become more apparent. If the papilla does not slough but remains free in the papillary region, a ring shadow is produced by contrast medium surrounding the necrotized papilla (Fig. 11.3). If the whole papilla has sloughed (papillary type) and passed down the ureter, (Fig. 11.4) renal colic and obstruction may result. If there is no obstruction the calyx from which the papilla has sloughed may then look blunt with loss of fornices.

Sudden increase in the serum creatinine levels in a patient with known papillary necrosis is usually an indication of obstruction due to sloughing of a papilla. A sloughed papilla passing down the ureter may or may not cause obstruction (Fig. 11.4). Sloughed papillae have been seen as radiolucent filling defects in nondilated ureters.

Papillary necrosis should not be confused with papillary stones. These stones account for 25% of passed kidney stones and have a definite microscopic appearance. Papillary stones are formed in the interstitium of the papilla and are 1–4 mm in size. They have a characteristic shape, convex on one side, concave on the other. On the concave side Randall's plaques form in over 70%. The concavity is produced by the papillary stone formation in

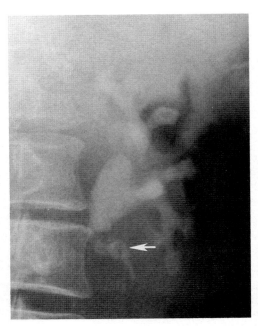

Figure 11.4.   Excretory urogram in a patient with analgesic abuse. Ring shadows are seen in the papillary region due to contrast medium surrounding sloughed papillae. A sloughed papilla in the proximal ureter (*arrow*) is seen as a radiolucent filling defect.

the interstitium against the cribriform plate. These stones are said to be formed by minute areas of ischemia that result in a small area of necrosis with the laying down of a calcium phosphate nidus on which calcium oxalate monohydrate (whewellite) deposits forming papillary stones. Papillary stones and Randall's plaques are extratubular and do not affect the collecting ducts, which function normally. There is no alteration in renal function.

MEDULLARY SPONGE KIDNEY (BENIGN TUBULAR ECTASIA)

Medullary sponge kidney (MSK) is the result of dysplastic dilatation of the collecting ducts (ducts of Bellini) that may be irregular in outline and cylindrically or saccularly dilated. The effect of these ectatic ducts is to enlarge the papilla, resulting in widening and flattening of the calyx. Occasionally the dysplasia results in ductal cysts that widen and deepen the calyx. The kidney is usually of normal size but is occasionally enlarged. In approximately 15% of cases, small calcifications are seen within the collecting ducts. Although the ductal openings into the cribriform plate of the calyces are normal, calcifications occasionally erode through the plate and cause renal colic. There is a slight tendency to an increased incidence of pyelonephritis.

First described on a histologic basis in 1908, the radiologic appearance was not described until 1939 and was not recognized as a disease entity until 1948. Since then,

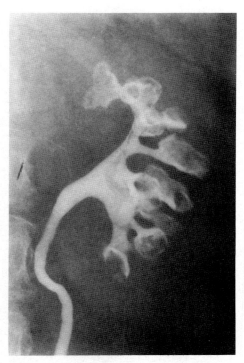

Figure 11.3.   Papillary necrosis. The papillae have sloughed but remain in the papillary region. They are seen as filling defects surrounded by contrast material.

numerous reports confirm the nature of the condition as clinically silent unless renal colic or infection supervene. Renal function is normal except for mild reduction in urinary concentration ability and a tendency to renal hypercalcemia in approximately 50% of patients. There is no association with cystic disease in the liver or pancreas. Numerous literature reports suggest an association with conditions including ipsilateral hemihypertrophy, cortical renal cysts, calyceal diverticula, medullary cystic disease, horseshoe kidney, renal ectopia, Ehlers-Danlos syndrome, adult-type polycystic disease, distal renal tubular acidosis, and more recently hyperparathyroidism due to parathyroid adenoma. The association of MSK and parathyroid adenoma has been noted in 25 cases, although the pathogenesis is obscure. The association may be a chance occurrence but the possibility of the parathyroid adenoma causing the MSK, or MSK with a renal leak hypercalcemia causing the parathyroid adenoma, has been considered. MSK is seen in approximately 0.5% of excretory urograms. It is very uncommon in children, probably because the disease is usually clinically silent and excretory urography is only done in symptomatic patients.

Radiology

The plain film is commonly normal, although occasionally multiple punctate calcifications are seen (Fig. 11.5). On excretory urography, MSK is seen as streaks of contrast medium extending from the cribriform plate of the calyx into the papilla (Fig. 11.6). These streaks of contrast medium outline ectatic collecting ducts, which with a magnifying glass are irregular in outline and of varying caliber (Fig. 11.7). The timing of this "paintbrush hair" visualization is important. In a urogram in which compression is applied after a 5-minute film, nor-

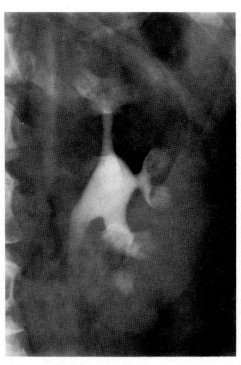

Figure 11.6.   Medullary sponge kidney. Contrast material is seen in several dilated collecting tubules in all calyceal regions. The rays are outside the interpapillary line.

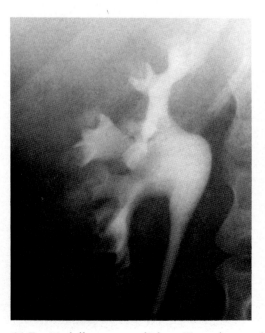

Figure 11.7.   Medullary sponge kidney. Normal cupped calyces with contrast medium seen in collecting tubules. Careful scrutiny reveals ectatic, irregular caliber of collecting tubules indicating medullary sponge kidney.

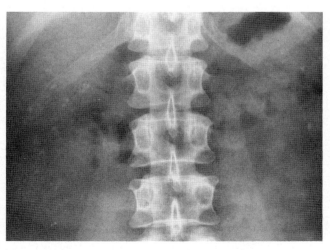

Figure 11.5.   The plain film in a patient with known medullary sponge kidney. Multiple punctate calcifications are seen in both kidneys.

mal collecting ducts can sometimes be seen as a blush in the papilla. When compression is removed the blush disappears. In MSK, the paintbrush hairs or blush is usually visible on the 5-minute film and persists through compression, release film, and postvoid films. MSK is therefore another cause of contrast medium collecting outside the calyx. The kidneys are smooth in outline and usually of normal size although they may be slightly enlarged. If a small calcification in a collecting duct has eroded through the cribriform plate, obstruction may ensue if the calcification is arrested in the ureter. In this case the calyces will be dilated and blunt with loss of the normal calyceal cup. Although contrast medium will be present in dilated collecting ducts, it may be obscured by the dilated calyx and the diagnosis cannot be made. Only after passage of the calcification and a follow-up urogram is obtained will the diagnosis be ascertained. Rarely massive collecting duct dilatation occurs. This may cause difficulty in differentiating polycystic disease, however, cysts in polycystic disease do not usually fill with contrast medium.

CALYCEAL DIVERTICULUM

A *calyceal diverticulum* is an outpouching of the calyx into the corticomedullary region. The diverticulum is a smooth-walled, mainly spherical lesion connected to the calyx by a thin channel (Fig. 11.8). When present they are more commonly seen extending from the fornix of a calyx in the upper or lower pole. A large diverticulum

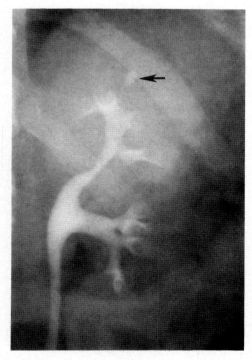

Figure 11.8. Calyceal diverticulum. A collection of contrast material (*arrow*) is seen outside the collecting system. The thin stalk connecting it to the fornix of the calyx cannot be seen.

may develop as an outpouching from the medial aspect of the renal pelvis and has been called pyelogenic cyst. A calyceal diverticulum is usually asymptomatic but may develop stones within it (Fig. 11.9). Passage of a stone through the narrow channel into the calyx may cause pain and microhematuria.

Radiology

On excretory urography the calyceal diverticulum is seen as a spherical collection of contrast medium adjacent to the papilla (Fig. 11.8). Occasionally the narrow connecting channel may be visualized, but often the channel is too narrow to be seen. On an upright film contrast medium and urine form a fluid level within a larger diverticulum which is diagnostic (Fig. 11.10). *Pyelogenic cyst* is a diverticulum that is in the central region of the kidney. These cysts are usually larger and may cause infundibular or calyceal compression and displacement. Calyceal diverticulae and pyelogenic cysts are asymptomatic until either stones or infection supervenes. They are readily recognized on ultrasound (US) or CT examination, both of which identify stones within a diverticulum.

RENAL TUBERCULOSIS

Renal tuberculosis is discussed in Chapter 7. However, there may occasionally be confusion in the differential diagnosis of tuberculosis, papillary necrosis, and MSK since all three conditions are causes of extracalyceal contrast medium. In tuberculosis sloughing of the caseous papillary lesions produces cavities in the papilla. These cavities are usually irregular in shape and produce an irregular cribiform plate. Healing of the granulomatous disease results in fibrosis leading to calyceal distortion, infundibular, and pelviureteric and ureterovesical stricture formation that usually leads to some degree of obstruction. Fibrosis in the suprahilar region and superior part of the renal pelvis results in narrowing of the renal pelvis and upward contraction producing a sharp pelvic angle known as "Kerr's kink" or "pursestring appearance" to the renal pelvis. Fibrosis in the infundibulum can result in "amputated calyx," in which the calyx is never seen, or late follow-up films may show faint contrast medium in the dilated calyx (Fig. 11.11). Fibrosis at the ureteropelvic junction (UPJ) or ureterovesical junction may result in the development of caseous pyonephrosis. This eventually calcifies, resulting in the classic autonephrectomy.

DIFFERENTIAL DIAGNOSIS OF EXTRACALYCEAL CONTRAST MEDIUM

Papillary necrosis, MSK, and tuberculosis all may result in contrast medium in the papilla outside the interpapillary line (Fig. 11.12). Differentiating papillary necro-

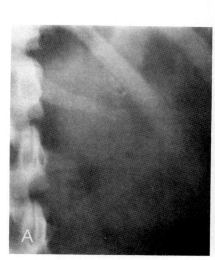

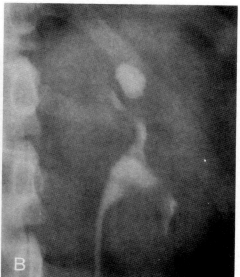

Figure 11.9.   Calyceal diverticulum. **A,** Several small calcifications are seen in the upper pole of the left kidney on the plain film of this 32-year-old man complaining of left upper quadrant pain. **B,** Excretory urogram. Stones seen on the preliminary film are within the diverticulum.

sis from MSK and tuberculosis may be difficult. Both papillary necrosis and MSK are more common in women. Patients with papillary necrosis may have a history of high analgesic ingestion. Both conditions may produce punctate nephrocalcinosis, more commonly bilateral in MSK. The dilated tubules of MSK may be confused with the early changes of partial papillary destruction. In both conditions a cupped calyx may be preserved, with streaks

of contrast medium in the papilla. However, the brush appearance of MSK is usually generalized in the papillae of both kidneys, unlike papillary necrosis, which is usually more apparent in one kidney and does not usually affect all papillae to the same degree. When the investigator uses a magnifying glass, a brush border is apparent in the papillae in sponge kidney. In papillary necrosis a brush border is not visualized, but usually one or two

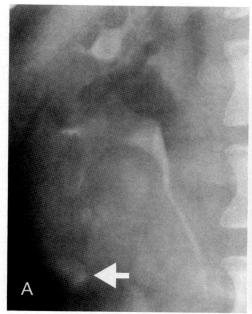

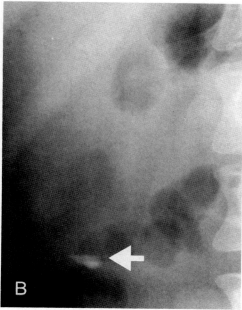

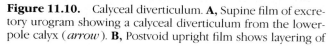

Figure 11.10.   Calyceal diverticulum. **A,** Supine film of excretory urogram showing a calyceal diverticulum from the lower-pole calyx (*arrow*). **B,** Postvoid upright film shows layering of contrast medium and urine producing a fluid level within the calyceal diverticulum (*arrow*).

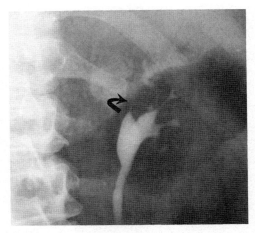

Figure 11.11. Tuberculosis. Late film from an excretory urogram showing dilated, partially obstructed calyx in the upper pole due to upper pole infundibular stricture (*arrow*). An irregular collection of contrast medium is also seen in the papilla of an adjacent calyx.

irregular collections of contrast medium are seen in one or two papillae. In spite of these distinguishing features, it may still be impossible to make the diagnosis radiologically. In this case a family history of sponge kidney may be helpful. Urine analysis and renal function studies are usually normal in MSK, unlike papillary necrosis in which some impairment of renal function is usually present and the urine invariably contains leukocytes.

When contrast medium is seen in a papilla outside a calyx, early renal tuberculosis should be considered. The collection of contrast medium is usually localized to one papilla and is probably more extensive and irregular. Although the calyx may remain normally cupped, more commonly the calyx and fornices are irregular or ragged in appearance. Unlike MSK there is always an abnormal urine examination, usually sterile pyuria. There may be more difficulty in distinguishing papillary necrosis from early renal tuberculosis radiologically but the patient's history is helpful. In renal tuberculosis the presenting features are commonly from the lower urinary tract. Some degree of renal impairment occurs in papillary necrosis. This is less likely in early renal tuberculosis. The diagnosis of a calyceal diverticulum is not usually difficult, although a solitary necrotic sloughed fragment

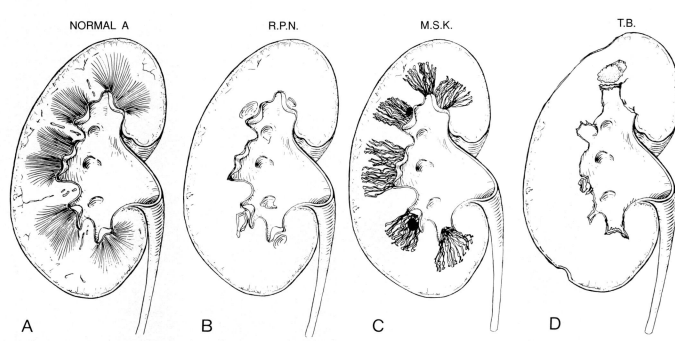

NORMAL A   R.P.N.   M.S.K.   T.B.

A   B   C   D

Figure 11.12. Normal. **A,** Diagrammatic representation of contrast medium seen in normal collecting tubules after the application of compression in excretory urography. The rays of contrast medium in collecting tubules are outside the interpapillary line. **B,** Papillary necrosis. Diagrammatic representation of necrotic papillae in papillary necrosis. The papilla may be completely (papillary type) or partially (medullary type) necrotic. The calyces are normally cupped unless the necrotic papilla has sloughed and passed into the collecting system in which case the calyx will appear to be blunt. **C,** Medullary sponge kidney. Diagrammatic representation of dilated collecting ducts some containing small calcifications. The collecting ducts are irregular in outline. The calyx is either normal or flattened. This is the classic appearance of medullary sponge kidney. **D,** Tuberculosis. Diagrammatic representation of intermediate renal tuberculosis. Contrast medium is seen in cavities in the papilla. These collections are irregular and extend toward the cortex. There may be associated scarring opposite the affected papilla. The associated calyx has a moth-eaten, ragged appearance.

in papillary necrosis may be present at the same site as a diverticulum. The small round shape of a diverticulum in a characteristic site, commonly the upper pole, is unlike the irregular space left by a sloughing fragment in papillary necrosis. The pelvicalyceal system may be affected by tumors. Parenchymal tumors may affect the calyces, infundibula, and renal pelves and are discussed in detail in Chapter 6.

BENIGN MASSES

Benign lesions of the pelvicalyceal system are exceedingly rare. These include papillomas, inverted papillomas, leukoplakia, and malacoplakia.

Inverted Papilloma

Inverted papillomas are uncommon; a little over 120 have been reported since 1963 when this entity was first described. Most of these lesions occur in the bladder. Twenty five percent of inverted papillomas occur in the renal pelvis. Although considered a benign lesion, approximately 20% of inverted papillomas have been associated with urothelial malignancy, either adjacent to the inverted papilloma or more distant with normal urothelium between. The associated malignancy may be in the contralateral renal pelvis or ureter. Although these lesions may be associated with urothelial malignancy, they are considered benign. Three reported cases recurred in the bladder. Resection of the recurrences were benign. No recurrence has been noted in the renal pelvis. However, the significant incidence of locally associated urothelial malignancy raises the possibility that inverted papilloma may be a premalignant condition. The pathogenesis of inverted papilloma is not fully understood, but it has been suggested that its development may be a reaction to inflammatory change. Grossly these lesions are small. Histologically they show an inverted configuration with a normal layer of transitional cell epithelium, microcystic formation, infrequent areas of squamous metaplasia, and absence of mitotic figures.

Benign Papilloma

Benign papillomas may occur in the renal pelvis and infundibulum. Although these have a benign histologic appearance they have a definite potential for malignant change.

Leukoplakia (Squamous Metaplasia)

The term *leukoplakia* refers to a white patch seen on the mucosal surface of an area of squamous metaplasia. A *cholesteatoma* is a mass of desquamated keratin within the renal collecting system. The term *keratinizing desquamative squamous metaplasia* has been proposed to include both entities.

Squamous metaplasia is associated with chronic infection but has a low malignant potential. Symptoms are nonspecific and are usually related to urinary tract infection. Squamous metaplasia is seen as prominent mucosal thickening giving a "corduroy" appearance on urography or retrograde pyelography.

Malacoplakia

Malacoplakia is a benign lesion associated with recurrent inflammatory processes usually due to *E. coli.* Seventy-five percent of cases of malacoplakia are associated with *E. coli.* A few cases have occurred in the renal pelvis and infundibulum. These lesions are usually small, up to 3 mm in diameter, and are commonly multiple. Grossly these lesions are smooth yellow plaques. Histologically, histiocytes contain the typical Michaelis-Guttmann bodies. Inflammatory cells always make up much of the plaque.

MALIGNANT TUMORS

Malignant tumors affecting the pelvicalyceal system are uncommon. Ninety percent of these tumors are transitional cell carcinoma. A few cases of adenocarcinoma within the renal pelvis have been reported. Rarely squamous metaplasia occurs in transitional cell carcinoma, resulting in squamous cell carcinoma.

Transitional Cell Carcinoma

Approximately 12% of all transitional cell carcinomas occur in the upper urinary tract. Most of these occur in the renal pelvis, but a few are present in the infundibulae. Rarely both may occur together. Up to 40% of patients with upper urinary tract transitional cell carcinomas have bladder transitional cell carcinomas at the time of diagnosis. Multicentricity of transitional cell carcinoma is well recognized. Multicentric lesions may occur anywhere in the urinary tract (Fig. 11.13). Bilateral lesions are present in 2% of cases. The incidence of transitional cell carcinoma in the renal pelvis is less than 1 per 100,000 population and accounts for only 4% of all renal tumors. There is a 60–70% recurrence rate on the ipsilateral side. Approximately 7% of transitional cell carcinomas develop a second transitional cell carcinoma in the contralateral pelvis at a later date.

Definite etiology associations have been established in upper urinary tract transitional cell carcinoma. These include analgesic abuse, cigarette smoking, cyclophosphamide therapy, radiation exposure, and chronic inflammatory change leading to pyelitis cystica and pyelitis glandularis. Calculi have been implicated in the past as a cause of transitional cell carcinoma of the upper urinary tract. However, urine cytology has shown tumor cell features in 7% of cases in which no transitional cell carcinoma was present or developed later. Cytologists are now wary of suggesting transitional cell carcinoma on

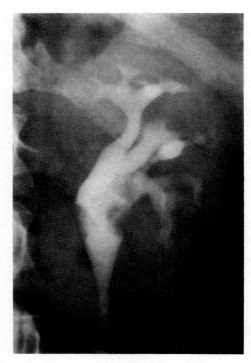

Figure 11.13. Transitional cell carcinoma. Multiple irregular filling defects in renal pelvis and calyces are most consistent with transitional cell carcinoma.

urine cytology when renal calculi are present. A recent report by Marchetto et al. indicates a familial tendency in reporting multiple urothelial tumors occurring in one family.

High analgesic ingestion produces renal papillary necrosis and there is a definite increase in the incidence of transitional cell carcinoma in the upper urinary tracts of these patients. Transitional cell carcinoma may also develop without any evidence of papillary necrosis in analgesic abuse patients. Histopathologic examination of renal pelvic transitional cell carcinoma resulting from analgesic abuse is said to show capillary sclerosis pathognomonic of analgesic abuse even when there is no papillary necrosis or history of analgesic abuse. Diabetes mellitus and sickle cell disease causing papillary necrosis have no known association with transitional cell carcinoma. Cigarette smokers have an increased incidence of transitional cell carcinoma, more commonly in the bladder, however, renal pelvic carcinoma has been reported as well. Cigarette smoking is said to interfere with tryptophan metabolism, producing orthoaminophenol which is carcinogenic. It requires at least 20 years of heavy cigarette smoking before the development of transitional cell carcinoma. The alkylating cyclophosphamide may also induce transitional cell carcinoma by the cytotoxic effects of its metabolites acrolein and phosphonamide.

Approximately 70% of renal pelvic carcinomas are invasive. Positive urine cytology is present in 70% of those with invasive renal pelvic tumors. Positive cytology may also be found in retrograde pelvic brushing or in renal pelvic aspiration fluid obtained during antegrade pyelography. Ileoconduit urine may also show positive cytology indicating upper tract carcinoma.

Staging of transitional cell carcinoma correlates well with tumor grading and generally is the same in the upper tract as in the lower urinary tract. At the time of diagnosis approximately 50% of transitional cell carcinomas are low stage (i.e., limited to the mucosa or lamina propria). Muscle invasion or spread through the muscle has occurred in the other 50%. Five-year survival rates for low-stage tumors are approximately 5–7 years, but fall to only approximately 1 year for high-stage tumors. Local recurrence, i.e., recurrence in a ureteral stump after nephroureterectomy, or local recurrence if only local removal has been performed, occurs in 25% of patients. Approximately 50% of patients eventually develop lung metastases. Rarely, transitional cell carcinoma of the renal pelvis invades the renal parenchyma before presenting clinically. The usual event is for transitional cell carcinoma to bleed and produce hematuria before it has invaded renal parenchyma. Invasion of renal parenchyma is an ominous event resulting in a prognosis of only a few months. Recent literature emphasizes the role of vesicoureteral renal reflux in patients with a recurrent bladder carcinoma who later develop renal pelvic carcinoma. In a series of 16 renal pelvic transitional cell carcinomas reported by Affre et al., six patients showed vesicoureteral reflux on voiding cystography and a further six were seen to reflux on cystoscopy. Three of the remaining patients had indirect evidence of reflux, namely, dilated ureters but did not have any direct evidence of reflux. It is suggested that repeated ablation of bladder tumors transurethrally may be the cause of reflux. Reports by Yousemetal and Booth and Kellett suggest that follow-up excretory urography, voiding cystography, and cystoscopy should be continued indefinitely following recurrent ablation of bladder tumors.

Adenocarcinoma

Adenocarcinoma of the renal pelvis is rare, accounting for less than 1% of renal pelvic tumors. Approximately 40 cases of mucinous adenocarcinoma occurring in the renal pelvis or ureter have been reported. Repeated infection, calculi, and long-standing hydronephrosis are associated and may be etiologic conditions. Chronic inflammatory change stimulates metaplastic cells (Von Brunn's nests) to form pyelitis cystica and glandularis in the renal pelvis, which progresses to mucin producing adenocarcinoma. These conditions may also be associated with adenocarcinoma in the bladder. The clinical presentation of upper urinary tract tumors is almost invariably hematuria, but loin pain or ureteral colic may also be present.

Radiology

Transitional cell carcinoma of the collecting system and renal pelvis is commonly diagnosed on excretory urography and retrograde pyelography. Both of these modalities localize the tumor, and together they show the extent of the lesion. Transitional cell carcinoma in an infundibulum or renal pelvis that does not cause obstruction can usually be visualized on urography as a filling defect at the site of the tumor (Fig. 11.13). Radiolucent filling defects can represent radiolucent stone, blood clot, or tumor. Blood clot may be adherent or loose in the collecting system. Retrograde pyelography may show movement within the collecting system or change of shape if the defect is blood clot. Transitional cell carcinoma is commonly sessile and not pedunculated and does not move. Radiolucent stones such as uric acid may also be mobile. However, the diagnosis of uric acid stone can be made on an unenhanced CT scan as the uric acid stone has a high density (100–600 HU). Transitional cell carcinoma is soft tissue density on CT scan rarely containing calcium and is shown as a fixed filling defect which may be identified as a sessile mass, infundibular or pelvic wall thickening (Fig. 11.14), or rarely a pelvic or infundibulum mass invading the parenchyma. Contrast-enhanced scans show the lesion as a filling defect displacing contrast medium. Transitional cell carcinoma may slightly enhance on dynamic CT scan.

A definite advantage of CT in transitional cell carcinoma is its ability to stage transitional cell carcinoma.

Low-stage lesions have not invaded the muscularis. High-stage lesions are seen to penetrate the infundibular or pelvic wall and enlarge localized lymph nodes. Stage IV disease with nodal enlargement may be understaged since involved nodes may be less than 1 cm and may present a normal appearance. The diagnosis of transitional cell carcinoma is more difficult when the lesion causes obstruction or when there is renal impairment.

If a pelvic lesion causes obstruction, US is helpful in showing dilated calyces and the site of obstruction. An isoechoic mass may be seen in the dilated renal pelvis, or, if the lesion is in the infundibulum, localized hydronephrosis is seen with the pelvis and remaining calyces being normal.

In arteriography, transitional cell carcinoma rarely visualizes tumor vessels unless the carcinoma has invaded the renal parenchyma or invaded through the renal pelvis (Fig. 11.15).

Ultrasound examination of the kidney is seldom helpful in the recognition of small transitional cell carcinomas. Ultrasound may demonstrate transitional cell carcinoma when it obstructs an infundibulum and extends into a dilated calyx (Fig. 11.16).

Occasionally there is difficulty on excretory urography and retrograde pyelography in distinguishing an intrapelvic from an extrapelvic filling defect. A tortuous renal artery or a renal artery aneurysm may cause a persistent defect in the renal pelvis. Views in the supine, prone, and oblique and upright positions may help clarify the defect

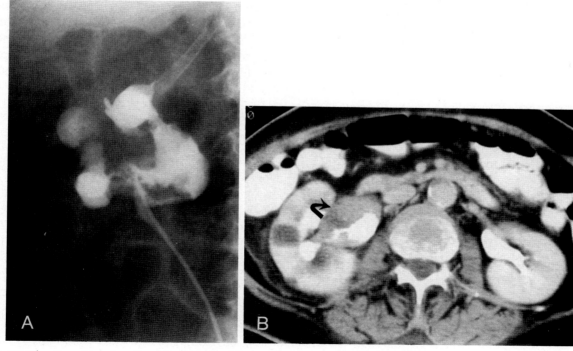

Figure 11.14. Transitional cell carcinoma. **A,** Retrograde pyelography demonstrates a large irregular filling defect in the renal pelvis. **B,** The soft tissue mass component (*arrow*) is shown on this enhanced CT examination.

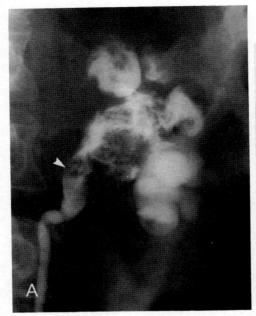
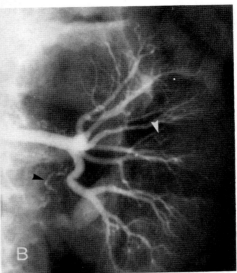

Figure 11.15. Transitional cell carcinoma. **A,** Excretory urogram in a patient with invasive transitional cell carcinoma. The tumor has extended into the calyces and through the renal pelvic wall (*arrowhead*). Much of the filling defect represents blood clot. **B,** Selective renal angiography shows small tumor vessels centrally (*white arrowhead*) and tortuous tumor vessels where the tumor has invaded the renal pelvis (*black arrowhead*). Tumor vessels are not commonly seen in transitional cell carcinoma.

since altering position may alter the appearance of the defect. Rarely it may be necessary to resort to angiography, which will identify the renal artery or renal artery aneurysm (Fig. 11.17).

Extrinsic defects may occur in the infundibulum or at the UPJ. Most of these are vascular and rarely cause compression on the infundibulum or ureteropelvic junction. Rarely these extrinsic vessels cause sufficient compression to produce obstruction, which is localized to one calyx if the vessel is across an infundibulum, (Fraley's syndrome), or the calyces and pelvis may be dilated if the vessel is across the UPJ. The degree of obstruction can be assessed by excretory urography, but a Lasix urogram may be required to prove significant obstruction. Angiography is generally requested for operative planning.

Pelvicalyceal filling defects cannot be adequately assessed by MRI at the present time. Small soft tissue lesions may not be seen because of limited spatial resolution and motion artifacts. Furthermore, calcified stones cannot be distinguished from soft tissue.

VESICOURETERAL REFLUX

The pelvicalyceal system may be severely affected by vesicoureteral reflux, which may be classified as high or low pressure. It occurs because of a defective vesicoureteral junction. The defect is thought to be the result of a short intramural segment of the ureter which is a common occurrence in infants and children. As growth proceeds into adulthood the intramural segment of the ureter lengthens and reflux no longer occurs, usually by the age of 5 years. This usually occurs as growth proceeds, but there are some children in whom reflux continues into adulthood.

Vesicoureteral reflux is graded according to the degree of dilatation of the ureter and how far up the ureter the reflux reaches. Thus, in Grade 1 reflux, refluxed urine extends into the lower half of the ureter. Grade 2

Figure 11.16. Transitional cell carcinoma. Ultrasound examination showing echogenic discrete mass in the lower pole calyceal region (*arrowhead*).

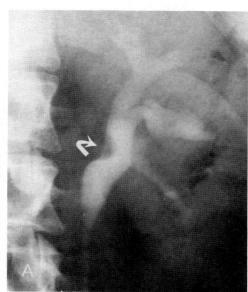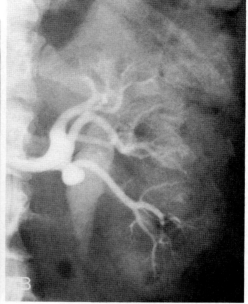

Figure 11.17.   Renal artery aneurysm. **A,** Excretory urogram showing renal pelvic defect (*arrow*). **B,** Selective renal arteri-ography shows a renal artery aneurysm in the exact position of the renal pelvic defect.

reflux exists when the whole ureter and pelvicalyceal system fill with refluxed urine. In Grade 3 reflux, the pelvicalyceal system and ureter are mildly dilated. However, a refluxing dilated ureter does not always appear dilated. When the bladder is empty, the Grade 3 refluxing ureter can look normal in caliber. There may be a few linear mucosal striations seen, which is a clue to a refluxing ureter. Grade 4 reflux includes more marked dilation of the intrarenal collecting system and tortuosity of the ureter.

Low-pressure reflux occurs with bladder filling. High-pressure reflux occurs when the intravesical pressure increases as in voiding. Naturally, in low-pressure reflux the pressure on the collecting system is greatly increased on voiding. The pressure on the pelvicalyceal system during voiding may therefore be sufficient to cause marked dilatation of the pelvicalyceal system and ureter, an appearance that resembles obstruction. Even on an upright postvoid film the large amount of refluxed contrast medium in the collecting system may still fill the system and ureter down to the ureterovesical junction making it difficult to exclude obstruction at the distal ureter. Consequently Grade 3 reflux may produce persistent hydronephrosis, which requires further investigation.

To aid in this differentiation two tests have evolved, the Lasix (furosemide) hydration urogram and the Whitaker test. The Lasix hydration urogram involves the administration of 2 mg/kg body weight in children or 20–40 mg of Lasix to adolescents or adults. The diuretic is given as a single intravenous injection during an excretory urogram after contrast medium has outlined the collecting system.

Since Lasix is a powerful diuretic the urine flow rate is greatly increased. If no obstruction is present, all of the contrast medium in the collecting system is washed out rapidly. If obstruction is present, contrast medium remains in the system which becomes more dilated due to the increased urine flow. This test is more simple than the Whitaker test, which involves a percutaneous nephrostomy and measurement of the urine flow rate through the suspected obstruction and measurement of the pressure in the bladder and the renal pelvis simultaneously (Chapter 14).

Vesicoureteral reflux in infants and young children may cause such high pressure on the calyces that intrarenal reflux occurs. Intrarenal reflux is more common in the upper and lower poles of the kidneys because the papillary orifices of compound calyces are spherical and more open allowing reflux into the papilla. Simple papillae have slit-like orifices into the cribriform plate and generally do not allow reflux. Intrarenal reflux occurs in young children usually before the age of 5 years. If bladder urine is infected, intrarenal reflux of infected urine causes an acute infection in the parenchyma invading the cortex adjacent or opposite a calyx, usually in the upper and lower pole. This acute inflammatory reaction heals by fibrosis, producing scars and retraction of the calyx which becomes blunt. This is the typical appearance of chronic pyelonephritis. A more descriptive term is reflux nephropathy, and this appearance of chronic pyelonephritis in adults may be the result of previous intrarenal reflux of infected urine when the patient was younger than 5 years. Therefore reimplantation of ureters to correct reflux should be done at an early age. It is said that most of the reflux nephropathy changes occur before the age of 2 years and reimplantation is required before this age for the operation to have any success in altering the development of the pathologic changes. Even when reflux continues into adulthood, the adult kidney appears to be significantly more resistant to intrarenal reflux and further pyelonephritic changes.

Patients with neurogenic bladder also have an increased incidence of vesicoureteral reflux and pyelonephritic scarring. The reflux results from outlet obstruction, usually due to distal sphincter dyssynergia and superimposed infection in the bladder. The resulting cystitis alters the shape of the ureteral orifice to allow reflux. Reflux is rare in patients with neurogenic bladder without bladder infection. The demonstration of reflux in patients with neurogenic bladder may be dangerous to the patient, since septic shock may occur with intrarenal reflux of infected urine. Reflux may also occur into the lower moiety of patients with double collecting systems. The ureter to the lower moiety has an abnormal insertion which allows reflux. It is not uncommon for the lower pole of a double collecting system to be smaller than expected. The lower pole may be scarred but more commonly is not. The hypoplastic lower pole may be the result of sterile intrarenal reflux either in utero or early in life.

Alteration of the ureterovesical junction is seen in patients who have had recurrent bladder tumor fulgarization. This is another possible cause of upper-tract transitional cell carcinoma which develops after reflux occurs.

Radiology

Excretory urography with tomography clearly defines the renal outline. Cortical atrophy and scarring, usually at the poles, is readily identified (Fig. 11.18). Polar compound calyces are blunted with loss of normal fornices. Simple calyces are usually normal. Persistent low- and high-pressure reflux may produce calyceal, pelvic and

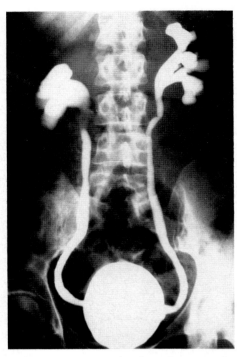

Figure 11.19. Vesicoureteral reflux. Cystogram in a female patient showing low-pressure Grade 3 reflux into dilated pelvicalyceal systems.

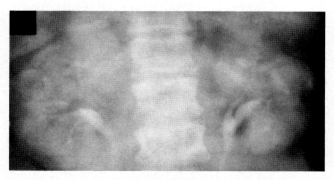

Figure 11.18. Reflux nephropathy. Excretory urogram with tomography in a 35-year-old woman, showing bilateral parenchymal scarring and blunted calyces in a patient who refluxed in early childhood.

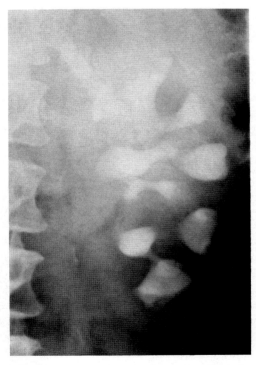

Figure 11.20. Congenital megacalyces. Romboid-shaped calyces are seen in an enlarged kidney, but there is no evidence of obstruction.

ureteric dilatation. If Grade 3 reflux is present, contrast medium is likely to be seen throughout the length of the dilated ureters and pelvicalyceal systems (Fig. 11.19) even on a postvoid upright film. Renal US is also helpful in the diagnosis of reflux nephropathy. A longitudinal scan clearly shows polar scarring and parenchymal loss. The corticomedullary junction is lost in the scarred area which may be hyperechoic. Computed tomography is not usually necessary for this diagnosis. Voiding cystography is mandatory to establish if vesicouretero reflux is still present. The demonstration of grades 2 and 3 reflux may require antibiotic therapy to maintain a sterile urine. Approximately 20% of young children with recurrent urinary tract infection develop renal scarring. All of these patients have ureterovesical reflux.

Grade 3 reflux into a lower-pole moiety of a double collecting system is rarely seen. When present the lower pole is scarred and the calyces are blunt.

Megacalyces is a congenital condition in which there are supernumerary (more than 20) enlarged calyces. The renal parenchyma is normal and creatinine clearance is normal. It is said that some degree of diminished concentrating ability is present. The infundibulae, renal pelvis, and ureter are normal.

Excretory urography reveals a characteristic appearance. The kidney is usually enlarged and the calyces are enlarged but not clubbed (Fig. 11.20). If megacalyces are unilateral, contrast medium appears in both kidneys simultaneously, therefore the concentrating ability is not sufficiently diminished to be seen radiologically.

SUGGESTED READINGS

Papillary Necrosis

Allen RC, Petty RE, Lirenman DS, et al: Renal papillary necrosis in children with chronic arthritis. *Am J Dis Child* 140:20, 1986.
Andriole GL, Bahnson RR: Computed tomographic diagnosis of ureteral obstruction caused by a sloughed papilla. *Urol Radiol* 9:45, 1987.
Delatte LC, Minon-Cifuentes JLR, Medina JA: Papillary stones: calcified renal tubules in Randall's plaques. *J Urol* 133:490, 1985.
Gong MB, Davidson AJ: Development and progression of renal papillary necrosis in SA hemoglobinopathy. *Urol Radiol* 2:55, 1980.
Henrich WL: Southwestern Internal Medicine Conference: analgesic nephropathy. *Am J Med Sci* 295:561, 1988.
Henry MA, Tange JD: Ultrastructural appearances of acute renal papillary lesions induced by aspirin. *J Pathol* 139:57, 1983.
Henry MA, Tange JD: Lesions of the renal papilla induced by paracetamol. *J Pathol* 151:11, 1987.
Maher JF: Analgesic nephropathy. Observations, interpretations, and perspectives on the low incidence in America. *Am J Med* 76:345, 1984.

Medullary Sponge Kidney

Gedroyc WMW, Saxton HM: More medullary sponge variants. *Clin Radiol* 39:423, 1988.

Megacalyces

Higashihara E, Munakata A, Hara M, et al: Medullary sponge kidney and hyperparathyroidism. *Urology* 31:155, 1988.
Mellins HZ: Cystic dilatations of the upper urinary tract: a radiologist's developmental model. *Radiology* 153:291, 1984.

Zawada ET, Sica DA: Differential diagnosis of medullary sponge kidney. *South Med J* 77:686, 1984.

Tuberculosis

Becker JA: Renal tuberculosis. *Urol Radiol* 10:25, 1988.
Goldman SM, Fishman EK, Hartman DS, et al: Computed tomography of renal tuberculosis and its pathological correlates. *J Comput Assist Tomogr* 9:771, 1985.
Premkumar A, Lattimer J, Newhuse JH: CT and sonography of advanced urinary tract tuberculosis. *AJR* 148:65, 1987.
Psihramis KE, Donahoe PK: Primary genitourinary tuberculosis: rapid progression and tissue destruction during treatment. *J Urol* 135:1033, 1986.

Benign Masses

Irby PB, Stoller ML, McAninch JW: Fungal bezoars of the upper urinary tract. *J Urol.* 143:447, 1990.
Renfer LG, Kelley J, Belville WD: Inverted papilloma of the urinary tract: histogenesis, recurrence and associated malignancy. *J Urol* 140:832, 1988.

Malignant Tumors

Affre J, Michel JR, de Peyronnet R, et al: Secondary foci of primary tumors of the bladder in the upper urinary tract. *Urol Radiol* 3:7, 1981.
Anselmo G, Rizzotti A, Felici E, et al: Multiple simultaneous bilateral urothelial tumours of the renal pelvis. *Br J Urol* 60:312, 1987.
Balfe DM, McClennan BL, AufderHeide JF: Multimodal imaging in evaluation of two cases of adenocarcinoma of the renal pelvis. *Urol Radiol* 3:19, 1981.
Baron RL, McClennan BL, Lee JKT, et al: Computed tomography of transitional cell carcinoma of the renal pelvis and ureter. *Radiology* 144:125, 1982.
Bree RL, Schultz SR, Hayes R: Large infiltrating renal transitional cell carcinomas: CT and ultrasound features. *J Comput Assist Tomogr* 14(3):381, 1990.
Brenner DW, Schellhammer PF: Upper tract urothelial malignancy after cyclophosphamide therapy: a case report and literature review. *J Urol* 137:1226, 1987.
Booth CM, Kellett, MJ: Intravenous urography in the follow up of carcinoma of the bladder. *Br J Urol* 53:246, 1981.
Highman WJ: Transitional carcinoma of the upper urinary tract: a histological and cytopathological study. *J Clin Pathol* 39:297, 1986.
Leder RA, Dunnick NR: Transitional cell carcinoma of the kidney and ureter. *AJR* (In Press).
Marchetto D, Li FP, Henson DE: Familial carcinoma of ureters and other genitourinary organs. *J Urol* 130:772, 1983.
Munechika H, Kushihashi T, Gokan T, et al: A renal cell carcinoma extending into the renal pelvis simulating transitional cell carcinoma. *Urol Radiol* 12:11, 1990.
Narumi Y, Sato T, Hori S, et al: Squamous cell carcinoma of the uroepithelium: CT evaluation. *Radiology* 173:853, 1989.
Oldbring J, Glifberg I, Mikulowski P, et al: Carcinoma of the renal pelvis and ureter following bladder carcinoma: frequency of risk factors and clinicopathologic findings. *J Urol* 141:1311, 1989.
Pollack HM: Long-term follow-up of the upper urinary tract for transitional cell carcinoma: how much is enough? *Radiology* 167:871, 1988.
Renfer LG, Kelley J, Belville WD: Inverted papilloma of the urinary tract: histogenesis, recurrence and associated malignancy. *J Urol* 140:832, 1988.
Tasca A, Zattoni F: The case for a percutaneous approach to transitional cell carcinoma of the renal pelvis. *J Urol* 143:902, 1990.
Yousem DM, Gatewood OMB, Goldman SM, et al: Synchronous and metachronous transitional cell carcinoma of the urinary tract: prevalence, incidence and radiographic detection. *Radiology* 167:613, 1988.

Vesicouretero Reflux

Hodson CJ: Reflux nephropathy: a personal historical review. *AJR* 137:451, 1981.
Rizzoni G, Perale R, Bui F, et al: Radionuclide voiding cystography in intrarenal reflux detection. *Ann Radiol* 29:415, 1986.

CHAPTER 12

URINARY TRACT TRAUMA

RENAL INJURIES

Clinical Features

Hematuria after blunt abdominal injury is common; significant injury to the kidney is, however, relatively uncommon. Hematuria after penetrating injury, however, is virtually always a sign of renal damage that requires surgical evaluation.

The amount of hematuria that should trigger radiologic investigation of the urinary tract after blunt trauma is controversial. Many authorities feel that any amount of hematuria should be investigated, as it is well known that significant urinary tract injury may be present in patients with little or even no hematuria. Furthermore, there is little correlation between the degree of hematuria and the amount of renal injury that is present. An oft-cited example is patients suffering from renal pedicle injury in whom hematuria is said to be absent in 25% of the cases.

As a result, screening studies of the urinary tract are often performed in virtually every patient after abdominal trauma. This low threshold for investigation has resulted in a relatively low yield for injury on radiologic screening studies. In a series of patients studied by McDonald et al. at a major trauma center, only 18 of 209 urograms performed for blunt trauma were considered abnormal (9%). Similar results have been reported from other major institutions.

As a result of these statistics, other investigators have sought to refine the criteria that should lead to investigation. Guice et al. found that no significant renal injury would be missed had investigation been limited to those with either gross or 4+ hematuria on dipstick urinalysis. Fortune et al., in a series encompassing 216 patients, found that in all but 1 of 20 patients with significant urographic abnormalities, hematuria greater than 50 red cells per high-power field was present and that all of the renal injuries present were associated with obvious abdominal injury. Similarly, Nicolaisen et al. found that significant renal injury was limited to the group of patients in whom shock and either gross or microscopic hematuria was present among 306 individuals analyzed retrospectively following blunt trauma. There were no significant renal injuries among the 221 patients who had microscopic hematuria, but were not suffering from shock. In patients in the same series who suffered penetrating injuries, however, no such discrimination was possible and the authors suggest radiologic evaluation be undertaken in all patients suffering penetrating injury and hematuria.

It can therefore be concluded that investigation of hematuria is warranted in those patients suffering penetrating injury, gross hematuria, and those individuals with microscopic hematuria with shock or other clinical indications suggesting that the urinary tract be evaluated.

Other clinical findings associated with the presence of a renal injury include a flank mass or hematoma on physical examination; the presence of a soft tissue mass on plain film studies; a scoliosis of the lumbar spine and fractures of the lower ribs (Fig. 12.1), lumbar vertebral bodies, or transverse processes. Loss of the psoas shadow is a nonspecific finding on which significant injury cannot be reliably diagnosed or excluded.

Most blunt renal injuries (75%) occur in patients suffering multisystem trauma. In a recent series from Cass et al. (1985), 241 of 831 patients had what were considered to be solitary renal injuries, however, the vast majority (98%) were minor injuries. Therefore, only five patients in the entire series suffered significant isolated renal injury. There were 33 significant renal injuries in the group of 590 patients with hematuria who suffered multisystem trauma. Other injuries associated with injury of the kidneys following multisystem blunt trauma include (in order of decreasing frequency): fractures of the extremities, thoracic injury, pelvic fracture, intraabdominal injury, head injuries, and diaphragmatic rupture. The liver and spleen are the abdominal organs most commonly associated with renal injury, followed by the pancreas, the colon, and the small bowel.

In most series, blunt trauma accounts for 80% of all renal injuries, but obviously the incidence reported depends on the referral pattern of the reporting institution. About three-quarters of the reported renal injuries occur in men under the age of 50 years. Motor vehicle accidents account for about one-half the reported cases; falls, altercations, industrial accidents, and sports injuries comprise the remainder.

Penetrating renal injuries fall into two categories—those related to gunshot wounds and those related to stabbings. Limited posterior stab wounds that do not penetrate the renal fossa may be managed conservatively by many surgeons. In the remainder, the mere demonstration that the kidney is in the path of the injury or the presence of hematuria is an indication for surgical exploration. More than 80% of gunshot wounds of the kidney are associated with other abdominal injuries, usually of the bowel, the pancreas, the diaphragm, or the liver and spleen.

Anatomy and Mechanism of Injury

The kidney is relatively protected from injury by the thoracic cage, the vertebral column, and the psoas muscles. In addition, the fascial coverings of the kidney and the retroperitoneal fat provide additional protection. Injury of the lower ribs or the vertebra is associated with a higher incidence of renal injury; an injury to the spleen

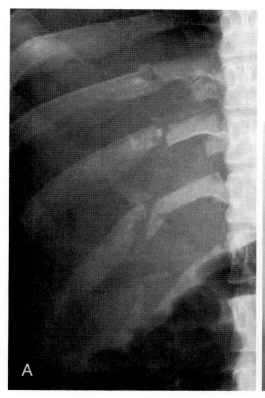
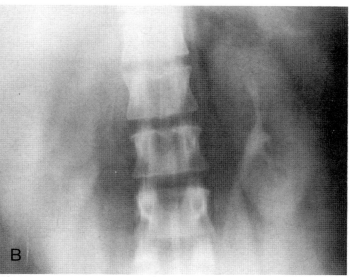

Figure 12.1. **A,** Scout radiograph demonstrates multiple lower right rib fractures. **B,** Tomogram from an IVP demonstrates a poorly defined renal outline, decreased contrast excretion, and poor filling of the collecting system of the right kidney indicative of a right renal injury.

frequently accompanies injury to the left kidney, while a liver injury accompanies injury of the right kidney. Each kidney is invested by a fascial covering known as Gerota's fascia. Bleeding from renal injuries is usually self-limiting as this fascial envelope provides a tamponade effect.

Bleeding within the substance of the kidney results in an intrarenal hematoma. Bleeding that occurs between the renal parenchyma and the renal capsule is termed a *subcapsular hematoma*. If the capsule is also torn, hemorrhage within the confines of Gerota's fascia is termed a *perinephric hematoma*. Rarely, hemorrhage may also extend beyond Gerota's fascia within the retroperitoneum.

Blunt injuries of the kidney occur either as a result of a direct blow to the flank or deceleration. With a direct blow, the kidney is crushed causing a laceration or lacerations of the renal parenchyma which results in subcapsular, intrarenal, or perinephric hematomas. With a deceleration injury, acute tension on the renal pedicle may produce a laceration of the renal vein or artery, an intimal tear in the vessel that generally results in secondary thrombosis, or rarely laceration of or avulsion of the ureteropelvic junction (UPJ). Penetrating injury generally results in direct injury of the renal parenchyma, the vascular pedicle, or the collecting system.

In patients with a preexisting renal abnormality, relatively minor trauma may cause disproportionate symptomatology that brings the patient to medical attention. Such underlying conditions include renal calculi, renal tumors, renal cystic disease, and some congenital conditions including UPJ obstruction and horseshoe kidney.

Classification

At present there is no universally accepted or uniformly applied classification of renal injuries. As such, comparison of data among various published series can be difficult or even misleading. For example, some investigators use the term *renal contusion* to denote any renal injury that results in hematuria even when the results of radiologic studies are normal. It is preferable, therefore, to use a functional classification in which injuries are grouped according to the severity of the injury and its therapeutic implications rather than classifying them by the use of descriptive terminology, the criteria of which are more subjective in nature. Renal injuries are therefore best classified as being minor, intermediate, or major. In addition, it is advisable to group renal injuries by their mechanism of injury, as this factor also has significant therapeutic implications.

Minor injuries are those that may be treated expectantly and rarely require surgical intervention. They are the most common form of renal injury, comprising 85% of injuries in most series. In patients suffering isolated renal injuries, minor injuries constitute an even higher percentage of the total number of injuries. In those suffering multisystem trauma, minor injuries still account for 75% of the total. The vast majority of minor renal injuries consist of small intrarenal hematomas and their associated renal lacerations, a complex that is often collectively referred to as *renal contusion* (Fig. 12.1). Other injuries that may be included in this group include small subcapsular (Fig. 12.2) or perinephric hematomas, small cortical lacerations, subsegmental renal infarcts, and rarely pyelosinus extravasation associated with blunt injury. In general, these injuries do not involve a break in the renal capsule.

Intermediate injuries constitute approximately 10% of the cases reported in most series. They are usually managed conservatively but may, on occasion, require surgical intervention, particularly if clinical deterioration develops. Injuries included in this category include major renal lacerations that extend beyond the renal capsule, with and without involvement of the renal collecting system. These lacerations, which when distracted are termed "fractures," may be sufficiently large to be visible radiographically or at the time of surgical exploration. Extensive perirenal hematomas are usually present and if the laceration involves the collecting system, they demonstrate extravasation of contrast material on radiologic examination (Fig. 12.3).

Vascular injuries involving the segmental renal vessels are usually included in this category. Lang has reported that traumatic occlusion of a segmental renal vessel is the most common vascular injury of the kidney following blunt renal trauma. Such occlusion results in segmental renal infarction. In the past, when this injury has been diagnosed, some authors have advocated either partial nephrectomy or attempted revascularization out of concern that it might result in the subsequent development of hypertension. Bertini et al. studied 24 such patients identified by angiography and found that in none of the 10 patients who were available for follow-up did sus-

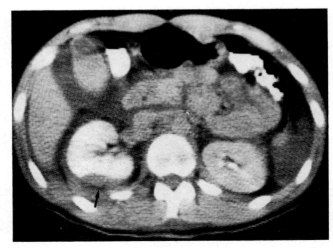

Figure 12.2. A small subcapsular hematoma is present on the posterior surface of the right kidney (*arrow*).

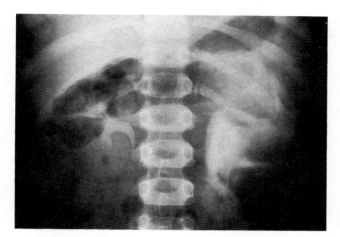

Figure 12.3. IVP demonstrates obvious contrast material extravasation from the left kidney. At surgery, a major laceration with involvement of the collecting system was present.

tained hypertension develop for periods ranging up to 5 years after injury.

Major renal injuries, which account for approximately 5% of all renal injuries, virtually always require surgical exploration either because of a threat to the viability of the kidney itself or because of life-threatening hemorrhage. In such situations, immediate surgical exploration and nephrectomy is frequently necessary. Major renal injuries include multiple renal lacerations (renal rupture) (Fig. 12.4) or injury of the renal pedicle including avulsion of one or more of the renal veins, thrombosis or laceration of the main renal artery, and avulsion of the ureteropelvic junction. With renal rupture or injury of the renal veins, large perinephric hematomas are the rule, and the tamponade effect of the renal fascia may be lost.

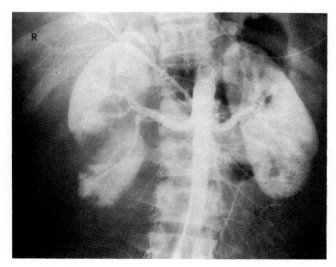

Figure 12.4. Abdominal aortogram demonstrates multiple right renal lacerations (renal rupture) in a patient who suffered a direct blow to the flank.

Isolated avulsion of the ureteropelvic junction (Fig. 12.5) is a rare injury that principally occurs in children when there is a deceleration injury of the renal pedicle. In such cases, the vascular supply of the renal pedicle remains intact; however, the UPJ is sheared from its attachment to the renal pelvis resulting in the formation of a urinoma that surrounds the kidney. While this injury may occur in adults, it is more common in children and adolescents, presumably owing to the great elasticity of the child's blood vessels which allows the renal vascular supply to remain intact at a force sufficient to cause disruption of the ureter. In addition, the smaller amount of retroperitoneal fat in children provides less cushioning of the kidney during sudden deceleration. Avulsion of the UPJ as a part of a total renal pedicle disruption is reported to be more common in adults than in children.

Radiologic Examination

Excretory Urography

Excretory urography is the basic screening study for the demonstration of a suspected renal injury. This study is readily available, inexpensive, and when normal, except after penetrating injury, obviates the need for further evaluation. The preference for the use of urography as a screening study for renal injuries is predicated on the fact that clinical signs of renal injury are relatively nonspecific and a large number of patients with hematuria must be screened in order to demonstrate those with significant renal injuries.

Urography for suspected renal injury should be performed by a thorough but quick routine designed to yield a maximum amount of information. The "one-shot IVP," so often referred to in the surgical literature, is unacceptable for the evaluation of a renal injury; such a study serves only to confirm the presence of functioning renal units but, when abnormal, gives the urologist insufficient information on which to base a decision about whether surgical management of a renal injury is necessary.

In general, urography for trauma should be performed with a higher dose of contrast material than might be used for an elective study in order to compensate for the large volume of fluid such patients generally receive. A contrast dose of 1–1.5 ml/lb generally yields a satisfactory study. Tomography is an extremely valuable adjunct in such patients and should be utilized whenever feasible. Needless to say, an adequate scout radiograph is absolutely mandatory.

Multiple series have shown that urography is very sensitive for the detection of blunt renal injury. Cass et al. (1986) found no patients with a renal injury greater than renal contusion among blunt trauma patients with normal urograms. Nicolaisen et al. reported similar findings in 214 patients in whom urograms were performed. Ber-

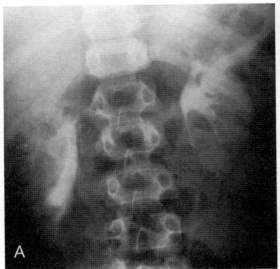
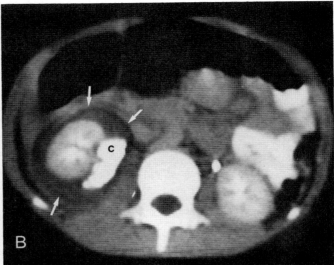

Figure 12.5. Isolated avulsion of the ureteropelvic junction in a child involved in a motor vehicle accident. **A,** IVP demonstrates extravasation of contrast material from the right kidney. No filling of the right ureter is seen. **B,** Computed tomography shows no evidence of a renal laceration. A large collection of extravasated contrast (c) as well as a perinephric urinoma (*arrows*) are present.

gren et al. reported there were no cases of renal pathology greater than contusion when the results of urography were reported as normal.

The sensitivity that urography displays as an indicator of blunt renal injury is unfortunately not the case in patients suffering penetrating injury. Wilson and Ziegler found renal injuries that required surgery in one-third of such patients whose urograms were thought to be normal. In Bergren's series, an alarming 75% of patients (9 of 12) whose urograms were thought to be normal had what the authors called serious renal pathology after penetrating injury. However, many of the urograms in this series were performed with a low dose of contrast material or were limited to a single exposure.

Most commonly the results of urography are normal in patients suffering from minor renal injuries. Urographic abnormalities indicative of renal injury include delayed opacification, incomplete visualization of the renal outlines, displacement of the kidney, poor or incomplete calyceal filling (Fig. 12.1), a diminished nephrogram that might be segmental, as well as nonvisualization of the affected kidney. These findings, however, are generally nonspecific and additional studies are generally required to define the specific renal injury that is present.

Some specific urographic findings may be present. A filling defect in the collecting system, in the setting of trauma, usually indicates the presence of clot. In some instances, a cleft in the renal parenchyma may be visualized indicating that there is a major renal laceration. Extravasation of contrast material (Fig. 12.3), when present, is generally an indication that a laceration extends into the renal collecting system.

In rare instances extravasation of contrast may be present in less significant injuries. Pyelosinus extravasation may be present from minor injuries or may be demonstrated in patients with preexisting renal calculi at the time of injury. In addition, patients with congenital renal anomalies such as horseshoe kidney or ureteropelvic junction obstruction may demonstrate pyelosinus extravasation when undergoing evaluation for suspected renal trauma. In such instances, computed tomography (CT) examination will demonstrate the extravasation but will not demonstrate a renal laceration. In most cases of benign extravasation following trauma, urography demonstrates some degree of caliectasis which suggests the presence of the preexisting condition. Extravasation of urine may also be found in major injuries when there is avulsion of the ureteropelvic junction.

The unilateral absence of excretion on urography (Fig. 12.6) suggests that a renal vascular injury is present. Stables studied 23 patients (20 following blunt trauma) who exhibited unilateral excretion on urography after abdominal injury and found that in 17 cases the cause for this finding was traumatic occlusion of the main renal artery. In only three patients was renal agenesis found to be responsible. Stables concluded that when such a finding is encountered in a patient who has suffered abdominal injury, a renal artery injury is the most likely etiology and immediate aortography should be undertaken. Cass and Luxenberg reported a series of 53 patients (47 after blunt trauma) in whom similar findings were present on urography. In their series, traumatic occlusion of the renal artery was present in 16 cases; the final diagnosis in the remaining patients were parenchymal laceration (12), renal rupture (12), renal contusion (8), branch arterial injury (1), and renal vein laceration (4).

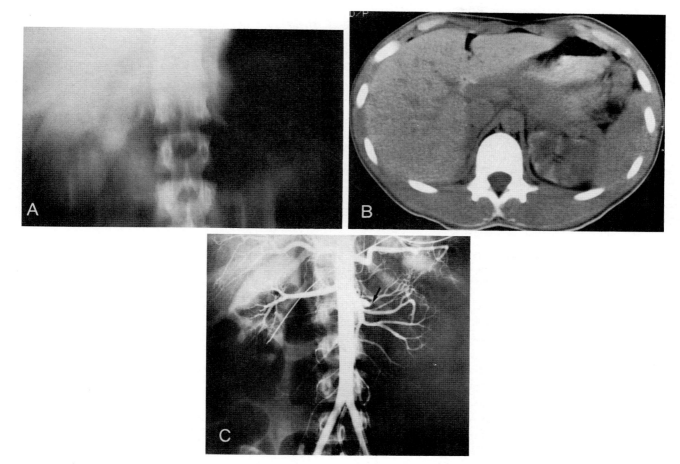

Figure 12.6.   Traumatic occlusion of the renal artery. **A,** IVP demonstrates no visible excretion from the left kidney. **B,** Computed tomography shows only a rim of enhancement of the outer cortex of the left kidney secondary to intact left renal capsular vessels. The majority of the renal parenchyma shows no contrast enhancement. **C,** Abdominal aortogram shows the characteristically tapered appearance of traumatic main renal artery occlusion (*arrow*).

Computed Tomography

The specific nature of an injury detected on urography can often be determined by CT. In 1977, Schaner et al. documented the ability of CT to display subcapsular and perinephric hematomas of the kidney after percutaneous renal biopsy. Not only was the presence of these injuries demonstrated by this study, but their location within the retroperitoneum was accurately defined. This was an important demonstration in that the previously utilized imaging studies, urography and angiography, are frequently "blind" to fluid collections located either directly anterior or directly posterior to the kidney. In separate reports, Federle et al. (1981) and Sandler (1981) documented the utility of CT in patients suffering from external injury of the kidney. It is now well established that CT is the imaging study of choice to define the nature and extent of suspected renal injuries.

Computed tomography for the detection of renal injuries should be performed in 10-mm intervals using 10-mm collimation. A scan time designed to minimize respiratory motion is desirable. In general, precontrast scans yield too little additional information to be of routine value. If contrast material has been administered more than 1 hour prior to the start of the study (i.e., for a preceding urogram), an additional bolus of contrast material should be utilized. Lang et al. (1985) have advocated the routine use of dynamic CT for the evaluation of renal injuries. With this technique, 6–10 CT sections are acquired in rapid sequence following the administration of a bolus of contrast material. The authors claim an increased sensitivity with this procedure for the detection of vascular injuries when compared with conventional CT.

The accuracy of CT staging of renal injuries has been compared with other imaging studies in several retrospective series. Cass and Vieira report that CT gave determinate diagnoses in 22 cases of suspected severe renal injuries, while urographic findings were indeterminate in 82% of the cases. Bretan et al. studied 85 patients with renal injuries using CT and a variety of other imaging techniques. Blunt trauma accounted for 87% of their

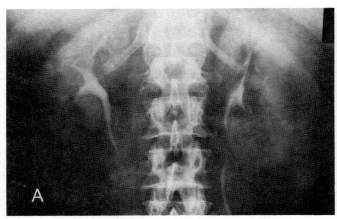

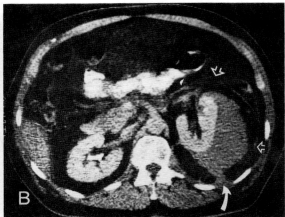

Figure 12.7. Subcapsular hematoma. **A,** IVP shows compression of the calyces of the left kidney and straightening of the lateral renal border. **B,** Computed tomography shows the renal margin to be indented by a large subcapsular hematoma. A small area of extension to the perinephric space is present (*curved arrow*). Gerota's fascia can also be identified (*open arrows*) confirming the subcapsular location of the hematoma.

cases while the remainder were secondary to penetrating injury. In 33 patients who subsequently underwent laparotomy, the CT diagnoses were confirmed; in contrast, the most common finding on urography, diminished opacification, was found to bear no relationship to the severity of the injury found at surgery. In the same series, angiography was found to have appreciably understaged the severity of the injury in one of five patients in whom this procedure was employed. In addition, CT has been found to have a great impact on the management of renal injuries; Erturk et al. reported that early CT evaluation allowed confident nonoperative management in 17 of 22 patients with renal injuries. Federle et al. (1987) have reported equally favorable results utilizing CT in patients suffering penetrating renal injuries.

The excellent results of these studies and others have led some authorities to advocate the use of CT as a screening method to detect renal injuries. These authors correctly suggest that CT is the only method by which multiple organ systems may be simultaneously evaluated and that CT has a greater sensitivity and specificity than other studies in detecting renal injuries. Most authorities, however, feel that CT screening for renal injuries is not cost effective and that urography should continue to be used as the principle screening method as the incidence of significant renal injuries is so low.

On CT, subcapsular hematomas appear as rounded or elliptical areas of decreased attenuation located between the renal cortex and the renal capsule (Fig. 12.7). Such hematomas indent the renal margins because of their subcapsular location. Intrarenal hematomas (Figs. 12.8 and 12.9) are seen as rounded or ovoid poorly margin-

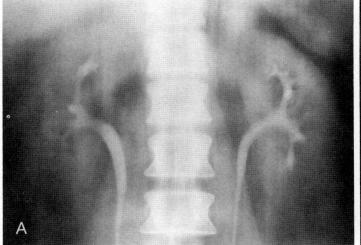

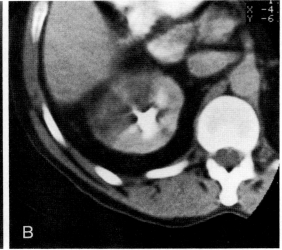

Figure 12.8. Intrarenal hematoma. **A,** IVP shows minimal indistinctness of the right renal outline. **B,** On CT, a poorly marginated area of decreased attenuation in the anterolateral aspect of the right kidney is present.

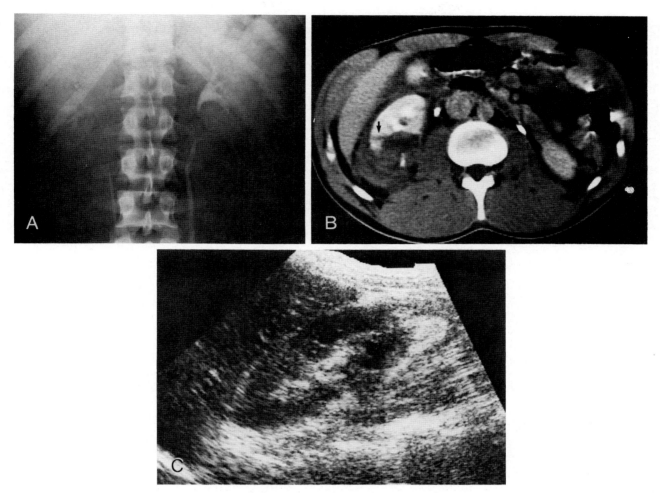

Figure 12.9. Intrarenal hematoma. **A,** IVP shows nonspecific findings including an indistinct right renal outline and poor calyceal filling. **B,** On CT, a large area of decreased density is present in the inferior portion of the right kidney. A small laceration extending into the hematoma is visualized (*arrow*). A small perinephric hematoma is present as well. **C,** Longitudinal ultrasound shows decreased echogenicity in the area of the hematoma and slight anterior displacement of the lower pole of the right kidney.

ated areas of decreased attenuation within the renal parenchyma; in some cases the small intrarenal lacerations with which they are associated may be visualized extending into the hematoma itself. Perinephric hematomas are located between the renal capsule and Gerota's fascia and are usually associated with an intrarenal hematoma (Fig. 12.10). Perinephric hematomas may be quite large and may extend inferiorly into the true pelvis following the cone of renal fascia, may displace the kidney anteriorly, or occasionally may be quite localized and simulate a subcapsular collection.

The attenuation coefficient of these hematomas depends on their age, with acute hematomas having a higher attenuation value than unenhanced renal parenchyma. With time, their attenuation value decreases due to liquification of the clot. In addition, the measured attenuation value of these perinephric hematomas may be lower than expected, reflecting their tendency to infiltrate the nor-

mal perinephric fat. This tendency also may produce a streaked or bubbled appearance in the retroperitoneum which should not be confused with abscess.

Major lacerations can be diagnosed on CT when a hematoma-filled cleft that extends through the renal capsule is visualized in the renal parenchyma. If the laceration extends into the renal collecting system, extravasation of opacified urine into the perinephric space will also be present. If the lacerated segment has become devitalized, this portion of the kidney will not enhance following contrast administration. Since this segment is surrounded by hematoma and does not enhance, it may be difficult to appreciate as a separate fragment.

Segmental or cortical infarcts are the most common vascular injury following blunt trauma. On CT, infarcts appear as sharply demarcated wedge-shaped areas of diminished or absent contrast enhancement that extend to the renal cortex (Fig. 12.11). Most commonly, they are

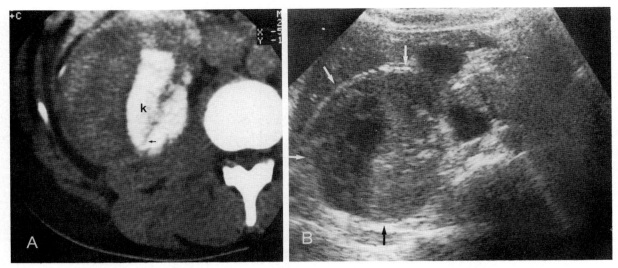

Figure 12.10. Perinephric hematoma. **A,** Computed tomography shows a large perinephric hematoma filling Gerota's fascia. The lateral margin of the right kidney (k) is compressed, thereby simulating a subcapsular collection. A small renal laceration is also present (*arrow*). **B,** Transverse sonogram also shows the large perinephric collection (*arrow*).

unassociated with a perinephric hematoma, thereby helping to distinguish them from intrarenal hematomas. The sensitivity of CT for the detection of such injuries can be enhanced with the use of dynamic scanning. Indeed, the ability of CT to reliably distinguish these injuries from hematomas is dependent on the contrast enhancement provided by the bolus of contrast material. If there has been too long an interval between the contrast administration and the CT study, their sharply marginated appearance will be lost because of collateral circulation.

In patients with isolated avulsion of the ureteropelvic junction, CT demonstrates contrast extravasation into a urinoma that collects predominantly in the medial perinephric space (Fig. 12.5). There will be no associated

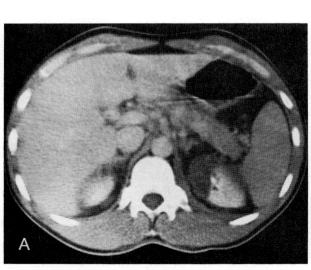

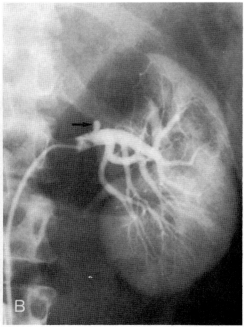

Figure 12.11. Segmental infarct. **A,** Computed tomography demonstrates a sharply marginated area of absent contrast enhancement in the left kidney. There is no associated perinephric hematoma. **B,** Selective left renal angiogram shows an amputated upper segmental artery (*arrow*). (From Sandler CM, Toombs BD: Computed tomographic evaluation of blunt renal injuries. *Radiology* 141:461, 1981.)

perinephric hematoma unless a coexisting parenchymal laceration is present. It is usually possible to identify the unopacified ureter within the area of contrast extravasation which confirms that the ureter has been completely avulsed.

Thrombosis of the main renal artery results in complete absence of contrast enhancement when studied shortly after injury. In some cases, and especially in those instances where the diagnosis of pedicle injury is delayed, a rim of enhancement in the outer renal cortex may be present owing to circulation from capsular and collateral vessels (Fig. 12.6). Similar findings are frequently present in patients with nontraumatic renal infarction. In the majority of patients with this injury, there will be no evidence of a perinephric or subcapsular hematoma unless this injury has been caused by a penetrating wound or is associated with injury of another organ. Retrograde opacification of the renal vein of the affected kidney has been reported as a secondary sign of this injury, especially if an infusion technique for contrast enhancement is utilized. While the CT appearance of renal artery thrombosis is characteristic, renal angiography is usually still required if a revascularization procedure is to be considered. The period of warm ischemia that can be tolerated by the kidney is controversial; many authorities feel that renal revascularization should not be attempted if a period of longer than 8–12 hours has elapsed since the original injury.

Angiography

The use of angiography in the evaluation of renal injuries has significantly declined since the advent of CT. However, angiography continues to be the primary method by which suspected renal vascular injuries are evaluated. In addition, in patients in whom angiography is required for another purpose (i.e., the evaluation of a suspected injury of the thoracic aorta), it may be utilized as a primary imaging technique in the evaluation of suspected renal injuries.

Angiographic assessment of renal injuries may be carried out by a variety of techniques. Film aortography or intraarterial digital subtraction aortography is sufficient to diagnose injury of the main renal artery; however, for precise demonstration of intrarenal vascular injuries, selective renal angiography is required.

Angiography is the only method capable of identifying certain traumatic lesions such as AV fistulae and pseudoaneurysms, and provides definitive diagnosis of traumatic arterial thrombosis and infarcts. The extent of the collateral vascular supply to the injured parenchyma can be directly evaluated. In addition to diagnosis, angiography provides a method by which traumatic renal hemorrhage (Fig. 12.12) can be directly diagnosed and treated through transcatheter embolization. Lang has suggested that angiography is an excellent method by which parenchymal viability, prior to surgery, can be assessed through an analysis of the vascular nephrogram.

The disadvantages and limitations of angiography must be recognized. The technique is invasive, time-consuming, and expensive and carries far greater risk of complications than do the noninvasive techniques. Some injuries, particularly perinephric hematomas, either anterior or posterior to the kidney, may be grossly underestimated. Thus, angiographic evaluation of renal injuries is best suited to those situations in which vascular injury is suspected (i.e., a nonvisualized kidney on urography),

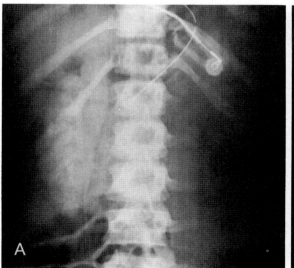
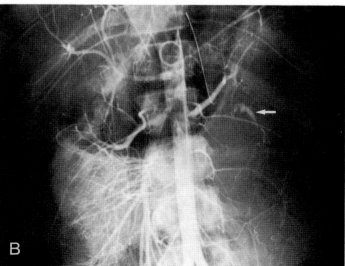

Figure 12.12. Traumatic renal hemorrhage. **A,** IVP shows nonvisualization of the left kidney in this child involved in an auto-pedestrian accident. **B,** On angiography, the left renal artery is intact, however, active bleeding from a segmental artery (*arrow*) is demonstrated.

the evaluation of suspected late complications of renal injury, and those patients in whom transcatheter therapy of renal injury may be necessary.

Angiographic findings in minor renal injuries include a slowing of arterial flow and evidence of cortical ischemia; these changes produce a striated appearance to the angiographic nephrogram. Intrarenal hematomas demonstrate displacement of the interlobar arteries and a diminished vascular nephrogram. Perirenal hematomas show displacement of the capsular arteries and the pelvic branch vessels. With subcapsular hematomas there is indentation of the renal margin similar to that seen on urography.

Major renal lacerations (Fig. 12.13) demonstrate a well-defined cleft in the nephrogram on angiographic examination. The degree of displacement of the lacerated segment and its viability can be assessed by an analysis of the nephrogram at the fracture margins. Multiple lacerations are a feature of renal rupture (Fig. 12.4).

Traumatic arteriovenous fistulae almost always result from penetrating renal injury. The vast majority occur after percutaneous renal biopsy, are not hemodynamically significant, and close spontaneously. Clinically, symptomatic lesions may present with hypertension, evidence of left heart failure, and there may be an audible bruit on physical examination. On angiography, opacification of the large draining veins is visible during the arterial phase of the study. The draining vein is usually saccular in appearance; with hemodynamically significant lesions, there may be decreased nephrographic staining and evidence of renal ischemia.

Traumatic arterial pseudoaneurysms are rare injuries that also almost always occur after penetrating trauma. While the diagnosis may be suspected by CT, definitive diagnosis always requires angiography.

Segmental renal infarcts are demonstrated as wedge-shaped areas of absent vascular perfusion. The occluded artery responsible for the infarct can usually be identified by its sharply cutoff appearance (Figs. 12.11 and 12.13). Collateral vascular supply through capsular branch vessels may also be identified angiographically.

Occlusion of the main renal artery usually occurs in its proximal one-third and has one sharply defined oblique edge (Fig. 12.6), the point where the intimal injury has occurred; if the occlusion is not acute, collateral supply to the kidney may be visualized on aortography. In kidneys supplied by more than one renal artery, supply through the unaffected vessels may prevent total renal infarction from occurring.

Radionuclide Scanning

Radionuclide scanning of the kidneys following trauma has been used to detect suspected renal injury as an alternative to urography. Such studies may be performed with either ^{99m}Tc-DTPA or ^{99m}Tc-glucoheptonate. For the detection of renal injury, perfusion studies should be acquired by computer for the first 1 minute followed by immediate static and a series of delayed static images. Views acquired with a pinhole collimator give the highest spatial resolution and are very helpful in detecting major renal lacerations.

One advantage of radionuclide scanning is the ability to acquire images even in relatively uncooperative patients and children. Radionuclide studies are also of value in patients with known sensitivity to contrast material. It should not be used in patients with a nonvisualized kidney on urography as this study cannot differentiate a congenitally absent kidney from renal artery thrombosis.

Analysis of the radionuclide perfusion curve in patients with renal injuries demonstrate a decrease in the kidney peak to plateau ratio and a delay in the peak of the activity in the kidney when the renal curve is normalized to that of the aorta. Static imaging reveals diminished uptake and excretion of the radiopharmaceutical in the affected kidney.

Studies reported in the literature have suggested that radionuclide imaging has a higher sensitivity than does urography for the detection of renal injuries. As with urography, the specificity of an abnormal radionuclide study is low.

Renal lacerations may be visualized as photon-deficient areas in the renal parenchyma. A laceration that

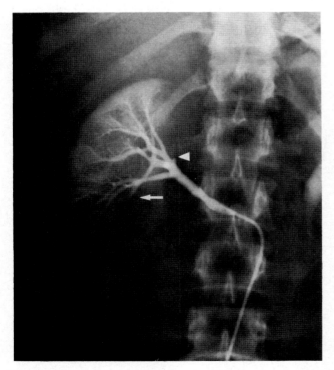

Figure 12.13.   Selective right renal angiogram demonstrates a major laceration involving the mid portion of the kidney. The lower pole is completely devitalized with traumatic occlusion of the lower pole segmental artery (*arrow*). There is also a segmental infarct involving the upper pole (*arrowhead*).

extends into the collecting system may demonstrate an area of tracer activity outside the kidney indicating extravasation of urine. Renal infarcts may be diagnosed as photon-deficient areas in the renal parenchyma, but differentiation of this injury from intrarenal hematomas is difficult. Large perinephric hematomas may be visualized as photopenic defects adjacent to the kidney. Urinomas are also present as photopenic areas, however, on delayed images, such areas accumulate activity indicating their uriniferous nature.

Occlusion of the renal artery is suggested by the absence of perfusion to one kidney. In such cases, a photopenic defect may be present in the renal fossa. Large perinephric hematomas that displace the kidney anteriorly may simulate this finding; in this instance an anterior image of the abdomen usually demonstrates the displaced kidney.

URETERAL INJURIES

Ureteral Injuries Secondary to External Violence

Aside from disruption of the ureteropelvic junction, which has been discussed in Renal Injuries, above, injuries of the ureter secondary to external violence virtually always occur secondary to penetrating trauma. As such, nearly all ureteral injuries are associated with injuries of other organs including the small bowel, liver, spleen, or a major blood vessel. Ureteral injuries include either partial or complete laceration and ureteral contusion, an injury of the ureter that produces ureteral wall damage, but not a frank laceration. Ureteral contusion is generally considered to result from the blast effect of the missile on the ureter (Fig. 12.14). A significant percentage of patients with ureteral injuries do not have hematuria.

The diagnosis of ureteral injury may be established by urography when extravasation of contrast material is present. The accuracy of urography in establishing this diagnosis is uncertain since most of the published series are small, and because of the nature of the associated injuries, many of the patients are taken to surgery prior to the performance of this study. Steers et al. report that the urogram was diagnostic of the injury in seven of eight patients with penetrating ureteral injury in whom this study was performed; Spirnak et al. report that the urogram was falsely normal in the one patient in the series in whom it was performed. In cases when radiologic studies are not performed prior to surgical exploration, the diagnosis may be established with the aid of intraoperative vital dyes that usually demonstrate the point of injury.

Iatrogenic Ureteral Injury

Surgical injury of the ureter may result from a variety of abdominal, pelvic, urological, and gynecologic procedures. The risk of surgical injury varies with the type of

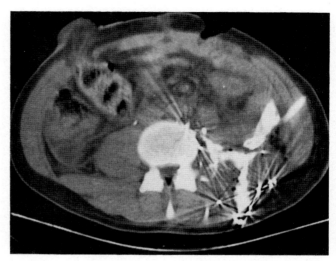

Figure 12.14.   Ureteral contusion with subsequent necrosis. Computed tomography demonstrates frank contrast material extravasation from the left ureter in a patient who suffered a shotgun wound of the left flank. No laceration had been identified at the time of exploratory surgery, however, after several days urine was noted emanating from a surgically placed Penrose drain prompting CT investigation.

surgery that is performed, with the highest risk occurring as a consequence of gynecologic procedures. With radical hysterectomy, ureteral injury may occur in as many as 10–30% of patients. The reported incidence of ureteral injury as a complication of abdominal hysterectomy varies between 1.5 and 2.5%, and it may occur less commonly during other pelvic operations including vaginal hysterectomy and cesarean section.

In these procedures, ureteral injury generally occurs when there is inadvertent ligation of the ureter. With radical hysterectomy, injury may occur because of ureteral ligation or when the blood supply of the distal ureters is stripped during dissection of periureteral lymphatics. Patients with this complication have either ureteral necrosis and the formation of a urinoma, or at a later stage the development of a long ureteral stricture.

Ureteral injury may complicate a number of urologic procedures including retrograde pyelography, ureteroscopy, ureteral stone basketing (Fig. 12.15), and ureterolithotomy. In most of these cases, the injury is a result of ureteral perforation. Ligation of the ureter may also occur during vesicourethral suspension.

Injury of the ureter may complicate other surgical procedures including abdominoperitoneal resection, enterolysis, resection of abdominal aortic aneurysm, and lumbar laminectomy. In such cases, the injuries consist of ureteral perforation, transection, ligation, or a crush injury associated with inadvertent clamping of the ureter.

Bilateral ureteral injuries are generally recognized in the immediate postoperative period because of anuria. Unilateral injury may be recognized at the time of the

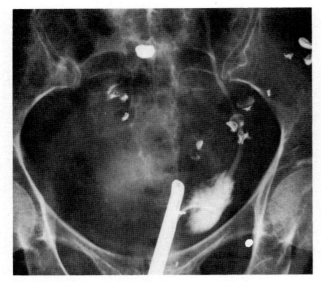

Figure 12.15. Retrograde pyelogram showing extravasation of contrast material following a traumatic ureteral stone basketing procedure.

original surgery, but more commonly it is not recognized until 10–30 days after surgery. Fever and ipsilateral flank pain are the most common symptoms. A significant number of cases go unrecognized until the development of a ureterovaginal (Fig. 12.16) or ureterocutaneous fistula. Dowling et al. reported this presentation in 9 of 23 patients (39%) in whom there was delayed recognition of

the ureteral injury. In all cases, the diagnosis of ureteral injury was established by urography.

Interventional uroradiologic procedures play an important role in the management of iatrogenic ureteral injury. Harshman et al. reported three patients with ureteral injury following gynecologic surgery who were successfully treated with percutaneous nephrostomy drainage alone. They postulated that the ureteral injury in these cases was secondary to suture ligation or entrapment of the ureter and that with time, there was resorption of the suture material allowing resolution of the ureteral obstruction. In Dowling et al.'s series, 11 of 15 ureteral injuries, including 6 of 7 cases that were believed to have resulted from ureteral ligation, were successfully treated with either percutaneous nephrostomy alone or with nephrostomy combined with antegrade ureteral stenting. Lang (1985) reported successful management of 15 ureteral fistulas with a combination of nephrostomy and stent placement for periods ranging between 30 and 45 days.

BLADDER INJURIES

Injury of the bladder may occur as a result of blunt, penetrating, or iatrogenic trauma. The susceptibility of the bladder to injury varies with its degree of filling at the time of the accident; a collapsed or nearly empty bladder is much less vulnerable to injury than is a distended organ.

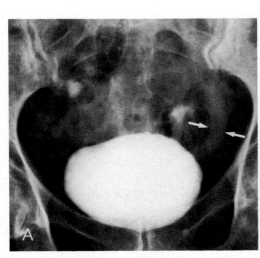

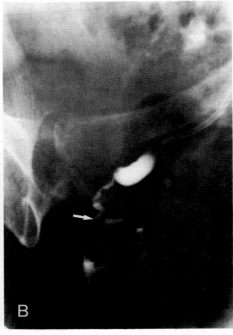

Figure 12.16. Iatrogenic ureteral ligation. **A,** Delayed film from an IVP shows a faintly opacified dilated distal left ureter (*arrow*) in a patient who complained of incontinence following vaginal hysterectomy. **B,** Contrast study made after advancing an end-hole nephrostomy catheter down the ureter demonstrates complete occlusion of the distal ureter and ureterovaginal fistula.

Clinical Features

Signs of bladder injury are relatively nonspecific. Suprapubic tenderness is usually present, however, the etiology of this discomfort may be manifold. Hematuria inevitably accompanies bladder rupture; in some of the reported series, gross hematuria was present in 95% of the cases of bladder rupture. The urge to void may be absent or normal; in some forms of bladder rupture the organ may still act as a reservoir and thus a normal urge to void may be present.

Radiologic Examination

Cystography is the examination of choice by which the presence of a bladder rupture is diagnosed. Although it is generally preferable to perform such an examination with fluoroscopic equipment, the procedure may be performed with fixed radiographic or even portable equipment when the clinical situation demands this be done. The method by which cystography is performed has been discussed in Chapter 3; however, some modification of the procedure may be necessary in the trauma patient. A minimum of 300 ml of diluted (30%) contrast material must be utilized in order that adequate bladder distention is achieved. The use of 14 × 17-inch films that cover the upper abdomen facilitates the diagnosis of intraperitoneal bladder rupture and therefore should be utilized for at least one of the radiographs. When fluoroscopic equipment is not used, an initial radiograph after instillation of approximately 100 ml of contrast material can be used to check for gross extravasation; if none is present, the remainder of the contrast material is then infused. The postdrainage radiograph is an essential component of the cystogram made for trauma and should not be omitted; the diagnosis of bladder rupture may be established by this film only in approximately 10% of the cases (Fig. 12.17).

The accuracy of cystography for the diagnosis of bladder injury varies from 85 to 100% in the reported series. Carroll and McAninch report, however, that the accuracy of cystography would have fallen from 100 to 79% in their series had careful technique not been followed. A false-negative cystogram may occur in patients who have suffered penetrating bladder injury, especially when caused by small caliber bullets. In such cases it is assumed that the bladder rent seals with hematoma or by the surrounding mesentery and thus results in a false-negative study.

While cystography is highly accurate in the diagnosis of bladder injury, the cystographic phase of the excretory urogram cannot be relied on to exclude bladder injury (Fig. 12.18). In the series reported by Carroll and McAninch (1983), cystographically verified bladder injuries were found in only 16% of the cases by urography. Computed tomography, while very accurate in the diagnosis of renal injury, cannot be substituted for cystography in patients with suspected bladder injury. In a prospective study, Mee et al. found conventional cystography superior to contrast enhanced CT for the diagnosis of bladder rupture.

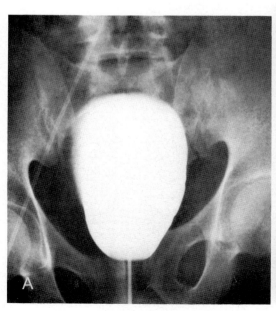
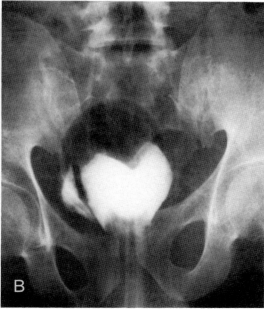

Figure 12.17.   A, Filled film from a cystogram demonstrates extrinsic compression of the right side of the bladder, but no evidence of extravasation. Catheter in right femoral artery is from an arteriogram performed just prior to the cystogram. **B,** Postdrainage film shows simple extraperitoneal rupture (Type 4a).

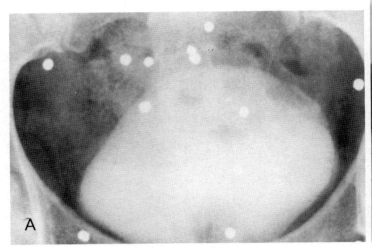

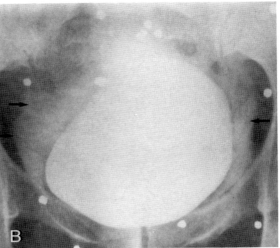

Figure 12.18.   **A,** Cystographic phase of an IVP in a patient suffering a gunshot wound of the pelvis shows no evidence of contrast extravasation. **B,** Cystogram performed a few minutes later shows obvious extravasation (*arrows*) indicating extraperitoneal bladder injury.

Bladder Injury in Blunt Pelvic Trauma

Major bladder injury occurs in approximately 10% of patients suffering a pelvic fracture. Injury of the bladder following blunt trauma may be classified as follows.

Type 1   Bladder contusion
Type 2   Intraperitoneal rupture
Type 3   Interstitial bladder injury
Type 4   Extraperitoneal rupture
    a   Simple
    b   Complex
Type 5   Combined bladder injury

Bladder contusion (Type 1) is an incomplete tear of the bladder mucosa following blunt injury. The injury results in an ecchymosis in a localized segment of the bladder wall. The results of cystography are normal. The diagnosis is usually established by exclusion in patients who have hematuria following pelvic trauma for which no other cause can be found. Cystoscopy is rarely performed for confirmation. Bladder contusion may be present in patients in whom extrinsic compression of the bladder (the so-called teardrop bladder) by a pelvic hematoma or hematomas is found.

Bladder contusion is generally regarded as the most common form of bladder trauma, however, it is not considered a major bladder injury.

Intraperitoneal bladder rupture (Type 2) accounts for approximately one-third of major bladder injuries. It occurs when there is a sudden rise in intravesicle pressure as a result of a blow to the lower abdomen in patients who have a distended bladder. This injury results in rupture of the weakest portion of the bladder wall, the dome, where the bladder is in contact with the peritoneal surface. Intraperitoneal rupture commonly occurs as a seat-belt or steering wheel injury. Approximately 25% of the cases occur in patients without a pelvic fracture. On cystography, contrast material is seen in the paracolic gutters and outlining the abdominal viscera and loops of small bowel (Fig. 12.19).

Interstitial bladder injury (Type 3) occurs as a result of an incomplete perforation of the serosal surface of the

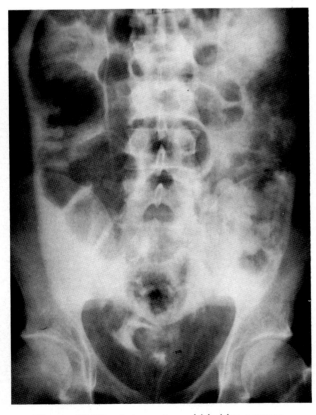

Figure 12.19.   Intraperitoneal bladder rupture.

bladder. On cystography, a mural defect in the bladder wall representing the site of injury is present, however, there is no extravasation of contrast material. This injury is rare but should be considered a major injury.

Extraperitoneal bladder rupture (Type 4) is associated with one or more fractures of the pubic rami or diastasis of the symphysis pubis in virtually every case. Classically, the injury occurs when there is a laceration of the extraperitoneal portion of the bladder wall by a bone spicule associated with the fracture. However, recent data have shown that cystograms in such patients often show the site of extravasation to be far removed from the site of pelvic fracture, suggesting that this injury can be caused by other mechanisms. One such explanation is that bladder injury results when stress is applied to the hypogastric wings or to the puboprostatic ligaments causing the bladder wall to tear. In still other cases, the injury may occur by a mechanism analogous to the intraperitoneal rupture.

In *simple extraperitoneal rupture*, contrast material extravasation on cystography is limited to the pelvic extraperitoneal space (Fig. 12.17B). With *complex extraperitoneal rupture*, the contrast extravasation extends beyond the perivesicle space to the thigh, the scrotum, the penis, or the perineum (Fig. 12.20). Complex extravasation implies that a disruption in the fascial boundaries of the pelvis has occurred as a result of the injury. Thus, extravasation into the perineum may be present with a bladder injury alone; the presence of such extravasation should not be mistaken as evidence of a coexisting urethral injury.

Combined bladder injury (Type 5) results in both intraperitoneal and extraperitoneal bladder rupture (Fig. 12.21). In Palmer et al.'s series, this injury occurred in approximately 0.5% of patients with pelvic fracture and represents approximately 5% of all major bladder injuries. On cystography both types of extravasation may be demonstrated, however, in some cases only one component is shown.

External Penetrating Bladder Injury

Penetrating injury of the bladder may occur as a result of a bullet wound or as a result of impalement of the bladder by various objects. Penetrating bladder injury may result in intraperitoneal rupture, extraperitoneal rupture, or combined bladder injury.

The diagnosis is usually suggested by cystography and confirmed at exploration; as in renal injuries the high association of injury to other viscera mandates surgical exploration in the majority of cases. Vascular injuries are especially commonly associated with bladder injuries following gunshot wounds; with knife wounds of the bladder there is a high incidence of associated colon injury.

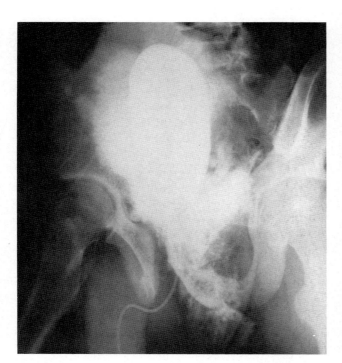

Figure 12.20. Complex extraperitoneal bladder rupture (Type 4b). Extravasated contrast material extends outside the confines of the pelvis into the perineum.

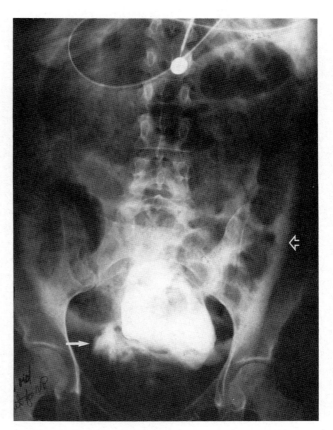

Figure 12.21. Combined bladder injury. The extraperitoneal component (*arrow*) and the intraperitoneal component (*open arrows*) are both demonstrated.

Iatrogenic and Obstetric Bladder Injury

Injury of the bladder may occur in virtually any type of obstetric, gynecologic, urologic, or pelvic surgery, or as the result of migration of surgically placed devices.

Obstetric bladder injury may result from laceration of the bladder during cesarean birth, injury secondary to trauma from obstetric forceps, or from pressure necrosis of the bladder wall during labor. Vesicouterine fistula is a rare, delayed complication of cesarean section. Such patients may present with menouria (Youseff's syndrome).

Injury to the bladder has been reported during dilatation and curettage of the uterus, laparoscopy, or during hysterectomy. Transurethral urologic procedures, especially transurethral biopsy of bladder tumors, not uncommonly result in bladder injury. Surgically placed instruments that may damage the bladder include intrauterine contraceptive devices, Foley catheters, orthopedic hip nails, Penrose drains, and ventriculoperitoneal shunt catheters.

Spontaneous Bladder Injury

Spontaneous bladder rupture refers to the occurrence of a bladder injury without known antecedent trauma. In most cases, an underlying pathologic condition of the bladder is thought to be responsible. Such conditions include bladder tumors, inflammatory conditions of the bladder, lesions that infiltrate the bladder from outside its walls, and lesions resulting in bladder outlet obstruction.

The term *idiopathic bladder rupture* is used to refer to the occurrence of bladder rupture when there is no known antecedent trauma and no underlying or adjacent bladder pathology. Most of these cases occur in alcoholics and it is postulated that the bladder injury results from relatively minor external trauma that the patient is unable to recall.

INJURY OF THE MALE URETHRA

Urethral Injury in Pelvic Fracture

Clinical Features

Urethral injury in pelvic fracture is a devastating injury because it may be associated with major complications including bulbomembranous urethral stricture, impotence, and urinary incontinence. It is generally agreed that the more severe the injury to the pelvic ring the more severe is the urethral injury. However, severe urethral injury may occur with relatively minor pelvic bone fracture, and posterior urethral rupture has been reported without pelvic fracture. Conversely, severe pelvic fracture may result in relatively minor urethral injury. Patients with urethral injury in pelvic fracture commonly have multisystem injuries. Mortality rates in these patients are reported as 9–33%. The reported incidence of urethral injury in pelvic fracture is 4–17%. The average age is approximately 30 years, but ranges from 4 to 80 years.

The single most important clinical sign of urethral injury is blood at the external meatus. There may be a high-riding prostate on rectal examination, but in young male patients it is often difficult to distinguish the prostate from a firm hematoma. The "pie in the sky" or inverted teardrop bladder on excretory urography is a good indication of urethral rupture. Urethral catheterization is condemned in suspected urethral injury, although the inability to pass a urethral catheter is considered evidence of urethral rupture. No attempt should be made to pass a catheter until the urethral injury is assessed by dynamic retrograde urethrography.

Mechanism of Injury and Classification

The urogenital diaphragm is attached to the medial surface of the inferior pubic rami. The prostate is attached to the pubis by the puboprostatic ligaments. Pubic ramus fracture with separation or displacement of the symphysis pubis may result in disruption of the urogenital diaphragm and puboprostatic ligaments causing proximal displacement of the prostate gland.

The classically described urethral injury is separation of the urethra at the prostatomembranous junction produced by a shearing effect at the time of injury. Less severe injury may result in a urethral tear, producing a hole in the urethra at this site. Although membranous urethral tear is still described in the literature as the classic injury, retrograde urethrography has shown that the most common injury occurs at the proximal bulbous urethra, below the urogenital diaphragm. This is consistent with the known anatomy of the region. The apex of the prostate intermingles with fibers of the external sphincter at the urogenital diaphragm, but it is not firmly fixed. When trauma occurs, the prostate readily separates and moves proximally, taking with it the prostatic and membranous urethras. The membranous urethra has the support of the urogenital diaphragm. The proximal bulbous urethra has no significant support—only fat and loose connective tissue. Consequently, in urethral rupture the prostate, the prostatic urethra, and the membranous urethra move proximally taking with them the unsupported proximal bulbous urethra where the urethral rupture most commonly occurs.

Dynamic retrograde urethrography using the Foley catheter method is performed. In suspected urethral injury, the film is exposed during injection of 10–20 ml of contrast medium. Too much contrast medium may produce a confusing radiograph with obliteration of landmarks (Fig. 12.22).

The radiologic classification of urethral injury is as follows (Fig. 12.23).

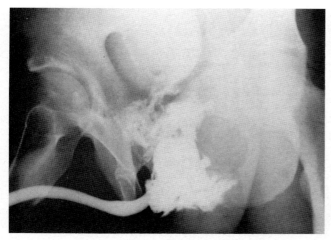

Figure 12.22. Dynamic retrograde urethrogram in a patient with urethral meatal blood following pelvic fracture. The radiograph is confusing. Too much contrast media has been injected obliterating the urethral landmarks and the site of urethral injury. Contrast medium has extravasated from the urethra into the perineum, but some contrast has entered the bladder indicating partial rupture. The excess contrast medium makes it difficult to decide whether this is a partial Type II or III injury. However contrast medium in the perineum favors Type III.

- Type I   The urethra remains intact but may be stretched and narrowed by proximal displacement of the prostate and the accumulation of hematoma elevating the bladder high in the pelvis. The urethra is compressed and may be contused (Fig. 12.24).
- Type II   The urethra is ruptured at the prostatomembranous junction above the urogenital diaphragm. This is the erroneously described classic injury. Retrograde injection of contrast medium shows extravasation of contrast medium into the true pelvis above the urogenital diaphragm. No contrast medium extravasates into the perineum (Fig. 12.25).
- Type III The prostate is dislocated proximally. The urogenital diaphragm is disrupted and the proximal displacement of the prostatomembranous urethra pulls the bulbous urethra proximally. The tear in the urethra occurs below the urogenital diaphragm. Retrograde injection of contrast medium shows extravasation into the perineum and often into the scrotum which may outline the testicle (Fig. 12.26).

Both the Type II and Type III urethral injuries may be partial or complete. In partial Type II, the hole in the urethra is above the urogenital diaphragm. Extravasation occurs into the true pelvis, however, some contrast medium will usually pass into the bladder. In partial Type III urethral injury, the hole in the urethra is below the uro-

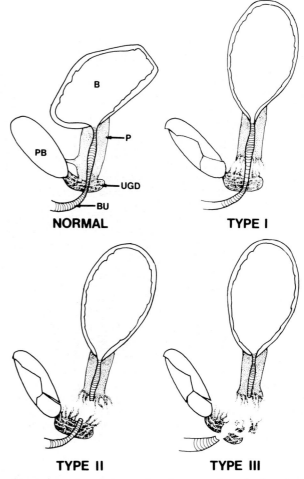

Figure 12.23. Radiologic classification of urethral injury in pelvic fractures. The diagrams describe the types of injury. Type III is the most common.

genital diaphragm and extravasation is into the perineum with some contrast passing into the bladder. Partial rupture is reported in between 27 and 52% of the cases.

Clinical Management

Two schools of thought have existed for many years. *Primary repair* of the urethral injury involves surgical intervention as soon as possible after the injury. The injury is approached suprapubically. The hematoma is evacuated and interlocking urethral sounds are used to approximate the torn ends of the urethra.

Delayed repair involves only the insertion of a suprapubic catheter for drainage without any attempt at urethral repair. The suprapubic catheter is left in place for approximately 3 months, after which the urethra is repaired by one- or two-stage urethroplasty. There has recently been a shift of emphasis toward delayed repair due to the decrease in the incidence of impotence and incontinence by using the delayed repair method. Most patients with urethral injury in pelvic fracture are young

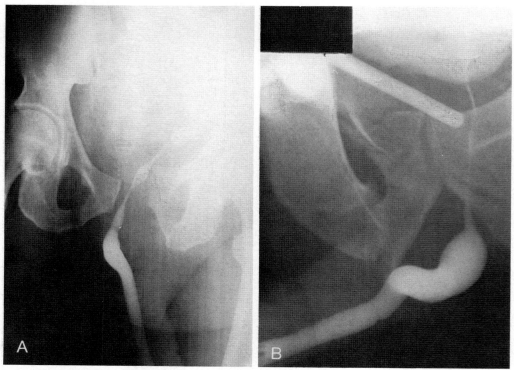

Figure 12.24. **A,** Dynamic retrograde urethrogram in a patient with pelvic fracture. The study shows an "inverted teardrop" bladder, large pelvic hematoma, intact but stretched urethra, and displacement of the prostate into the pelvis. Type I injury. **B,** Dynamic retrograde urethrogram in a patient with pelvic fracture. The urethra is narrowed and stretched but intact. Type I injury. (**A** from McCallum RW, Colapinto V: *Urological Radiology of the Adult Male Urinary Tract.* Springfield, IL, Charles C Thomas, 1976.)

males. The incidence of impotence after primary repair approaches 40% although there is controversy whether the initial injury or the primary surgical repair or both cause the impotence. The incidence of impotence drops to less than 10% when delayed repair is used. The rate of incontinence drops from 30 to 2%. However, in delayed repair, 100% of cases result in urethral stricture.

The initial urethrogram indicates the site of injury and commonly whether the injury is partial or complete. However, a partial injury may appear to be complete and no contrast medium enters the bladder. This appearance in partial rupture is likely due to the presence of blood clot blocking the urethra. If delayed repair is the chosen method, a repeated urethrogram 7–10 days later usually demonstrates that the urethral tear is partial. A second or third urethrogram is necessary in delayed repair immediately before the urethroplasty is performed. In this study, the bladder is filled through the suprapubic cystostomy tube and a retrograde urethrogram is done at the same time as a voiding study (Fig. 12.27). This examination outlines the full extent of the stricture, provided the patient is able to open the bladder neck. Rarely the bladder neck does not open because the bladder capacity is small and the bladder neck has not opened for 3 months due to the suprapubic drainage. In this instance, the surgery

should be delayed until a voiding study through the suprapubic tube combined with a dynamic retrograde urethrogram can be obtained. The suprapubic catheter should be clamped for 6–8 hours before attempting a second voiding study. The combined retrograde and voiding study delineate the length of the stricture (Fig. 12.27). Type III urethral injuries treated by delayed repair have a stricture several centimeters long and extend from the site of the bulbous urethral tear proximally, usually up to the verumontanum. After 3 months, the pelvic hematoma is usually resorbed and the prostate and bladder neck have returned to a more normal position.

Type II urethral injuries show a much shorter stricture on the preoperative retrograde and voiding study since resorption of the pelvic hematoma allows the prostate, prostatic urethra, and torn membranous urethra to move back to a normal position with approximation of the torn ends of the urethra.

Type I urethral injuries generally require no surgical intervention. The initial urethrogram showing an intact urethra allows the careful insertion of a small, well-lubricated catheter into the bladder. The bladder can be filled through this catheter and a voiding study obtained with the patient voiding around the catheter. The bladder is assessed for concomitant bladder tear. If no extravasation

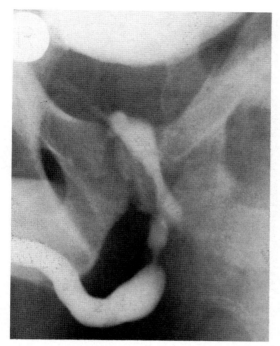

Figure 12.25.   Acute urethral injury. The dynamic retrograde study shows a partial Type II injury. The injury has disrupted the urogenital diaphragm and the urethra is stretched but continuous. Contrast medium enters the bladder and extravasates into the pelvis from the hole in the urethra. No contrast medium extravasates into the perineum or scrotum. The bladder base is elevated by hematoma and the prostate is elevated into the pelvis.

occurs from the bladder, the catheter can be removed and the patient allowed to void at will. Repeat retrograde and voiding urethrogram in 3 months demonstrate resorption of the pelvic hematoma and return of the bladder and prostate to a normal position.

Surgical Approach

If primary repair is performed in Type II or III urethral injuries, a suprapubic approach allows evacuation of the pelvic hematoma and realignment of the scarred urethra over a stent catheter. The incidence of urethral stricture following primary repair is reported in from 50 to 100% of cases. It is likely that successful primary repair without subsequent stricture are all Type II injuries, which is not common. It is to be expected that a suprapubic approach to a Type III urethral injury (the most common) will result in bulbomembranous stricture which would account for the high incidence of stricture following primary repair.

Straddle Injury

Straddle injury most commonly occurs when a male patient falls astride a hard object such as the crossbar of a bicycle, a steel or wooden beam, or the edge of a manhole cover. Kicks to the perineum may also injure the bulbous urethra. The urethra and corpus spongiosum are compressed between the hard object and the inferior aspect of the pubis. This may result in urethral contusion with an intact urethra or partial or complete rupture of

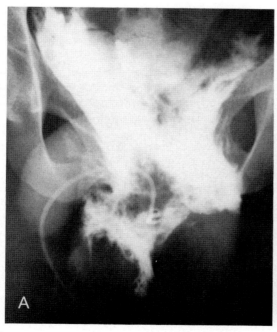

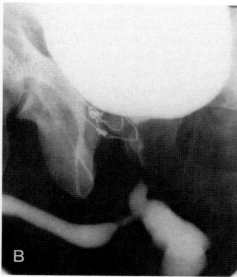

Figure 12.26.   **A,** Acute urethral injury in pelvic fracture. Attempted bladder catheterization. Injection of a large amount of contrast medium shows the catheter in the scrotum. Contrast extravasates into the perineum and obliterates the normal landmarks. The excess contrast medium appears to be in the pelvis, but has tracked up the anterior abdominal wall behind Scarpa's fascia. **B,** Dynamic retrograde urethrogram 3 months following primary repair. The resulting stricture and large diverticulum have developed well below the urogenital diaphragm in the bulbous urethra.

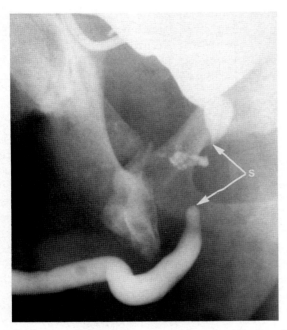

Figure 12.27.   Simultaneous retrograde and voiding urethrogram 3 months following pelvic fracture. A suprapubic catheter was inserted into the bladder at the time of urethral injury. The bladder is filled through the suprapubic cystostomy and the patient attempts to void at the same time as a dynamic retrograde injection is done. The bladder neck is open, and the proximal prostatic urethra is filled. A small amount of extravasation has occurred. The retrograde injection defines the distal end of the stricture. Between the distal end of the visualized prostatic urethra and the proximal visualized bulbous urethra is hard fibrous scarring (S). This is repaired from below by transperineal urethroplasty.

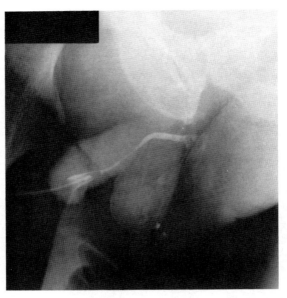

Figure 12.28.   Straddle injury. Dynamic retrograde urethrogram with a small amount of contrast medium shows complete blockage in the mid-bulbous urethra (bulbar sump) with a little extravasation into the scrotum.

the sump of the bulbous urethra. Straddle injury is not generally related to any bony injury.

In minor straddle injury to the urethra there is usually no blood at the external meatus although the urethra may be contused. The hematoma is usually confined to Buck's fascia and the tunica albuginea of the corpus spongiosum. More violent straddle injury commonly ruptures Buck's fascia and the hematoma spreads to involve the perineum and scrotum and is usually well delineated by Colles' fascia bilaterally at its junction with the ischial bones. In such injuries blood is commonly present at the external meatus.

In minor straddle injury, the retrograde urethrogram may show an intact urethra and the patient can be allowed to void normally. If the urethra is compressed or distorted by hematoma, but intact, and there is no extravasation, a small, well-lubricated catheter may be carefully inserted into the bladder and left for a few days. In more severe straddle injuries, the retrograde urethrogram generally shows partial or complete rupture (Fig. 12.28). If a partial rupture is present, attempted catheterization may complete the rupture. Suprapubic cystostomy tube insertion is recommended and repeat urethrog-

raphy is performed 2–3 weeks later. Small partial ruptures may heal without stricture, but the patient should have follow-up urethrography 6 months to 1 year later. Large partial or complete ruptures in the bulbous urethra show extensive extravasation, and if Buck's fascia is lacerated, contrast medium extravasates into the scrotum and may outline the testicle. Excess injection of contrast medium may show contrast medium passing up the anterior abdominal wall beneath Scarpa's fascia. When suprapubic cystostomy is used, large partial and complete rupture results in stricture. Such strictures are usually short (Fig. 12.29) and scarring does not extend to the membranous urethra. Such strictures can be repaired by anterior urethroplasty using a patch or pedicle graft.

Penetrating Injuries

Penetrating injuries to the urethra are uncommon. They result from gunshot or knife wounds and more commonly affect the anterior urethra. Penetrating urethral injuries generally require immediate surgical exploration and antibiotic therapy to contain superimposed infection. Knife wounds to the perineum can generally be treated by anastomosis of the cut bulbous urethra. Gunshot wounds may destroy some urethra, and patch or pedicle grafting may be necessary either as a one-stage urethroplasty or as the first stage of a two-stage urethroplasty.

Combined Bladder and Urethral Injury

In pelvic fracture, up to 20% of male patients with urethral injury have an associated bladder tear (Fig.

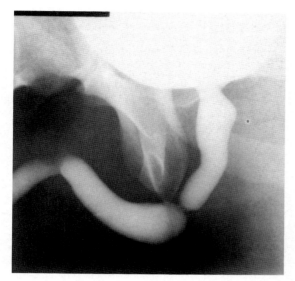

Figure 12.29. Dynamic retrograde and voiding cystourethrogram 3 months after partial rupture from straddle injury. The bladder is filled through a suprapubic cystostomy tube. The stricture is short and well defined.

12.30). Type I injury in which the urethra is intact allows contrast medium to fill the bladder and the bladder can be assessed for extravasation of contrast medium. Partial Type II and Type III urethral ruptures allow some contrast medium to enter the bladder, but bladder filling in these cases should not be attempted since much of the contrast medium injected will extravasate through the

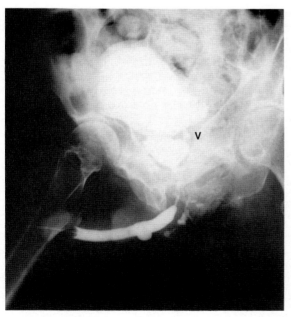

Figure 12.30. Partial Type III urethral injury and tear in the bladder base. Retrograde injection shows some extravasation into the perineum through a small hole in the proximal bulbous urethra. The verumontanum is visualized (V). Contrast fills the bladder and extravasates into the pelvis through a tear in the bladder base.

hole in the urethra. If delayed repair is to be used, cystography should be performed following placement of the suprapubic catheter. If primary repair is attempted for partial or complete Type II or Type III injuries, the bladder must be carefully inspected at surgery to exclude bladder tear.

INJURY OF THE FEMALE URETHRA

Clinical Features

Traumatic rupture of the female urethra is rare. It is usually the result of instrumentation, vaginal operation, or obstetric complications. Approximately 1% of urethral injuries in females are due to pelvic fracture. Most reported cases have occurred in female children or young adult females. The rarity of this lesion is likely due to the shortness of the urethra and to its mobility since the female urethra is only loosely fixed by the urogenital diaphragm. In pelvic fracture, rupture of the female urethra should be suspected when deep vaginal lacerations are present. There is inability to void or inability to pass a catheter. The urethra may be avulsed at the bladder neck or 1 or 2 cm below the bladder neck. Rupture may be partial or complete. Avulsion at the bladder neck requires a suprapubic approach with anastomosis of the separated urethral ends over a stenting catheter. More distal urethral rupture may be approached transvaginally with end-to-end urethral anastomosis over a stenting catheter.

Radiologic Evaluation

Excretory urography and cystourethrography are the best methods of assessment. In avulsion of the urethra at the bladder neck, the extravasation of contrast medium from the bladder base into the retroperitoneal space may be apparent on excretory urography. Similarly, attempted voiding cystography after the insertion of a suprapubic catheter will show extravasation when the urethrovesical junction is disrupted. The obvious complication in such cases is urinary incontinence, but the incidence of incontinence is not significant. More distal urethral ruptures extravasate into the vagina on voiding cystourethrography. In such cases, care must be taken to actually visualize the point of extravasation since contrast medium refluxing into the vagina is not an uncommon finding on cystourethrography in normal females. The other complication is urethral stricture, which is usually managed by urethral dilatation, usually with metal sounds. Balloon dilatation of urethral stricture in females has been reported in cases of chronic recurrent stricture.

INJURY OF THE PENIS

Rupture of the corpus cavernosum ("fracture of the penis") is an uncommon injury that generally occurs during strenuous sexual activity. Cavernosography may be useful for the preoperative evaluation of such injuries. In fracture of the erect penis, the tunica albuginea is torn and cavernosography may show the exact site and extent of the tear. This may be useful as the site of a tunica albuginea tear may not be obvious at operation. Urethrocavernous fistula may also occur in the fractured penis and the fistula can be demonstrated on cavernosography.

SUGGESTED READINGS

General References—Renal Trauma

Heyns CF, de Klerk DP, de Kock MLS: Stab wounds associated with hematuria—a review of 67 cases. *J Urol* 130:228, 1983.

Peters RC, Bright TC III: Management of trauma to the urinary tract. *Adv Surg* 10:197, 1976.

Pollack HM, Wein AJ: Imaging of renal trauma. *Radiology* 172:297, 1989.

Sagalowsky AI, McConnell JD, Peters TC: Renal trauma requiring surgery: an analysis of 185 cases. *J Trauma* 23(2):128, 1983.

Clinical Features and Excretory Urography

Bergren CT, Chan FN, Bodzin JH: Intravenous pyelogram results in association with renal pathology and therapy in trauma patients. *J Trauma* 27(5):515, 1987.

Bright TC, White K, Peters TC: Significance of hematuria after trauma. *J Urol* 120:445, 1978.

Cass AS: Immediate radiological evaluation and early surgical management of genitourinary injuries from external trauma. *J Urol* 122:772, 1979.

Cass AS, Bubrick M, Luxenberg BE, et al: Renal trauma found during laparotomy for intra-abdominal injury. *J Trauma* 25(10):997, 1985.

Cass AS, Luxenberg M, Gleich P, et al: Management of perirenal hematoma found during laparotomy in patients with multiple injuries. *Urology* 26(6):546, 1985.

Cass AS, Luxenberg M, Gleich P, et al: Type of blunt renal injury rather than associated extravasation should determine treatment. *Urology* 26(3):249, 1985.

Cass AS, Luxenberg M, Gleich P, et al: Clinical indications for radiographic evaluation of blunt renal trauma. *J Urol* 136:370, 1986.

Fortune JB, Brahme J, Mulligan M, et al: Emergency intravenous pyelography in the trauma patient. *Arch Surg* 120:1056, 1985.

Hardeman WS, Husmann DA, Chinn GKW, et al: Blunt urinary tract trauma: identifying those patients who require radiological diagnostic studies. *J Urol* 138:99, 1987.

Kisa E, Schenk WG: Indications for emergency intravenous pyelography (IVP) in blunt abdominal trauma: a reappraisal. *J Trauma* 26(12):1086, 1986.

Mee SL, McAninch JW, Robinson AL, et al: Radiographic assessment of renal trauma: a 10-year prospective study of patient selection. *J Urol* 141:1095, 1989.

Nicolaisen GS, McAninch JW, Marshall GA, et al: Renal trauma: re-evaluation of the indications for radiographic assessment. *J Urol* 133:183, 1985.

Roberts RA, Belitsky P, Lannon SG, et al: Conservative management of renal lacerations in blunt trauma. *Can J Surg* 30(4):253, 1987.

Wilson RF, Ziegler DW: Diagnostic and treatment problems in renal injuries. *Am Surg* 53(7):399, 1987.

Computed Tomography of Renal Trauma

Bretan PN, McAninch JW, Federle MP, et al: Computerized tomographic staging of renal trauma: 85 consecutive cases. *J Urol* 136:561, 1986.

Cass AS, Vieira J: Comparison of IVP and CT findings in patients with suspected severe renal injury. *Urology* 24(5):484, 1987.

Cates JD, Foley WD, Lawson TL: Retrograde opacification of the renal vein: a CT sign of renal artery avulsion. *Urol Radiol* 8:92, 1986.

Fanney DR, Casillas J, Murphy BJ: CT in the diagnosis of renal trauma. *RadioGraphics* 10:29, 1990.

Federle MP, Brown TR, McAninch JW: Penetrating renal trauma: CT evaluation. *J Comput Assist Tomogr* 11(6):1026, 1987.

Federle MP, Kaiser JA, McAninch JW, et al: The role of computed tomography in renal trauma. *Radiology* 141:455, 1981.

Glazer GM, Francis IR, Brady TM, et al: Computed tomography of renal infarction: clinical and experimental observations. *AJR* 140:721, 1983.

Kenney PJ, Panicek DM, Witanowski LS: Computed tomography of ureteral disruption. *J Comput Assist Tomogr* 11(3):480, 1987.

Lang EK, Sullivan J, Frentz G: Renal trauma: radiological studies. *Radiology* 154:1, 1985.

Lis LE, Cohen AJ: CT cystography in the evaluation of bladder trauma. *J Comput Assist Tomogr* 14(3):386, 1990.

Lupetin AR, Mainwaring BL, Daffner RH: CT diagnosis of renal artery injury caused by blunt abdominal trauma. *AJR* 153:1065, 1989.

Peitzman AB, Makaroun MS, Slasky BS, et al: Prospective study of computed tomography in initial management of blunt abdominal trauma. *J Trauma* 26(7):585, 1986.

Rhyner P, Federle MP, Jeffrey RB: CT of trauma to the abnormal kidney. *AJR* 142:747, 1984.

Sandler CM, Toombs BD: Computed tomographic evaluation of blunt renal injuries. *Radiology* 141:461, 1981.

Schaner EG, Balow JE, Doppman JL: Computed tomography in the diagnosis of subcapsular and perirenal hematoma. *AJR* 129:83, 1977.

Sclafani SJA, Becker JA: Radiologic diagnosis of renal trauma. *Urol Radiol* 7:192, 1985.

Steinberg DL, Jeffrey RB, Federle MP, et al: The computerized tomography appearance of renal pedicle injury. *J Urol* 132:1163, 1984.

Yale-Loehr AJ, Kramer SS, Quinlan DM, et al: CT of severe renal trauma in children: evaluation and course of healing with conservative therapy. *AJR* 152:109, 1989.

Renovascular Injuries

Bertini JE, Flechner SM, Miller P, et al: The natural history of traumatic branch renal artery injury. *J Urol* 135:228, 1986.

Cass AS, Luxenberg M: Unilateral nonvisualization on excretory urography after external trauma. *J Urol* 132:225, 1984.

Cass AS, Luxenberg M: Traumatic thrombosis of a segmental branch of the renal artery. *J Urol* 137:1115, 1987.

Cass AS, Susset J, Khan A, et al: Renal pedicle injury in the multiple injured patient. *J Urol* 122:728, 1979.

Halpern M: Angiography in renal trauma. *Surg Clin North Am* 48(6):1221, 1986.

Lang EK: The role of arteriography in trauma. *Radiol Clin North Am* 14(2):353, 1976.

Lang EK, Trichel BE, Turner RW, et al: Arteriographic assessment of injury resulting from renal trauma, an analysis of 74 patients. *J Urol* 106:1, 1971.

Radionuclide Studies

Rosenthall L, Ammann W: Renal trauma. *Semin Nucl Med* 13(3):238, 1983.

Uthoff LB, Wyffels RL, Adams CS, et al: A prospective study comparing nuclear scintigraphy and computerized axial tomography in the initial evaluation of the trauma patient. *Ann Surg* 98(5):611, 1983.

Ureteral Injuries

Beamud-Gomez A, Martinez-Verduch M, Estorness-Moragues F, et al: Rupture of the ureteropelvic junction by nonpenetrating trauma. *J Pediatr Surg* 21(8):702, 1986.

Bright TC III, Peters PC: Ureteral injuries secondary to operative procedures. *Urology* 11(1):22, 1977.

Cass AS: Blunt renal pelvic and ureteral injury in multiple injured patients. *Urology* 22(3):269, 1983.

Dowling RA, Corriere JN Jr, Sandler CM: Iatrogenic ureteral injury. *J Urol* 135:912, 1986.

Fry DE, Milholen L, Harbrecht PJ: Iatrogenic ureteral injury. *Arch Surg* 118:454, 1983.

Harshman MW, Pollack HM, Banner MP, et al: Conservative management of ureteral obstruction secondary to suture entrapment. *J Urol* 127:121, 1982.

Sieben DM, Howerton L, Amin H, et al: The role of ureteral stenting in the management of surgical injury of the ureter. *J Urol* 119:330, 1978.

Spirnak JP, Persky L, Resnick MI: The management of civilian ureteral gunshot wounds: a review of 8 patients. *J Urol* 134:733, 1985.

Steers WD, Corriere JN Jr, Benson GS, et al: The use of indwelling ureteral stents in managing ureteral injuries due to external violence. *J Trauma* 25(10):1001, 1985.

Bladder Injuries

Carroll PR, McAninch JW: Major bladder trauma: the accuracy of cystography. *J Urol* 130:887, 1983.

Carroll PR, McAninch JW: Major bladder trauma: mechanisms of injury and unified method of diagnosis and repair. *J Urol* 132:254, 1984.

Corriere JN Jr, Sandler CM: Management of the ruptured bladder: seven years experience with 111 cases. *J Trauma* 26(9):830, 1986.

Corriere JN Jr, Sandler CM: Mechanisms of injury, patterns of extravasation and management of extraperitoneal bladder rupture due to blunt trauma. *J Urol* 139:43, 1988.

Eisenkop SM, Richman R, Platt LD, Paul RH: Urinary tract injury during cesarean section. *Obstet Gynecol* 60(5):591, 1982.

Huffman JL, Schraut W, Baley DH: Atraumatic perforation of bladder. *Urology* 22(1):30, 1983.

Mee SL, McAninch JW, Federle MP: Computerized tomography in bladder rupture: diagnostic limitations. *J Urol* 137:207, 1987.

Palmer JK, Benson GS, Corriere JN Jr: Diagnosis and initial management of urological injuries associated with 200 consecutive pelvic fractures. *J Urol* 130:712, 1983.

Sandler CM, Hall JT, Rodriguez MB, et al: Bladder injury in blunt pelvic trauma. *Radiology* 158:633, 1986.

Sandler CM, Phillips JM, Harris JD, et al: Radiology of the bladder and urethra in blunt pelvic trauma. *Radiol Clin North Am* 19(1):195, 1981.

Shumaker BP, Pontes JE, Pierce JM Jr: Idiopathic rupture of the bladder. *Urology* 15(6):566, 1980.

Urethral Injuries

Casselman RC, Schillinger JF: Fractured pelvis with avulsion of the female urethra. *J Urol* 117:385, 1977.

Colapinto V, McCallum RW: Injury to the male posterior urethra in fractured pelvis: a new classification. *J Urol* 118:575, 1977.

Netto NR, Ikari O, Zuppo VP: Traumatic rupture of the female urethra. *Urology* 22:601, 1983.

Sandler CM, Harris JH, Corriere JN, et al: Posterior urethral injuries after pelvic fracture. *AJR* 137:1233, 1981.

CHAPTER 13

THE ADRENAL GLAND

ANATOMY

Along with the kidneys, the adrenal glands lie within the perinephric space. In most patients, there is sufficient perinephric fat that they are easily seen on computed tomography (CT) examination (Fig. 13.1). The right adrenal gland lies anteromedial to the upper pole of the right kidney and immediately posterior to the inferior vena cava. The left gland is anteromedial to the upper pole of the left kidney and posterior to portions of the splenic vein and artery. The right adrenal gland consistently extends above the upper pole of the kidney while the left is more often at the level of the left upper pole and may extend to the renal hilus.

Both adrenal glands have an inverted Y configuration with the tail of the Y pointing anteromedially. The angle between the two arms is more acute in the cephalad portion and widens inferiorly as the gland tends to straddle the upper pole of the kidney (Fig. 13.2). In patients with renal agenesis or ectopy, the ipsilateral adrenal gland has a more linear shape rather than the inverted Y configuration (Fig. 13.3).

The adrenal glands weigh only about 5 g each and vary from 3 to 6 mm in width. This small size makes it difficult to distinguish a normal from an atrophic or hyperplastic gland on the basis of size.

The arterial supply to the adrenal glands is from many small arterial branches from one of three main feeding arteries. This produces a comb-like appearance with small arteriae comitantes arising from one of three dominant vessels (Fig. 13.4). The arteries supplying the superior portion of the gland come from the superior adrenal artery which is usually a branch of the inferior phrenic artery. The middle adrenal artery arises directly from the aorta and provides vessels for the midportion of the gland. The inferior aspect of the adrenal gland is supplied by branches of the inferior adrenal artery which most often branches from the renal artery.

Each adrenal gland is drained by a single central vein. On the right side the adrenal vein enters directly into the posterior aspect of the vena cava (Fig. 13.5). Occasionally, however, it may join an accessory hepatic vein before entering the cava. The left adrenal vein enters the inferior phrenic vein before joining the left renal vein. The right adrenal vein is shorter and has a smaller diameter than the left adrenal vein. This explains the increased difficulty in obtaining a venous sample from the right adrenal vein as compared to the left.

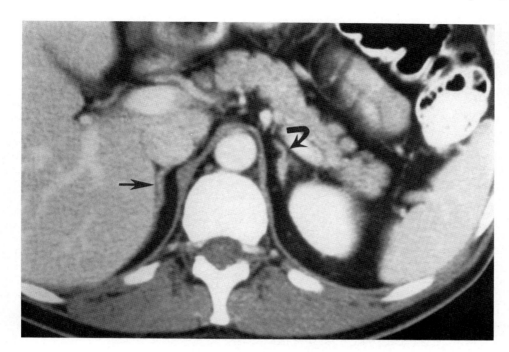

Figure 13.1. Normal adrenal glands. The right adrenal (*arrow*) lies behind the inferior vena cava and medial to the liver. The left adrenal (*curved arrow*) is anteromedial to the upper pole of the left kidney.

FUNCTIONAL DISEASES

The adrenal glands are small, and patients seldom present with pain or a palpable adrenal mass. Since the adrenal gland is an active site of synthesis of a variety of hormones, patients usually present with symptoms of hormone excess or, less likely, hormone deficiency. Thus, we will discuss adrenal diseases as those hyperfunctional disorders in which excess hormone is produced, disorders of adrenal insufficiency and those diseases in which adrenal function is normal. Since these hormones can be readily measured, there is seldom doubt as to which category a patient belongs.

Cushing's Syndrome

Cushing's syndrome is the manifestation of excess glucocorticoids. These steroids may come from either exogenous or endogenous sources. Exogenous Cushing's syndrome is seen in patients being treated with large doses of steroids. Endogenous Cushing's syndrome is due to overproduction of cortisol by the adrenal cortex. This can be due to an autonomous adrenal tumor, benign or malignant, or due to adrenal hyperplasia from unregulated ACTH production.

Cushing's disease refers to bilateral adrenal hyperplasia due to excess ACTH production by a pituitary adenoma. However, the pituitary gland is not always the source of ACTH in patients with adrenal hyperplasia, as a variety of other tumors, such as oat cell carcinoma, bronchial adenoma, and tumors of the ovary, pancreas, thymus, and thyroid may also secrete ACTH.

The characteristic appearance of a patient with Cushing's syndrome includes truncal obesity, hirsutism, abdominal striae, and muscle atrophy. Hypertension is a common finding as is glucose intolerance. The diagnosis of Cushing's syndrome may be confirmed by measuring plasma or urinary 17-hydroxycorticosteroids which are elevated.

The most common etiology of endogenous Cushing's syndrome is bilateral adrenal hyperplasia, which accounts for approximately 70% of cases. The vast majority of these patients also have a pituitary adenoma secreting increased amounts of ACTH. Ectopic sources of ACTH cause the other 10% of cases.

A few patients with adrenal hyperplasia have macronodules that can be seen in the adrenal glands on CT examination. These macronodules usually measure less than 3 cm and may be less than 1 cm in diameter. Macronodular hyperplasia is due to an ACTH-secreting pituitary microadenoma in the majority of cases. A benign but autonomous adrenal cortical adenoma is the etiology of 20% of cases of endogenous Cushing's syndrome, and a primary adrenal cortical carcinoma is responsible for about 10% of cases.

Conn's Syndrome

Conn's syndrome, or primary aldosteronism, is the result of excess aldosterone produced by the adrenal glands. As with Cushing's syndrome, it may be caused by either adrenal hyperplasia or as a primary adrenal tumor. A benign but unregulated aldosterone secreting adenoma is the most common etiology of primary aldosteronism, being responsible for almost 80% of cases. Bilateral adrenal hyperplasia accounts for 20% of cases. Rarely does a primary adrenocortical carcinoma secrete

Figure 13.2. Normal adrenal glands. **A,** At the level of the celiac axis a Y-shaped left adrenal (*arrow*) is appreciated but only the anteroposterior limb of the right adrenal (*curved arrow*) is present. **B,** At lower levels the right adrenal (*curved arrow*) becomes Y-shaped while only a portion of the lateral limb of the left adrenal (*arrow*) is identified.

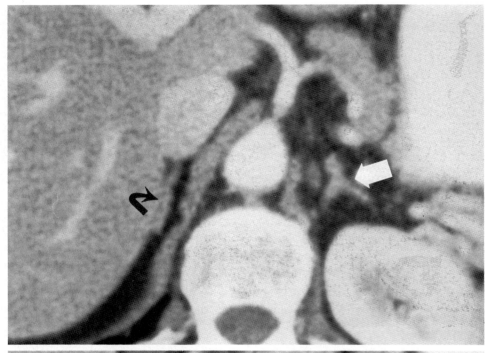

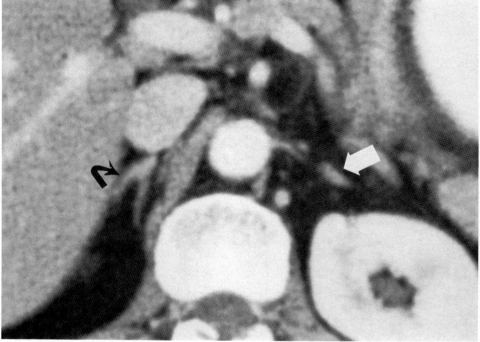

enough aldosterone to cause a recognizable clinical syndrome.

The syndrome Conn described in 1955 includes hypokalemia, hypertension, elevated serum aldosterone but low serum renin levels. Excess levels of aldosterone cause sodium retention, an increase in the plasma volume, and hypertension. Since potassium is exchanged for sodium in the distal tubule, sodium retention creates hypokalemia.

Aldosteronism also occurs in patients with renovascular hypertension. However, this form of secondary aldosteronism is distinguished from primary aldosteronism by measuring the serum renin which is low in Conn's syndrome.

Laboratory tests can also be used to help distinguish between hyperplasia or an adenoma, as the etiology of primary aldosteronism. However, these tests are not entirely accurate and radiographic confirmation is usually

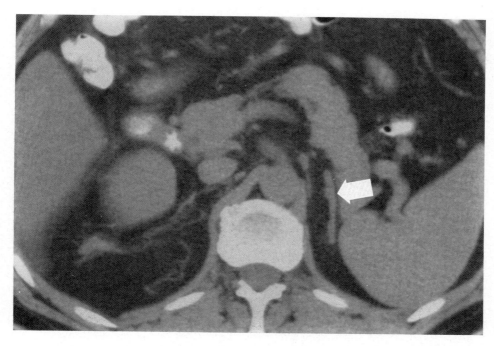

Figure 13.3. Left renal agenesis. The left adrenal gland (*arrow*) has a linear rather than an inverted **Y** configuration.

obtained. Furthermore, if an adenoma is present, radiographic techniques are needed to localize the tumor.

Adrenogenital Syndromes

These syndromes are the result of an inborn error in the adrenal enzyme system which blocks or impairs the

synthesis of cortisol or aldosterone. Low serum levels of cortisol stimulate ACTH secretion by the pituitary gland, while inadequate concentrations of aldosterone lead to increases in renin and angiotensin. Each of the six different enzyme deficiencies results in a different form of congenital adrenal hyperplasia. The clinical manifesta-

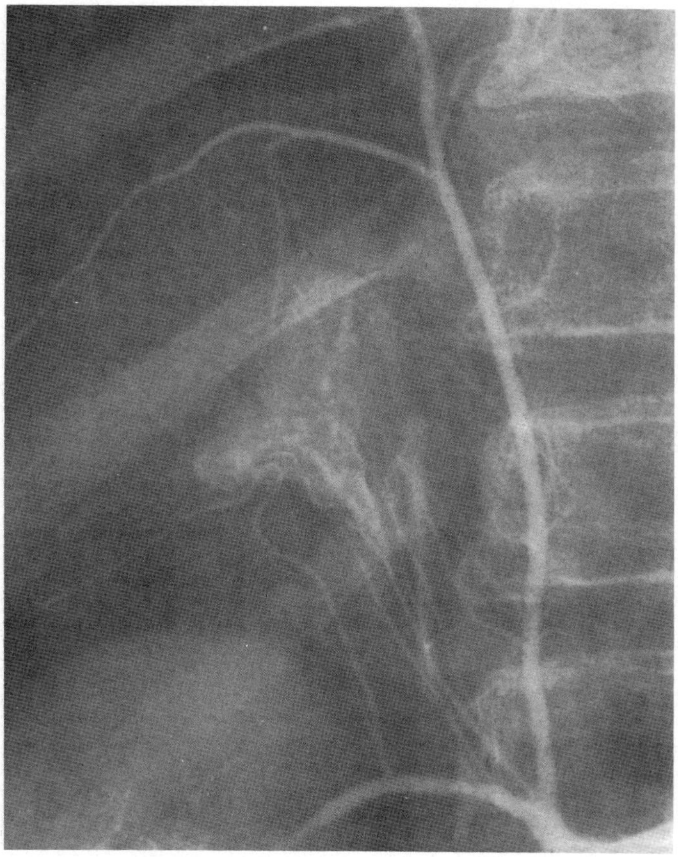

Figure 13.4. Adrenal arteries. The adrenal gland is supplied by many small arterial branches which arise from the inferior phrenic artery, aorta, and renal artery.

Figure 13.5. Adrenal vein. A single draining right adrenal vein (*arrow*) enters directly into the inferior vena cava.

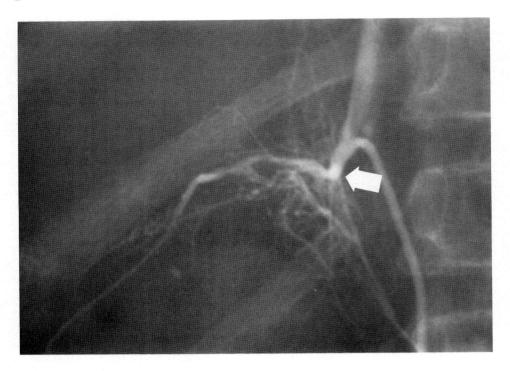

tions are determined by the degree of deficiency of cortisol or aldosterone and by the biologic properties of the biochemical intermediates that are formed and secreted in excess.

Deficiencies of either 21-hydroxylase or 11B-hydroxylase are the most common forms of congenital adrenal hyperplasia. Insufficient 21-hydroxylase impairs production of both cortisol and aldosterone. Since androgens do not require 21-hydroxylase for their synthesis, they are overproduced in response to high levels of ACTH. The clinical manifestation depends on the sex of the patient and the age at which the androgen excess appears. Virilization is seen in women and precocious puberty is found in young boys.

When a deficiency of 11B-hydroxylase exists, cortisol secretion is impaired. This results in an increase in ACTH and the precursor 11-deoxycortisol is oversecreted. This precursor is a mineralocorticoid that induces hypertension. Since androgens do not require 11B-hydroxylation, virilization, or precocious puberty may result.

Virilizing Tumors

Androgen-producing tumors are rare, may be benign or malignant, and occur in either males or females at any age. Patients whose virilization is due to a tumor usually present at a later age than those with congenital adrenal hyperplasia.

The typical clinical manifestations include amenorrhea, hirsutism, enlargement of the clitoris, and deepening of the voice. Elevated testosterone levels are also frequently found in adrenal tumors so a high testoster-

one level cannot be used to distinguish a gonadal from an adrenal tumor.

Feminizing Tumors

Feminizing tumors are quite rare. They are usually seen in men but have been reported in prepubertal girls and postmenopausal women. Gynecomastia is the predominant clinical manifestation.

Adrenal Insufficiency

Adrenal insufficiency may result from inadequate stimulation by ACTH (secondary) or may be due to tissue destruction of the adrenal glands (primary). Since normal adrenal function depends on ACTH, any disorder that impairs the ability of the pituitary gland to secrete ACTH may lead to adrenal hypofunction. With decreased ACTH activity, cortisol and adrenal androgen secretion diminish, but aldosterone secretion remains relatively intact. Thus, patients with hypopituitarism can tolerate sodium deprivation better than patients with primary adrenal insufficiency. Furthermore, hypopituitary patients do not develop mucocutaneous hyperpigmentation, as this depends on excessive ACTH secretion.

Primary adrenal insufficiency, or Addison's disease, occurs only after at least 90% of the adrenal cortex has been destroyed. Idiopathic adrenal atrophy is the most common cause in the United States and is most likely an autoimmune disorder. The other common cause of Addison's disease is destruction of the adrenal glands by a granulomatous disease, usually tuberculosis. However, other causes such as infarction, amyloidosis, hemorrhage, or destruction by histoplasmosis, blastomycosis, disseminated fungal infection, lymphoma, and metastatic tumor have been reported.

The clinical onset of Addison's disease is usually gradual and may be difficult to recognize. Manifestations are primarily a function of cortisol and aldosterone deficiency. Since cortisol deficiency results in increased pituitary secretion of ACTH and other melanocyte stimulating hormones, patients with Addison's disease develop a characteristic hyperpigmentation. Treatment includes cortisol and aldosterone replacement as well as saline to correct extracellular fluid depletion.

The radiographic manifestations of adrenal insufficiency depend on the cause of adrenal dysfunction. The plain abdominal radiograph may reveal adrenal calcification, commonly seen in tuberculosis or histoplasmosis.

The most useful examination is CT, which defines the size and shape of the adrenal glands. In idiopathic Addison's disease there is severe cortical atrophy such that the adrenal glands may be difficult to detect.

Granulomatous involvement by either tuberculosis or histoplasmosis is usually bilateral. The glands are enlarged but often maintain a normal configuration. Calcification is common.

If adrenal hemorrhage is acute, it may be recognized by the increased density of the recent hemorrhage. As the density of the hematoma decreases, it becomes indistinguishable from other adrenal masses. Although adrenal metastases are common, adrenal insufficiency rarely occurs. This is because so much of the adrenal cortex must be destroyed before insufficiency ensues.

RADIOLOGY

Urography

The plain radiograph is usually unrewarding in patients with hyperfunctioning adrenal cortical disease, although large masses can often be recognized. Calcification may be present in an adrenal carcinoma, but this is a nonspecific finding. Excretory urography will be normal unless the adrenal mass displaces the kidney. Since the adrenal glands lie anteromedial to the upper pole of the kidneys, an adrenal mass will push the upper renal pole laterally creating a more vertical renal axis. If the adrenal lesion is huge, the ipsilateral kidney will also be displaced inferiorly.

Ultrasound

Although the normal adrenal gland may be difficult to image with US, tumors larger than 2 cm can often be detected (Fig. 13.6). The right adrenal gland is usually easier to study because the liver provides a good acoustic window. As with other areas, obese patients are more difficult due to the higher sound attenuation of fat.

In patients with hyperfunction of the adrenal glands ultrasound (US) has two major uses. Large functioning tumors, such as an adrenal carcinoma, may be difficult to distinguish from adjacent organs, such as the kidney or liver. The multiple scan projections that can be used with US may allow a tissue plane to be distinguished that could not be seen with CT. Some hyperfunctioning adenomas may have sufficient fat within them to appear as low-density (near-water) masses. Computed tomography is unable to differentiate a small homogeneous adenoma

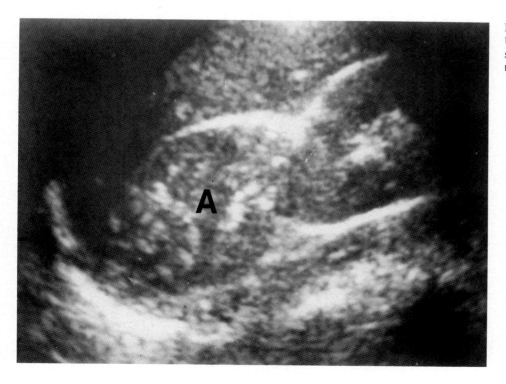

Figure 13.6. Adrenal tumor. Ultrasound demonstrates a solid suprarenal mass (A) easily distinguished from an adrenal cyst.

Figure 13.7. Adrenal adenoma. A small right adrenal adenoma (*arrow*) is detected by CT.

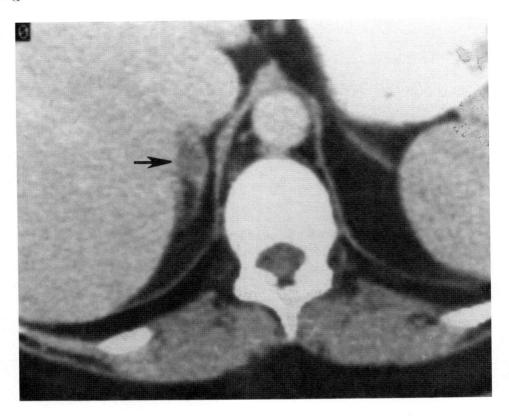

from an adrenal cyst. Ultrasound may be valuable in demonstrating the solid nature of the adenoma.

Computed Tomography

The single most valuable modality in examining the adrenal glands is CT. The perinephric fat present in most patients allows the adrenal gland to be clearly displayed, and tumors as small as 5 mm in diameter can be identified (Fig. 13.7). The adrenal glands must be carefully examined using contiguous 5-mm collimated slices. Intravenous contrast material is not usually needed but may be used to distinguish an adrenal mass from the upper pole of the kidney.

The adenomas in Conn's syndrome are usually the most difficult to detect because they tend to be the small-

Figure 13.8. Adrenal adenoma. An aldosterone-secreting adenoma (*arrow*) is seen in the left adrenal gland.

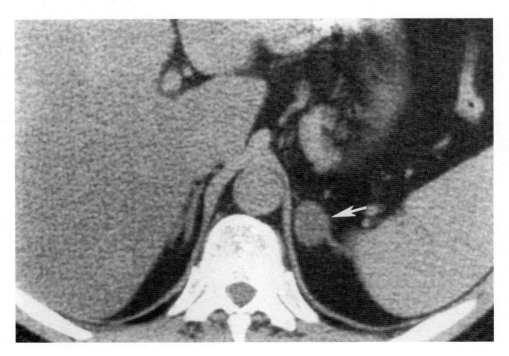

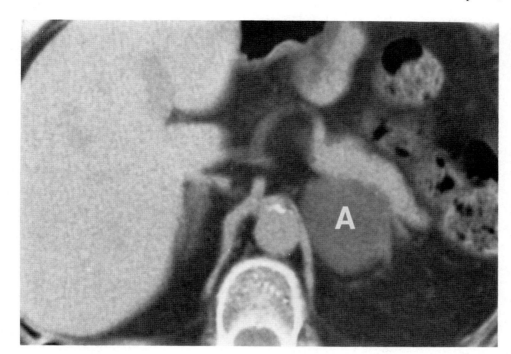

Figure 13.9. Adrenal adenoma. Cortisol secreting adenomas (A) are easy to detect because of the abundant retroperitoneal fat.

est, averaging less than 2 cm in diameter. Careful study of the adrenal gland is required and repeat, narrowly collimated sections may be needed. The left adrenal gland, which is often thicker in the crotch of the **Y**, may be particularly troublesome (Fig. 13.8).

Cushing's syndrome, on the other hand, is relatively easy to examine by CT. The tumors in these patients are larger than those causing Conn's syndrome and the adrenal glands are clearly depicted by the abundant retroperitoneal fat (Fig. 13.9). Tumors that are greater than 4 cm in diameter or demonstrate central necrosis are suspicious for malignancy and may be instances of a primary adrenocortical carcinoma rather than an adenoma.

Bilateral adrenal hyperplasia is seen as enlargement of the entire adrenal gland, but without a focal mass. The limbs of the adrenal are both thicker and longer, and they are seen over a larger series of CT sections (Fig. 13.10). On the right side, the false impression of a fatty adrenal mass may be created as the horizontal arm is forced posteriorly by the liver. The normal perinephric fat seen between the two arms may be misinterpreted as a myelolipoma.

Enlargement of the adrenal gland is usually more obvious in patients with Cushing's syndrome than Conn's syndrome. However, there is significant overlap with the appearance of normal adrenal glands, and hyperplasia should not be diagnosed by morphology alone.

Arteriography

Adrenal arteriography is seldom used in the evaluation of functional adrenal diseases. Computed tomography is a superior method of detecting both adrenal hyperplasia or an adrenal tumor. Occasionally arteriogra-phy is used to identify the tissue of origin of a large upper quadrant mass and delineation of the vessels supplying the mass defines the organ from which it arose.

Venous Sampling

Although venography can be used to detect an adrenal mass, it is more often employed to provide samples of blood from the adrenal veins for hormone analysis. Venous sampling can be valuable in patients with Conn's syndrome as the aldosterone secreting adenoma is often less than 1 cm and may be too small to be detected by CT. It is rarely needed in Cushing's syndrome but may be applied to patients suffering from masculinizing or feminizing tumors.

Bilateral adrenal venous samples are obtained and compared with each other and with a sample obtained from the inferior vena cava below the renal veins. ACTH may be administered to the patient before drawing the venous samples in an effort to increase hormone output and make side-to-side differences more pronounced.

Catheterization of the left adrenal vein is relatively easy and satisfactory adrenal venous samples can reliably be obtained. The right adrenal vein is smaller and more difficult to find. Once the catheter has cannulated this vessel, it is difficult to obtain the 7–10 ml of blood required for hormone analysis. The catheter often falls out of the right adrenal vein and the sample is diluted with blood from the vena cava.

This problem of dilution can be offset by measuring an adrenal hormone that is unaffected by the presence of an adrenal tumor. In the case of Conn's syndrome, measurement of cortisol will demonstrate how "pure" the adrenal vein sample is. Thus, an aldosterone/cortisol ra-

Figure 13.10. Bilateral adrenal hyperplasia. Both adrenal glands (*arrows*) are thick and elongated in this patient with Cushing's disease.

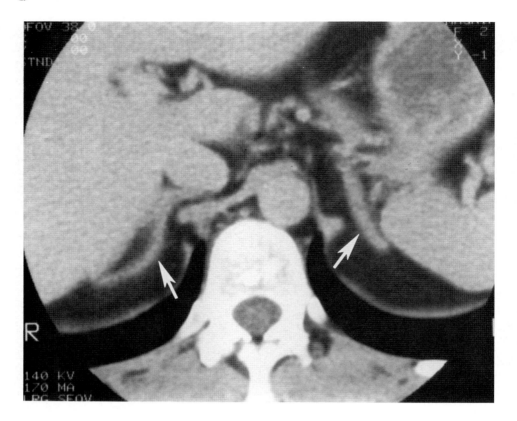

tio is obtained and compared with similar ratios from the contralateral adrenal vein and the inferior vena cava (IVC).

In experienced vascular laboratories the technique of adrenal venous sampling is quite accurate and provides tumor localization that may not be obtained with other imaging techniques. However, these syndromes are relatively uncommon and few laboratories have sufficient experience to maintain a high level of experience.

An additional venous sampling technique is occasionally used in patients with Cushing's syndrome due to bilateral adrenal hyperplasia. In these patients the source of the ACTH is usually a pituitary adenoma but may be from an ectopic source, such as a lung tumor. In this situation blood samples are obtained from the right and left petrosal sinuses and ACTH is measured.

Venography

Since each adrenal gland is drained by a central vein, the entire gland can be visualized with a single contrast injection. An adenoma is detected as a focal mass that displaces intraadrenal veins (Fig. 13.11). However, the veins, especially the right, are small and catheterization may be difficult. Both adrenal veins are approached from the right femoral vein. A catheter with a double-curve configuration is usually chosen for the left adrenal vein that joins the inferior phrenic vein and then the left renal vein in a rather constant position. The catheter is introduced into the left renal vein and the superior margin is

probed for the entrance of the inferior phrenic vein. Once in this position, care must be taken not to advance the catheter too far and pass the entrance of the adrenal vein.

The right adrenal vein is smaller and more difficult to catheterize. A downward-seeking catheter tip, which may be found in a "cobra" or Mikaelson configuration, is useful. The right adrenal vein usually enters the posterior aspect of the inferior vena cava at the level of the 11th or 12th rib.

Adrenal venography should be performed with hand injections as the vessels are small and it is easy to cause extravasation. This usually results in back pain that is self-limited and without sequelae. Occasionally this sequence of events may damage the adrenal gland and adrenal insufficiency has been reported. However, attempts to ablate aldosterone containing adrenal glands in this manner were unsuccessful, and adrenal venography is generally safe. The few major complications reported are usually due to clot formation, which can be avoided with heparinization.

Magnetic Resonance Imaging

The perinephric fat provides excellent contrast for magnetic resonance imaging (MRI) as well as CT. Although the spatial resolution of MRI is still inferior to that of CT, the additional parameters that are available, especially to distinguish benign from malignant lesions, may prove quite useful. For most patients with hyperfunction of the adrenal cortex, MRI does not provide additional information after a CT examination.

Radioisotope Scanning

Cortical imaging agents have been developed that can localize hyperfunctioning adrenal cortical tumors, particularly in patients with Cushing's syndrome. The labeling agent [131]I-19-iodocholesterol is given intravenously and scans obtained after a delay of 2–14 days. However, the success of CT in localizing these adrenal tumors has made this examination unnecessary in most centers.

ADRENAL MEDULLA

Pheochromocytoma

Pheochromocytomas are tumors comprised of chromaffin cells and are usually located in the adrenal medulla. Extraadrenal pheochromocytoma (paragangliomas) may lie anywhere between the base of the brain and the epididymis but usually lie along the sympathetic chain in the retroperitoneum. They are rare tumors and account for less than 1% of patients with systemic hypertension.

Patients may present complaining of episodes of headaches associated with palpitation and diaphoresis. If the pheochromocytoma is located in the bladder wall, micturation may induce a symptomatic episode.

Hypertension is the most common finding and is present in over 90% of patients. A pheochromocytoma may be difficult to distinguish from renovascular or essential hypertension, however, patients with a pheochromocytoma are more likely to have labile hypertension with discrete paroxysmal attacks. These patients are also prone to have hypertensive attacks during anesthesia induction.

Pheochromocytomas are associated with other endocrine tumors. The multiple endocrine neoplasia (MEN) syndrome, Type 2A, includes medullary carcinoma of the thyroid and parathyroid hyperplasia as well as pheochromocytoma. The MEN syndrome, Type 2B, is comprised of pheochromocytoma, medullary carcinoma of the thyroid, and the mucocutaneous manifestations of mucosal neuromas, intestinal ganglioneuromatosis, and a marfanoid habitus. The majority of patients with the MEN 2A or MEN 2B syndromes have pheochromocytomas that are bilateral and almost always intraadrenal. All manifestations of the syndrome may not occur at the same time. Thus, a careful history of a previous endocrine abnormality should be obtained in evaluating patients who may fall into these categories. These syndromes are inherited in an autosomal dominant fashion.

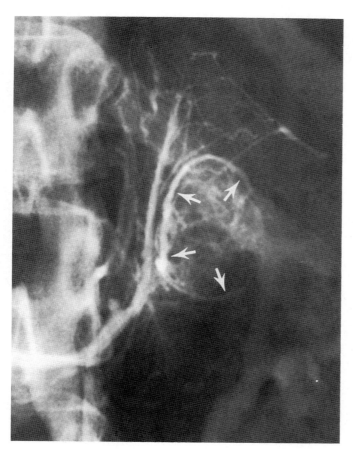

Figure 13.11. Adrenal adenoma. An adrenal adenoma is defined by the displacement of adrenal veins (*arrows*) in this patient with Conn's syndrome.

Pheochromocytoma is associated with neurofibromatosis and the von Hippel-Lindau syndrome. There is also a syndrome of familial pheochromocytomas not associated with other endocrine tumors.

Although 90% of all pheochromocytomas are located in the adrenal medulla, there is a striking difference between sporadic tumors and those associated with the MEN syndromes. The sporadic pheochromocytomas are located outside the adrenal gland in as many as 25% of cases, while those associated with the MEN 2 syndromes are virtually always intraadrenal. Pheochromocytomas found in MEN 2 patients are usually multicentric and involve both adrenal glands in more than 80% of cases.

Pheochromocytomas are usually benign but approximately 13% demonstrate malignant behavior. The histologic appearance is also different in sporadic and MEN 2– associated cases. The tumor is well encased in sporadic cases with normal adjacent medulla. In MEN 2 patients the medulla is hyperplastic and the tumor may be multicentric.

If a pheochromocytoma is suspected, the diagnosis can be made by measuring elevated levels of serum or urine catecholamines. Urinary metanephrines or vanillylmandelic acid (VMA) is elevated in over 90% of patients when measured on 24-hour urine collections. Epinephrine, norepinephrine, and dopamine can be measured by liquid chromatography which further aids in the diagnosis. Several separate determinations should be made because of the episodic hormone secretion found in these patients. Furthermore, patients taking medications such as methyldopa or mandelamine may have falsely high catecholamine levels.

In the past, provocative tests using an adrenal stimulator such as glucagon have been used. Although an occasional patient may still benefit from this procedure it has largely been abandoned. Since glucagon may induce a hypertensive crisis, it should not be used in patients undergoing an abdominal CT scan to identify a suspected pheochromocytoma. Fortunately, motion artifact from bowel peristalsis is seldom a limiting factor in the currently used scanners.

The treatment of patients with pheochromocytoma is surgical resection. Biochemical confirmation of the diagnosis and accurate preoperative radiologic localization have made these operations much safer. Nevertheless, patients undergoing surgical resection must still receive adrenergic blockade prior to the induction of anesthesia as well as careful monitoring during the operation to treat any crises. Both an α-adrenergic blocker (phenoxybenzamine) as well as a β-blocker (propranolol) are advocated while nitroprusside may be used to treat hypertensive episodes. This same regimen may be used in patients requiring invasive radiologic procedures such as arteriography, venography, or percutaneous biopsy.

Radiology

ULTRASOUND.   Sonography may be used to localize an intraadrenal pheochromocytoma (Fig. 13.12) but may also identify ectopic tumors lying in the paraaortic area. Pheochromocytomas tend to be more echogenic than normal adrenal tissue, possibly due to the hypervascularity they usually exhibit. By varying the angle of the transducer, US may be able to detect a tissue plane not seen with CT and determine the organ of origin of a large upper quadrant mass. Sonography is also often helpful in children when the relative lack of retroperitoneal fat makes CT evaluation difficult.

COMPUTED TOMOGRAPHY.   As with tumors of the adrenal cortex, CT is the primary localizing examination (Fig. 13.12). Most intraadrenal pheochromocytomas are detected and a sensitivity of 95% can be expected. Care must be taken when examining patients with the MEN syndrome, however, as the tumors in these patients are often smaller (Fig. 13.13).

MAGNETIC RESONANCE IMAGING.   Pheochromocytomas are both identified and characterized by MRI. T1-weighted sequences are used to identify the mass while the high signal intensity seen on T2-weighted images helps to characterize it as a pheochromocytoma (Fig. 13.14). This intense T2-weighted signal helps to distinguish a pheochromocytoma from an adrenal adenoma.

MRI is another potentially useful modality for the detection of pheochromocytomas. The spatial resolution achieved by MRI is inferior to that of CT, so routine scanning of the adrenal glands and retroperitoneum to look for a pheochromocytoma is still best done by CT. However, MRI can be quite valuable in the identification of lesions in areas that may be a problem for CT. Tumors in the wall of the urinary bladder or the paracardiac region are often problematic on CT but clearly recognized with MRI. Also postoperative patients in whom retroperitoneal tissue planes are disrupted may be difficult to examine with CT.

Chemotherapy has not proven to be useful for pheochromocytoma, but radiation therapy or high dose I-131-labeled metaiodobenzylguanidine (MIBG) may be used to control inoperative tumors.

NUCLEAR MEDICINE.   MIBG is an analogue of guanethidine that is taken up by adrenergic tissue. When MIBG is labeled with a radionuclide, pheochromocytomas can be localized (Fig. 13.15). Iodine-131 is the most commonly used isotope, but iodine-123 has been advocated as having better detection efficiency and superior dosimetry.

The overall accuracy of MIBG is similar to that of CT and MRI, however, scintigraphy has several advantages. With a single injection of radionuclide the entire body can be scanned. This is particularly helpful for ectopic tumors or in the detection of metastatic deposits. MIBG can also detect medullary hyperplasia, which is seen in

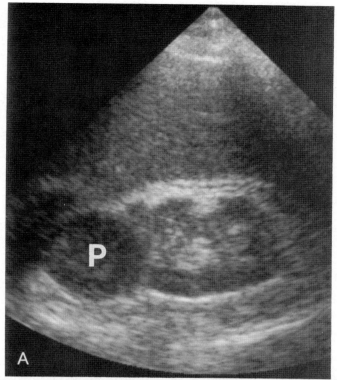

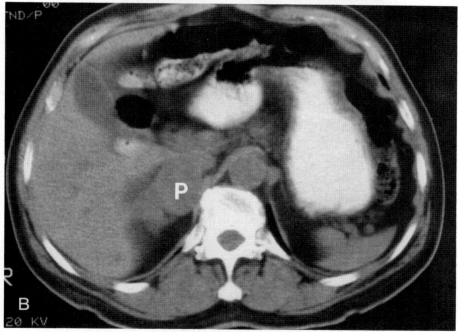

Figure 13.12. Pheochromocytoma. **A,** Ultrasound demonstrates a right adrenal mass (P). **B,** The right adrenal mass mentioned in (A) is confirmed (P) on an unenhanced CT examination.

patients with MEN syndromes and may be an early manifestation of a developing pheochromocytoma.

However, MIBG is not widely used to detect or localize pheochromocytomas. ^{131}I-MIBG has not gained FDA approval, and is not universally available. Furthermore, the spatial resolution is poor and studies require 1–3 days to complete.

Neuroblastoma

Neuroblastomas are primitive tumors that arise from sympathetic nervous system tissue. They may occur in the neck, thorax, abdomen, and pelvis, but no definite primary site can be found in a significant minority of patients. The most common location is the adrenal gland, which accounts for approximately 35% of patients.

Figure 13.13. Pheochromocytoma. This CT examination was performed to detect hepatic metastases in this patient with medullary carcinoma of the thyroid. The left adrenal mass (P) was found to be a pheochromocytoma.

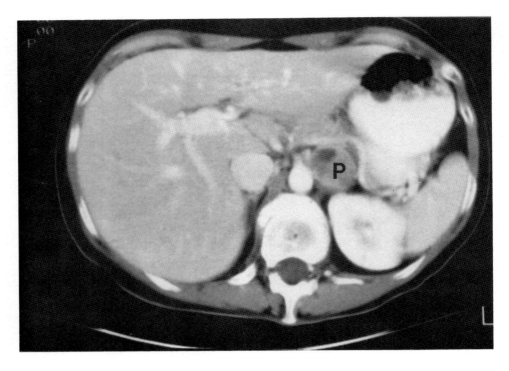

Neuroblastomas usually occur in young children. Approximately 25% of cases occur in the first year of life and as many as 60% occur by the age of 2 years.

Although neuroblastoma is the most common extracranial malignant tumor in childhood, its incidence is only one to three cases per 100,000 children per year. An increased incidence is seen in neurofibromatosis and familial associations have been reported.

Some neuroblastomas spontaneously mature into benign ganglioneuromas. Histologically, neuroblastomas contain densely packed small round cells that may be difficult to differentiate from other tumors, such as Ewing's sarcoma, lymphoma, or rhabdomyosarcoma. Other tumors may contain more mature ganglion cells mixed with neuroblasts and are classified as ganglioneuroblastomas. A mature ganglioneuroma is benign, but careful evaluation of the entire tumor is necessary as there may be marked variation in different parts of the tumor.

The most common presentation of a child with a neu-

Figure 13.14. Adrenal pheochromocytoma. 2000/40 spin echo image showed a hyperintense left adrenal mass (*arrow*) (T2 relaxation time = 82 msec). (From Baker ME, Blinder R, Spritzer C, Leight GS, Herfkens RJ, Dunnick NR: MR evaluation of adrenal masses at 1.5 T. *AJR* 153:307, 1989.)

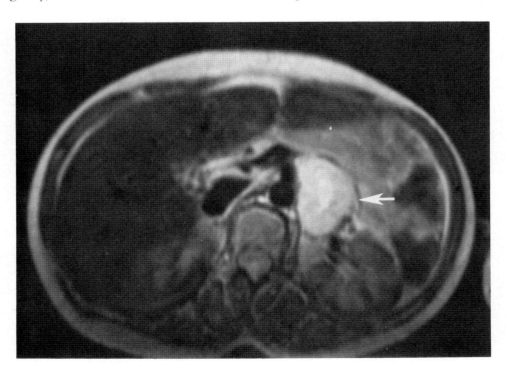

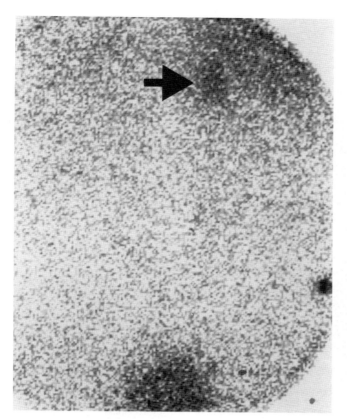

Figure 13.15. Pheochromocytoma. Increased radionuclide activity in the region of the right adrenal gland (*arrow*) on this MIBG scan helps to localize a pheochromocytoma.

roblastoma is with an abdominal mass discovered by a parent. Other presenting symptoms include opsoclonus and myoclonus, paresis due to tumor extension through the neural foramina, Horner's syndrome, or bone pain due to metastatic disease. Most patients have elevated urinary catecholamines when measured as catechol excretion per milligram of creatinine. More than half of patients excrete high levels of VMA and up to 90% of patients have an elevation of either VMA or homovanillic acid.

Radiology

UROGRAPHY. The plain abdominal radiograph may demonstrate a pattern of stippled calcification that helps distinguish a neuroblastoma from a Wilms' tumor. Evidence of bone metastases or widened neuroforamina may also be detected with plain radiographs.

Excretory urography may be useful to distinguish an extraadrenal tumor from an intrarenal Wilms' tumor. The kidney is often displaced inferiorly by an adrenal neuroblastoma. It is also important to evaluate the contralateral kidney, as the adjacent kidney may be compromised or removed as the neuroblastoma is excised.

ULTRASOUND. Sonography and CT are replacing urography as the primary modalities for evaluating a patient with a suspected neuroblastoma. Ultrasound is especially valuable in small children who have a paucity of retroperitoneal fat. A mass of heterogeneous echogenicity is usually seen in the region of the adrenal gland (Fig. 13.16). The margins are poorly defined and a capsule is not present. A sonographic "lobule" of homogeneous increased echogenicity consisting of an aggregate of cells separated from the surrounding tumor by collagen deposition has been described in a minority of patients. Sonography can also be used to detect involvement of adjacent vascular structures, such as the inferior vena cava.

COMPUTED TOMOGRAPHY. Unenhanced CT scans are more sensitive than plain radiographs in detecting the mottled calcification commonly seen in neuroblastoma (Fig. 13.17). Intravenous contrast material is commonly used to distinguish a renal from an extrarenal mass (Fig. 13.18). Computed tomography may be used to identify neuroblastomas in the abdomen, pelvis, or chest. Involvement of adjacent organs or retroperitoneal lymph nodes can be detected. However, its usefulness is limited by the lack of retroperitoneal fat in these young patients.

MAGNETIC RESONANCE IMAGING. MRI is a useful study in children with neuroblastoma if the child is sedated and motion artifact reduced or eliminated. The tumor has a signal intensity slightly lower than liver or renal cortex on T1-weighted images. On T2-weighted sequences the intensity is higher than liver but similar to kidney (Fig. 13.19).

The ability to scan in any plane is especially helpful. Using the coronal plane and T1-weighted sequences the neuroblastoma can be distinguished from the kidney and liver. T2-weighted images have superior contrast differentiation and are used in differentiating the extent of the tumor from adjacent normal tissue.

NUCLEAR MEDICINE. Since neuroblastomas commonly metastasize to bone, radionuclide bone scans are useful. In addition, many primary tumors demonstrate tracer uptake.

TREATMENT

Surgical excision is indicated in patients with Stage I or II disease (Table 13.1), as well as Stage II disease originating in the mediastinum. In patients with more advanced disease, chemotherapy is used first to reduce the size of the primary tumor and control metastases. Irradiation may also be used in combination with chemotherapy.

NONFUNCTIONAL DISEASES

Adenoma

Benign, nonhyperfunctioning adrenal adenomas are commonly encountered on abdominal CT examinations. Commons and Callaway found adenomas greater than 3 mm in 2.86% of 7437 autopsies. The incidence of adeno-

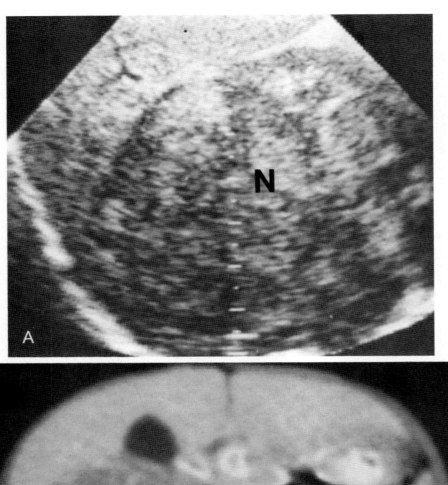

Figure 13.16. Neuroblastoma. **A,** A large neuroblastoma (N) with heterogeneous echogenicity is defined by US. **B,** Although there is very little retroperitoneal fat, the tumor (N) is easily detected on CT due to its large size.

mas was higher among older patients and those with diabetes or hypertension.

Adenomas consist of cords of clear cells separated by fibrovascular trabeculae. It is often difficult to distinguish a benign adenoma from an adrenal cortical carcinoma. Although carcinomas are more likely to have hemorrhage, necrosis, pleomorphism, and giant cells, these features may also be seen in benign adenomas.

Nonhyperfunctioning adenomas are almost always de-tected as an incidental finding. Occasionally, they are large enough to cause pain or compress adjacent structures. Rarely does hemorrhage into an adenoma occur.

Radiology

Calcification may occasionally be seen on an abdominal radiograph, and large adenomas may displace the ipsilateral kidney. Ultrasound can detect adrenal adenomas when they reach 2 to 3 cm in diameter. Furthermore,

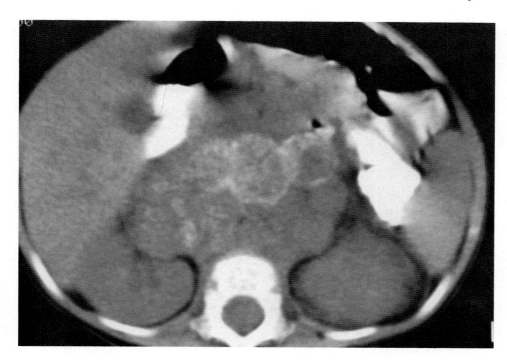

Figure 13.17. Neuroblastoma. Calcification is seen in this malignant tumor involving paraaortic lymph nodes.

US may be helpful in distinguishing a solid tumor from a cyst.

Most adenomas are detected during a CT examination of the upper abdomen. Typically, the nonhyperfunctioning adenoma is a well-defined, rounded, homogeneous mass (Fig. 13.20). Calcification may occur but is uncommon. Central necrosis or hemorrhage is rare. The density ranges from approximately 0 to 30 HU; a higher lipid content is presumably responsible for the lower-density lesions.

MRI can detect adrenal masses larger than 1.5 cm almost as well as CT. Furthermore, MRI may be used to characterize adrenal masses, but these data are still incomplete. Nonhyperfunctioning adenomas seem to be less intense than adenomas secreting aldosterone or cortisol. However, this is seldom a clinical problem as adrenal hyperfunction can be assessed by measuring serum hormone levels.

More importantly, MRI may be useful in distinguishing a nonhyperfunctioning adrenal adenoma from metastatic tumor. Metastases typically have a higher signal intensity on T2-weighted sequences (Fig. 13.21). Several methods have been employed to demonstrate this difference. Since the normal adrenal gland is small, it is difficult to measure the signal from normal adrenal cortex. Thus, a ratio of the intensity of the adrenal tumor and adjacent fat, muscle, or liver have been employed. Data from several studies suggest there are cutoff points below which all lesions are adenomas and above which all lesions are metastases. However, this leaves an overlap group which contains 21–31% of cases. Others have used calculated T2 values to distinguish benign from malignant masses, but similar overlap has been observed.

Radionuclide imaging with a cortical labeling agent such as NP59 may also be useful. Studies with NP59 show that these nonhyperfunctioning adenomas accumulate the radiopharmaceutical. Thus, radionuclide uptake indicates a benign lesion. Absence of radionuclide activity suggests a metastatic tumor, but is also consistent with an adrenal cyst or hematoma.

Carcinoma

Primary adrenal cortical carcinoma is an uncommon malignancy that occurs with a frequency of approximately one case per million population. Men and women are affected equally, but functional tumors are more common among females. Although the median age at presentation is the 5th decade, patients aged from 1 to 80 years have been reported.

Table 13.1
Neuroblastoma Staging

I	Confined to organ or origin
II	Contiguous extension beyond organ of origin but not beyond midline. Regional ipsilateral lymph nodes may be involved.
III	Contiguous extension beyond midline. Regional lymph nodes may be involved bilaterally.
IV	Remote disease involving skeleton, parenchymatous organs, soft tissues, or distant lymph nodes
IVs	Stage I or II disease and remote disease confined to one or more of the following sites: liver, skin, or bone marrow

Figure 13.18. Neuroblastoma. **A,** Paraaortic masses are present but difficult to distinguish on an unenhanced CT examination. **B,** After contrast injection the kidneys and large retroperitoneal vessels are clearly defined.

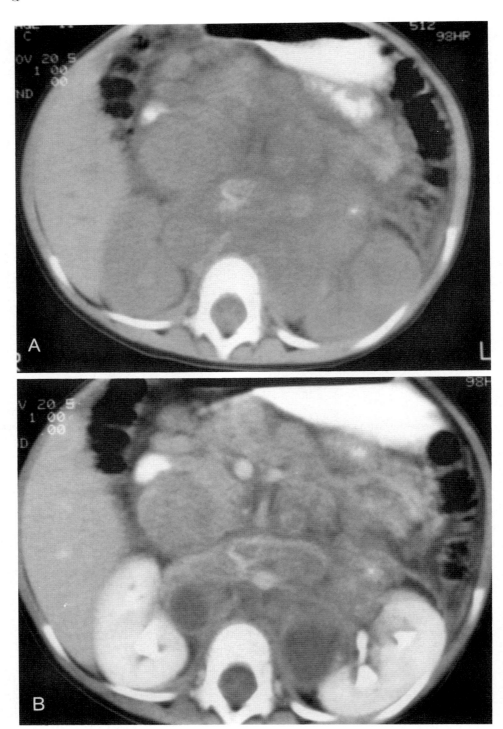

Adrenal carcinomas occur more commonly in the left gland than the right, and up to 10% may be bilateral. They are usually quite large at presentation, although a tumor as small as 1 cm has been reported. They have a nodular surface and are incompletely encapsulated. Central tumor necrosis and hemorrhage are common.

The microscopic appearance is variable. Some carcinomas are well differentiated such that differentiation from an adenoma is difficult. In other more frankly malignant lesions, highly abnormal cells with giant nuclei, multinucleation, and atypical mitoses are found.

The most common presentation of patients with an adrenal carcinoma is abdominal pain or a palpable mass. Approximately half of these tumors are functional and may be detected by the manifestations of excess hormone production. Cushing's syndrome is most frequent

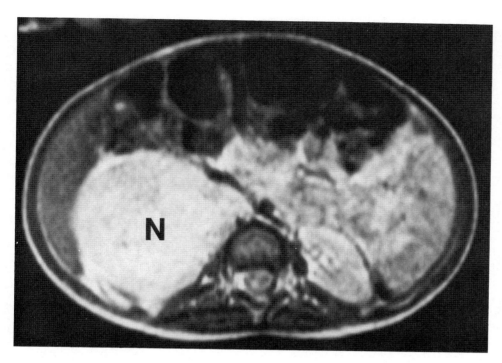

Figure 13.19. Neuroblastoma. A large right neuroblastoma (N) is easily seen on this T2-weighted (TR 2000, TE 35) MR image.

followed by virilization and feminization. Hyperaldosteronism is rarely due to carcinoma.

Many of the "nonfunctional" carcinomas may produce hormones that do not cause a clinical syndrome. This can be most easily demonstrated by measurement of urinary 17-ketosteroid levels.

Surgical excision is the only effective therapy. Chemotherapy with ortho para DDD (OP' DDD) and radiation therapy may be given for palliation, but it does not improve survival.

Radiology

A large upper abdominal mass may be detected on plain abdominal radiographs. Although calcification is common, it is much easier to detect on CT than on a plain film. The urogram is usually abnormal. The ipsilateral kidney is displaced inferolaterally by the adrenal mass. Since the adrenal gland lies medial to the upper pole of the kidney, the renal axis is more vertical than normal. The kidney itself is normal unless there is involvement of the left renal vein or direct extension into the kidney.

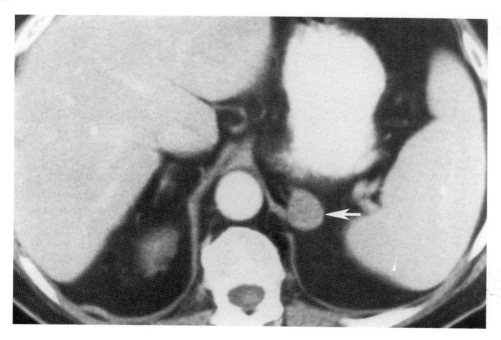

Figure 13.20. Benign adenoma. A left adrenal mass (*arrow*) was found to be a nonhyperfunctioning adenoma at autopsy.

Figure 13.21. Benign adenoma. **A,** The left adrenal mass (A) is well defined on T1- (TR 500, TE 25) weighted images. **B,** The relatively low signal intensity on T2-weighted (TR 2500, TE 80) images distinguishes this benign tumor from an adrenal metastasis.

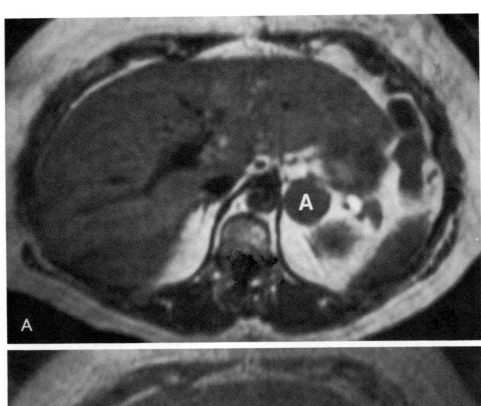

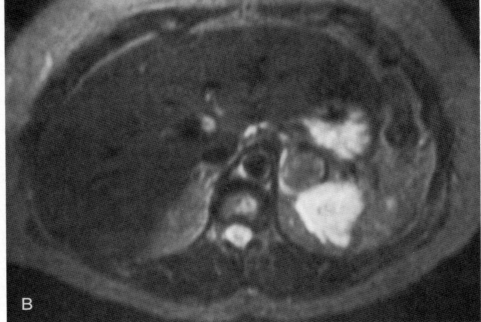

Ultrasound can demonstrate a suprarenal mass. Smaller lesions, up to 6 cm, are often homogeneous, while larger tumors have a heterogeneous texture with scattered echopenic areas representing tumor necrosis or hemorrhage. The tumors are characteristically well defined. Venous extension may occasionally be demonstrated.

The typical CT appearance of adrenal carcinoma is a large mass with central areas of low attenuation representing tumor necrosis (Fig. 13.22). Calcification is seen in approximately 30% of cases. Evidence of hepatic or regional lymph node metastases may also be seen on CT. Extension of tumor into the left renal vein or inferior vena cava may also be detected by CT. If a bolus technique is used for contrast injection, the CT scan may define the extent of tumor thrombus. If this delineation is not clear, additional studies such as cavography or MRI may be needed.

The most difficult area for CT staging of adrenal carcinoma has been the detection of direct hepatic extension.

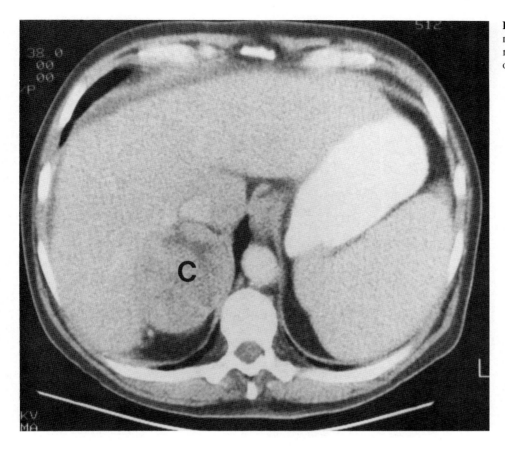

Figure 13.22. Adrenal carcinoma. A large heterogeneous right adrenal mass (C) is seen on an enhanced CT scan.

If a fat plane exists between the tumor and the liver, there is no hepatic involvement. However, if there is no fat plane, it is impossible to predict the presence or absence of liver invasion.

Although there are many indications for arteriography, it is not often needed in the evaluation of patients with suspected adrenal carcinoma. In patients with a huge mass in the region of the adrenal gland, it may be difficult to determine the tissue of origin. The adrenal gland may not be identified due to compression by the huge mass and fat planes no longer separate it from adjacent organs such as the kidney and liver. Selective arteriography can identify the primary vascular supply and determine the organ of origin of the mass. Selective renal, inferior phrenic, and celiac or hepatic artery injections should be performed. If possible, selective injection of the middle adrenal artery may also be helpful.

Adrenocortical carcinomas are typically hypovascular with large areas of central necrosis. The most vascular portion of the tumor is usually the periphery and the inferior phrenic artery provides the majority of the tumor vessels (Fig. 13.23).

Selective hepatic arteriography may also be useful in predicting tumor extension to the liver. If tumor vessels are opacified on the hepatic arteriogram, the liver is involved.

Arteriography provides an anatomic map for the urologist contemplating resection and may help to plan the surgical approach. Any time vascular interventional techniques are used, a diagnostic study should be performed.

The primary value of venography is delineation of intravenous tumor extension. If there is obstruction of the vena cava, the standard cavogram from a groin access may demonstrate only caval occlusion. In such cases, an additional run "from above" with the catheter inserted in the arm may be required.

MRI is often used to evaluate a suspected adrenal carcinoma. The high signal intensity on T2-weighted images further supports the malignant diagnosis (Fig. 13.24). The sagittal projection may be helpful in determining whether or not there is hepatic invasion. Venous extension can also be detected. Limited flip angle techniques are most useful for this purpose.

Radionuclide examinations are seldom used for adrenal carcinoma. A cortical agent such as NP59 can detect the large tumor mass but does not add additional information.

Myelolipoma

A *myelolipoma* is a benign tumor comprised of mature adipose cells and hematopoetic tissue. The gross appearance resembles fatty tissue but may contain patchy

Figure 13.23. Adrenal carcinoma. **A and B,** A selective right inferior phrenic arteriogram demonstrates the peripheral vascularity of this adrenal carcinoma. Note the lateral displacement of the upper pole of the right kidney.

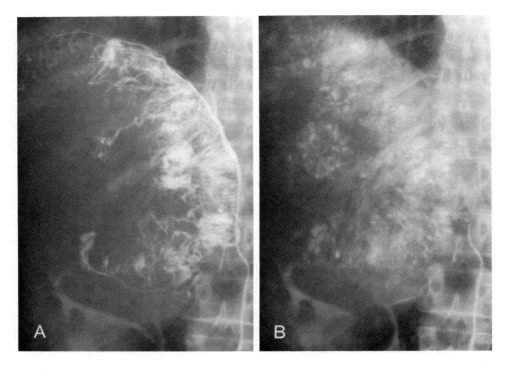

red areas of blood-forming cells. It is an uncommon lesion with only approximately 250 cases reported in the literature.

The tumors are functionally inactive and are usually detected as an incidental finding. Occasionally large tumors may cause pain or present with displacement of adjacent organs. Retroperitoneal hemorrhage has been reported. The most common age at detection is the sixth decade. There is no sex predilection, and both glands are equally affected. Although some reports suggest an association with obesity, hypertension, or chronic illness, this probably reflects the patients being studied.

Radiology

The plain radiograph is not helpful except in large tumors where the low-density fatty mass may be detected. Calcification may be present but is nonspecific. Similarly, the excretory urogram will be normal unless the kidney is displaced by the adrenal mass.

Ultrasound reveals a highly echogenic mass (Fig. 13.25). If the tumor is 4 cm or larger, a propagation speed artifact may be present. This appearance is suggestive of a myelolipoma, however, it cannot be clearly distinguished from a retroperitoneal lipoma or liposarcoma. If the tumor is small or the patient has abundant retroperitoneal fat, the myelolipoma may be difficult to distinguish from perirenal fat.

The most definitive radiographic examination is CT (Fig. 13.26). A fatty adrenal mass is virtually diagnostic of a myelolipoma. Unenhanced scans are usually adequate to make the diagnosis. Masking of the fat density of a

myelolipoma by intravenous contrast injection may occur. Although not yet reported, an adrenal lipoma or liposarcoma could mimic this appearance. A case of metastatic adenocarcinoma to the adrenal gland simulating myelolipoma has been reported. MRI can also image myelolipomas but does not add information not gained with CT.

Treatment of myelolipomas is usually conservative. The clear diagnosis of this benign lesion does not usually require further confirmation although diagnosis by fine-needle aspiration has been reported. Symptomatic lesions should be excised. Large asymptomatic lesions are sometimes removed to avoid potential complications such as retroperitoneal hemorrhage.

Hemorrhage

Adrenal hemorrhage may be spontaneous, traumatic, or related to anticoagulation. Spontaneous adrenal hemorrhage often occurs in patients with septicemia, hypertension, renal vein thrombosis, or adrenal pathology, such as a tumor. It more commonly involves the right than the left adrenal gland.

Adrenal hemorrhage is more common in the newborn than in older children or adults. It may be due to the trauma of delivery, asphyxia, septicemia, or abnormal clotting factors. It is bilateral in only about 10% of cases. If the hemorrhage is large, a palpable mass, anemia, or prolonged jaundice may occur. Adrenal insufficiency is rare in the neonate. Hemorrhage can usually be distinguished from a tumor such as neuroblastoma and surgery avoided. Most adrenal hematomas will be resorbed, but some may liquify and persist as an adrenal pseudocyst.

When adrenal hemorrhage occurs in the older child or adult, it is often due to trauma or associated with systemic illness or anticoagulation. It has been seen with hypertension, septicemia, renal vein thrombosis, seizures, surgery, or treatment with ACTH, insulin, or corticosteroids. When related to anticoagulation therapy, it usually occurs during the first 3 weeks of therapy. However, it is not due to excessive anticoagulation, as associated hemorrhage does not occur in other areas.

Adrenal hemorrhage may occur in up to 25% of severely traumatized patients and approximately 20% of cases are bilateral. The right adrenal gland is involved much more commonly than the left. This may be due to an acute rise in venous pressure, which is more directly transmitted to the right adrenal gland since the right adrenal vein enters the inferior vena cava directly. The hematoma is usually found in the adrenal medulla with stretching of the surrounding cortex.

Most adrenal hemorrhage is clinically silent. Only rarely is the endocrine function of the gland sufficiently impaired to cause adrenal insufficiency, although this is more likely to occur if both glands are affected.

Radiology

Large hematomas may be seen as a soft tissue mass on the plain radiograph, and the ipsilateral kidney may be

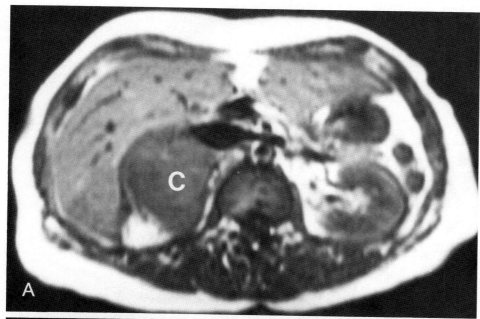

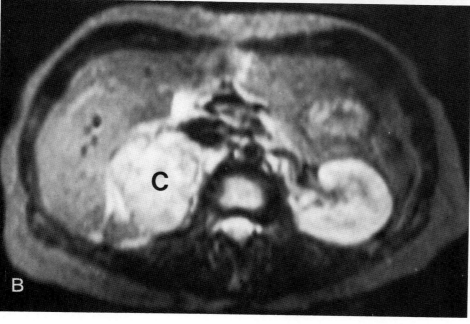

Figure 13.24.   Adrenal carcinoma. **A,** A large right adrenal mass (C) is seen on T1-weighted (TR 500, TE 25) images. **B,** The high signal intensity (C) on T2-weighted (TR 2000, TE 80) images is indicative of malignancy.

Figure 13.25. Myelolipoma. A highly echogenic adrenal mass (M) suggests a myelolipoma.

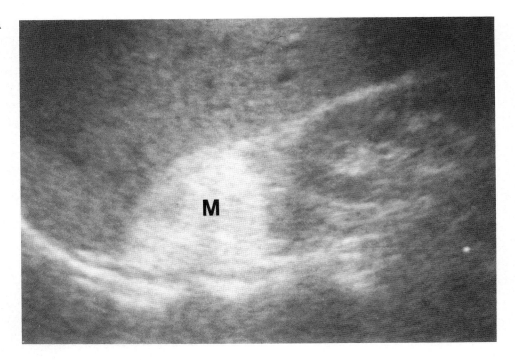

displaced downward. The axis of the kidney becomes more vertical and the upper pole may even be lateral to the lower pole.

An adrenal mass can usually be seen with US (Fig. 13.27). The echogenicity varies with the state of the hematoma and may be hypoechoic, mixed, or moderately echogenic.

The most reliable method of identifying adrenal hem-

orrhage is CT (Fig. 13.28). Initially the hematoma has a high density, 50–90 HU. Follow-up studies usually show resorption of the hematoma and a gradual decrease in density to near water.

MRI of adrenal hemorrhage has also been reported. The magnetic resonance appearance reflects the evolution from acute to chronic stages with hemoglobin breakdown.

Figure 13.26. Myelolipoma. The macroscopic fat seen on CT is the most reliable sign of a myelolipoma. Bilateral myelolipomas (*arrows*) demonstrate both fat and peripheral calcifications.

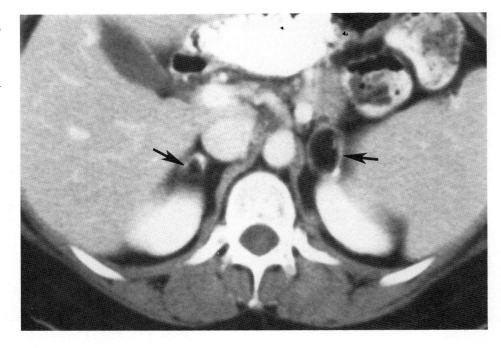

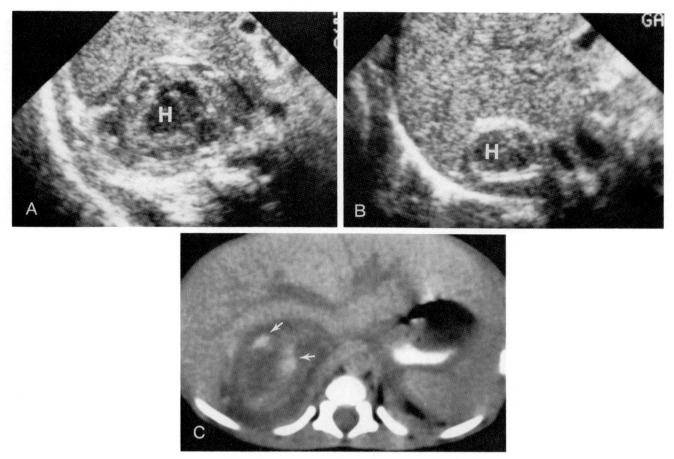

Figure 13.27.   Adrenal hemorrhage. **A,** A large mass (H) of mixed echogenicity is seen in the right adrenal gland. **B,** Six weeks later the hematoma (H) is much smaller as it has started to resorb. **C,** Calcification (*arrows*) can be seen in the hematoma on CT. (Case courtesy of Kate Feinstein, M.D.)

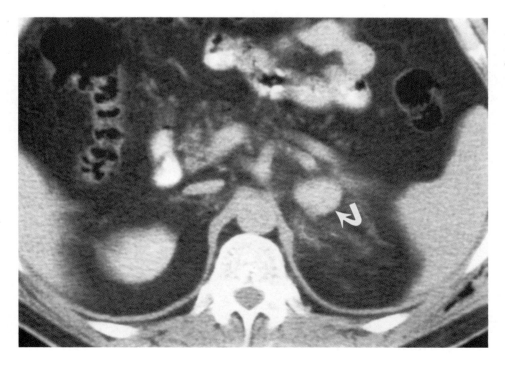

Figure 13.28.   Adrenal hemorrhage. The high density indicates hemorrhage (*curved arrow*) in this patient after left flank trauma.

Cysts

Adrenal cysts are uncommon lesions that may occur at any age. They involve the right and left glands equally but have a 3:1 female predilection.

Most adrenal cysts are asymptomatic and found either at autopsy or as incidental findings. Large cysts may cause dull pain or symptoms due to compression on the stomach or duodenum.

There are several recognized etiologies of adrenal cysts. Endothelial cysts are the most common, accounting for approximately 45% of all adrenal cysts. They have an endothelial lining and may be lymphatic or angiomatous in origin. Lymphangiomatous cysts are more common and probably arise from blockage of a lymph duct.

Epithelial cysts are quite uncommon, as they comprise only 9% of adrenal cysts. They have a cylindrical epithelium and include cystic adenomas.

Parasitic cysts are the least common variety, comprising only 7% of the total. They are usually echinococcal in origin and are associated with widespread disease.

Pseudocysts are the second most common variety, as they comprise 39% of adrenal cysts. They are probably due to adrenal hemorrhage into either a normal or abnormal gland. The lining is not covered by epithelium. Pseudocysts are most commonly detected radiographically, as they tend to be larger than endothelial cysts.

Radiology

The abdominal radiograph will be revealing only if the cyst is calcified or very large. When present, calcification is curvilinear in the cyst wall. Urography is useful to exclude a renal origin.

Ultrasound demonstrates a cystic suprarenal mass (Fig. 13.29). Unlike renal cysts, adrenal cysts often exhibit a thick wall. Pseudocysts may also demonstrate internal septations. If a soft tissue mass–like component is present, surgery may be required to exclude a neoplasm.

Similar findings are detected with CT. The density of the fluid can be measured, and calcification is easier to detect with CT than US. However, it may still be difficult to exclude malignancy. Cyst aspiration can be helpful if the fluid is clear and the cytology benign.

Hemangioma

Adrenal hemangioma is a rare tumor of the adrenal cortex. Pathologically, adrenal hemangiomas are similar to hemangiomas of other organs. The vessels are lined with a vascular endothelium and they may undergo degenerative changes including thrombosis, hemorrhage, and necrosis. They range in diameter from 2 to 22 cm. Patients have ranged in age from 25 to 79 years. The tumors more often involve the right adrenal gland and show a female preponderance. None of the hemangiomas reported have shown evidence of hyperfunction although one case of adrenal insufficiency has been seen.

Most patients are asymptomatic, and the tumor is found either at autopsy or during evaluation for another process. However, a dull pain and vague upper gastrointestinal symptoms may be present in very large lesions.

An abdominal mass may be seen either on a plain radiograph or may displace the ipsilateral kidney at urography. Calcification is common and may be either phlebolith-like or have an irregular stellate appearance.

Ultrasound demonstrates a complex mass and may reveal cystic areas. The CT appearance also depends on the tumor morphology. Typically, a large mass with a thick irregular wall and hypodense center is seen. There is patchy enhancement of the peripheral zone. Calcification is easily seen with CT.

The angiographic appearance of a hypovascular mass with contrast pooling and prolongation of the vascular stain is similar to hemangiomas in other organs. However, the radiographic findings are often not sufficiently characteristic and surgical resection is often performed.

Metastases

The adrenal glands are a common site of metastatic disease. In a series of 1000 consecutive postmortem examinations of patients with an epithelial malignancy, Abrams et al. found 27% to have adrenal metastases. The incidence of adrenal metastases from the two most common primary tumors was even higher. Carcinoma of the breast metastasized to the adrenal glands in 54% of cases while 36% of patients with lung carcinoma had adrenal metastases.

The radiographic appearance of adrenal metastases is not specific. They may be large or small, unilateral, or bilateral. A metastasis is a solid mass, and when less than 3 cm in diameter, is usually homogeneous (Fig. 13.30). Larger lesions may demonstrate central necrosis or areas of hemorrhage (Fig. 13.31). Thus, an adrenal metastasis cannot be clearly distinguished from benign lesions such as an adenoma, hematoma, pseudocyst, or inflammatory mass on the basis of its morphology.

Nevertheless, several investigators have tried to identify criteria that would allow the diagnosis of a benign or malignant etiology based on CT criteria. Features that suggest a malignant lesion include a large size (>3 cm), poorly defined margins, invasion of adjacent structures, inhomogeneous attenuation, and a thick irregular enhancing rim. Small ovoid lesions with a thin rim and homogeneous density are more likely to be benign.

In many patients there is evidence of widespread metastatic disease involving the lungs, liver, and retroperitoneal lymph nodes as well as the adrenal glands (Fig. 13.32). In these patients it is relatively unimportant

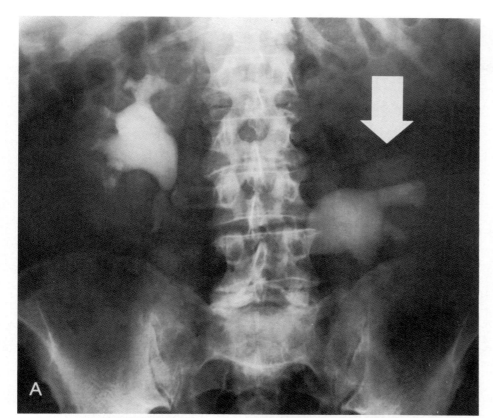

Figure 13.29. Adrenal cyst. **A,** A large left adrenal mass is displacing the kidney inferiorly (*arrow*). **B,** Ultrasound demonstrates its cystic (C) nature.

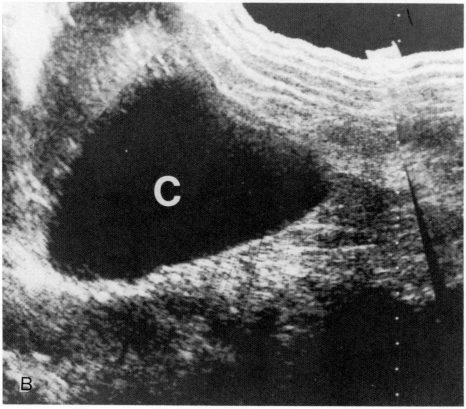

Figure 13.30. Adrenal metastasis. This right adrenal metastasis (*arrow*) from an underlying hepatoma is small, well defined, and homogeneous.

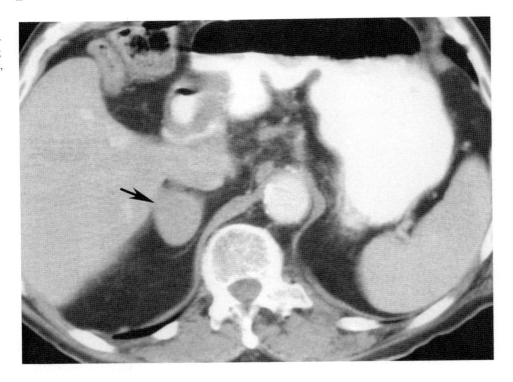

whether or not the adrenal mass represents metastatic tumor. However, in some patients an adrenal mass may be the only evidence of metastatic disease. This can be a critical distinction as it may change the therapy from an attempt at cure to palliation.

There are several radiographic procedures that can be used in this setting.

The nature of an adrenal mass can be predicted with MRI. As was discussed in "Adenoma" above, either a calculated T2 relaxation time or signal intensity ratios may be used to predict a benign or malignant nature of an adrenal mass (Fig. 13.33). However, this has met with limited success. Furthermore, the wide variety of magnets, operating field strengths, and the multiple examination se-

Figure 13.31. Adrenal metastasis. This large left adrenal metastasis (M) demonstrates central necrosis.

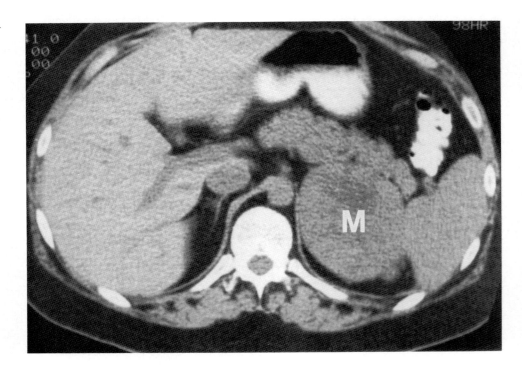

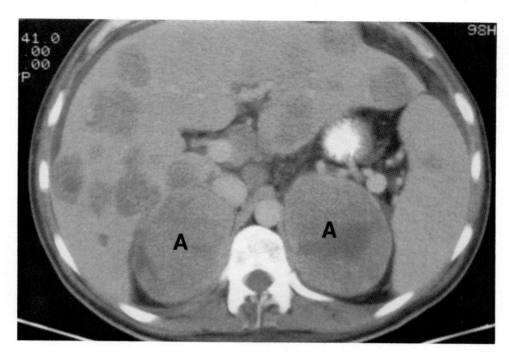

Figure 13.32. Adrenal metastases. Widespread metastatic disease is evidenced by involvement of both adrenal glands (A) as well as liver, spleen, and lymph nodes.

quences that can be used make it difficult to apply data obtained at one site to another clinical setting. It is hoped that further work will refine the MRI techniques to make the determination more reliable.

Adrenal cortical scintigraphy has also been applied to this problem. Since benign adenomas take up a cortical labeling agent such as NP59, they can be distinguished from nonadenomatous masses. Absence of uptake is not specific, however, as neither a cyst, hematoma, nor inflammatory mass will take up the radionuclide. Thus, these benign masses cannot be distinguished from a metastasis with this examination.

Francis et al. applied NP59 scintigraphy to 28 oncologic patients who had a unilateral adrenal mass. Each of 14 patients with increased radionuclide uptake had an adenoma. None of the 11 patients with decreased uptake on the side of the mass had an adenoma; 9 had metastases and 2 had cysts. Uptake was indeterminant in three patients. Despite these encouraging results, adrenal scintigraphy is not used widely to distinguish benign from malignant adrenal masses.

Percutaneous aspiration biopsy is the most definitive method of confirming metastatic disease (Fig. 13.34). With experienced cytopathologists, the positive predictive value approaches 100%. A negative aspiration is not as diagnostic, as sampling error or an inadequate specimen may preclude a confident diagnosis. The overall accuracy reported for percutaneous adrenal biopsy ranges from 80 to 100%. The results vary with the patient population and types of lesions aspirated. Positive results indicate malignancy. Negative aspirations can be repeated to increase the confidence that the lesion is benign.

Adrenal biopsy is an invasive procedure and complications may occur. The most common complication is pneumothorax. These pneumothoraces are usually small and resolve spontaneously. Large or symptomatic pneumothoraces should be treated with a small chest tube that can be placed by the radiologist under fluoroscopic guidance. Tumor seeding of the needle tract and bacteremia are rare. Pancreatitis may occur and can be a serious complication. Thus, the pancreas should be avoided if possible. Many patients will have a small amount of bleeding but this is seldom symptomatic.

The most worrisome complication of percutaneous needle biopsy of an adrenal mass is precipitation of a hypertensive crises by a pheochromocytoma. This complication may be fatal despite regaining control of the blood pressure. Screening catecholamines may be useful in hypertensive patients but may not be elevated in a nonfunctioning pheochromocytoma.

Lymphoma

Involvement of the adrenal gland by malignant lymphoma is more common with non-Hodgkin lymphoma than Hodgkin's disease. Most patients have a diffuse rather than a nodular form of lymphoma. In a review of 173 patients with non-Hodgkin lymphoma, Paling and Williamson, using CT, found evidence of adrenal involvement in seven (4%) patients during some portion of the course of their disease.

The adrenal glands are seldom an isolated site of disease, although other involvement may be distant. In most patients, however, retroperitoneal lymphoma is also

Figure 13.33. Adrenal metastasis. **A,** The adrenal mass (A) is well defined on CT. **B,** The high signal intensity on T2-weighted (TR 2500, TE 80) images indicates its malignant nature. (From Dunnick NR: CT and MRI of adrenal lesions. *Urol Radiol* 10:12, 1988.)

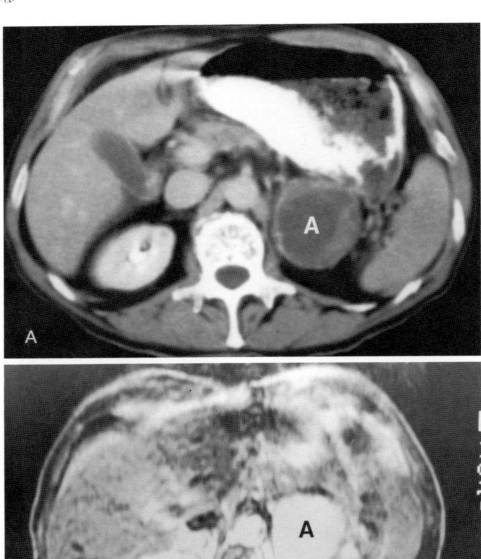

present. Bilateral adrenal involvement is seen in about half the cases. Even with extensive disease, adrenal insufficiency is rare. The modalities in which adrenal lymphoma can be identified are ultrasound, CT, and MRI. On US, lymphoma appears as a well-defined, relatively echopenic homogeneous tissue mass. If extensive retroperitoneal disease is present, it may be difficult to identify the adrenal glands.

Computed tomography provides the best morphologic delineation (Fig. 13.35). The adrenal glands are enlarged with either a rounded mass or more symmetric enlargement, preserving the basic glandular configuration. The tissue is usually homogeneous and demonstrates contrast enhancement. There is, however, no pathognomonic pattern to indicate lymphomatous involvement.

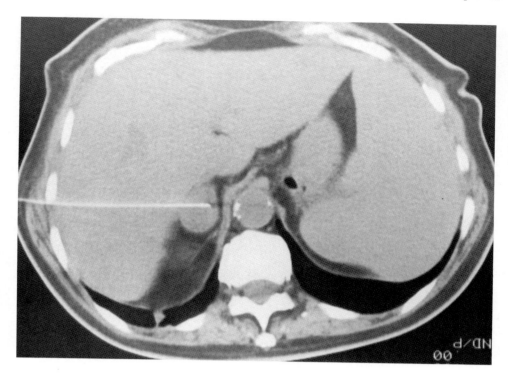

Figure 13.34. Adrenal biopsy. Computed tomography is the most useful modality for directing percutaneous adrenal biopsies, particularly for small tumors. (From Dunnick NR: The adrenal gland. In Tavaras JM, Ferrucci JT (eds): *Radiology: Diagnosis, Imaging, Intervention.* Philadelphia: JB Lippincott.)

Pseudotumors

Retroperitoneal fat provides the contrast needed to demonstrate the adrenal glands. When there is a paucity of fat in the perirenal space, the adrenal glands are difficult to evaluate. Furthermore, large masses may compress the normal adrenal gland such that it is impossible to determine its organ of origin.

Abnormalities in the upper abdomen may simulate an adrenal mass. In addition to creating diagnostic confusion, percutaneous biopsy may be attempted. An appreci-

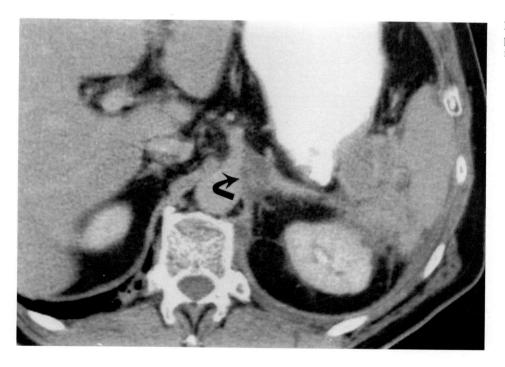

Figure 13.35. Adrenal lymphoma. The adrenal gland is involved (*curved arrow*).

Figure 13.36. Adrenal pseudotumor. Gastric varices (V) may mimic an adrenal mass but can be differentiated by their serpiginous configuration and vascular enhancement.

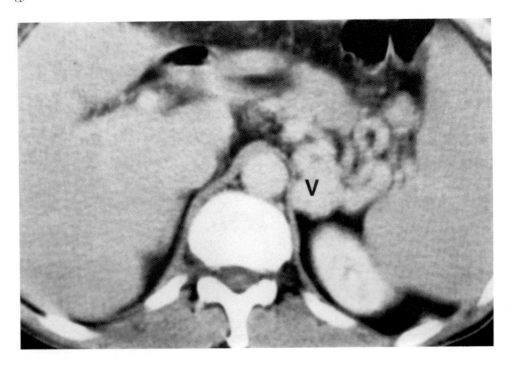

ation of some of the etiologies of an adrenal pseudotumor may help avoid these pitfalls.

Lesions that may simulate an adrenal mass on either side include an exophytic renal mass. A right-sided adrenal mass may be mimicked by an hepatic mass, interposition of the colon into the hepatorenal recess, or a dilated inferior vena cava.

Left-sided adrenal pseudotumors are more common.

They include splenic lobulations, an accessory spleen, varices (Fig. 13.36), tortuous splenic vessels and a splenic artery aneurysm. The tail of the pancreas may extend to the adrenal area and mimic a left adrenal lesion. While the stomach should be clearly distinguished by oral contrast material, a gastric diverticulum may present a diagnostic problem (Fig. 13.37).

Careful attention to the adrenal glands and the use of

Figure 13.37. Pseudotumor. A mass (*arrow*) is seen in the region of the left adrenal gland. Subsequent barium study demonstrated this to be a gastric diverticulum.

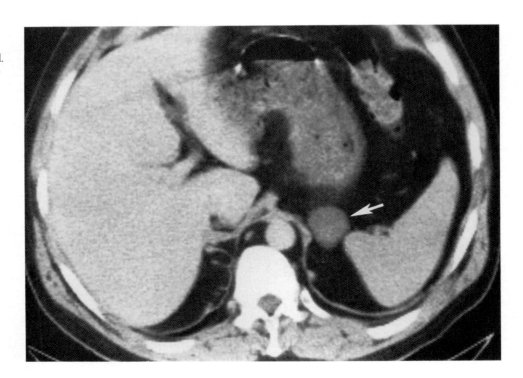

oral contrast should distinguish most confusing structures. A bolus injection of intravenous contrast material should further delineate vascular structures. Repeat sections with narrow collimation may also help to elucidate the true nature of these lesions. If the diagnosis is still in doubt, however, an additional study such as US or MRI may be needed for a confident diagnosis.

SUGGESTED READINGS

Functional Diseases

Conn JW: Primary aldosteronism. *J Lab Clin Med* 45:661, 1955.

Doppman JL, Miller DL, Dwyer AJ, et al: Macronodular adrenal hyperplasia in Cushing disease. *Radiology* 166:347, 1988.

Doppman JL, Nieman L, Miller DL, et al: Ectopic adrenocorticotropic hormone syndrome: localization studies in 28 patients. *Radiology* 172:115, 1989.

Dunnick NR: Adrenal imaging: current status. *AJR* 154:927, 1990.

Dunnick NR: The Adrenal Gland. In Tavaras JM, Ferrucci JT (eds): *Radiology: Diagnosis, Imaging, Intervention.* Philadelphia: JB Lippincott, 1988.

Dunnick NR, Doppman JL, Gill JR, et al: Localization of functional adrenal tumors by computed tomography and venous sampling. *Radiology* 142:429, 1982.

Dunnick NR, Doppman JL, Mills SR, et al: Preoperative diagnosis and localization of aldosteronomas by measurement of corticosteroids in adrenal venous blood. *Radiology* 133(2):331, 1979.

Geisinger MA, Zelch MG, Bravo EL, et al: Primary hyperaldosteronism: comparison of CT, adrenal venography and venous sampling. *AJR* 141:299, 1983.

Glazer GM, Francis IR, Quint LE: Progress in clinical radiology. *Invest Radiol* 23:3, 1988.

Kenney PJ, Streeten DP, Anderson GH: Difficulties in the prospective diagnosis of functional adrenal diseases by CT. *Urol Radiol* 8:184, 1986.

Mitty HA, Gendal ES: Modern approach to adrenal masses. *Curr Opinion Radiol* 1:248, 1989.

Miyake H, Maeda H, Tashiro M, et al: CT of adrenal tumors: frequency and clinical significance of low-attenuation lesions. *AJR* 152:1005, 1989.

Moulton JS, Moulton JS: CT of the adrenal glands. *Semin Roentgenol* 23(4):288, 1988.

Adrenal Insufficiency

Doppman JL, Gill JR, Nienhius AW, et al: CT findings in Addison's disease. *J Comput Assist Tomogr* 6(4):757, 1982.

Eason RJ, Croxson MS, Perry MC, et al: Addison's disease, adrenal autoantibodies and computerized adrenal tomography. *NZ Med J* 95(714):569, 1982.

Ling D, Korobkin M, Silverman PM, et al: CT demonstration of bilateral adrenal hemorrhage. *AJR* 141:307, 1983.

Seidenwurm DJ, Elmer EB, Kaplan LM, et al: Metastases to the adrenal glands and the development of Addison's disease. *Cancer* (Phila) 54:552, 1984.

Wilson DA, Muchmore HG, Tisdal RG, et al: Histoplasmosis of the adrenal glands studied by CT. *Radiology* 150:779, 1984.

Pheochromocytoma

Cho KJ, Freier DT, McCormick TL, et al: Adrenal medullary disease in multiple endocrine neoplasia type II. *AJR* 134:23, 1980.

Reinig JW, Doppman JL, Dwyer AJ, et al: Adrenal masses differentiated by MR. *Radiology* 158:81, 1986.

Swensen SJ, Brown ML, Sheps SG, et al: Use of ^{131}I-MIBG scintigraphy in the evaluation of suspected pheochromocytoma. *Mayo Clin Proc* 60:299, 1985.

Welch TJ, Sheedy PF, II, van Heerden JA, et al: Pheochromocytoma: value of computed tomography. *Radiology* 148:501, 1983.

Neuroblastoma

Amundson GM, Trevenen CL, Mueller DL, et al: Neuroblastoma: a specific sonographic tissue pattern. *AJR* 148:943, 1987.

Dietrich RB, Kangarloo H, Lenarsky C, et al: Neuroblastoma: the role of MR imaging. *AJR* 148:937, 1987.

Adenoma

Bernardino ME: Management of the asymptomatic patient with a unilateral adrenal mass. *Radiology* 166:121, 1988.

Chang A, Glazer HS, Lee JKT, et al: Adrenal gland: MR imaging. *Radiology* 163:123, 1987.

Chezmar JL, Robbins SM, Nelson RC, et al: Adrenal masses: characterization with T1-weighted MR imaging. *Radiology* 166:357, 1988.

Commons RR, Callaway CP: Adenomas of the adrenal cortex. *Arch Intern Med* 81:37, 1948.

Glazer GM, Woolsey EJ, Borrello J, et al: Adrenal tissue characterization using MR imaging. *Radiology* 158(1):73, 1986.

Glazer HS, Weyman PJ, Segal SS, et al: Nonfunctioning adrenal masses: incidental discovery on computed tomography. *AJR* 139:81, 1982.

Katz RL, Shirkhoda A: Diagnostic approach to incidental adrenal nodules in the cancer patient. *Cancer* 55:1995, 1985.

Mitnick JS, Bosniak MA, Megibow AJ, et al: Nonfunctioning adrenal adenomas discovered incidentally on computed tomography. *Radiology* 148:495, 1983.

Reinig JW, Doppman JL, Dwyer AJ, et al: MRI of indeterminate adrenal masses. *AJR* 147:493, 1986.

Remer EM, Weinfield RM, Glazer GM, et al: Hyperfunctioning and nonhyperfunctioning benign adrenal cortical lesions: characterization and comparison with MR imaging. *Radiology* 171:681, 1989.

Carcinoma

Bodie B, Novick AC, Pontes JE, et al: The Cleveland Clinic experience with adrenal cortical carcinoma. *J Urol* 141:257, 1989.

Dunnick NR, Doppman JL, Geelhoed GW: Intravenous extension of endocrine tumors. *AJR* 135:471, 1980.

Dunnick NR, Heaston D, Halvorsen R, et al: CT appearance of adrenal cortical carcinoma. *J Comput Assist Tomogr* 6(5):978, 1982.

Fishman EK, Deutch BM, Hartman DS, et al: Primary adrenocortical carcinoma: CT evaluation with clinical correlation. *AJR* 148:531, 1987.

Hamper UM, Fishman EK, Hartman DS, et al: Primary adrenocortical carcinoma: sonographic evaluation with clinical and pathologic correlation in 26 patients. *AJR* 148:915, 1987.

Hutter AM, Kayhoe DE: Adrenal cortical carcinoma. *Am J Med* 41:572, 1966.

Smith SM, Patel SK, Turner DA, et al: Magnetic resonance imaging of adrenal cortical carcinoma. *Urol Radiol* 11:1, 1989.

Myelolipoma

Dieckmann KP, Hamm B, Pickartz H, et al: Adrenal myelolipoma: clinical, radiologic and histologic features. *Urology* 29(1):1, 1987.

Gould JD, Mitty HA, Pertsemlidis D, et al: Adrenal myelolipoma: diagnosis by fine-needle aspiration. *AJR* 148:921, 1987.

Greene KM, Brantly PN, Thompson WR: Adenocarcinoma metastatic to the adrenal gland simulating myelolipoma: CT evaluation. *J Comput Assist Tomogr* 9(4):820, 1985.

Musante F, Derchi LE, Zappasodi F, et al: Myelolipoma of the adrenal gland: sonographic and CT features. *AJR* 151:961, 1988.

Vick CW, Zeman RK, Mannes E, et al: Adrenal myelolipoma: CT and ultrasound findings. *Urol Radiol* 6:7, 1984.

Hemorrhage

Bowen A, Kesler PJ, Newman B, Hashide Y: Adrenal hemorrhage after liver transplantation. *Radiology* 176:85, 1990.

Itoh K, Yamashita K, Satoh Y, et al: MR imaging of bilateral adrenal hemorrhage. *J Comput Assist Tomogr* 12(6):1054, 1988.

Khuri FJ, Alton DJ, Hardy BE, et al: Adrenal hemorrhage in neonates: report of 5 cases and review of the literature. *J Urol* 124:684, 1980.

Ling D, Korobkin M, Silverman PM, et al: CT demonstration of bilateral adrenal hemorrhage. *AJR* 141:307, 1983.

Murphy BJ, Casillas J, Yrizarry JM: Traumatic adrenal hemorrhage radiologic findings. *Radiology* 169:701, 1988.

Cysts

Cheema P, Cartagena R, Staubitz W: Adrenal cysts: diagnosis and treatment. *J Urol* 126:396, 1981.

Ghandur-Mnaymneh L, Slim M, Muakassa K: Adrenal cysts: pathogenesis and histological identification with a report of 6 cases. *J Urol* 122:87, 1979.

Johnson CD, Baker ME, Dunnick NR: CT demonstration of an adrenal pseudocyst. *J Comput Assist Tomogr* 9(4):817, 1985.

Tung GA, Pfister RC, Papanicolaou N, Yoder IC: Adrenal cysts: imaging and percutaneous aspiration. *Radiology* 173:107, 1989.

Hemangioma

Derchi LE, Rapaccini GL, Banderali A, et al: Ultrasound and CT findings in two cases of hemangioma of the adrenal gland. *J Comput Assist Tomogr* 13(4):659, 1989.

Metastases

Abrams HL, Spiro R, Goldstein N: Metastases in carcinoma: analysis of 1,000 autopsied cases. *Cancer* (Phila) 3:74, 1950.

Baker ME, Blinder R, Spritzer C, et al: MR evaluation of adrenal masses at 1.5 T. *AJR* 153:307, 1989.

Berland LL, Koslin DB, Kenney PJ, et al: Differentiation between small benign and malignant adrenal masses with dynamic incremented CT. *AJR* 151:95, 1988.

Bernardino ME, Walther MM, Phillips VM, et al: CT-guided adrenal biopsy: accuracy, safety and indications. *AJR* 144:67, 1985.

Casola G, Nicolet V, vanSonnenberg E, et al: Unsuspected pheochromocytoma: risk of blood-pressure alterations during percutaneous adrenal biopsy. *Radiology* 156:733, 1986.

Dunnick NR: CT and MRI of adrenal lesions. *Urol Radiol* 10:12, 1988.

Francis IR, Smid A, Gross MD, et al: Adrenal masses in oncologic patients: functional and morphologic evaluation. *Radiology* 166:353, 1988.

Kier R, McCarthy S: MR characterization of adrenal masses: field strength and pulse sequence considerations. *Radiology* 171:671, 1989.

Koenker RM, Mueller PR, vanSonnenberg E: Interventional radiology of the adrenal glands. *Semin Roentgenol* 22(4):314, 1988.

Oliver TW Jr, Bernardino ME, Miller JI, et al: Isolated adrenal masses in nonsmall-cell bronchogenic carcinoma. *Radiology* 153:217, 1984.

Pagani JJ: Non-small cell lung carcinoma adrenal metastases: computed tomography and percutaneous needle biopsy in their diagnosis. *Cancer* (Phila) 53:1058, 1984.

Whitney W, Dunnick NR: Biopsy techniques in uroradiology. *Radiology Rep* 2:302, 1990.

Lymphoma

Paling MR, Williamson BRJ: Adrenal involvement in non-Hodgkin lymphoma. *AJR* 141:303, 1983.

Pseudotumors

Berliner L, Bosniak MA, Megibow A: Adrenal pseudotumors on computed tomography. *J Comput Assist Tomogr* 6(2):281, 1982.

THE URETER

The ureter is a thin-walled muscular organ whose principal function is the transport of urine from the kidney to the bladder. Radiologic studies are the primary method by which suspected morphologic abnormalities of the ureter are evaluated and also play an important role in the evaluation of functional abnormalities of the ureter.

BASIC PHYSIOLOGY

Transport of urine through the ureter is a result of both active and passive forces. Passive transport occurs as a result of hydrostatic pressure in the collecting system generated as a result of glomerular ultrafiltration. Active urine transport occurs because of peristalsis. Peristaltic activity in the renal collecting system arises at pacemaker sites located at the junction of the minor and major calyces. In the renal pelvis, there is a gradual rise in intrapelvic pressure that peaks when the electrical activity generated at the calyceal pacing sites spreads to the renal pelvis. At normal urine production rates, however, further spread of the pelvic contraction is blocked at the ureteropelvic junction (UPJ). This mechanism is thought to protect the renal pelvis and kidney from the pressure effects of ureteral peristalsis as the bolus of urine is transported down the ureter.

The existence of a discrete pacemaker center in the proximal ureter remains controversial. It is known, however, that there is electrical activity in the proximal ureter that results in peristaltic activity. As renal pelvic pressure increases, urine is expelled into the proximal ureter, which is initially in a collapsed state. Urine is then formed into a bolus between two successive contractile waves and is propelled down the ureter in this form.

A baseline pressure that varies between 0 and 5 cm of water is present in the ureter. Superimposed on this baseline pressure is the pressure of each peristaltic wave, which varies between 20 and 60 cm H_2O. The ureterovesicle junction acts as a one-way valve, allowing urine to enter the bladder, but not in reverse. As the rate of urine flow increases, there is an increase in both the frequency of the peristaltic waves and in the volume of each bolus, however, the speed of the individual contractile waves does not increase. At high urine flow rates, urine transport in the form of discrete boluses ceases, but instead becomes a continuous column. At this point, the mean intraluminal ureteral pressure rises, so that it equals the peak pressure in the peristaltic wave. A rise in renal pelvic pressure follows. Urine transport through the ureter becomes inadequate when either too much fluid per unit time enters the ureter or too little fluid per unit time exits the ureter. In either case, stasis and subsequent dilatation of the ureter occur. A dilated ureter in turn cannot generate as efficient a contractile wave as can a nondilated ureter. A minor degree of obstruction will cause more dilatation at a high flow rate than at a lower flow rate.

While ureteral peristalsis is known to occur in a denervated state, there is evidence that ureteral peristalsis is modulated by the influence of the autonomic nervous system, however, the exact role the nervous system plays in ureteral function is not known.

ACUTE OBSTRUCTION

Pathophysiology

The degree to which renal function is permanently impaired by ureteral obstruction depends on the degree of the obstruction, the length of time the obstruction has been present, and the degree to which other factors, such as infection, complicate the obstruction. Initially, there is a rise in renal blood flow that is followed by a rise in ureteral pressure; as obstruction continues, both renal blood flow and ureteral pressure decline. There is a corresponding decrease in the glomerular filtration rate (GFR), as it is dependent on the difference between the glomerular capillary pressure and the sum of the colloid osmotic pressure of the plasma and the intratubular pressure.

The development of hydronephrosis is strong evidence that there is continued urine formation even in the face of complete ureteral obstruction. The primary mechanism by which the kidney allows the continued formation of new urine is the resorption of already formed urine. This resorption, termed *renal backflow*, has four major components, *pyelolymphatic backflow, pyelovenous backflow, pyelotubular backflow,* and *pyelosinus backflow*.

Pyelovenous backflow (Fig. 14.1) is thought to represent the most important route of backflow quantitatively in acute ureteral obstruction. Experimentally, renal pelvic pressures in excess of 100 cm H_2O are needed to establish this route of urine resorption, however, once established, much lower pressures are required to maintain it. Pyelovenous backflow is thought to occur at the fornices of the calyces where formed urine enters the venous plexus that surrounds the calyx. According to Hinman, after the second week of obstruction, histologic changes occur in the fornices that diminish the role of

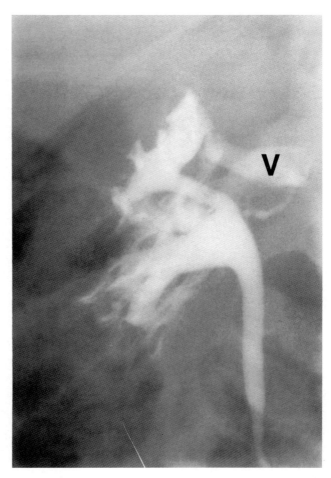

Figure 14.1. Pyelovenous backflow. Contrast is seen in the renal vein (V) as well as the lymphatics and renal sinus during this retrograde pyelogram.

pyelovenous backflow, at which time pyelotubular backflow becomes relatively more important as a protective mechanism for the kidney. Pyelovenous backflow is rarely demonstrated on urography or retrograde pyelography because the high flow rate in the veins dilutes the contrast material too quickly for it to be visualized.

Pyelotubular backflow (Fig. 14.2) begins to occur after the onset of hydronephrosis is well established. High intrapelvic pressures allow opening of the normally closed papillary ducts and thus the flow of urine back into the renal tubules. Pyelotubular backflow may be demonstrated on retrograde pyelography and urography when high intrapelvic pressures are present.

Pyelolymphatic backflow (Fig. 14.3) may occasionally be visualized on retrograde pyelograms as small serpiginous channels that course toward the renal hilus. Pyelolymphatic backflow is thought to supplement pyelovenous backflow, but in smaller volumes. *Pyelosinus backflow* (Figs. 14.4 and 14.7) can be readily observed on retrograde pyelography or on urography in the presence of acute ureteral obstruction. This phenomenon occurs when there is rupture of a fornix or fornices of the minor

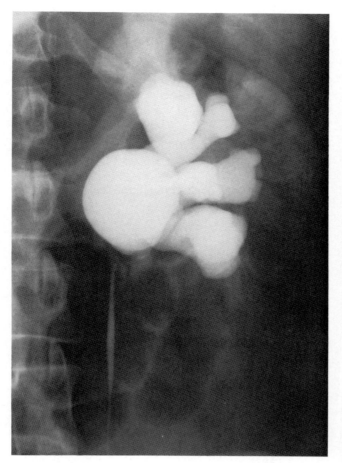

Figure 14.2. Pyelotubular backflow. A retrograde pyelogram demonstrates streaky collections of contrast material in the distal collecting ducts extending from the minor calyces.

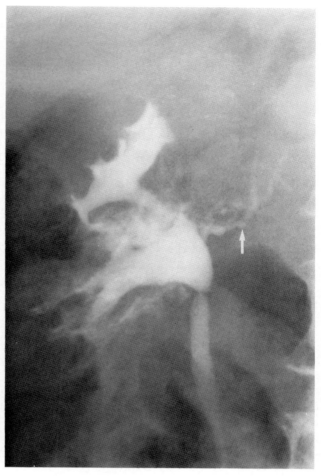

Figure 14.3. Pyelolymphatic backflow. Retrograde pyelogram demonstrating filling of lymphatic channels (*arrow*).

Figure 14.4. Pyelosinus extravasation. A CT scan demonstrates a collection of extravasated contrast material (*arrow*) adjacent to the renal pelvis in a patient with distal ureteral obstruction.

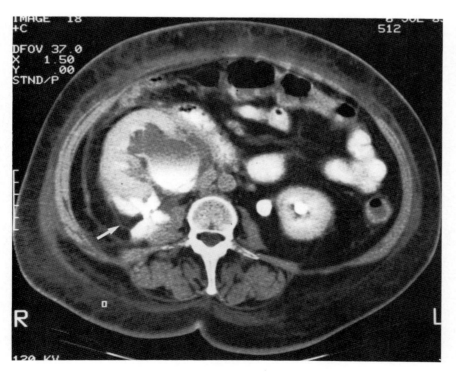

calyces and is demonstrated as a collection of contrast material that surrounds the renal hilus in the perinephric space. Occasionally, pyelosinus extravasation is demonstrated when tight ureteral compression is utilized during urography. Pyelosinus extravasation serves to decompress the renal pelvis when urine escapes into the perinephric space, where resorption takes place. Occasionally, a uriniferous pseudocyst (urinoma) (Fig. 14.5) forms as a result of this extravasation.

Imaging Studies

Elkin has investigated radiologic findings during urography in patients with acute ureteral obstruction. The affected kidney is usually enlarged. Initially, there is a diminished nephrogram, but on delayed radiographs there is a striking progressively intensifying nephrogram that is much more intense than normal. This phenomenon has been referred to as the "obstructive nephrogram." In some cases the nephrogram has a striated appearance thought to be related to increased opacification of the medullary rays—the loops of Henle and the cortical collecting ducts (Fig. 14.6). The appearance of contrast material in the collecting system is delayed, sometimes for as long as 24 hours after the injection of the contrast material. When the pyelogram is visualized, dilatation of the calyces and pelvis is usually present, even when the obstruction is of relatively short duration.

In studies on patients with acute obstruction secondary to ureteral calculi, Elkin was not able to relate the intensity of the nephrogram or the degree to which filling of the collecting system was delayed to the length of time that the obstruction was present. He speculated that this inability was related to the fact that judging the time of onset of the obstruction from the time the patient first experiences ureteral colic is unreliable.

In animal experiments performed in rabbits with surgically induced ureteral ligation, Elkin et al. were able to demonstrate that the obstructive nephrogram was still intense when the radiologic studies were performed as much as 6 hours after the onset of obstruction and that there was a progressive diminution in the intensity of the nephrogram as the period of ureteral obstruction increased. After 20 days of obstruction, only a faint nephrogram was produced in this animal model.

The pathophysiology responsible for the obstructive nephrogram has not been completely explained. Some authorities believe that increasing tubular distention that allows an increase in the volume of contrast material within each tubule is primarily responsible for this phenomenon. Others cite the fact that sodium and water resorption in the proximal tubule is increased during ureteral obstruction; this in turn increases the concentration of the contrast in the tubular lumen.

Ultrasound (US) has not proven to be as reliable as urography for the detection of acute ureteral obstruction. In a study of 20 patients with proven acute ureteral obstruction secondary to ureteral calculi, Laing et al. found that sonography depicted the collecting system as being normal in 35% (Fig. 14.7). In a prospective study, Hill et al. found that urography achieved a correct diagnosis in 85% of patients with acute flank pain; sonography was correct in 66%. The inaccuracy of sonography in this regard is related to the purely anatomic nature of the US study; in early obstruction caliectasis may not as yet have

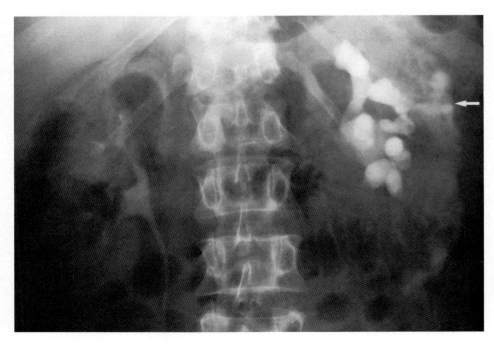

Figure 14.5. Urinoma. A discrete extracalyceal collection of contrast material (*arrow*) is present in this patient with ureteral obstruction secondary to a calculus.

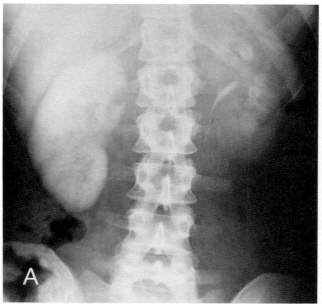

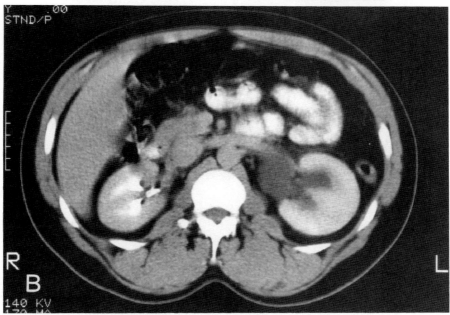

Figure 14.6. Obstructive nephrogram. **A,** A delayed film from an IVP demonstrates an obstructive nephrogram on the right with a striated appearance related to increased opacifica-tion of the medullary rays. **B,** Computed tomography scan showing an obstructive nephrogram on the left with nonopaci-fied urine filling the calyces and renal pelvis.

developed and thus the sonogram is falsely negative. Urography has the advantage of demonstrating both ana-tomic and functional information in patients with acute ureteral obstruction; furthermore, the diuresis produced by the contrast material enhances the amount of dilata-tion detected on the urographic study.

The precise length of time that the kidney can tolerate periods of acute ureteral obstruction without permanent loss of function is not known. Vaughn and Gillenwater demonstrated that in dogs complete return of function was possible with periods of ureteral obstruction ranging up to 7 days; after 28 days of obstruction, renal function recovered to only 30% of its baseline value. The corre-sponding periods in humans are not known; however, in patients suffering iatrogenic ureteral injury, return of re-nal function has been described for periods of obstruc-tion ranging up to several months.

Etiology of Acute Obstruction

The most common cause of acute ureteral obstruction is a calculus lodged in the ureter. These calculi, which are formed in the kidney, tend to obstruct at the UPJ; the

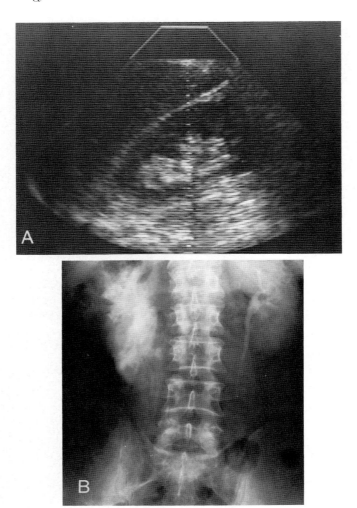

Figure 14.7. **A,** An ultrasound examination shows no evidence of right hydronephrosis. **B,** An IVP performed a few hours later demonstrates extensive pyelosinus extravasation in a patient with acute ureteral obstruction secondary to a ureteral calculus.

pelvic brim, where the ureter crosses the iliac blood vessels; or at the ureterovesical junction (UVJ) (Fig. 14.8). The UVJ is the most common site at which calculi become lodged as it is the narrowest part in the ureter; this region must be carefully scrutinized so small stones are not overlooked. With passage of the stone, there is almost immediate resolution of the evidence of acute obstruction on urography; the persistence of the obstructive nephrogram even when the calculus can no longer be identified is strong evidence of ongoing acute obstruction. Passage of a small calculus during urography is not uncommon as the diuretic effect of the contrast facilitates its passage. Under such circumstances, the patient reports the sudden resolution of the pain associated with the calculus and on a delayed radiograph, sudden resolution of the previously present obstructive nephrogram. There may be filling of the entire ureter with contrast material on such a film; this has been attributed to a transient decrease in ureteral peristalsis associated with the stone's passage.

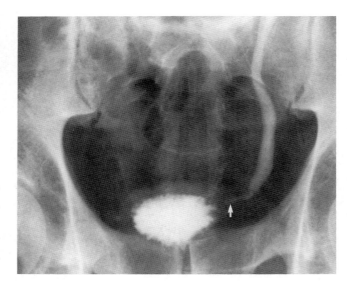

Figure 14.8. Distal ureteral calculus. A film of the bladder shows a dilated left ureter from a stone (*arrow*) impacted at the ureterovesicle junction.

Blood clots that form in the kidney may cause acute ureteral obstruction in a fashion similar to that produced by calculi. In these cases, the findings are identical to those produced by a nonopaque calculus. Other intraluminal filling defects that may cause acute ureteral obstruction include sloughed papillae and fungus balls.

Acute ureteral trauma, especially iatrogenic ureteral injury, may produce acute ureteral obstruction. These injuries are discussed in Chapter 12.

CHRONIC OBSTRUCTION AND OBSTRUCTIVE RENAL ATROPHY

As obstruction continues for periods of weeks or months, there is a reversal of many of the physiologic changes associated with acute ureteral obstruction. There is a reduction in renal blood flow and a concomitant reduction in glomerular filtration pressure. This and the decompressive mechanisms described earlier lead to progressive reduction in intraluminal pressures such that, in chronic obstruction, baseline intraluminal pressure is once again present. Ureteral peristalsis returns, albeit in a less forceful state. This reduction in peristalsis, coupled with dilatation of the ureter, makes coaptation of the ureteral walls during peristalsis difficult and there is a decreased rise in intraluminal pressure associated with each contraction. To some extent, these factors may be partially offset by hypertrophy of the smooth muscle of the ureter.

As obstruction continues, there is progressive atrophy of the renal parenchyma as a result of increased backpressure. The ureter becomes progressively more dilated, tortuous, and elongated. When sufficient renal function is present to excrete contrast material on urography, the cortex may be demonstrated as a thin rim of opacified parenchyma surrounding dilated, nonopacified calyces. This finding is frequently referred to as the "rim" sign. A "crescent" of increased density may be present adjacent to the dilated calyces representing contrast material in dilated, displaced collecting ducts. On delayed films, excretion of the contrast material into the calyces results in the obliteration of the crescents. The appearance of the unopacified calyces adjacent to the rims of enhanced parenchyma is sometimes referred to as representing a "negative pyelogram" (Fig. 14.9**A**).

Sonography has proven to be highly reliable in the detection of chronic ureteral obstruction by the demonstration of hydronephrosis (Fig. 14.9**B**). Ellenbogen et al. demonstrated a sensitivity of 98% for this modality in the detection of hydronephrosis when compared to urography. When patients with relatively acute obstruction were excluded, the sensitivity of ultrasonography in this setting was 100%; however, the false-positive rate was 26%. In a separate study, patients with azotemia were screened for the presence of obstruction with sonog-

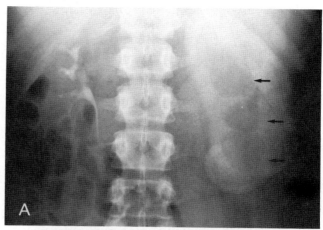

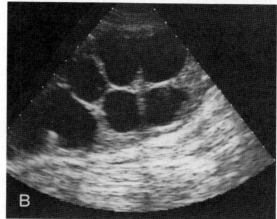

Figure 14.9. Negative pyelogram. **A,** An IVP demonstrates large, relatively radiolucent defects (*arrows*) in the nephrogram of a patient with chronic ureteral obstruction representing dilated but unopacified calyces. **B,** An ultrasound scan confirms that marked hydronephrosis is present.

raphy. Ninety-three percent of the obstructed kidneys were correctly identified with US; the false-positive rate was 7%. False-positive studies indicating the presence of obstruction, when none in fact is present, have been reported by Amis et al. in 10–26% of patients in whom hydronephrosis is detected sonographically. This is not surprising since a variety of conditions, i.e., vesicoureteral reflux, a parapelvic renal cyst, or an extrarenal pelvis may produce or mimic dilatation of the renal collecting system in the absence of acute obstruction. In addition, cases of obstruction producing renal failure in the absence of detectable hydronephrosis by sonography have occasionally been reported.

Angiography demonstrates compression of the interlobar arteries and the arcuate arteries become stretched by the adjacent calyceal dilatation. The main renal artery may have a diminished diameter related to the loss of cortex, however, the orifice of the artery retains a normal caliber. The extent of the angiographic changes depend on the degree and duration of the obstruction. These changes, however, lead to progressive renal ischemia which is a component of backpressure atrophy.

The radiologic features of postobstructive renal atrophy have been described by Hodson and Craven. There is a loss of renal cortex associated with calyceal clubbing which is relatively uniform throughout the kidney (Fig. 14.10). There is a variable degree of dilatation of the renal pelvis and ureter, which is largely dependent on the length of time the obstruction was present. In addition, patients with extrarenal pelves generally demonstrate more dilatation than do those with intrarenal pelves. The overall size of the kidney is reduced and there is a variable amount of excretion on urography which largely depends on the amount of renal damage that is present. This process may be difficult to separate

from pyelonephritic scarring, but the latter process is generally much more focal in nature, while postobstructive atrophy tends to affect the calyces more uniformly.

There are numerous causes of chronic ureteral obstruction (Table 14.1). Some of these conditions are discussed in the remainder of this chapter, while others are found in Chapters 2, 15, and 16.

While urography and retrograde ureteral studies are usually sufficient to establish the etiology of chronic ureteral obstruction, Bosniak et al. have shown that CT is very helpful in those cases where the etiology of the obstruction remains obscure. In a series of 33 such cases, CT established the correct diagnosis in almost 92%. Most of the cases in this series involved obstruction secondary to a variety of metastatic neoplasms, but in addition such studies were of value in a variety of benign diseases as well.

THE DILATED URETER

A variety of different terms have been applied to the finding of abnormal caliber of the ureter including megaloureter, megaureter, dilatation of the ureter, and the

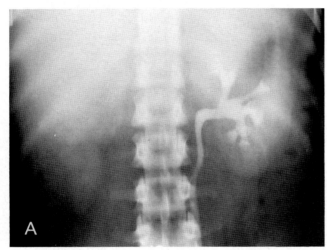

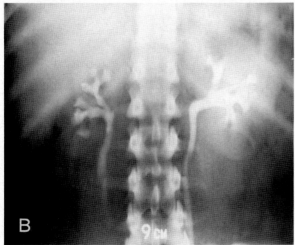

Figure 14.10. Obstructive atrophy. **A,** An IVP demonstrates a faint nephrogram on the right in a patient with long-standing ureteral obstruction. **B,** A follow-up IVP 1 year following relief of the obstruction shows global shrinkage of the right kidney with a minor degree of dilatation of the right collecting system and ureter.

Table 14.1
Etiology of Chronic Ureteral Obstruction

Congenital lesions
    Ureteropelvic junction obstruction
    Ectopic Ureterocele
Inflammatory conditions
    Tuberculosis
    Schistosomiasis
    Crohn's disease
    Pelvic inflammatory disease
    Pelvic abscess
Trauma
Tumors
    Primary ureteral tumors
    Retroperitoneal tumors
    Lymphadenopathy
    Metastases
Miscellaneous
    Ovarian vein syndrome ($\pm$)
    Primary megaureter
    Pregnancy
    Retroperitoneal fibrosis
    Lymphocele
    Urinoma
    Calculus
    Iliac artery aneurysm
    Uterine prolapse
Lower urinary tract conditions
    Bladder tumor
    Neurogenic bladder
    Inflammatory lesions of the bladder
    Benign prostatic hypertrophy
    Prostate cancer
    Pelvic lipomatosis
    Urethral obstruction

widened ureter. King has suggested the use of the term *megaureter* to describe any ureter that is found to be dilated. The generic term, megaureter, is then divided into three etiologic categories: (*a*) the *refluxing megaureter*, (*b*) the *obstructed megaureter*, and (*c*) the *non-refluxing-nonobstructed megaureter*. Each of these major categories is then further divided into primary and secondary subgroupings.

Primary refluxing megaureter is the term used to describe a wide ureter secondary to vesicoureteral reflux, when an abnormality of the ureteral orifice is the cause of the reflux. This entity, therefore, represents the usual form of vesicoureteral reflux, found primarily in children. Vesicoureteral reflux is discussed in detail in Chapter 11. A *secondary refluxing megaureter* may occur when the reflux is thought to be related to an abnormality of the bladder or urethra, such as reflux secondary to neurogenic bladder disease.

Primary obstructed megaureter, also known as *primary megaureter*, is thought to be related to an intrinsic abnormality of the distal ureter, such that a functional obstruction may be present. A *secondary obstructed megaureter* is present when there is any cause of ureteral obstruction not related to an adynamic ureteral segment; the various etiologies of secondary ureteral obstruction have been discussed in the preceding sections.

The *primary nonrefluxing-nonobstructed megaureter* is uncommon, but the term may be utilized to characterize a dilated ureter not related to either obstruction or reflux; an example is the dilatation of the ureter typically present in patients with Eagle-Barrett syndrome. Secondary nonrefluxing-nonobstructed megaureters are also uncommon but include those ureters that remain dilated after correction of the pathology that was initially responsible for the ureteral dilatation. A widened ureter that remains after surgical correction of vesicoureteral reflux, for example, can be considered to represent a secondary nonrefluxing-nonobstructed megaureter. Ureteral dilatation that occurs secondary to an increased urine flow rate, such as that seen in patients with diabetes insipidus, is also classified in this category.

There is an occasional patient in whom this classification fails. Patients have been described in whom obstruction demonstrated by ureteral perfusion studies and vesicoureteral reflux are present at the same time.

The *primary obstructed megaureter* (PM) is of particular interest. This entity is known by a variety of different, often confusing synonyms, including primary megaureter, primary megaloureter, and congenital megaureter. In some series, the entity is referred to as primary *non*obstructive megaureter, a reference to the fact that no anatomic cause for the obstruction is present, and there is no resistance to the passage of a retrograde catheter on cystoscopic cannulation of the ureteral orifice. There is, however, a functional obstruction of the juxtavesicle ureter, with failure to transmit normal peristalsis. There is a characteristic beak-like configuration of the distal ureteral segment on radiographic examination. Typically there is dilatation of the ureter proximal to the adynamic segment. Because the abnormal segment is the aperistaltic normal-caliber distal ureter, and the dilatation of the proximal ureter is a response of the normal ureter to this functional obstruction, the abnormalities in the ureter have been compared to Hirschsprung's disease in the colon. Pfister and Hendren have classified such cases on the basis of the degree of dilatation of the proximal ureter that is present. In Grade 1 (Fig. 14.11), the dilatation is limited to the distal ureteral segment; in Grade 2 (Fig. 14.12), the dilation extends into the proximal ureter and there may be mild caliectasis; in Grade 3 (Fig. 14.13), the entire ureter is dilated proximal to the adynamic segment and there is moderate to severe caliectasis. In contrast to ureters with secondary obstruction, there is characteristically no tortuosity of the ureter in cases of PM, despite the dilatation.

Primary megaureter has been reported in both children and in adults. In mild cases, the patient is typically asymptomatic and the diagnosis is established when urography is performed for another indication. In those with symptoms referable to the urinary tract, infection, pain, and hematuria have been reported in association with PM. In Pfister and Hendren's series, other urinary anomalies including contralateral UPJ obstruction, renal agenesis or ectopia, and ureteral duplication were present in 40% of the cases. Ipsilateral ureteral calculi may be the presenting complaint in adults. The abnormality was unilateral in approximately two-thirds of the cases; the remaining patients had bilateral PMs. In most

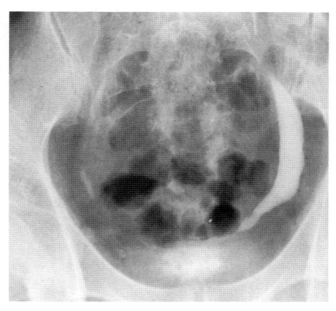

Figure 14.11. Primary megaureter—Grade 1.

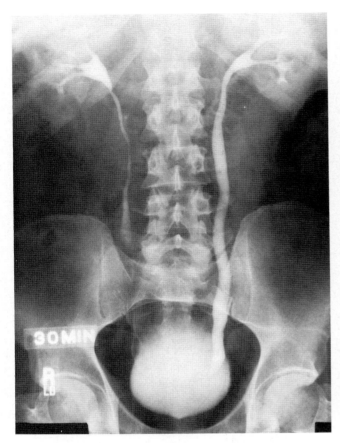

Figure 14.12. Primary megaureter—Grade 2.

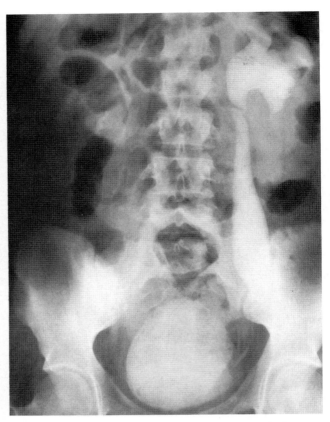

Figure 14.13. Primary megaureter—Grade 3.

such cases, there is equal severity of involvement on the two sides. Approximately two-thirds of the reported patients have been males; however, in one of the reported series there was a female predominance.

The diagnosis of PM is usually established by urography. In mild cases, there is prompt filling of the ureter which demonstrates the characteristic beak-like configuration of the distal ureteral segment. When this segment is not visualized or there is confusion with secondary ureteral obstruction, the abnormal segment may be visualized on retrograde pyelography. Voiding cystourethrography should be performed in every case to exclude dilatation secondary to vesicoureteral reflux. Radionuclide diuretic renography may also be performed to establish whether functionally significant ureteral obstruction is present. Ureteral perfusion studies typically demonstrate normal or minimally abnormal findings in cases of mild PM; in more severe cases, abnormal perfusion pressures are typically present with gradients between renal pelvic and bladder pressures as high as 35–40 cm H_2O. In addition to the radiologic studies, most urologists feel that cystoscopy should be performed; this can be done in conjunction with retrograde pyelography, when indicated.

TUMORS

Tumors may arise from any of the constituent components of the ureter or may involve the ureter secondary to a neoplasm elsewhere. Primary ureteral tumors are relatively rare, accounting for approximately 1% of all urinary tract tumors. Primary ureteral tumors either arise from the ureteral epithelium or from nonepithelial (mesodermal) tissue; each may present with either malignant or benign neoplasms. Ureteral neoplasms occur twice as frequently in males as in females; the right ureter, for unexplained reasons, is more commonly involved than the left. Most primary neoplasms involve the distal one-third of the ureter and are found in patients between the ages of 50 and 80 years.

Epithelial Tumors

Epithelial neoplasms account for 75% of all primary ureteral neoplasms. The most common of these lesions is *transitional cell carcinoma*, which is usually divided according to its histologic characteristics into papillary and nonpapillary subtypes.

Papillary tumors (80%) tend to be multicentric, producing multiple filling defects in the ureter. In 40% of the patients, the tumor may be found to have extended into the periureteral tissues at the time of presentation; metastases to the regional lymph nodes or hematogenous spread to distant sites, including the liver or the bones, may also occur. An associated transitional cell carcinoma of the bladder is found in 25% of the patients, however, as many as 70% have a history of an antecedent or a subsequent urothelial lesion elsewhere in the urinary tract. It is for this reason that complete nephroureterectomy is the standard therapy for lesions that are resectable at the time of diagnosis. The nonpapillary varieties tend to be solitary lesions but almost always are found to have infiltrated the submucosa at the time of presentation.

Transitional cell carcinomas of the ureter are staged as follows: *stage I*, the tumor is limited to the urothelial mucosa; *stage II*, invasion to the level of the ureteral muscle; *stage III*, invasion of the periureteral tissues; *stage IV*, distant metastasis. In addition to surgical stage of the lesion, the prognosis also depends on histologic characteristics of the tumor according to Broder's classification (see Chapter 15).

Pain and hematuria are the most common presenting features. As many as 40% of the patients are said to present with a nonfunctioning kidney on urography because of long-standing ureteral obstruction. When there is excretion of sufficient contrast medium to demonstrate the ureter, the lesion is present as a solitary filling defect in the lumen of the ureter (Fig. 14.14) or as a series of

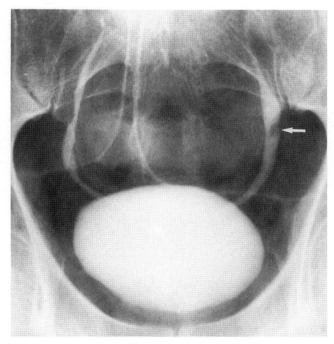

Figure 14.14. Transitional cell carcinoma of the ureter. A solitary defect (*arrow*) is present in the distal left ureter in this patient with a history of previous transitional cell carcinoma of the bladder.

polypoid discrete masses within the lumen separated by what appears to be normal ureteral mucosa. The solitary lesions frequently demonstrate slight dilatation of the ureter distal to the lesion (Bergman's sign), which helps differentiate the lesion from such benign filling defects as calculi or blood clots. This finding is said to occur because peristaltic waves cause the lesion to migrate distally on its stalk with each ureteral contraction. The lesion may produce a localized expansion of the ureter which resembles a "champagne glass" or "wine goblet" on retrograde ureterography. When urography fails to demonstrate the lesion, either antegrade or retrograde pyelography allows its demonstration. When the lesion infiltrates the submucosa of the ureter, fixation of the ureter occurs and the lesion will demonstrate an irregular narrowing of the lumen of the ureter with sharp margins which resemble an apple core lesion of the colon. In still other cases, the lesion may resemble a benign stricture of the ureter.

Kenney and Stanley have shown that computed tomography (CT) may be of value in the diagnosis of ureteral neoplasms, particularly in those patients in whom urography or retrograde pyelography is unsuccessful. Computed tomography may also be used to distinguish ureteral tumors from nonopaque ureteral calculi.

Computed tomography is also of value in the preoperative staging of transitional cell carcinoma of the upper urinary tract. Baron et al. showed that CT staging was accurate in demonstrating the absence of periureteral invasion by the tumor in patients with Stage I or II tumors.

Squamous cell carcinoma is the most malignant of the epithelial tumors of the ureter, however, they comprise less than 10% of the malignant ureteral tumors. The lesion is frequently associated with chronic urinary tract infection, and calculi are present in approximately one-half the cases. Most commonly, this tumor presents as a solitary filling defect within the ureter, but there is frequent periureteral invasion, which may be demonstrable by CT, at the time of presentation.

Adenocarcinoma of the ureter is extremely rare. The lesion is thought to arise from the cell nests of von Brunn, the basal layer of the urothelium.

Benign tumors of the urothelium constitute approximately 20% of ureteral neoplasms. The most common of these, the *benign papilloma*, is actually considered to represent a low-grade malignancy by many pathologists. Papillomas generally present as solitary filling defects and are attached to the ureteral wall by a small stalk. A variant of the papilloma, the *inverted papilloma*, is so named because the central core of the lesion is composed of a transitional epithelium rather than the connective tissue stroma of the benign papilloma. The malignant potential of this lesion is not known.

Nonepithelial Tumors

The most common of the nonepithelial tumors of the ureter is the *benign fibrous polyp*, also known as a fibroepithelial polyp. The lesion actually represents a core of fibrous tissue which is covered with normal transitional epithelium. While the lesion is most commonly solitary, multiple polyps within the same ureter have been reported. The tumor has been reported to occur in association with chronic urinary tract infection and, therefore, may be thought of as representing a form of inflammatory polyp. Flank pain and hematuria are common presenting complaints. Typically, on urography, the lesion is mobile owing to its long stalk (Fig. 14.15), and causes a variable degree of ureteral obstruction. Fibrous polyps vary in size from a few millimeters to those that reach up to 13 cm in length. Most have a smooth cylindrical appearance, but on occasion a multilocular or frond-like appearance of the lesion projecting from its stalk has

been reported. In contrast to other ureteral tumors, fibrous polyps are most commonly found in the proximal one-third of the ureter, and typically occur in the 20- to 40-year age group. Other benign mesenchymal ureteral tumors that have been reported include *leiomyomas, hemangiomas*, and *neurofibromas*.

Nonepithelial primary malignant tumors of the ureter are extremely rare; reticulum cell sarcoma, leiomyosarcoma, Hodgkin's disease, melanoma, and carcinosarcoma have all been reported.

Metastatic lesions (Fig. 14.16) involving the ureter are much more common than primary ureteral neoplasms. In most cases obstruction of the ureter occurs because of direct extension of the neoplasm from such primary sites as the ovary, the prostate, and the cervix. Ureteral obstruction may also occur because of adjacent retroperitoneal lymph node enlargement from lymphoma or primary tumors in the gastrointestinal tract, lung or breast. In addition, some tumors invoke an intense periureteral desmoplastic reaction which obliterates the soft tissue planes that normally surround the ureter. In such cases, imaging studies may demonstrate extrinsic compression of the ureter by a soft tissue mass, similar in appearance to retroperitoneal fibrosis. In other instances, however, a

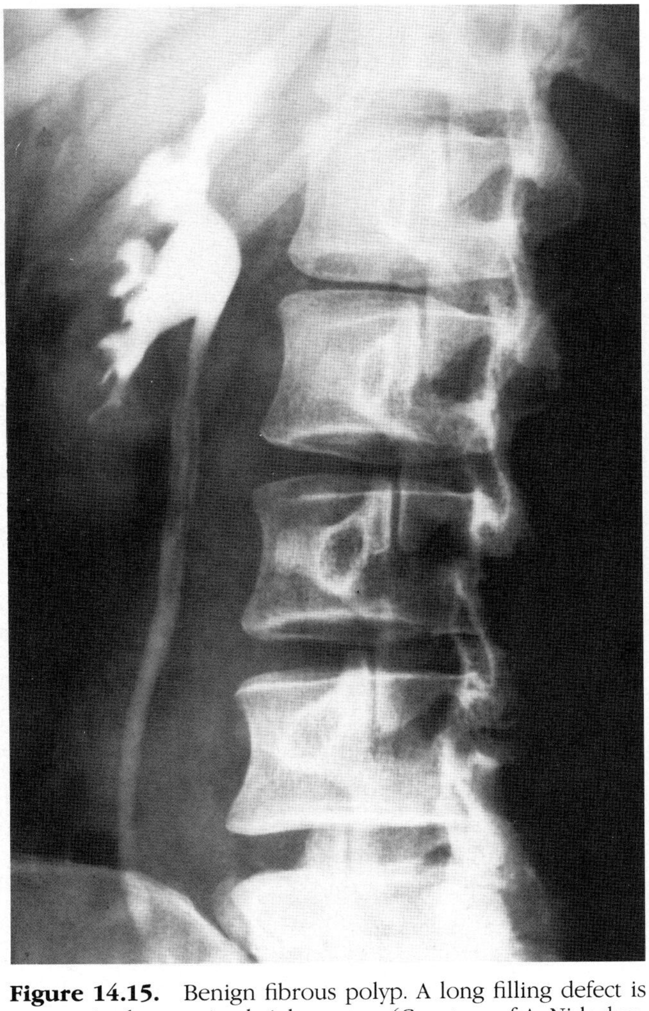

Figure 14.15. Benign fibrous polyp. A long filling defect is present in the proximal right ureter. (Courtesy of A. Nidecker, M.D.)

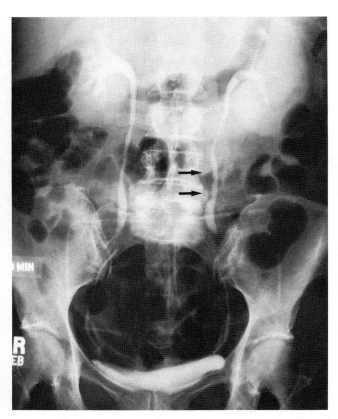

Figure 14.16. Metastatic disease of the ureter. A scalloped appearance of the proximal left ureter representing metastases from a primary gastric cancer is present.

well-defined mass cannot be demonstrated by CT. Barbaric and MacIntosh have shown that CT-guided periureteral biopsy, at the point at which the obstruction is demonstrated, even in the absence of a well-defined mass, may establish the correct diagnosis in some of these patients, but the majority require open surgical exploration.

Much less commonly, a hematogenous metastasis to the ureter, presenting as a solitary filling defect simulating a primary ureteral tumor, will occur. Carcinoma of the breast is the most common primary lesion to metastasize in this manner; however, melanoma, renal cell carcinoma, bronchogenic carcinoma, prostate carcinoma, and multiple myeloma may also present in this fashion.

INFLAMMATORY CONDITIONS

Leukoplakia

Leukoplakia is a rare inflammatory condition of the ureter. Ureteral involvement generally occurs in the proximal one-third of the organ and is almost invariably associated with involvement of the renal pelvis. Leukoplakia of the urinary tract more commonly occurs in the bladder and may also occur in the urethra. The lesion results from squamous metaplasia of the urothelium frequently in association with chronic urinary tract infection, however recent data has shown that squamous metaplasia may develop spontaneously in the absence of underlying urinary tract pathology. There is keratinization and desquamation of the involved epithelium with proliferation of the lower squamous epithelial layers. The condition has classically been thought of as a precursor of squamous cell carcinoma, however, this association has been poorly documented in the upper urinary tract and only one case of the simultaneous occurrence of leukoplakia and squamous cell carcinoma in the ureter has been reported. Some authorities, therefore, now believe that there is no association between leukoplakia and the subsequent development of squamous cell carcinoma, except in the urinary bladder. More than one-half of the cases of leukoplakia are associated with concurrent or antecedent renal or ureteral calculi. Bilateral involvement occurs in 10% of the cases. When the keratinized epithelium forms a soft tissue mass, the condition is often referred to as a *cholesteatoma*.

Leukoplakia occurs equally in middle-aged patients of both sexes. Hematuria is present in about one-third of the cases. In the typical case, symptoms of chronic urinary tract infection and calculi have been present for years. The pathognomonic feature of leukoplakia is a history of passage of pieces of desquamated epithelium in the urine as pieces or flakes of white chalky material. The passage of these fragments can in themselves cause renal colic.

Radiographic features of ureteral involvement include the demonstration of diffuse irregular filling defects in the upper ureter in association with a similar filling defect or defects in the renal pelvis. There may be ridging of the mucosa of the ureter with evidence of ureteral obstruction. The radiologic appearance is nonspecific and differentiation from transitional cell carcinoma and malacoplakia is difficult.

Malacoplakia

Malacoplakia is another uncommon inflammatory condition of the ureter associated with chronic urinary tract infection. Malacoplakia has never been considered to be a premalignant condition. The lesion is characterized by the presence of smooth yellow or brown submucosal nodules composed of inflammatory cells (histiocytes) that contain a basophilic staining material known as Michaelis-Gutmann bodies. Many investigators feel that these inclusions contain phagocytized bacteria or bacterial fragments. A history of urinary tract infection caused by *E. coli*. is present in a high percentage of patients who develop malacoplakia, and it is now felt by many that the development of malacoplakia represents a defect in intracellular digestion of the bacteria.

The bladder is the most common site of urinary tract involvement followed by the ureter, the renal pelvis, and the urethra. Cases involving the renal parenchyma, the testes and the prostate have also been described. The majority of cases have been reported in middle-aged women with nonspecific complaints, including dysuria, flank pain, and occasionally hematuria. On urography, the lesion is demonstrated as a series of filling defects characteristically involving the distal ureter. A variable degree of ureteral obstruction is present. Differentiation of this condition from ureteritis cystica or transitional cell carcinoma is difficult, based on its radiologic appearance alone. Ureteral involvement may also lead to frank stricture formation.

Ureteritis Cystica

This condition results in the development of multiple subepithelial fluid-filled cysts in the ureter. These cysts, which radiologically are seen as filling defects in the ureter, are typically small, 2–3 mm in diameter, but may be as large as 2 cm in size in the renal pelvis. The pathogenesis of these cysts has been postulated by von Brunn to be related to degeneration of the central cells of the basal layer of the urothelium, which results in a downward proliferation of the surface epithelial cells. These cells become isolated from the surface as a result of scar tissue; this leads to the formation of fluid-filled cysts that subsequently project into the lumen of the ureter. The stimulus for this degeneration appears to be chronic inflammation, usually related to urinary tract infection. The diagnosis is almost always established radiologically, as there are no symptoms other than those associated with urinary infection.

The condition is slightly more common in women and while it has been reported in all age groups, it usually is seen between the ages of 50 and 60 years. The condition may affect the ureter, the renal pelvis, or the bladder alone or in combination. In approximately one-half of the cases of ureteritis cystica, bilateral involvement has been reported.

The typical radiographic appearance is that of multiple small rounded radiolucent filling defects (Fig. 14.17), which cause scalloping of the ureteral margins when seen in profile on urography or retrograde pyelography. These findings are considered characteristic of ureteritis cystica; occasionally suburothelial hemorrhage from a bleeding diathesis such as Henoch-Schönlein purpura or aplastic anemia may produce similar changes. Ureteritis cystica most commonly affects the ureter in its proximal one-third. The cysts may regress or disappear with treatment of the underlying urinary infection, but in some cases may persist for months or years after successful therapy of the infection. No sequelae of persistent ureteritis cystica have been reported, although there are several cases reported in which malignant urinary tract tumors have been present in patients with coexisting ureteritis cystica. The condition has been reported to occur in association with ureteral shistosomiasis and has recently been reported to be associated with prolonged ureteral stenting.

Ureteral Pseudodiverticulosis

Ureteral pseudodiverticulosis is a rare acquired lesion that results in the development of multiple small (4 mm or less in diameter) ureteral diverticula. Less than 75 cases of the disorder have been described in mostly scattered case reports, with the largest series of 23 cases reported by Wasserman et al.

The condition results in multiple small ureteral outpouchings (between three and eight per ureter) generally involving the proximal two-thirds of the ureter (Fig. 14.18). Bilateral ureteral involvement was present in 73% of the cases. A history of urinary tract infection is the most consistent underlying disorder, however, ureteral pseudodiverticulae may be found in patients with a wide range of urinary tract pathology, including calculi, benign prostatic hypertrophy, and transitional cell carcinoma. Hematuria is present in one-third of the cases. Of primary importance was the finding by Wasserman et al. that there was an association of a history of urothelial malignancy in 30% of the patients with ureteral pseudodiverticulosis and that cytologic examination of ureteral washings revealed cellular atypia in 50% of the cases.

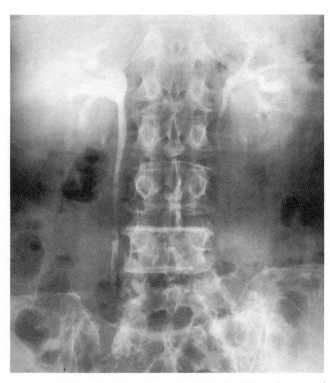

Figure 14.17. Ureteritis cystica. Multiple bilateral ureteral filling defects are present.

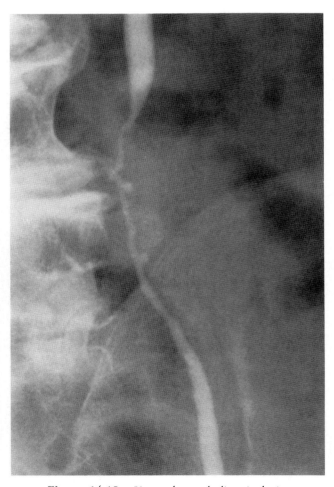

Figure 14.18. Ureteral pseudodiverticulosis.

Endometriosis

Endometriosis may involve the urinary tract by direct extension from the pelvis, from embryonic rests in the ureter or bladder wall, or by "metastases" via hematogenous or lymphatic routes to involve the bladder and ureter indirectly. Iatrogenic implantation has also been suggested as a mechanism for ureteral involvement in patients who have undergone previous surgery. The reported incidence of urinary tract involvement in patients with endometriosis is 1%, however, some authors have suggested that urinary tract involvement is more common than is generally appreciated, owing to incomplete urinary tract investigation in patients in whom this diagnosis is established at surgery. The bladder is the most commonly involved organ, followed by the ureter. Ureteral involvement generally occurs in patients with widespread pelvic disease, although isolated cases in the ureter have been reported. Clinically, flank pain and hematuria that may or may not be cyclic are clues to ureteral disease. Endometriosis generally occurs in women between the ages of 25 and 50 years, however, ureteral involvement in postmenopausal women has also been reported.

Two forms of ureteral involvement in endometriosis have been described. With intrinsic ureteral disease, there is direct invasion of the ureter; with extrinsic involvement, the ureter is affected by extrinsic disease in the pelvis. Extrinsic involvement is four times as common as intrinsic involvement. Pathologically, extrinsic involvement is characterized by the presence of endometrial elements in the adventitia of the ureter, while with intrinsic disease the endometrial tissue lies within the lamina propria or muscular layers of the ureter.

Ureteral involvement results in hydronephrosis, narrowing of the pelvic ureter, and occasionally, the development of intraureteral masses. Such involvement results in a short- to medium-length ureteral stricture (usually less than 2.5 cm) that affects the distal one-third of the ureter (Fig. 14.19). Pollack and Wills report that the involved ureteral segment is usually within 3 cm of the inferior aspect of the sacroiliac joint in the region where the uterosacral ligaments attach to the sacrum. The stricture is characteristically smooth, but abruptly tapered, and there may be sharp medial angulation of the ureter in the region of the narrowed segment. The ureter distal to the site of involvement is normal. Pollack and Wills were unable to determine whether the involvement was extrinsic or intrinsic by its radiographic appearance alone. Because of severe obstruction and the resultant impairment of contrast material excretion, the findings were usually better demonstrated on retrograde pyelography than on urography. In fact, in the majority of the reported cases, there has been nonvisualization of the collecting system on the involved side. Computed to-

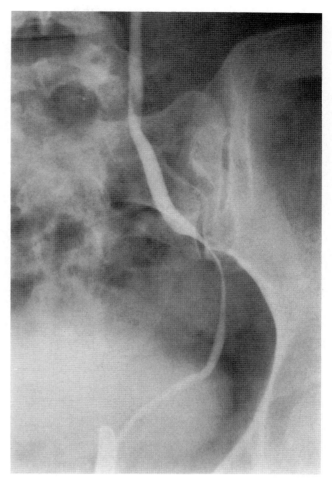

Figure 14.19.   Ureteral endometriosis. A retrograde pyelogram shows a medium-length stricture at the pelvic brim.

mography may demonstrate envelopment of the ureter by a soft tissue mass, particularly in those with the extrinsic form of ureteral involvement. The differential diagnosis of the ureteral lesions in endometriosis includes other causes of distal ureteral strictures, including primary and secondary ureteral tumors and other intrinsic or extrinsic inflammatory lesions that may affect the ureter. Because many of these patients have undergone prior pelvic surgery, the possibility of iatrogenic injury of the ureter must also always be considered when a distal ureteral stricture is encountered in a patient with endometriosis.

Amyloidosis

Amyloidosis is a disorder characterized by infiltration of the affected organ by a variety of insoluble proteins or protein-polysaccharide complexes. The disease is usually systemic or accompanies another systemic disorder, such as multiple myeloma. In a small percentage of the cases, amyloidosis may be localized to a specific organ. As of 1976, only 11 cases of localized amyloidosis of the ureter have been reported. In these cases, there was a slight female predominance, and the majority of patients have been elderly. The lower one-third of the ureter has been the most common site of involvement, although it has been reported in the upper ureter and in the renal pelvis. The clinical features of amyloidosis of the ureter are non-specific; symptoms of urinary tract obstruction are the presenting feature. The radiographic features are also nonspecific; a localized stricture of the ureter (Fig. 14.20), indistinguishable from those caused by primary or secondary ureteral tumors is the usual finding. Sub-mucosal calcification, which has been described in primary amyloidosis of the renal pelvis, has not been described in patients with isolated ureteral involvement.

Polyarteritis Nodosa

Polyarteritis nodosa is a systemic vasculitis that affects the kidneys in a high percentage of patients and commonly results in renal infarction and ultimately in renal failure. Ureteral involvement is considered rare, however, two distinct syndromes of ureteral involvement have been described. In the first instance, acute ureteral obstruction may be associated with acute systemic symptoms of fever, muscle pain, and the recent onset of hypertension. In the second instance, a stricture, presumably from involvement of the ureteral blood supply, may be present.

Eosinophilic Ureteritis

Inflammatory lesions characterized histologically by an infiltration of eosinophils may occur in a variety of organ systems. The majority of cases in the urinary tract involve the bladder. Fewer than 60 cases involving the ureter have been reported under a variety of names, including nonspecific granuloma of the ureter, eosinophilic granuloma of the ureter, and eosinophilic ureteritis.

The lesion may be found at multiple levels of the ureter and presents as a nodular defect within the ureteral lumen. There may be high-grade ureteral obstruction as demonstrated on retrograde pyelograms. Some of the reported cases have also been associated with urinary tract calculi.

Inflammatory Bowel Disease

Genitourinary complications of inflammatory bowel disease may occur in 4–23% of patients. Ureteral obstruction is the second most common finding after nephrolithiasis. In most patients, urinary tract involvement becomes evident after the gastrointestinal disease has been present for many years; rarely, urinary pathology may be the initial manifestation of the disorder.

The reported incidence of ureteral obstruction varies from 0.3 to 25.5% and occurs almost exclusively at the

Figure 14.20. Amyloidosis of the ureter. (Courtesy of J. Hodson, M.D.)

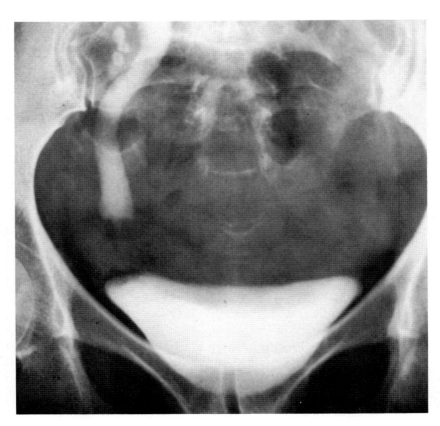

pelvic brim. In patients with Crohn's disease, the etiology of this process has been postulated to involve extension of the intestinal inflammatory process to the ureter by way of lymphatic communications. Others have found a fistula between an involved bowel segment and the retroperitoneum, sometimes leading to frank abscess, to be present in such cases. In Crohn's disease, unilateral involvement of the right ureter is the rule when the intestinal disease is limited to the terminal ileum and right colon (Fig. 14.21); left ureteral involvement may occur in those patients with granulomatous colitis or Crohn's disease involving the jejunum. The ureteral involvement is usually found incidentally as symptoms related to the urinary tract are frequently absent. When a retroperitoneal abscess is present, symptoms of ipsilateral psoas irritation may be present.

On urography, the involved ureter is found to have a sharply tapered smooth area of obstruction which generally involves a 4- to 5-cm segment, characteristic of obstruction from an extrinsic process. A soft tissue mass may or may not be demonstrated on urography but can usually be demonstrated by CT. The abnormal bowel segment responsible for the ureteral abnormality may also be imaged with this technique, thus providing a clue to the nature of the process. When secondary to an acute exacerbation of the inflammatory bowel disease, the ureteral obstruction usually resolves with resolution of active bowel inflammation or surgical bypass of the abnormal segment. When the process has become chronic, however, a dense periureteral fibrosis requiring ureterolysis may be present.

Other inflammatory processes of the bowel including appendicitis and sigmoid diverticulitis may also result in ureteral obstruction or fistula.

Pelvic Inflammatory Disease

Pelvic inflammatory disease and tubo-ovarian abscesses may produce extrinsic ureteral obstruction as a result of a periureteral inflammatory process that surrounds the ureter. This complication is unlikely to occur

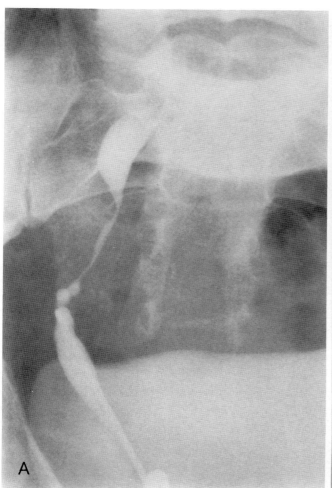
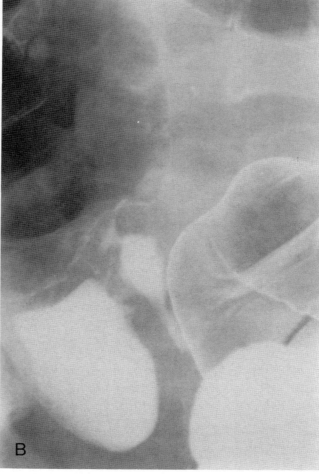

Figure 14.21. Crohn's disease. **A,** A retrograde pyelogram shows a long ureteral stricture involving the right ureter at the level of the pelvic brim. **B,** Barium enema shows characteristic changes of Crohn's disease involving the terminal ileum.

in the acute stage of the disease, however, in cases of chronic or recurrent pelvic inflammation, it occurs more commonly. The ureteral obstruction generally occurs at the pelvic brim, and its radiologic appearance is similar to that produced by inflammatory bowel disease. In some cases the ureteral obstruction associated with pelvic inflammatory disease will resolve after conservative therapy, however, when prominent scarring and fibrosis are present, ureterolysis is often necessary.

Schistosomiasis

Infection of the urinary tract caused by the fluke, *Schistosoma haematobium*, is endemic in many parts of the world including the Middle East, India, and Central and South Africa. While the disorder most commonly affects the bladder, ureteral involvement is present in up to 30% of the cases. The disorder primarily affects individuals under 30 years of age and is much more common in males than in females. Symptoms of ureteral involvement may be absent or limited to the presence of flank pain. The ureteral disease is almost always bilateral, but asymmetric involvement is the rule. The disorder most commonly involves the distal ureters, but lesions at the level of the L3 vertebral body and rarely, the UPJ may also be present. The ureteral disease is produced by hematogenous dissemination of the fluke with the ova being found in the submucosal and muscular layers of the ureter. This invasion results in varying degrees of ureteral stenosis, thickening, and dilatation. In addition to the disease caused by the presence of ova in the ureters, ureteral obstruction may be produced by the disease in the bladder.

Radiologic findings of urinary bilharziasis are characteristic of the disorder. Calcification, most commonly involving the pelvic portions of the ureters, is present in three-quarters of the cases. The calcification is usually linear (Fig. 14.22), or "tram-track," but may also be punctate, patchy, curvilinear, or diffuse in appearance. There is a characteristic deformity of the distal ureters resulting from medial and cephalic displacement of the ureters, which resembles a cow's horn. There are varying degrees of dilatation and stenosis of the ureters. In early cases, only mild fullness of the distal ureters may be present, but in more advanced cases, a beaded appearance of the ureters secondary to multiple ureteral strictures reminiscent of ureteral tuberculosis is found. The ureteral obstruction is generally produced by fibrosis of the intravesical portion of the ureters, however, abnormalities of ureteral peristalsis may also contribute to this finding. Although dilated, the ureters are not tortuous; in fact there is straightening of the midportion of the ureters presumably secondary to periureteral fibrosis. Because of fibrotic changes in the distal ureters, vesicoureteral reflux is commonly present. Solitary or multiple ureteral filling defects, termed *bilharzial polyps*, may be present.

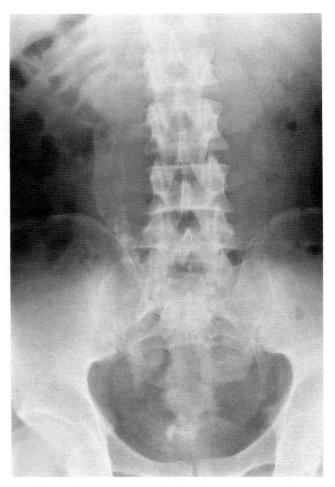

Figure 14.22. A diffusely calcified right ureter is present in this patient with urinary bilharziasis.

These polyps have been reported in as many as 17% of the cases. Although bilharziasis of the bladder predisposes the patient to the subsequent development of bladder carcinoma, this complication is very rare in the ureters. As discussed, ureteritis cystica may be present in patients with ureteral bilharziasis. Calcification in the cysts as a result of hemorrhage may occur in males resulting in a stippled appearance of the ureters, termed *ureteritis calcinosa*.

Tuberculosis

Urinary tract infection with *Mycobacterium tuberculosis* is the result of hematogenous dissemination of the organisms to the kidneys from a distant site, usually the lungs. Although it is generally believed that both kidneys are affected, the disease usually progresses in only one. Ureteral involvement is the direct result of infection within the kidneys with subsequent downward spread. The bladder, seminal vesicles, and prostate may also become affected.

The typical patient with urinary tract tuberculosis is age 40 years or older. Hematuria, sometimes gross, may be the initial presenting symptom, however, symptoms of lower urinary disease (frequency, dysuria, suprapubic pain) also commonly herald urinary tract involvement.

Radiographically demonstrable ureteral lesions are found in approximately 50% of patients with renal tuberculosis. The findings may be demonstrated on excretory urography if renal function is sufficient; otherwise, retrograde or antegrade pyelography is generally diagnostic (Fig. 14.23). Because of the bladder disease that is typi-

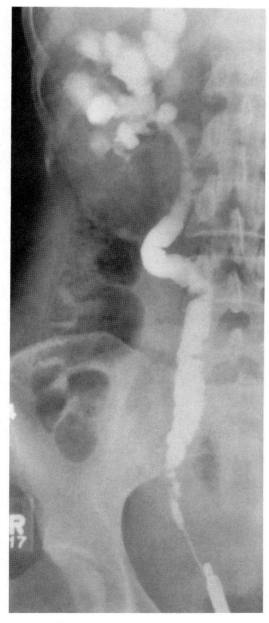

Figure 14.23. Ureteral tuberculosis. A retrograde pyelogram shows multiple ureteral strictures, as well as characteristic calyceal changes in this patient with proven urinary tract tuberculosis.

cally present, however, retrograde pyelography may be technically difficult or impossible to perform.

Ureteral infection produces ulceration, fibrosis, stricture, and calcification. The dilatation usually involves the entire ureter and is generally associated with hydronephrosis. The dilatation is frequently related to a stricture in the distal ureter associated with vesicle tuberculosis, but tuberculous ureteritis may also play a role. Early ulceration may produce a ragged appearance of the ureters, which if superficial may heal without sequela. Healing of deeper mucosal ulcerations results in ureteral fibrosis, so that there are alternating segments of dilatation and stricture; this produces a beaded appearance that is characteristic of ureteral tuberculosis. The ureter typically is shortened and straightened due to periureteral fibrosis that occurs in the healing phase of the disease. This finding has been referred to as representing a "pipe stem" ureter. Calcification in the ureters is much less common in tuberculous ureteritis than in tuberculosis of the kidney or in bilharzial ureteritis; when present, it is usually of the linear variety and confined to the pelvic portions of the ureters. Ureteral filling defects, usually multiple, secondary to mucosal granulomas may be present.

Inflammatory Strictures/Balloon Dilatation of the Ureter

Strictures of the ureter, not associated with a known pathogen or neoplasm, are commonly the result of some form of ureteral injury, either iatrogenic, following radiation therapy, or as the result of external violence. The stricture is caused by damage to the blood supply of the ureter with resultant fibrosis. Inflammatory strictures may also occur as a consequence of a calculus that has been impacted in the ureter for a long period of time. Such a stricture results in ureteral obstruction even after the stone has been removed. Approximately 10% of patients who undergo ureteroileal conduit diversion following cystectomy will develop a benign stricture at the ureteroileal anastomosis.

Antegrade transluminal dilatation now offers an attractive alternative to surgical therapy for the treatment of such strictures (Fig. 14.24). Following percutaneous nephrostomy, a floppy-tipped guidewire is passed down the ureter through the area of the stricture. A high-pressure angioplasty balloon catheter is then advanced over the guidewire through the stricture and the balloon inflated for a period of 30–60 seconds. Successful dilatation occurs when the "waist" of the balloon caused by the stricture disappears upon balloon inflation. Balloons ranging in size from 4 to 8 mm have been employed for this purpose; for ureteroileal strictures larger balloons (8–10 mm) are generally employed. In those cases where it is not possible to pass the balloon catheter through the stricture, initial dilatation with a tapered teflon (Van An-

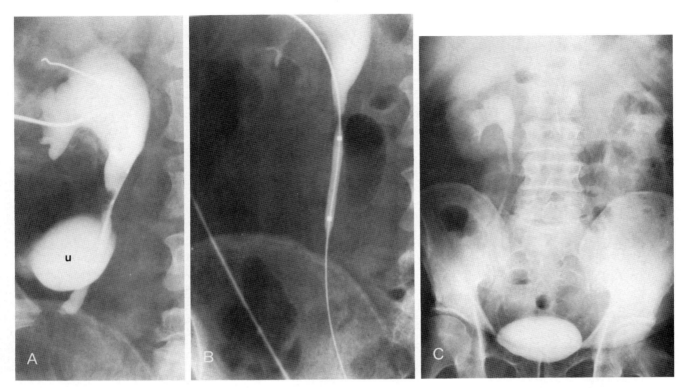

Figure 14.24.   Balloon dilatation of a ureteral stricture. **A,** Antegrade pyelogram demonstrates complete occlusion of the midportion of the right ureter associated with a large urinoma (u) in a patient who underwent a traumatic mid-ureteral stone basketing. Following a period of nephrostomy drainage, the urinoma resolved. **B,** A guidewire has been advanced through the stricture and a 6-mm balloon catheter inflated to dilate the stricture. A ureteral stent was then placed for 6 weeks. **C,** Follow-up urogram shows patency of the ureter with minimal residual fullness of the right collecting system.

del) catheter may facilitate passage of the balloon catheter. Following successful dilatation, a double pigtail ureteral stent (8–10 French) is placed for periods ranging from 2 to 6 weeks.

The long-term results of balloon catheter dilatation of ureteral strictures have been reported in several series. Johnson et al. report that for strictures less than 7 months old, an approximate 65% success rate was achieved; in strictures that have been present for longer than 7 months, however, there were no successful balloon ureteroplasties. Lang reported an overall success rate of 50% for long-term patency. In this series also, strictures of short duration and those not associated with a compromised vascular supply of the ureter (i.e., following radiation therapy) were associated with a higher success rate. Shapiro et al. have reported, however, that long-term success with the subgroup of patients having ureteroileal stricture dilatation is only 16% in patients followed for at least 1 year.

MISCELLANEOUS CONDITIONS

Retroperitoneal Fibrosis

Retroperitoneal fibrosis (RF) is a disease of unknown etiology in which a fibrous soft tissue mass envelops the retroperitoneum usually between the kidneys and the pelvic brim. As a result of this location, the ureters and the great blood vessels are the organs most commonly affected by the disease. A number of underlying conditions may be responsible for the development of retroperitoneal fibrosis including the ingestion of methysergide (Sansert); the presence of an abdominal aortic aneurysm; radiation therapy; retroperitoneal hematomas, tumors, infection, or urinomas; and previous retroperitoneal surgery. In more than 70% of the cases, however, the etiology of the condition is unclear; such cases are termed *idiopathic retroperitoneal fibrosis.*

The ingestion of methysergide is one of the most specific conditions that predispose to the development of retroperitoneal fibrosis. The disease in such cases occurs after therapy with the drug for several months; it may regress when such therapy is stopped. Some authorities have recommended that methysergide therapy be interrupted for a month or 2 each year to prevent the development of this complication.

Retroperitoneal fibrosis associated with the presence of an abdominal aortic aneurysm is also of interest (Fig. 14.25). Although it was initially postulated that blood from leaking aneurysms might be the factor responsible for the development of RF, several authors have con-

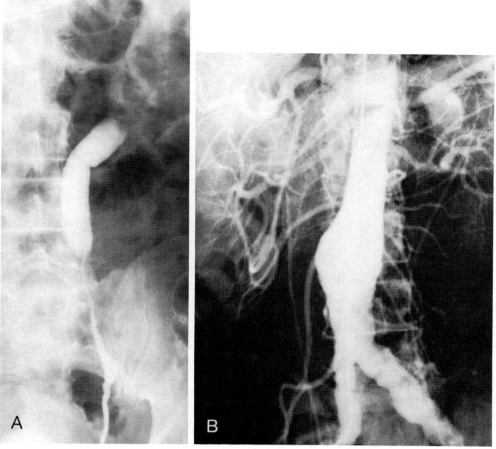

Figure 14.25. Retroperitoneal fibrosis. **A,** A retrograde pyelogram shows obstruction of the left ureter just above the pelvic brim. **B,** Abdominal aortogram shows an abdominal aortic aneurysm.

cluded that leakage is not a necessary precondition in the evolution of retroperitoneal fibrosis as hemosiderin-laden macrophages are generally not found on retroperitoneal biopsy. Some authors have suggested that the fibrotic reaction is an exaggerated extension of the inflammatory process that normally takes place in the wall of the aneurysm.

The pathogenesis of idiopathic retroperitoneal fibrosis is unknown; it has been speculated that it is either a type of collagen disease, a hypersensitivity angiitis in response to an unknown antigen, or the result of a viral infection. Many authorities feel that retroperitoneal fibrosis is a periaortitis that may be immunologically based. It is for this reason that therapy with corticosteroids has been advocated as a major form of treatment; however, a combination of ureterolysis and steroid therapy is generally used for patients in whom the disease has not progressed to the point of irreversible renal damage.

The disease classically presents in patients between the ages of 50 and 70 years; males are more commonly affected than females in a ratio of 3:1. Flank or back pain, weight loss, nausea and vomiting, oliguria, and malaise are the most frequent presenting symptoms. In some cases, symptoms of lower-extremity venous obstruction or claudication are present. Clinically, hypertension, anemia, uremia, and an elevated erythrocyte sedimentation rate are commonly found. On pathologic examination, a plaque-like soft tissue mass 2–6 cm thick composed primarily of fibrous tissue infiltrated in varying degrees by mononuclear cells and other blood elements extending from the level of the renal pelvis to the pelvic brim is found. In some cases, the mass may be confined to the true pelvis. The mass surrounds, but does not invade, the adjacent hollow organ structures, muscles, and nerves of the retroperitoneum. It is said to exert its effect through a restriction of the lumen of the involved structures as a result of contraction of the collagen fibers. Because the ureters are more sensitive to such compression than are the nerves, arteries, and veins, it is generally the effect of the process on the urinary tract that brings the condition to light.

The diagnosis of RF is almost always established on radiologic examination. On urography, the ureters are found to be encased and there is a variable degree of proximal dilatation; in many cases only mild or moderate caliectasis is present. Classically, the degree of renal failure that is present is greater than would be expected based on the amount of proximal dilatation that is found. This fact lends credence to the supposition that interference with ureteral peristalsis rather than mechanical compression of the ureters is primarily responsible for the renal impairment that is present. The obstruction usually involves the middle one-third of the ureters, and there may be medial deviation of the ureter in the involved segment. Some authors, however, have emphasized that the medial displacement may merely represent a variation in the course of the normal ureter, and the absence of this finding does not preclude the diagnosis of retroperitoneal fibrosis. In three-quarters of the cases, bilateral ureteral involvement is evident, but the degree to which this occurs is variable; there may be a considerable degree of asymmetry in the amount of ureteral obstruction that is present. When the degree of renal impairment precludes satisfactory urographic visualization, retrograde or antegrade pyelography is necessary to demonstrate the characteristic ureteral changes. As in primary megaureter, there is said to be little resistance to the passage of the retrograde catheter on cystoscopic cannulation of the ureteral orifice.

On sonography, the retroperitoneal mass is readily demonstrated; it is typically poorly marginated and virtually anechoic, reflecting its homogeneous nature. In a recent report from Rubenstein et al., 11 of 12 fibrous lesions were found to be either echo free or hypoechoic on sonography. The accompanying hydronephrosis is readily demonstrated by sonography, as well. If the process is related to an abdominal aortic aneurysm, the aneurysmal segment of the aorta is demonstrated. The diagnosis may be obscured, however, in obese patients or those with an abundance of intestinal gas.

Computed tomography demonstrates the mass to be homogeneous, usually with a sharp anterior margin. The mass envelops the aorta, the vena cava, and the ureters (Fig. 14.26), but in contrast to other retroperitoneal tumors such as lymphoma, does not displace them. Rubenstein et al. have emphasized that the density of the typical fibrous lesion on CT is either uniformly or focally denser than the adjacent soft tissue structures. On postcontrast studies, this difference is even more pronounced; the typical case of retroperitoneal fibrosis shows marked enhancement after contrast administration. The authors postulated that this pattern of enhancement was related to the abundant capillary network of retroperitoneal fibrosis. It must be emphasized, however, that some retroperitoneal tumors, particularly those associated with a dense desmoplastic reaction may have similar CT characteristics, therefore definitive diagnosis requires biopsy, particularly for suspected idiopathic retroperitoneal fibrosis.

On magnetic resonance imaging (MRI), retroperitoneal fibrosis appears as a soft tissue mass of intermediate intensity with less signal than retroperitoneal fat but a higher intensity than that of the psoas muscle, when imaged with a spin echo technique. Because no signal is

Figure 14.26. Retroperitoneal fibrosis. Computed tomography shows a large retroperitoneal mass which envelops the aorta and the vena cava. Bilateral hydronephrosis, worse on the right, is present.

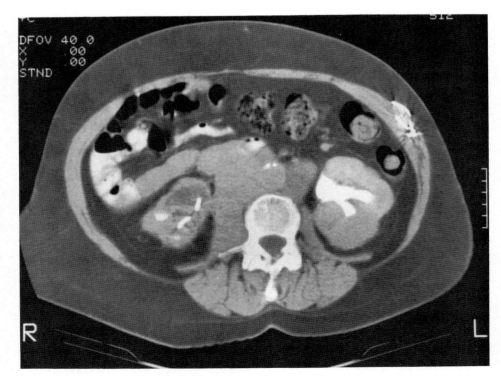

received from flowing blood, MRI is an excellent tool to study the effect of retroperitoneal fibrosis on retroperitoneal blood vessels.

Ovarian Vein Syndrome and Vascular Impressions

The right ovarian vein crosses the ureter at the level of the third lumbar vertebra but does not normally cause a distinct vascular impression. In cases of dilatation or thrombosis of the vein, however, an oblique impression on the ureter secondary to this phenomenon may be present. Several cases of ureteral dilatation and hydronephrosis, sometimes in association with urinary tract infection, attributed to obstruction of the right ovarian vein have been reported. Symptoms of flank pain and urinary tract infection are typical presenting complaints. The syndrome typically occurs in young women who have had one or more pregnancies and has been implicated as the cause of the flank pain that sometimes occurs during the mid and later stages of pregnancy. Some authorities, however, have questioned whether ovarian vein syndrome should be considered a distinct clinical entity as identical findings may be present in patients with no symptoms. Occasionally, varicosities of the ovarian vein may produce multiple notched defects on the ureter during urography.

Other vascular structures may produce impressions on the ureters including those produced by tortuosity or aneurysms of the iliac vessels. Notching of the proximal one-third of the ureter is often attributed to prominent ureteral collaterals, usually in association with renal artery stenosis or occlusion. Venous collaterals associated with inferior vena cava obstruction, vascular malformations, or congenital anomalies of venous drainage may also be found. Rarely, impressions on the ureters related to dilated lymphatics may also be found. Such cases occur in association with lymphatic obstruction or lymphangiectasis.

Pregnancy Dilatation

Physiologic dilatation of the upper urinary tract occurs during pregnancy. The etiology of this dilatation has been a matter of dispute for many years, with opinion divided between those who believe it to be primarily a hormonal effect on the ureters and those who believe the phenomenon to be primarily obstructive in etiology. The weight of opinion has supported the obstructive theory. The changes of pregnancy dilatation on urography are characteristic; the dilatation involves the proximal two-thirds of the ureters, with the more pronounced changes being present on the right side. The distal ureters are normal in caliber. It has been shown that the ureteral dilatation ends where the ureters cross the iliac arteries at the pelvic brim (Fig. 14.27); the affected ureter shows an

oblique impression on its lumen from this vascular structure. It has further been postulated that as the left ureter crosses the iliac artery at a less acute angle than on the right side, the effect of the compression is less pronounced on the left. The changes in pregnancy, therefore, are presumed to be related to compression by the gravid uterus of the ureters against the iliac arteries where they cross the pelvic brim. Dure-Smith has suggested that the changes occur in every pregnancy and once present may persist in varying degrees thereafter. Support for this theory has come from the observation that pelvic masses in both men and women (i.e., uterine leiomyomata) can produce changes in the ureters identical to that produced by pregnancy.

Pseudoureterocele

"True" ureteroceles are thought to represent a congenital cystic dilatation of the submucosal segment of the intravesicle ureter (Chapter 15). The term *pseudoure-*

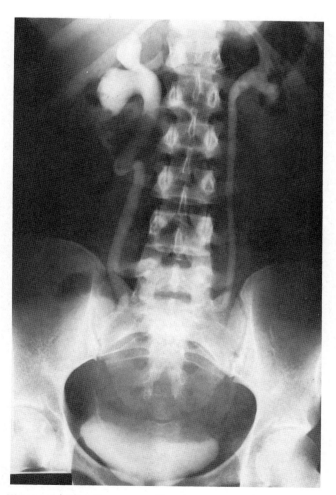

Figure 14.27. Pregnancy dilatation. An IVP shows bilateral ureterectasis, worse on the right, in this recently pregnant patient. The soft tissue mass in the pelvis represents the still enlarged uterus.

terocele is used to denote a lesion that has a similar radiologic appearance to a simple ureterocele, but actually represents an acquired lesion. In the majority of such cases, the acquired lesion is found to represent a calculus impacted in the ureterovesicle junction, transitional cell carcinoma of the bladder, radiation cystitis, or invasion of the trigone of the bladder by a secondary malignancy.

Thornbury et al. have defined characteristics of pseudoureteroceles that allow differentiation of this lesion from the congenital variety. While both groups had a "halo" sign, or a zone of lucency, surrounding the ureteral orifice and are associated with dilatation of the terminal portion of the ureter (Fig. 14.28), in patients with pseudoureteroceles, the dilated segment tended to be larger, and there was accompanying proximal dilatation of the upper ureter which was not present in true ureteroceles. In addition, there tended to be asymmetry of the dilated segment. The authors of this study also described a series of patients with *"false" ureteroceles*; cases in which there was radiologic evidence of a ureterocele, but in whom cystoscopy revealed no pathology. No explanation of this phenomenon was offered, however, it was noted that the false ureteroceles tended to be visible on the initial radiographs made during an excretory urogram, but either disappeared or decreased in size as bladder filling occurred; true simple ureteroceles tended to be visible throughout the study.

Procidentia

Prolapse of the uterus is an uncommon cause of bilateral ureteral obstruction, that in severe cases leads to azotemia and progressive renal failure. The patients are generally elderly females with third-degree uterine prolapse. Upright radiographs of the bladder during urography demonstrate the abnormality as well as the proximal ureteral obstruction. The mechanism by which ureteral obstruction is produced is poorly understood; ureteral kinking, obstruction produced by the uterine artery, pressure related to the levator ani muscles, and mechanical deformity of ureteral meati in the bladder have all been proposed as possible mechanisms.

Ureteral Fistula

Ureteral fistula may develop as a result of trauma to the ureter from external violence, iatrogenic injury of the ureter during the course of surgery for an unrelated condition, or as a complication of a urinary tract procedure. In other cases, ureteral fistula may develop as a result of involvement of the ureter by malignant or inflammatory disease originating in an adjacent organ. Ureteral fistula developing after radiation therapy may be especially difficult to manage.

Most ureteral fistula present with an associated urinary tract infection, flank pain, or with the leakage of urine. Traumatic ureteral fistula are discussed in Chapter 12 and

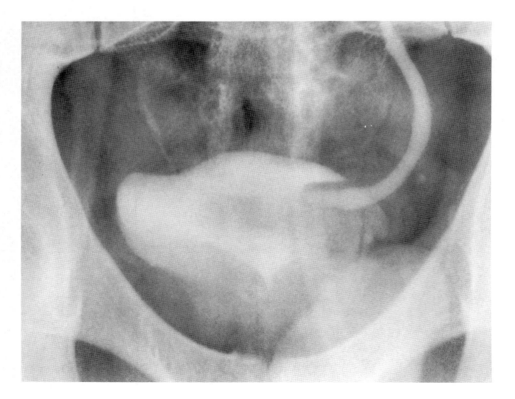

Figure 14.28. Pseudoureterocele. A dilated left ureter with a "halo sign" surrounding the ureteral orifice is present in this patient with a calculus impacted at the ureterovesicle junction.

the inflammatory conditions associated with ureteral fistula are covered elsewhere in this chapter. Rarely, fistula between the ureter and a blood vessel may result in massive gross hematuria.

The diagnosis of a ureteral fistula is usually established by imaging studies of the urinary tract that demonstrate extravasation or intravasation of contrast material outside the confines of the ureter. Imaging studies that may be useful in this regard include excretory urography, antegrade or retrograde pyelography, and CT. Rarely, contrast studies of the gastrointestinal tract in patients with ureteroenteric fistula demonstrate a communication with the ureter.

Interventional uroradiologic procedures using a variety of catheters and guidewires to cross the segment of ureter containing the fistula and subsequent antegrade ureteral stenting now play a major role in the management of such fistulas. Mitty et al. reported successful healing of all six ureteral fistulas in whom the procedure was technically successful among a series of 24 patients who underwent antegrade stenting for a variety of lesions. Similar excellent results have been reported by Lang in a series of 50 patients with a variety of ureteral leaks or fistulas. In 41 of the cases, the injured area of the ureter was successfully crossed, however, in only 30 cases (60%) was renal function preserved for at least 6 months.

DEVIATION OF THE URETER

The ureter exits the renal pelvis opposite the L_1-L_2 interspace and descends to the true pelvis within the confines of the perirenal space. The initial course of the ureter is roughly parallel to the psoas muscle; it exits Gerota's fascia at approximately L_4-L_5 where it crosses anterior to the iliac artery at the pelvic brim and then takes a gentle lateral course to the area of the ischial spine. At this point, the pelvic ureter curves medially to enter the bladder. Deviations from this expected course of the ureter on urography were formerly the major method by which retroperitoneal pathology was diagnosed; with the advent of cross-sectional imaging techniques, urography has been relegated to a secondary role for initial diagnosis. It is nonetheless necessary to recognize pathologic deviations of the course of the ureter and not to confuse normal variations in this course with pathology. Many congenital malformations of the ureter and postoperative changes may cause deviation and may therefore also be a source of confusion.

Lateral deviation of the proximal two-thirds of the ureter should be considered when the ureter is found to lie more than 1 cm lateral to the margin of the transverse processes of the lumbar vertebral bodies; medial deviation is present when the ureter overlaps or is projected medial to the pedicles of these vertebrae. For the pelvic portion of the ureter, medial deviation should be considered when the normal convexity of this portion of the ureter is lost; any focal lateral bulge should be considered as lateral deviation.

Urograms showing possible ureteral displacement must be interpreted with caution. Some racial and sexual variations in the course of the ureters may be one source of confusion. In black patients, the ureters may take a more medial course than in whites; this is especially true at the lower lumbar and upper sacral levels where the ureter may be normally found overlapping the pedicle of the vertebral bodies. In women, the pelvic portion of the right ureter may have a more straightened appearance than does the left ureter because of the normal placement of the uterus slightly to the left of the midline. A distended urinary bladder may also cause similar findings in women. Psoas hypertrophy that has been described in Chapter 3 may also cause lateral, or rarely, medial displacement of the proximal ureters. Hypertrophy of the iliopsoas muscles may explain medial deviation of the lower portion of the ureter (Fig. 14.29).

Pathologic Ureteral Deviations

Pathologic deviations of the ureter are customarily grouped according to whether the displacement affects the proximal, middle, or distal one-third of the ureter.

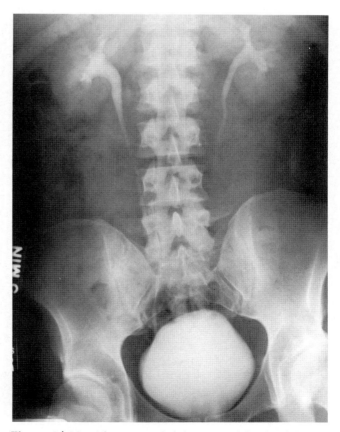

Figure 14.29.   There is medial deviation of the distal third of the right ureter secondary to iliopsoas hypertrophy.

Lateral displacement of the proximal one-third of the ureter is most commonly secondary to enlarged retroperitoneal lymph nodes (Fig. 14.30). Lateral deviation of this segment is also usually present with a malrotated kidney. Rarely, dilatation of the renal collecting system accompanying long-standing hydronephrosis may also cause this finding.

Medial displacement of the proximal one-third of the ureter is uncommon; when present, it is usually related to a mass in the lower pole of the ipsilateral kidney; in such cases, the cause of the displacement is readily apparent.

The most common cause of lateral displacement of the middle one-third of the ureter is retroperitoneal lymph node enlargement. The presence of an abdominal aortic aneurysm may also cause lateral displacement of the middle one-third of the ureter particularly on the left side, however, the same process may rarely also deviate the ureter medially.

Medial deviation of the middle one-third of the ureter may be related to retroperitoneal fibrosis, retrocaval ureter, and to the presence of retroperitoneal tumors that arise lateral to the ureter. Large retroperitoneal fluid collections, i.e., a hematoma secondary to a renal injury, may

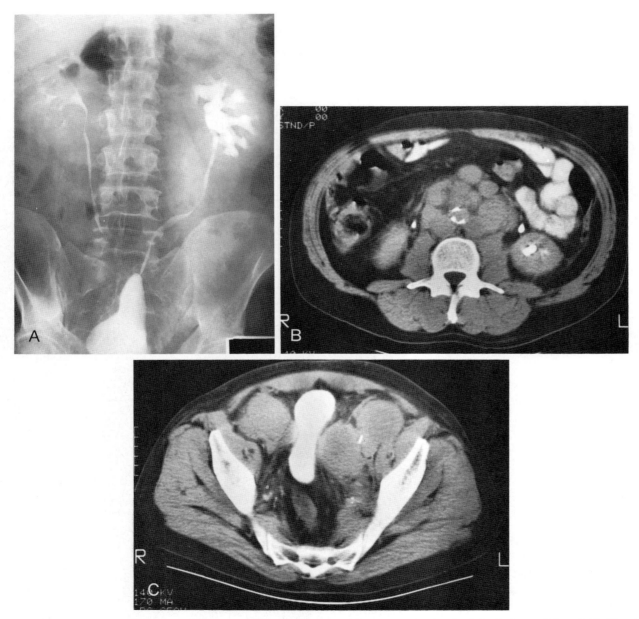

Figure 14.30. A, An IVP shows *lateral* deviation of the proximal one-third of the left ureter and *medial* deviation of the distal third of the ureter on the same side. Computed tomography scans at the level of the kidneys **(B)** and bladder **(C)** demonstrate massive retroperitoneal lymphadenopathy.

also cause medial displacement of this segment of the ureter. In such cases, the ureter may have a slightly compressed appearance, as well.

Deviations of the distal one-third of the ureter are more common and can usually be related to their specific etiology. The most common cause of medial deviation of the pelvic portion of the ureter is the presence of a posterior or posterolateral bladder diverticulum (Fig. 14.31). In such cases, the deviation commonly extends to the level of the ureterovesicle junction. At the pelvic brim, tortuosity or frank aneurysms of the iliac arteries (Fig. 14.32) may deviate and medially displace the ureter. In this instance, vascular calcification is usually present as a clue to the correct diagnosis. Enlargement of the iliac lymph nodes is another common cause for medial dislocation of the distal one-third of the ureter (Fig. 14.30). A variety of other processes, including pelvic lipomatosis, uterine prolapse, and following abdominoperineal resection for rectal carcinoma may also be associated with medial deviation of the distal ureters. In the latter case, the normal support for the pelvic ureters is lost following the surgery; there is bilateral medial deviation and straightening of the ureters toward the midline. Pelvic extraperitoneal hematomas, such as those accompanying fractures of the bony pelvis, may cause medial deviation of the ureter in the acute setting.

Lateral displacement of the pelvic ureter may accompany a variety of central pelvic masses, particularly those of gynecologic origin, such as uterine leiomyomata. Lateral deviation of the ureter may occur in patients with either femoral or inguinal hernias where the affected segment of the ureter is trapped by the hernia.

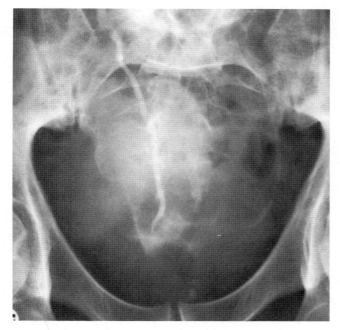

Figure 14.31. There is medial deviation of the distal right ureter secondary to a large bladder diverticulum.

FUNCTIONAL STUDIES

Ureteral Perfusion Studies

Differentiation of dilated, but unobstructed renal collecting systems from those with functionally significant obstruction is a difficult clinical problem. Ureteral perfusion studies are considered the most definitive procedure by which the dilated, but unobstructed upper urinary tract can be differentiated from those with functionally significant upper tract obstruction. The procedure for such perfusion studies was initially described by the English urologist, Robert Whitaker, and the study is therefore referred to as the *Whitaker test*. This procedure measures the resistance of the ureter to a known flow rate during perfusion of the renal pelvis.

To perform ureteral perfusion studies, needle puncture of the collecting system is performed, usually with a 22-gauge Chiba needle. The needle is connected to an infusion pump capable of providing a continuous infusion of diluted contrast material at a rate that is varied between 5 and 20 ml/min. A manometer connected to a three-way stopcock is placed in series with the infusion line. At the end of a specific period of infusion, the pressure in the renal pelvis is recorded. Pressure in the urinary bladder is simultaneously measured by a manometer connected to a Foley catheter. Alternatively, perfusion studies may be performed through a percutaneous nephrostomy or by the use of a dual-needle technique that allows continuous recording of the renal pelvic pressure during the actual infusion. In Whitaker's original description in 1973, an infusion rate of 10 ml/min was utilized; a pressure differential between the kidney and the bladder greater than 15 cm H_2O was considered indicative of obstruction. Vesicoureteral reflux must be excluded before ureteral perfusion studies are performed as the presence of reflux invalidates the results of the procedure.

The technique of ureteral perfusion has been expanded and modified by Pfister et al. (1979) at the Massachusetts General Hospital. He used variable perfusion rates and showed that some equivocal cases of obstruction could only be demonstrated with perfusion rates of 15–20 ml/min. Pfister felt that at perfusion rates of 10 ml/min or lower, differential pressures of less than 12 cm H_2O were normal; pressures between 12 and 14 cm H_2O were equivocal; and pressures greater than 15 cm H_2O were indicative of functionally significant obstruction. Other investigators have suggested that the equivocal range should be broader, but most agree that if the pressure differential is greater than 25–30 cm H_2O, moderate or severe obstruction is present. At higher flow rates, however, absolute renal pressure may rise and there is a corresponding rise in differential pressure. Pfister (1982) has indicated that a pressure differential of 18 cm H_2O is

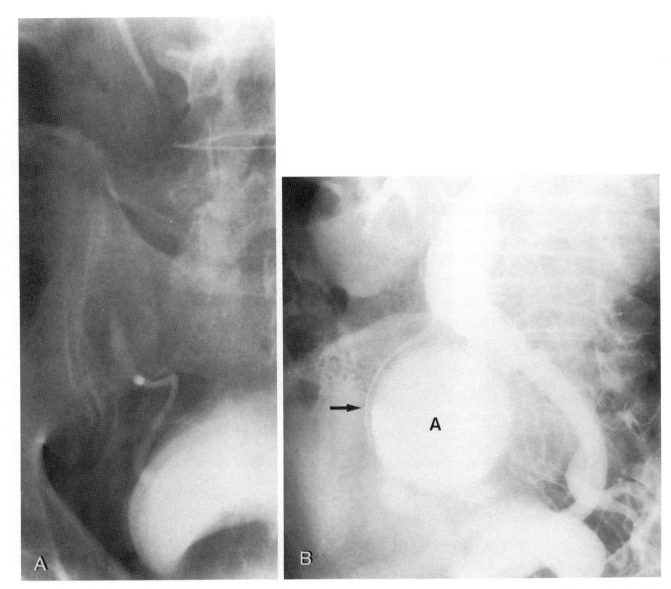

Figure 14.32.   A, IVP demonstrates toruosity and medial deviation of the right ureter. **B,** Oblique film from a pelvic angiogram shows a large right iliac aneurysm (A). Note the displacement of the right ureter (*arrow*).

normal at a flow of 15 ml/min and at 20 ml/min the pressure difference may normally reach 21 cm H_2O. He also indicated that the perfusion studies should be performed with the patient's urinary bladder both empty and filled, as some cases of significant obstruction are only evident after bladder filling. This circumstance may be seen following ureteroneocystostomy using the Leadbetter-Politano technique. The high insertion of the ureteroneocystostomy may result in kinking of the reimplanted ureter when the bladder is distended; therefore, ureteral obstruction is present only when the bladder is filled. Similar findings may be seen in patients with hypertonic neurogenic bladder disease. Under normal circumstances, as the bladder fills, intravesicle pressure naturally rises and there is a rise in renal pelvic pressure;

however, the differential pressure between the bladder and the renal pelvis decreases.

The accuracy of ureteral perfusion studies in assessing urinary tract obstruction has not been addressed because there is lacking a standard against which the results of perfusion can be compared. Whitaker (1979) reported 170 perfusion studies in which clinical and radiographic criteria were used to assess results. There were only six cases in which indeterminate results were obtained.

Diuretic Renography

The use of the radionuclide renogram supplemented by the administration of a diuretic to assess the functional significance of dilatation of the upper urinary tract was initially described in the late 1970s by English investigators. Subsequently, the technique was modified for use with a gamma camera by Koff et al. (1979) from the University of Michigan. These authors also suggested the use of the radiopharmaceutical ^{99m}Tc-DTPA for such studies because of its excellent imaging characteristics and its relatively low radiation dose. Time-activity curves are acquired for both kidneys simultaneously with the patient in the sitting position following injection of the tracer. When the activity in the collecting system peaks (usually 10–20 minutes after the tracer is administered), a dose of furosemide (Lasix) is administered and the "washout" of the activity from the collecting system is monitored. The recommended dose of furosemide is 0.5 mg/kg or 20–40 mg for an adult. Three patterns for the resultant renogram curves were described; the normal pattern, the dilated but nonobstructed pattern (Fig. 14.33), and the obstructed pattern. These patterns were assessed by visual inspection of the renogram curves. In patients with nonsignificant dilatation, there is a prompt decline in the tracer activity within the collecting system as demonstrated by the time-activity curve. With obstruction, there is an increase in the activity in the collecting system following administration of the diuretic (Fig. 14.34).

In their initial series, Koff (1979) reported the obstructed pattern correlated with significant urinary tract obstruction at surgery. Moreover, postoperative studies in these same patients showed a return to an unobstructed pattern. Thus, the authors concluded that the examination provided a valuable tool for preoperatively predicting a positive surgical outcome.

Other investigators have also reported similar excellent results from diuretic renography. Meller and Eckstein reported an overall sensitivity of 0.87 and a specific-

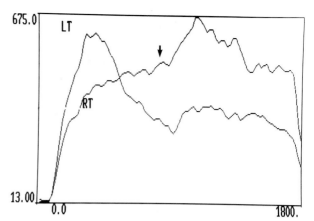

Figure 14.34.   Diuretic renogram showing obstruction. Following administration of the diuretic (*arrow*), the tracer activity in the right kidney shows an ascending slope.

ity of 0.93 in a series of 426 dilated upper urinary tracts in children. Shore et al. reported almost identical results in a series of 20 children.

Despite these excellent results, the pitfalls and limitations of diuretic renography must be recognized. When renal function is severely compromised, a definite response of the renogram curve to the administration of the furosemide may not be apparent. In such cases, the study is indeterminate; no assessment of the possible contribution of the obstruction to the compromised function can be made. The precise level of renal function at which the test is unreliable is variable; most investigators feel that with a GFR below 30 ml/min, diuretic renography is unreliable. Indeterminate results may also occur from a variety of other factors including technical errors, dehydration, and as a result of a relatively low-grade obstruction. In addition, false-negative studies have been reported when too low a dose of furosemide has been administered or when obstruction is intermittent— present at high urinary flow rates only. The presence of a distended urinary bladder or vesicoureteral reflux may also invalidate the results of the procedure.

Several modifications of the original technique have been suggested by other investigators in an attempt to overcome some of these limitations. Some authors have suggested that the diuretic be administered *before* the radiopharmaceutical to ensure that a high urine flow rate is present. This same objective can be accomplished by the active hydration of the patient through the administration of fluids intravenously 30 minutes prior to the examination. Krueger et al. suggested that the results of the diuresis be quantified by the time required to clear one-half the activity from the collecting system ($T\frac{1}{2}$). These investigators suggested that a $T\frac{1}{2}$ of more than 20 minutes be considered to be indicative of significant obstruction. A commonly utilized modification of this

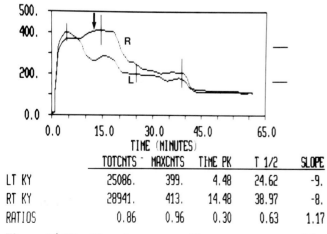

	TOTCNTS	MAXCNTS	TIME PK	T 1/2	SLOPE
LT KY	25086.	399.	4.48	24.62	-9.
RT KY	28941.	413.	14.48	38.97	-8.
RATIOS	0.86	0.96	0.30	0.63	1.17

Figure 14.33.   Diuretic renogram. The renogram curve of the right kidney shows an ascending slope; however, following administration of the diuretic (*arrow*) there is a prompt decline in tracer activity. The left kidney shows the normal response to the diuretic.

scheme is as follows: a T$\frac{1}{2}$ of 10 minutes of less is considered normal, a T$\frac{1}{2}$ of 10–20 minutes is considered indeterminate, and a T$\frac{1}{2}$ of greater than 20 minutes indicates obstruction.

The results of diuretic renography and ureteral perfusion studies have been compared in several series. Whitaker (1984) found disagreement between the two studies in 39% of the cases in whom equivocal urinary obstruction was present. Of these, five of 28 were considered to be false-positive renograms while six of 28 renograms were considered to be false-negative. In another series, Hay et al. found that 32 of 45 symptomatic patients with normal renograms showed obstruction according to Whitaker's criteria (pressure differential greater than 22 cm H$_2$O). When the renogram suggested obstruction, however, there was good correlation with the perfusion study. Senac et al., however, reported much more comparable results between the two studies; they reported that the Whitaker test correlated with "clinical correctness" in 86% of the cases while the renogram was correct in 85%.

SUGGESTED READINGS

General References

Bergman H (ed): *The Ureter*, ed 2. New York, Springer-Verlag, 1981.
Fein AB, McClennan B: Solitary filling defects of the ureter. *Semin Roentgenol* 21(3):201, 1986.
Pfister RC, Newhouse JH: Radiology of ureter. *Urology* 12(1):15, 1978.
Williamson B Jr, Hartman GW, Hattery RR: Multiple and diffuse ureteral filling defects. *Semin Roentgenol* 21(3):214, 1986.

Basic Ureteral Physiology

Griffiths DJ: Ureteral mechanics. *Semin Urol* 5(3):155, 1987.
Weiss RM: Ureteral function. *Urology* 12(2):114, 1978.
Weiss RM: Physiology of the upper urinary tract. *Semin Urol* 5(3):148, 1987.

Acute Ureteral Obstruction

Elkin M: Radiological observations in acute ureteral obstruction. *Radiology* 81:484, 1963.
Elkin M, Boyarsky S, Martinez J, et al: Physiology of ureteral obstruction as determined by roentgenologic studies. *Radiology* 92(2):291, 1964.
Hill MC, Rich JI, Mardiat JG, et al: Sonography vs. excretory urography in acute flank pain. *AJR* 144:1235, 1985.
Hinman F Jr: The pathophysiology of urinary obstruction. In Campbell MF, Harrison JH (eds): *Urology*, ed 3. Philadelphia, WB Saunders, vol 1, 1970.
Laing FC, Jeffrey RB Jr, Wing VW: Ultrasound versus excretory urography in evaluating acute flank pain. *Radiology* 154:613, 1985.
Vaughan ED Jr, Gillenwater JY: Recovery following complete chronic unilateral ureteral occlusion: functional radiographic and pathological alterations. *J Urol* 106:27, 1971.

Chronic Ureteral Obstruction and Obstructive Renal Atrophy

Amis ES, Cronan JJ, Pfister RC, et al: Ultrasonic inaccuracies in diagnosing renal obstruction. *Urology* 19(1):101, 1982.
Bosniak MA, Megibow AJ, Ambos MA, et al: Computed tomography of ureteral obstruction. *AJR* 138:1107, 1982.
Hodson CJ, Craven JD: The radiology of obstructive atrophy of the kidney. *Clin Radiol* 17:305, 1966.
Kamholtz RG, Cronan JJ, Dorfman GS: Obstruction and the minimally dilated renal collecting system: US evaluation. *Radiology* 170:51, 1989.

Lee JKT, Baron RL, Melson GL, et al: Can real-time ultrasonography replace static B-scanning in the diagnosis of renal obstruction? *Radiology* 139:161, 1981.
Maillet PJ, Pelle-Francoz D, Laville M, et al: Nondilated obstructive acute renal failure: diagnostic procedures and therapeutic management. *Radiology* 160:659, 1986.
Naidich JB, Rackson ME, Mossey RT, et al: Nondilated obstructive uropathy: percutaneous nephrostomy performed to reverse renal failure. *Radiology* 160:653, 1986.
Talner LB, Scheible W, Ellenbogen PH, et al: How accurate is ultrasonography in detecting hydronephrosis in azotemic patients? *Urol Radiol* 3:1, 1981.

The Dilated Ureter

Blickman JG, Lebowitz RL: The coexistence of primary megaureter and reflux. *AJR* 143:1053, 1984.
Hamilton S, Fitzpatrick JM: Primary non-obstructive megaureter in adults. *Clin Radiol* 38:181, 1987.
King LR: Megaloureter: definition, diagnosis and management. *J Urol* 123:222, 1980.
Pfister RC, Hendren WH: Primary megaureter in children and adults. *Urology* 12(2):160, 1978.
Sherwood T: The dilated upper urinary tract. *Radiol Clin North Am* 17:333, 1979.

Ureteral Tumors

Abulafi A, Leese T, Osborn DE: Inverted papilloma of the ureter. *Br J Urol* 59(5):480, 1987.
Ambos MA, Bosniak MA, Megibow AJ, et al: Ureteral involvement by metastatic disease. *Urol Radiol* 1:105, 1979.
Anderstrom C, Johnsson SL, Pettersson S, et al: Carcinoma of the ureter: a clinicopathologic study of 49 class. *J Urol* 142:280, 1989.
Banner MP, Pollack HM: Fibrous ureteral polyps. *Radiology* 130:73, 1979.
Barbaric ZL, MacIntosh PK: Periureteral thin-needle aspiration biopsy. *Urol Radiol* 2:181, 1981.
Baron RL, McClennan BL, Lee JKT, et al: Computed tomography of transitional cell carcinoma of the renal pelvis and ureter. *Radiology* 144:125, 1982.
Corkill M, Srigley J, Graham R, et al: Inverted papilloma: an uncommon benign cause of a ureteral filling defect. *Urol Radiol* 9:165, 1987.
Hughes FA, Davis CS: Multiple benign ureteral fibrous polyps. *Radiology* 126(4):723, 1976.
Kenney PJ, Stanley RJ: Computed tomography of ureteral tumors. *J Comput Assist Tomogr* 11(1):102, 1987.
Pollack HM: Long-term follow-up of the upper urinary tract for transitional cell carcinoma: how much is enough? *Radiology* 167:871, 1988.
Winalski CS, Lipman JC, Tumeb SS: Ureteral neoplasms. *RadioGraphics* 10:271, 1990.
Witters S, Vereecken RL, Baert L, et al: Primary neoplasm of the ureter: a review of twenty eight cases. *Eur Urol* 13:256, 1987.
Yousem DM, Gatewood OMB, Goldman SM, et al: Synchronous and metachronous transitional cell carcinoma of the urinary tract: prevalence, incidence, and radiographic detection. *Radiology* 167:613, 1988.

Leukoplakia

Benson RC Jr, Swanson SK, Farrow GM: Relationship of leukoplakia to urothelial malignancy. *J Urol* 131:507, 1984.
Hertle L, Androulakakis R: Keratinizing desquamative squamous metaplasia of the upper urinary tract: leukoplakia-cholesteatoma. *J Urol* 127:631, 1982.
Willis JS, Pollack WM, Curtis JA: Cholesteatoma of the upper urinary tract. *AJR* 136:941, 1981.

Malacoplakia

Arap S, Denes FT, Silva J, et al: Malakoplakia of the urinary tract. *Eur Urol* 12:113, 1986.

Stanton MJ, Maxted W: Malacoplakia: a study of the literature and current concepts of pathogenesis, diagnosis and treatment. *J Urol* 125:139, 1981.

Ureteritis Cystica

Loitman BS, Chiat H: Ureteritis cystica and pyelitis cystica. A review of cases and roentgenologic criteria. *Radiology* 68:345, 1957.

Thompson JS, McAlister WH: Subepithelial hemorrhage in the renal pelvis and ureter simulating pyeloureteritis cystica. *Pediat Radiol* 3:156, 1975.

Ureteral Pseudodiverticulosis

Parker MD, Rebsamen S, Clark RL: Multiple ureteral diverticula: a possible radiographically demonstrable risk factor in development of transitional cell carcinoma. *Urol Radiol* 11:45, 1989.

Wasserman NF, Pointe SL, Posalaky IP: Ureteral pseudodiverticulosis. *Radiology* 155:561, 1985.

Wasserman NF, Posalaky IP, Dykoski R: The pathology of ureteral pseudodiverticulosis. *Invest Radiol* 23(8):592, 1988.

Eosinophilic Ureteritis

Uyama T, Moriwaki S, Aga Y, et al: Eosinophilic ureteritis. *Urology* 18(6):615, 1981.

Endometriosis

Ball TL, Platt MA: Urologic complications of endometriosis: *Am J Obst Gynecol* 84(1):1516, 1962.

Plous RH, Sunshine R, Goldman H, et al: Ureteral endometriosis in postmenopausal women. *Urology* 26(4):408, 1985.

Pollack HM, Wills JS: Radiographic features of ureteral endometriosis. *AJR* 131:627, 1978.

Amyloidosis

Davis PS, Babaria A, March DE, et al: Primary amyloidosis of the ureter and renal pelvis. *Urol Radiol* 9:158, 1987.

Lee KT, Deeths TM: Localized amyloidosis of the ureter. *Radiology* 120:60, 1976.

Robinson CR, Fowler JE Jr: Localized amyloidosis of the ureter. *J Urol* 131:112, 1984.

Inflammatory Bowel Disease

Banner MP: Genitourinary complications of inflammatory bowel disease. *Radiol Clin North Am* 25(1):199, 1987.

Schistosomiasis

Al-Ghorab MM: Radiological manifestations of genito-urinary bilharziasis. *Clin Radiol* 19:100, 1968.

Emerah BC: The less familiar manifestations of schistosomiasis of the urinary tract. *Br J Radiol* 50:105, 1977.

Young SW, Khalid KH, Farid Z, et al: Urinary tract lesions of schistosoma haematobium. *Radiology* 111:81, 1974.

Tuberculosis

Friedenberg RM, Ney C, Stachenfeld RA: Roentgenographic manifestations of tuberculosis of the ureter. *J Urol* 99:25, 1968.

Kollins SA, Hartman GW, Carr DT, et al: Roentgenographic findings in urinary tract tuberculosis. *AJR* 121(3):487, 1974.

Roylance N, Penry JB, Davies ER, et al: The radiology of tuberculosis of the urinary tract. *Clin Radiol* 21:163, 1970.

Inflammatory Strictures/Balloon Dilatation of the Ureter

Beckmann CF, Roth RA, Bihrle W III: Dilation of benign ureteral strictures. *Radiology* 172:432, 1989.

Johnson CD, Oke EJ, Dunnick NR, et al: Percutaneous balloon dilatation of ureteral strictures. *AJR* 148:181, 1987.

Lang EK, Glorioso LW III: Antegrade transluminal dilatation of benign ureteral strictures: long term results. *AJR* 150:131, 1988.

Shapiro MJ, Banner MP, Amendola MA, et al: Balloon catheter dilatation of ureteroenteric strictures: long term results. *Radiology* 168:385, 1988.

Retroperitoneal Fibrosis

Abbott DL, Skinner DG, Yalowitz PA, et al: Retroperitoneal fibrosis associated with abdominal aortic aneurysms: an approach to management. *J Urol* 109:987, 1973.

Alexopoulos E, Memmos D, Bakatselos S, et al: Idiopathic retroperitoneal fibrosis: a long term follow up study. *Eur Urol* 13:313, 1987.

Baker LRI, Mallinson WJW, Gregory MC, et al: Idiopathic retroperitoneal fibrosis: a retrospective analysis of 60 cases. *Br J Urol* 60:497, 1988.

Broders AC: Epithelioma of the genitourinary organs. *Ann Surg* 75:574, 1922.

Degesys GE, Dunnick NR, Silverman PM, et al: Retroperitoneal fibrosis: use of CT in distinguishing among possible causes. *AJR* 146:57, 1986.

Fagan CJ, Amparo EG, Davis M: Retroperitoneal fibrosis. *Semin Ultrasound* 3(2):123, 1982.

Fagan CJ, Larrieu AJ, Amparo EG: Retroperitoneal fibrosis: ultrasound and CT features. *AJR* 133:239, 1979.

Graham JR, Suby HI, LeCompte PR, et al: Fibrotic disorders associated with methysergide therapy for headache. *N Engl J Med* 274(7):359, 1966.

Hricak H, Higgins CB, William RD: Nuclear magnetic resonance imaging in retroperitoneal fibrosis. *AJR* 141:35, 1983.

Inaraja L, Franquet T, Caballero P, et al: CT findings in circumscribed upper abdominal idiopathic retroperitoneal fibrosis. *J Comput Assist Tomogr* 10(6):1063, 1986.

Labardini MM, Ratliff RK: The abdominal aortic aneurysm and the ureter. *J Urol* 98:590, 1967.

Lalli AF: Retroperitoneal fibrosis and inapparent obstructive uropathy. *Radiology* 122:339, 1977.

Rubenstein WA, Gray G, Auh YH, et al: CT of fibrous tissues and tumors with sonographic correlation. *AJR* 147:1067, 1986.

Ovarian Vein Syndrome and Vascular Impressions

Cleveland RH, Fellows KE, Lebowitz RL: Notching of the ureter and renal pelvis in children. *AJR* 129:837, 1977.

Derrick FC Jr, Rosenblum RR, Frensilli FJ: Right ovarian vein syndrome. Six year critique. *Urology* 1:383, 1973.

Derrick FC Jr, Rosenblum RR, Lynch KM Jr: Pathological association of the right ureter and right ovarian vein. *J Urol* 97:633, 1967.

Dykhvizen RF, Roberts JA: The ovarian vein syndrome. *Surg Gynecol Obstet* 130:443, 1970.

Pregnancy Dilatation

Dure-Smith P: Pregnancy dilatation of the urinary tract. *Radiology* 96:545, 1970.

Pseudoureterocele

Thornbury JR, Silver TM, Vinson RK: Ureteroceles vs. pseudoureteroceles in adults. *Radiology* 122:81, 1977.

Procidentia

Chapman RH: Ureteric obstruction due to uterine prolapse. *Br J Urol* 47:531, 1975.

Stabler J: Uterine prolapse and urinary tract obstruction. *Br J Radiol* 50:493, 1977.

Ureteral Fistula

Lang EK: Diagnosis and management of ureteral fistulas by percutaneous nephrostomy and antegrade stent catheter. *Radiology* 138:311, 1981.

Lang EK: Antegrade ureteral stenting for dehiscence, strictures and fistulae. *AJR* 143:795, 1984.

Mitty HA, Dan SJ, Train JS: Antegrade ureteral stents: technical and catheter-related problems with polyethylene and polyurethane. *Radiology* 165:439, 1987.

Mitty HA, Train JS, Dan SJ: Antegrade ureteral stenting in the management of fistulas, strictures and calculi. *Radiology* 149:433, 1983.

Deviations of the Ureter

Adams EJ, Desai SC, Lawton G: Racial variations in normal ureteric course. *Clin Radiol* 36:373, 1985.

Cunat JS, Goldman SM: Extrinsic displacement of the ureter. *Semin Roentgenol* 21(3):188, 1986.

Ney C, Friedenberg RM: *Radiographic Atlas of the Genitourinary System.* Philadelphia, JB Lippincott, 1981, p 1295.

Saldino RM, Palubinskas AJ: Medial displacement of the ureter: a normal variant which may simulate retroperitoneal fibrosis. *J Urol* 107:582, 1972.

Ureteral Perfusion Studies

Newhouse JH, Pfister RC, Hendren WH, et al: Whitaker test after pyeloplasty: establishment of normal ureteral perfusion pressures. *AJR* 137:223, 1981.

Pfister RC, Newhouse JH: Interventional percutaneous pyeloureteral techniques: I. Antegrade pyelography and ureteral perfusion. *Radiol Clin North Am* 17:341, 1979.

Pfister RC, Newhouse JH, Hendren WG: Percutaneous pyeloureteral urodynamics. *Urol Clin North Am* 9:41, 1982.

Pfister RC, Yoder IC, Newhouse JH: Percutaneous uroradiologic procedures. *Semin Roentgenol* 16:135, 1981.

Whitaker RH: Diagnosis of obstruction in dilated ureters. *Ann R Coll Surg* 53:153, 1973.

Whitaker RH: Investigating wide ureter and ureteral pressure flow studies. *J Urol* 116:81, 1976.

Whitaker RH: An evaluation of 170 diagnostic pressure flow studies of the upper urinary tract. *J Urol* 121:602, 1979.

Diuretic Renography

Hay AM, Normal WJ, Rice ML, et al: A comparison between diuresis renography and the Whitaker test in 64 kidneys. *Br J Urol* 56:561, 1984.

Howman-Giles R, Uren R, Roy LP, et al: Volume expansion diuretic renal scan in urinary tract obstruction. *J Nucl Med* 28:824, 1987.

Koff SA, Thrall JA, Keyes JW: Diuretic radionuclide urography: a noninvasive method for evaluating nephroureteral dilatation. *J Urol* 122:451, 1979.

Koff SA, Thrall JA, Keyes JW: Assessment of hydroureteronephrosis in children using diuretic radionuclide urography. *J Urol* 123:531, 1980.

Krueger RP, Ash JA, Silver MM, et al: Primary hydronephrosis: assessment of diuretic renography, pelvis perfusion pressure, operative findings and renal and ureteral histology. *Urol Clin North Am* 7:231, 1980.

Meller ST, Eckstein HB: Renal scintigraphy: quantitative assessment of upper urinary tract dilatation in children. *J Pediatr Surg* 16(2):126, 1981.

Senac MO Jr, Miller JH, Stanley P: Evaluation of obstructive uropathy in children: radionuclide renography vs. the Whitaker test. *AJR* 143:11, 1984.

Shore RM, Uehling DT, Bruskewitz R, et al: Evaluation of obstructive uropathy with diuretic renography. *Am J Dis Child* 137:236, 1983.

Thrall JH, Koff SA, Keyes JW: Diuretic radionuclide renography and scintigraphy in the differential diagnosis of hydroureteronephrosis. *Semin Nucl Med* 11(2):89, 1981.

Upsdell SM, Leeson SM, Brooman PJC, et al: Diuretic-induced urinary flow rates at varying clearances and their relevance to the performance and interpretation of diuresis renography. *Br J Urol* 61:14, 1988.

Wacksman J, Brewer E, Gelfand MJ, et al: Low grade pelviureteric junction obstruction with normal diuretic renography. *Br J Urol* 58:364, 1986.

Whitaker RH, Buxton-Thomas MS: A comparison of pressure flow studies and renography in equivocal upper urinary tract obstruction. *J Urol* 131:446, 1984.

CHAPTER 15

THE URINARY BLADDER

BENIGN INTRAVESICLE LESIONS

Filling Defects

Blood clot within the bladder may arise from a bleeding renal, ureteric, or bladder lesion. On excretory urography, blood clot is usually an irregular mobile filling defect but occasionally may appear to be relatively fixed in position and may not be distinguishable from a tumor. Ultrasound (US), however, shows that the echogenicity in blood clot is unlike that of bladder tumor in which the echogenicity is the same as the bladder wall or other soft tissue. Computed tomography (CT) may help to distinguish blood clot from tumor but is mainly useful to exclude a radiolucent stone.

Edema

Mucosal edema of the bladder may result from a stone impacted in the ureterovesicle junction, or the recent passage of such a stone (Fig. 15.1). Mucosal edema may also result from bladder irritation from acute appendicitis, Crohn's disease, or sigmoid diverticulitis. Mucosal edema may result from hemorrhagic cystitis, in which the whole bladder mucosa is edematous.

Excretory urography shows the irregularity of the bladder wall (Fig. 15.2**A**) when the bladder is filled with

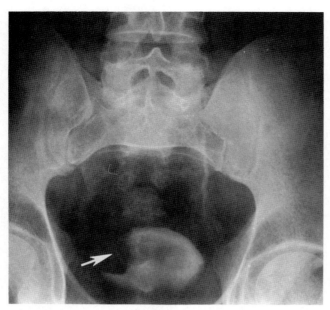

Figure 15.1. Excretory urogram in a patient with severe right renal colic. There is a faintly opacified stone (*arrow*) at the right UV junction. The filling defect in the bladder outline represents edema. (From McCallum RW, Colapinto V: *Urological Radiology of the Adult Male Lower Urinary Tract.* Springfield, IL, Charles C Thomas, 1976, p 271.)

contrast medium, however, the etiology of the edema cannot be ascertained on excretory urography or a similar appearance may be produced by malignant bladder infiltration. Pelvic and bladder ultrasound is capable of showing the edematous nature of the filling defects. It may also show an extravesicle cause for localized bladder edema, such as an appendiceal abscess, diverticular abscess, or a mass due to Crohn's disease. If no localized extravesicle mass is seen, care should be taken to visualize the bladder wall for localized thickening, which may indicate a bladder tumor causing localized edema. Computed tomography may likewise show an associated extravesicle mass. The density of the edematous mucosa is only slightly less than that of soft tissue and presents as a filling defect within the bladder producing an irregular outline to the contrast medium within the bladder. Computed tomography is unlikely to distinguish edema from any intravesicle cause of bladder wall thickening including the presence of infiltrating bladder tumor (Fig. 15.2**B** and **C**).

Foreign Bodies

Foreign bodies within the bladder are most commonly the result of self-insertion. Hair clips, pens, pencils (Fig. 15.3), matches, wire, tubing, and string have all been seen within the bladder. Rarely they are the result of penetrating wounds (bullets) or a nasocomial cause. Broken or shorn catheter fragments have been seen within the bladder. Bladder catheterization may introduce pubic hair into the bladder. These may become encrusted with calcification (Fig. 15.4**A** and **B**).

Most foreign bodies within the bladder are radiopaque. Long-standing intravesicle radiolucent foreign bodies commonly have a deposit of encrusted calcium and may become apparent on plain film. Intravenous tubing may be seen as faintly radiopaque on plain film. Foreign bodies are usually well seen on excretory urography but ultrasound is the method of choice for the identification of any bladder foreign body. The mobility, shape, and acoustic shadowing are well seen.

Acute Infection

Infectious cystitis is present when over 100,000 bacteria are present in 1 ml of fresh urine. This may result in transient, acute, or chronic cystitis. Most bacteria causing cystitis enter the bladder via the urethra. *Escherichia coli* is the most common infection, but other agents include *Staphylococcus aureus* and *Staphylococcus albus*, *Streptococcus faecales*, *Proteus*, *Pseudomonas*, *Aerobacter aerogenes*, and *Candida albicans*. Infections entering the bladder in an antegrade fashion from the kidney include tuberculosis.

There is a natural resistance to bladder infection per urethra that must be overcome before bladder infection occurs. The natural resistance to bladder infection consists of four factors: (a) the intact bladder mucosa is resistant to invasion by infection; (b) bladder emptying washes out bacteria; (c) the mucous secretion of the periurethral glands traps bacteria; and (d) prostatic secretions have a bacteriocidal action. Therefore bladder infection is almost invariably the result of interference with these factors. The bladder mucosa may be damaged by trauma, stone, or tumor. Outlet obstruction results in residual urine so that bacteria are not completely washed out. Bladder catheterization or instrumentation may introduce infection bypassing the natural prostatic secretions. Any cause of residual urine such as obstruction, neurogenic bladder, or residual urine in a bladder diverticulum may result in infection.

Transient cystitis is an acute episode of cystitis that may result in frequency, dysuria strangury, or microhematuria. Inflammatory changes are usually confined to the trigone. It is more common in young females. Adequate antibiotic therapy and increased fluid intake are sufficient to eradicate the condition without permanent effects on the bladder. Radiologically the bladder is normal. The condition does not tend to recur.

Acute cystitis with virulent organisms gives rise to similar symptoms as transient cystitis but is more severe and may produce gross hematuria. Inflammatory changes involve the bladder mucosa producing mucosal thicken-

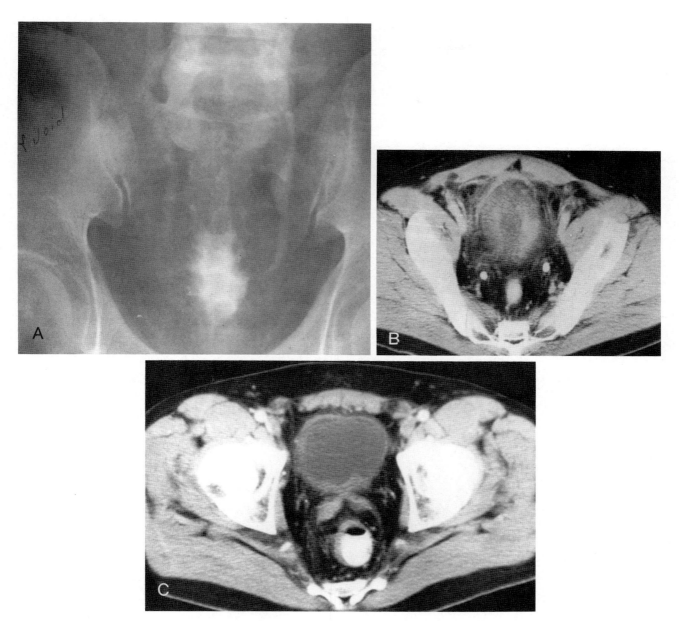

Figure 15.2. **A,** Excretory urogram in a patient with acute fulminating cystitis and severe bladder edema. Note the markedly reduced bladder capacity due to edema. **B,** Computed tomography of the same patient showing marked bladder wall thickening. **C,** Computed tomography 1 month later. The edema has subsided but the bladder wall remains irregularly thickened. Multiple bladder biopsies showed infiltrating transitional cell carcinoma. (Courtesy P. Poon, M.D.)

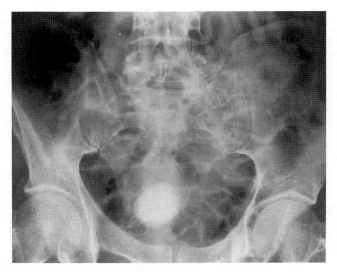

Figure 15.3. Small pencil inserted into the bladder per urethra. The pencil has had continuous encrustations presenting as a bladder stone. (From McCallum RW, Colapinto V: *Urological Radiology of the Adult Male Lower Urinary Tract.* Springfield, IL, Charles C Thomas, 1976, p 266.)

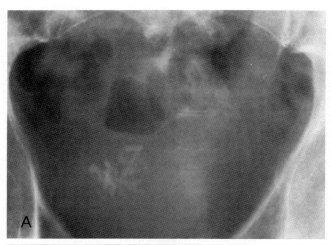

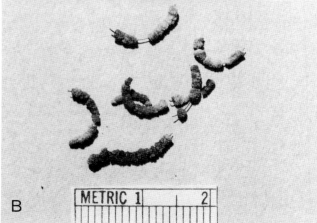

Figure 15.4. **A,** A plain film of the pelvis showing multiple irregular elongated calcifications within the bladder outline. **B,** Gross specimen on calcific encrusted hairs after removal at cystoscopy. (From Amendola MA, et al: *AJR* 141:751, 1983.)

ing and a cobblestone appearance. The excretory urogram is usually normal with a normal filled bladder appearance. The cobblestone appearance may be apparent on a postvoid film if some residual contrast medium is present (Fig. 15.2**A**). Acute cystitis usually responds well to antibiotic therapy and increased fluid intake. Recurrence of acute cystitis should raise the possibility of an underlying causative lesion, and cystoscopy is indicated.

Chronic Infection

Chronic cystitis and the persistence of bladder infection in spite of adequate management should raise the possibility of descending infection such as tuberculosis. However, the possibility of underlying bladder tumor or residual urine due to outlet obstruction or bladder diverticulum should be excluded. Transabdominal ultrasound is helpful in excluding bladder diverticulum, but transrectal ultrasound may be necessary for best assessment of the prostate and bladder neck. The posterior lip of the bladder neck may be hypertrophied due to chronic outlet obstruction. The hypertrophied posterior bladder lip may contribute to outlet obstruction. Thickened bladder mucosal folds may also be seen in chronic cystitis, and when these are close to the bladder neck, they may contribute to outlet obstruction. Infiltrating bladder carcinoma may cause thickening of the bladder wall, which is usually localized but may be generalized. Cystoscopy and biopsy are necessary to exclude this.

Chronic cystitis due to tuberculosis is an interstitial cystitis, initially causing mucosal edema, later causing bladder wall thickening and fibrotic contraction with reduced bladder capacity. Excretory urography usually reveals evidence of renal tuberculosis. Rarely there is evidence of calcification in the vas deferens and seminal vesicles, prostate, and epididymis. Calcification in the ampulla of the vas deferens is more commonly found as a result of diabetes mellitus. The effect of tuberculosis on the bladder may be nil in early tuberculosis. More advanced bladder involvement may show a small contracted, thick-walled bladder with an irregular outline and rarely calcification (Fig. 15.5). Multiple filling defects within the bladder on urography or cystoscopy are usually the result of associated cystitis cystica or cystitis glandularis, both of which are the result of chronic inflammation. Cystitis cystica is the result of transitional epithelial rests producing serous filled cysts that are usually small but can attain a size of 2 cm. Cystitis glandularis is the result of mucin-secreting glandular hypertrophy within the bladder mucosa. This produces multiple cyst-like filling defects along the bladder mucosa. The chest radiograph shows evidence of pulmonary tuberculosis in approximately 50% of patients. Stricture formation of the ureterovesicle junction results in dilated ureters. Occasionally the bladder contraction causes widening of the ureterovesicle junction resulting in vesicoureteral reflux, however, this occurs in less than 5% of cases of urinary tuberculosis.

Emphysematous cystitis or cystitis emphysematosa is a rare condition. True emphysematous cystitis is gas within the bladder *and gas within the bladder wall,* which is almost pathognomonic of diabetes mellitus. This is a true infectious cystitis most often due to *Escherichia coli,* which ferments urine glucose to produce carbon dioxide and hydrogen. This occurs in poorly controlled diabetes together with an ascending coliform infection. True cystitis emphysematosa may also occur in patients with long-standing urinary stasis such as outlet obstruction, neurogenic bladder, or bladder diverticulum. However, these causes of cystitis emphysematosa are extremely rare.

Gas within the bladder but not in the bladder wall is usually not a true cystitis, but the result of a vesicocolic fistula or the iatrogenic insertion of air per urethra. Gas within the bladder is sometimes erroneously called cystitis emphysematosa or emphysematous cystitis, although there is usually no associated infection.

True cystitis emphysematosa causes dysuria, hematuria, and pneumaturia. The pneumaturia may go unnoticed for sometime since the gas bubbles within the urine are small and occur mainly at the end of micturition. True cystitis emphysematosa on cystoscopic examination reveals a red and edematous mucosa with multiple blebs that rupture easily, releasing gas.

The plain film shows gas within the bladder and irregular streaky radiolucencies within the bladder wall (Fig.

15.6). Gas may also enter proximally up the ureters, which should raise the possibility of vesicoureteral reflux, although it is possible for gas to pass through a competent vesicoureteral junction. On plain film examination, air within the bladder should not be mistaken for rectal air (Fig. 15.7). Air within the bladder conforms to the bladder shape, i.e., round, and in central position low in the pelvis. The radiolucency of bladder air is usually slightly less than rectal air due to the presence of urine layering behind the bladder air on the supine plain film. The excretory urogram outlines the contrast medium containing bladder with an air-fluid level on upright films. True cystitis emphysematosa is managed adequately by stabilizing the patient's diabetes mellitus and instituting antibiotic therapy. Cystitis emphysematosa due to other causes may require surgical intervention.

Gas within the bladder due to vesicocolic fistula requires investigation to elicit the fistula. Both cystography and barium enema are disappointing in demonstrating vesicocolic fistula (Fig. 15.8). The success rate of fistula visualization is only 35% when diverticulitis of the colon is the cause of the fistula. Colonic carcinoma causing vesicocolic fistula is less common but is usually demonstrated on barium enema. A history of recent bladder catheterization or instrumentation may indicate an iatrogenic cause. Vesicocolic fistula requires surgical intervention. Computed tomography may clearly show diverticulitis and air in the bladder although the fistulous tract may not be obvious (Fig. 15.9). Barium and air may enter the bladder from a coloureteric fistula, which is rare (Fig. 15.10).

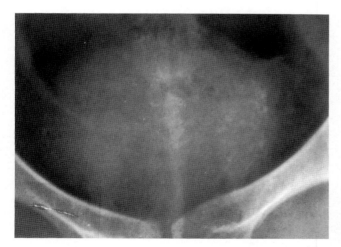

Figure 15.5.   Early film of excretory urogram in a patient with renal tuberculosis. Very little contrast medium has entered the bladder at this time. Multiple densities in the left bladder outline represent bladder tuberculous calcifications. (Courtesy of G. Hartman, M.D.)

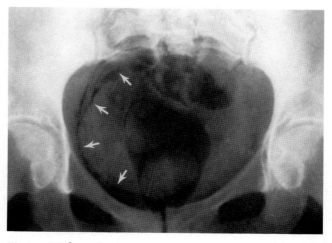

Figure 15.6.   Emphysematous cystitis. Linear collections of gas within the bladder wall (*arrows*) indicate infection in this patient with diabetes mellitus.

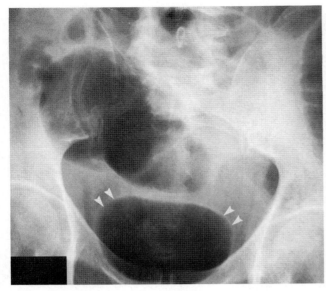

Figure 15.7.   Gas within the bladder outline (*arrows*) resulting from colovesicle fistula. (Modified from McCallum RW, Colapinto V: *Urological Radiology of the Adult Male Lower Urinary Tract.* Springfield, IL, Charles C Thomas, 1976, p. 302.)

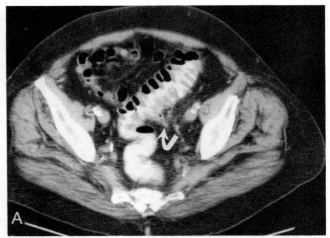

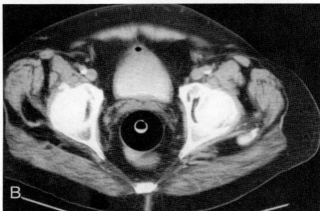

Figure 15.9.   **A,** Computed tomography examination in a patient with diverticulitis and paracolic abscess. The examination clearly shows evidence of diverticulitis and an irregular leak of barium (*arrow*) from the sigmoid colon. **B,** Same patient showing small pocket of air within the bladder.

Bilharziasis (Schistosomiasis) of the Bladder

Three types of Schistosoma exist, but two, *Schistosoma japonicum* and *Schistosoma mansoni,* usually affect the GI tract. *Schistosoma haematobium* affects the urinary tract. Bilharziasis is a parasitic infection endemic in many countries but most prevalent in North Africa, the Nile Valley, and Egypt. It is not known to occur in North America and European countries. The definitive host is human. The intermediate host is usually freshwater snails. In the human, *Schistosoma* lives within the liver and portal system. Eggs are excreted in feces and urine. Excretion of *Schistosoma haematobium* is predominantly in the urine. The *Schistosoma haematobium* eggs hatch in fresh water, invade the intermediate host, and produce larvae that are excreted. These larvae then penetrate the skin of humans; and vessels and lymphatics carry the larvae to the liver where they survive and produce millions of eggs. Excretion of eggs in the urine begins the cycle again. Many of the eggs are not excreted in the urine but become trapped in the ureteric and bladder mucosa producing a

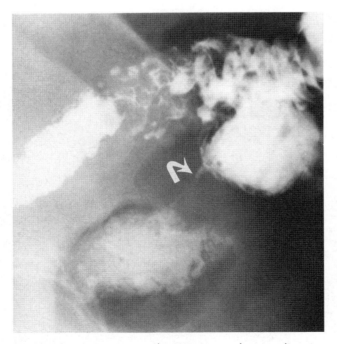

Figure 15.8.   Air contrast barium enema showing diverticulitis, a paracolic abscess, and a fistulous tract (*arrow*) from the sigmoid colon to the bladder. The bladder contains air and barium.

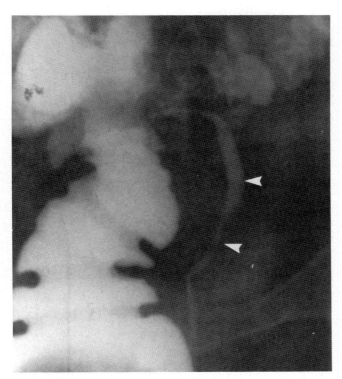

Figure 15.10. Barium enema in a patient with pneumaturia. The study shows a coloureteric fistula with barium outlining the ureter (*arrows*).

severe granulomatous reaction. Eggs penetrate the submucosa of the ureter and bladder, causing granulomatous reaction, fibrosis, and death of the eggs. The dead eggs calcify causing fine linear streaks of calcium in the ureteric and bladder walls. Large conglomerations of eggs in the bladder wall produce masses known as bilharzioma, which may eventually calcify.

The clinical presentation of urinary bilharziasis is dysuria, hematuria, and frequency. Patients from the Middle East presenting with these symptoms in North America should always raise the possibility of bilharziasis. In initial stages the bladder mucosa is edematous and hemorrhagic, and cystitis cystica may be present. Later the bladder is fibrotic with a reduced volume. Cystoscopic examination is mandatory to exclude bladder cancer, which has a markedly increased incidence in bilharziasis. Biopsy may be necessary to distinguish bilharzioma from carcinoma, although carcinoma usually presents as a later complication. It is to be emphasized that unlike tuberculosis, in which bladder involvement follows renal involvement, bladder involvement occurs before renal involvement in bilharziasis. Bilharziasis rarely affects the kidneys or collecting systems except by obstruction due to ureteric and bladder disease.

Radiologic findings in early bilharziasis may show an irregular bladder outline due to edema and granulomatous reaction. No bladder or ureteric calcification is evi-

dent. Later in the disease the plain film finding may be spectacular, showing calcification in the bladder wall, bladder stones and ureteric calcification (Figs. 15.11 and 15.12). The ureterovesicle junction (UVJ) is likely to be affected initially causing ureteric dilatation. Later the dilated ureter may show significant calcification within the dilated ureteric walls. Excretory urography in well-developed cases usually shows obstructive dilatation of the pelvicalyceal system, dilated ureters, and a small partly calcified contracted bladder. Bilharziasis may also affect the prostate and urethra. The disease is destructive and results in fistula formation and cavitation within the prostate. Fistulae may drain into the perineum, scrotum, suprapubic skin, or buttocks. Fistulous formation in the urethra occurs initially followed by urethral stricture usually in the bulbous urethra. This is in direct opposition to other fistulous urethral disease, which is secondary to urethral stricture. Consequently excretory urography in well-developed cases is likely to show a dilated pelvicalyceal system, dilated ureters that may be calcified, patchy linear or crescentic calcification within the bladder wall, and fistulous tracts from the bladder base and prostate with extravasation of contrast medium into the fistulous tracts. Occasionally bladder stones are present.

All of the above findings can be assessed by ultrasound. The presence of calcifications in the distal ureters and bladder wall are seen as bright echoes with or without acoustic shadowing. Ultrasound is an excellent method of follow up in patients with urinary bilharziasis. If treated early with antischistosomal drugs, the pathologic changes may be reversible. Advanced changes are irreversible.

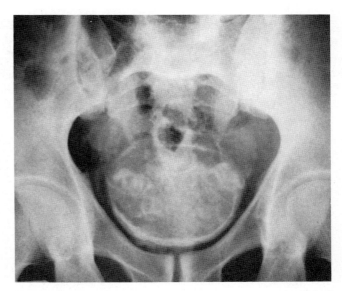

Figure 15.11. Plain film of the pelvis showing marked bladder wall calcification. Seminal vesicle calcification is also seen through the bladder outline. (Courtesy S. Sejeni, M.D.)

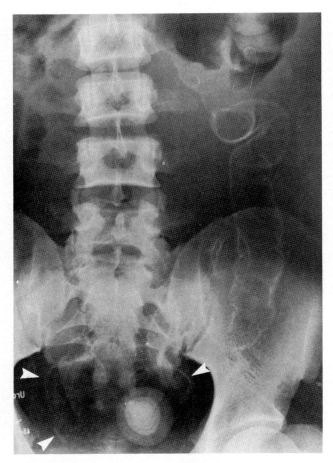

Figure 15.12. Plain film in a patient with schistosomiasis. Crescentic calcifications are seen in the bladder wall (*arrows*). There is a large laminated stone within the bladder. The ureter is dilated and calcified. (Modified from McCallum RW, Colapinto V: *Urological Radiology of the Adult Male Lower Urinary Tract.* Springfield, IL, Charles C Thomas, 1976, p 272.)

Computed tomography is more sensitive than excretory urography in visualizing faint calcifications in the ureters and bladder walls. With the patient's geographic history such calcification is pathognomonic. The presence of associated bladder cancer can be suspected when a mass is present interrupting the linear or crescentic calcification.

Candidiasis

Candidiasis or bladder fungus ball has been reported. This is most commonly a complication of poorly controlled diabetes and when present is seen as a laminated, gas-containing filling defect within the bladder. The complications of chronic bladder infection include the development of cystitis cystica, cystitis glandularis, malacoplakia, granulomatous cystitis, bladder stones, and bladder carcinoma.

Inflammatory Conditions

Radiation Cystitis

Bladder cancer is responsive to radiation therapy but may result in radiation cystitis in up to 15% of patients. It may also occur in 3–5% of patients treated for cervical cancer. Radiation cystitis may occur when a dose of 6500–7500 R is given in a six to eight week period. This may be an acute cystitis in which edema and hemorrhage occur, followed by mucosal ulceration, fibrosis, and a small capacity bladder. Rarely calcification is seen in the bladder wall. Hemorrhage may be severe and angiographic embolization may be necessary to control bleeding. Cystography and excretory urography show filling defects in the bladder wall due to edema, indistinguishable from other causes of bladder mucosal edema (Fig. 15.13).

Cyclophosphamide Cystitis

Up to 40% of patients treated with cyclophosphamide may develop an acute cystitis. Marked bladder edema and hemorrhage occur. Hemorrhage may be so severe that angiographic embolization may be required. Uncontrolled bleeding may require cystectomy. There is a marked increased in the incidence of bladder carcinoma in patients being treated with cyclophosphamide (Fig. 15.14). Bladder edema and hemorrhage may subside and the bladder can return to normal if cyclophosphamide is discontinued early in cystitis. Edema and hemorrhage may not be severe, and continued therapy with cyclophosphamide results in fibrosis and a small capacity bladder. Irregular bladder wall calcification may occur.

Eosinophilic Cystitis

Eosinophilic cystitis occurs in patients with severe allergic conditions and is more common in women. Rarely

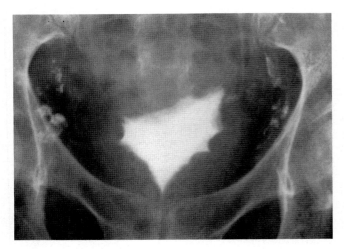

Figure 15.13. Radiation cystitis. Bladder irradiation has resulted in marked thickening of the bladder wall with edema.

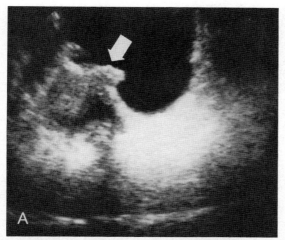

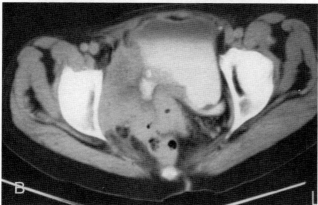

Figure 15.14. **A,** This 38-year-old female had renal transplant and was treated with cyclophosphamide. The ultrasound study shows a bladder mass (*arrow*) at the UVJ which proved to be transitional cell carcinoma. **B,** Computed tomography on the same patient. The transitional cell carcinoma extends through the bladder wall producing a large extravesicle mass.

it is seen in elderly men in association with chronic outlet obstruction. Eosinophilic infiltration of the bladder mucosa and submucosa results in edema, hemorrhage and ulceration.

Interstitial Cystitis

Interstitial cystitis is rare and seen only in females, usually after menopause. The mucosa is hemorrhagic, and Hunner's ulcerations are often present in the dome. The condition results in fibrosis and a small capacity bladder. There is no known etiology and no associated conditions have been identified.

Malacoplakia

Malacoplakia of the bladder is of unknown etiology but is associated with chronic disease such as pulmonary tuberculosis, chronic osteomyelitis, and long-standing malignant disease elsewhere in the body. It has been suggested that there is also an association with coliform

bladder infection. The bladder mucosa contains multiple yellow-gray plaques. Biopsy of these plaques show histiocytes, lymphocytes, and plasma cells. Michaelis-Gutmann bodies in the biopsy specimen are diagnostic. These inflammatory noninfective conditions of the bladder have similar clinical presentations. Bladder pain, dysuria, and frequency are common to all. Radiation and cyclophosphamide cystitis also result in hemorrhage. Radiologic investigation including excretory urography ultrasound and CT are all nonspecific. Each shows filling defects at the bladder wall due to edema and hemorrhage, or a thick-walled, contracted bladder. The definitive diagnosis is made on historical, clinical, and cystoscopic findings.

Infiltrating Lesions

Amyloidosis

Amyloidosis of the bladder is rare. It may be primary or secondary and associated with amyloidosis elsewhere. The patient presents with hematuria and frequency. Cystoscopy shows irregular infiltrating defects in the mucosa and submucosa that bleed readily. Biopsy is necessary for diagnosis. Excretory urography, ultrasound, and CT may show multiple filling defects projecting into the bladder from the bladder wall, but the appearance is nonspecific and cannot be distinguished from other mucosal filling defects. Rarely bladder wall calcification develops within the submucosal infiltrations.

Endometriosis

Endometriosis affecting the bladder is rare. Endometrial tissue may infiltrate through the bladder muscle and produce filling defects projecting into the bladder. This results in hematuria that is more prominent at menstruation. The diagnosis is based on historical and cystoscopic findings. Ultrasound may be helpful in showing mucosal defects within the bladder and also extravesicle endometrial masses in the pelvis and peritoneal space.

Miscellaneous Lesions

Bladder diverticulum occurs as a result of outlet obstruction. Rarely a congenital deficiency in bladder musculature adjacent to the ureterovesicle junction causes a diverticulum adjacent to the ureteric orifice. This is a "Hutch" diverticulum and is commonly associated with ipsilateral vesicoureteral reflux.

Bladder diverticulum from outlet obstruction is rare in children but may occur because of urethral valves or congenital urethral stricture. In adult males it may occur because of urethral stricture (Fig. 15.15), prostatitis, prostatic abscess (Fig. 15.16), prostatic hypertrophy, or prostatic carcinoma. In females urethral diverticulum and urethral carcinoma may cause outlet obstruction.

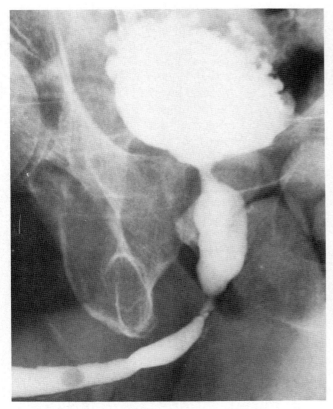

Figure 15.15. Severe bulbous urethral stricture causing outlet obstruction. Multiple bladder diverticulae and saccules are seen.

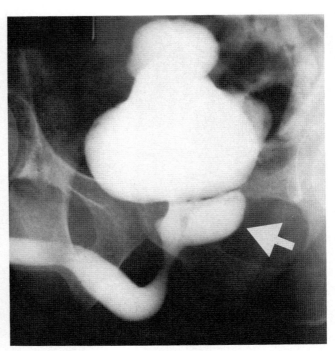

Figure 15.16. Retrograde urethrocystogram in a patient with known tuberculosis. Contrast fills a prostatic cavity (*arrow*), the end result of an old prostatic abscess. Bladder diverticulae are seen at the dome and at the left of the bladder due to long-standing outlet obstruction from prostatitis and prostatic abscess.

Multiple bladder diverticulae are not uncommon, usually arising from the lateral walls and rarely arising near the bladder dome. A wide-necked diverticulum empties readily when the bladder empties (Fig. 15.17). A narrow-necked diverticulum empties slowly as the bladder empties and is therefore more likely to have residual urine and urinary stasis. A large bladder diverticulum may displace the bladder to the opposite side, and a diverticulum larger than the bladder has been recorded.

The plain film is usually not helpful. Excretory urography commonly shows a diverticulum well (Fig. 15.18), but occasionally a narrow-necked diverticulum does not fill with contrast medium and can be overlooked. Anteroposterior and oblique views should be obtained and Chassard-Lapine (squat shot) views may best visualize a diverticulum and the neck of the diverticulum. Films should be obtained before voiding. If a bladder diverticulum is not visualized but suspected, cystography is indicated. Cystography may be performed with a catheter in the bladder, but retrograde urethrography with the balloon of the catheter in the fossa navicularis can give information as to the cause of outlet obstruction and fill the bladder to show the diverticulum. For better assessment of the bladder and diverticulum mucosa, double contrast

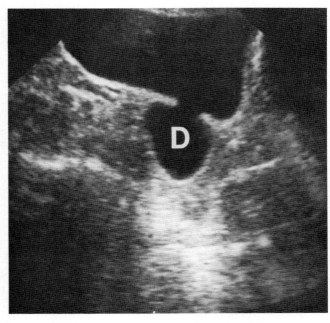

Figure 15.17. Transabdominal ultrasound showing the urine-filled bladder with a urine-filled wide-necked diverticulum (D).

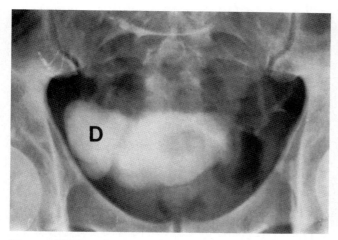

Figure 15.18. Bladder diverticulum. The irregular contour of the bladder is easily distinguished from the smooth contours of the diverticulum (D) on this excretory urogram.

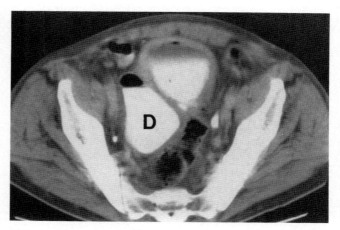

Figure 15.19. Bladder diverticulum. Contrast defines a thick-walled bladder. Gas and contrast (D) are seen in a smooth-walled diverticulum.

cystography is indicated. Tumors within the diverticulum can be assessed in this fashion. The contrast medium used for coating the bladder is dilute barium, 6 ounces of barium to 100 ml of saline. Gas contrast can be provided by the injection of air, nitrous oxide, or carbon dioxide. Most of the barium is removed after rotating the patient, thus coating the bladder and diverticulum mucosa. The bladder and diverticulum is then distended by injection of gas or air. In a series of 142 examinations by double-contrast cystography, Lang found 3.5% of diverticula contained tumor and 26% contained stones.

Ultrasound is also effective in the assessment of bladder diverticulum and has replaced excretory urography and cystography as the method of choice. Echo-free out-pouchings from the bladder are readily seen (Fig. 15.17), and filling defects within the diverticulum such as stones or tumor are also visible. Tumor within the diverticulum may present only as a thickening of the diverticulum wall, but this is easily assessable by ultrasound. Stones within the diverticulum are also readily visible as echogenic areas with acoustic shadowing.

Computed tomography is also an excellent method of assessing bladder diverticulum (Fig. 15.19) but is usually unnecessary. The neck of the diverticulum is usually well visualized. Stones are seen on CT without contrast medium, and a tumor may be seen as a filling defect in the contrast medium–filled diverticulum (Fig. 15.20).

Herniation of the bladder through the inguinal canal presents as an increasing swelling in the groin or scrotum as the urinary bladder fills and subsides as the patient voids. This may cause painful, partly obstructed micturition since the trigourethral area remains in normal position, resulting in a sharp angle at the inguinal canal. Bladder herniation can be seen readily when the bladder is full of contrast medium during excretory

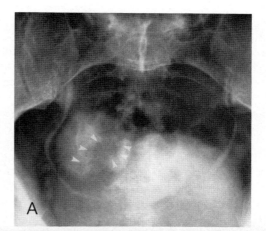

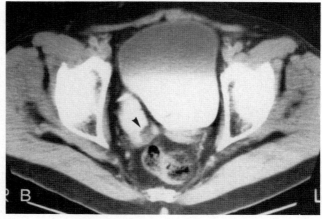

Figure 15.20. **A,** Excretory urogram showing a bladder diverticulum containing a lobulated filling defect (*arrows*). **B,** Computed tomography clearly showing the filling defect within the contrast medium filled diverticulum (*arrow*). Proven transitional cell carcinoma.

urography or cystography (Fig. 15.21), but a pre- and postvoid ultrasound examination is the method of choice for examination of suspected bladder herniation.

Cystocele occurs almost exclusively in multiparous women. Prolapse of the anterior vaginal wall, slackness of the pelvic floor muscles including the external sphincter due to stretching, and lengthening of these muscles during childbirth contribute to lack of support to the posteroinferior bladder wall that prolapses along with the anterior vaginal wall. Patients with cystocele and some postchildbirth patients may complain of stress incontinence, which is urine loss on increased intraabdominal pressure, without detrusor contraction. This implies damage or weakness of the smooth muscle sphincters controlling passive continence and also damage or weakness of the external sphincter, which should contract reflexly on increased intraabdominal pressure to inhibit stress incontinence. The weakening or damage effects to these muscles is almost invariably due to vaginal childbirth. The best method of assessing stress incontinence in the female is by bladder and urethral pressure profiles. However, static chain cystourethrography is still used and may be an adjunct to pressure profile studies, although many gynecologists and radiologists are of the opinion that static chain cystourethrography is of little value. Films are obtained in the lateral position while the patient is resting and repeated while the patient is straining. The anterior angle of inclination, i.e., the angle between the vertical and the urethra is measured and should not be more than 40%. The posterior vesicourethral angle should not be more than 100° (Fig. 15.22). An abnormal posterior vesicourethral angle and a normal anterior angle of inclination represents a Green Type 1 deformity. If both angles are abnormal a Green Type 2 deformity is present. Green Type 1 deformity is generally repaired per vagina by colporrhaphy; Green Type 2 deformity usually requires a suprapubic Marshall-Marchetti type operation.

BLADDER TUMORS

Benign bladder tumors are rare, and the definitive diagnosis is cystoscopic and pathologic rather than radiologic. Most benign bladder tumors are mesenchymal in origin. Leiomyomas are the most common with approximately 160 being reported in the medical literature. Other benign bladder lesions include neurofibroma hamartoma, nephrogenic adenoma, hemangioma, lymphangioma, paraganglioma, pheochromocytoma chemodectoma, arteriovenous malformation (AVM), and fibrous polyp. A few of these tumors require special mention.

Urinary Bladder Leiomyoma

Leiomyoma is most commonly found in females aged 30–50 years. It usually arises at the trigone but may be found on the lateral or posterior walls. The dome and

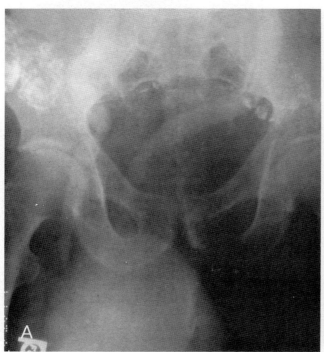
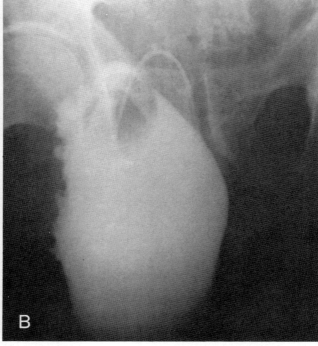

Figure 15.21.   A, Excretory urogram showing dilated distal ureters and contrast medium filling the bladder which is within a scrotal hernia. (Courtesy A. J. Davidson, M.D.). **B,** Cystogram showing a Foley catheter at the bladder base and the herniated bladder inverted.

CHAIN CYSTOURETHROGRAPHY

GREEN'S CLASSIFICATION OF STRESS INCONTINENCE

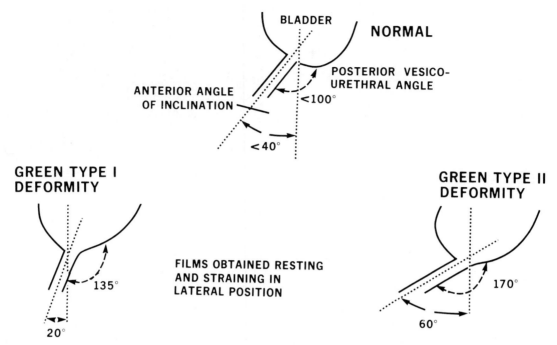

Figure 15.22. Diagrammatic representation of normal and abnormal angles in the assessment of stress incontinence.

anterior bladder wall are infrequent sites. Over 60% project intravesically, but 30% project peripherally from the bladder wall and are extravesicle. The remainder have both intra- and extravesicle components. The intravesicle leiomyoma commonly presents with hematuria and irritative cystitis symptoms. Outlet obstruction due to trigonal leiomyoma at the bladder neck has been reported. Extravesicle leiomyomas are usually asymptomatic until they reach a large size and present as a lower abdominal mass.

Radiologic Diagnosis

Intravesicle leiomyomas may present as a fixed filling defect within the bladder if the lesion is 1–2 cm or more in diameter. Extravesicle leiomyoma presents as an extrinsic mass distorting the bladder outline.

Transabdominal, transrectal, and intravesicle ultrasound are the most useful noninvasive methods of assessing bladder lesions. Transabdominal ultrasound is the most commonly used method. The urine-filled bladder is well visualized. A fixed intravesicle mass can be visualized but cannot be distinguished from other intravesicle fixed lesions. Extravesicle leiomyoma is seen as an extrinsic mass and care must be taken to elicit the origin of the

mass as that of the bladder wall. It may be difficult to distinguish from uterine leiomyomata. If the ultrasound examination shows both an intravesicle and extravesicle component, leiomyoma should be considered in the differential diagnosis, but bladder carcinoma may give a similar appearance, although it is less likely to produce a large extravesicle mass.

Contrast medium is generally necessary to visualize a bladder filling defect on CT. Extravesicle leiomyoma is seen as a soft tissue mass adjacent to the bladder, but it may be difficult to separate the mass from the uterus in female patients if no fat plane is present.

Bladder Hamartoma

The few cases of bladder hamartoma that have been reported are associated with hamartomas elsewhere, especially in the intestinal tract as found in Peutz-Jeghers syndrome. Malignant change is well recognized in the intestinal hamartomas of Peutz-Jeghers syndrome, but no malignant potential has been recorded in bladder hamartomas. Local excision appears to be adequate therapy. The few reported cases have occurred in children or young adults. The lesion arises submucosally and the overlying urothelium is commonly ulcerated.

Nephrogenic Adenoma (Adenomatoid Tumor, Nephrogenic Metaplasia)

Nephrogenic adenoma is associated with a metaplastic process resulting from chronic urinary tract infection, bladder stones, an indwelling catheter, previous bladder trauma, and interstitial cystitis. Nephrogenic adenoma occurs as a localized polypoid lesion after a latent period of some years after the initial bladder insult. Unsuspected neoplastic processes such as adenocarcinoma and transitional cell carcinoma may be concomitantly present and patients with nephrogenic adenoma require close follow-up. Radiologic examination is nonspecific and indistinguishable from other polypoid lesions.

Fibrous Polyp (Fibroepithelial Polyp)

A fibrous polyp is a small solitary polypoid lesion on a stalk consisting of a fibrovascular core covered by normal or slightly hyperplastic urothelium. The lesion is rare but is found in children and young adults. The length of the stalk may allow the polyp to prolapse into the vesicourethral orifice causing intermittent outlet obstruction or difficulty in micturition. The lesion is benign without malignant potential.

Bladder Papilloma

Bladder papilloma is epithelial in origin and is felt by many to be Stage 0 bladder cancer. There are, however, a few patients who have had papillary lesions lined by transitional cells that are normal on cytology examination without the presence of mitosis. The lesions are benign at the time of local resection but have a recurrence rate approximating 50%, and 10% of patients develop transitional cell carcinoma. Fifty percent of females and 30% of males with bladder papilloma will develop malignancy in a nonurologic site.

Pheochromocytoma

The bladder is an uncommon location for an ectopic pheochromocytoma. These tumors arise from chomaffin cells of the sympathetic plexus in or near the bladder wall. Most are found in the dome of the bladder or the trigone. During cystoscopy, they are seen as a small bulge in the bladder wall covered by transitional epithelium. A 3:2 female predilection is reported.

Most patients are hypertensive, and many have characteristic attacks of palpitations, sweating, headache, and blurred vision on micturition. The diagnosis should be suspected by this typical history and can be confirmed by measuring serum catecholamines.

An intramural mass may be detected on excretory urography. On CT examination, a soft tissue mass is seen in the wall of the bladder (Fig. 15.23). Since these tumors have a high signal intensity on T2-weighted images, they are readily identified on MRI as well. Often, only moder-

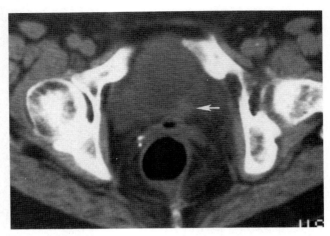

Figure 15.23. Pheochromocytoma. A small tumor mass (*arrow*) is seen in the bladder wall.

ately T2-weighted images are needed to distinguish the pheochromocytoma from urine.

MALIGNANT LESIONS

Transitional Cell Carcinoma

Primary transitional cell carcinoma of the bladder affects males to females in the ratio of 3:1. Bladder cancer accounts for 3% of all malignant deaths and the incidence is increasing. Ninety percent occur over the age of 50 years. The white/black ratio is 4:1. Ninety percent of bladder cancers are transitional cell carcinomas. Squamous cell carcinoma represents 8% of bladder cancers and adenocarcinoma the remaining 2%. The male:female ratio in squamous cell carcinoma is less than in transitional cell carcinoma. This is probably because squamous cell carcinoma is associated with chronic irritation and infection that is more common in females. The risk factor for transitional cell carcinoma in cigarette smokers is 2–5 times that in the nonsmoking population. A variety of sarcomas may affect the bladder, the commonest being sarcoma botryoides. This lesion occurs in childhood when the male:female ratio is 2:1.

Etiology of Transitional Cell Carcinoma

EXOGENOUS CAUSES. Analine dye workers and employees in the cable, plastic, synthetic rubber, leather, metal, and paint industries have increased risk of transitional cell carcinoma of the bladder. Transitional cell carcinoma is an acquired lesion resulting from the formation of the carcinogen orthoaminophenol of which there are two, 3-hydroxykinurenine, and 3-hydroxyanthranilic acid. Bladder cancer results from the production of three aromatic amines, 2-naphthylamine, benzidine, and paraxenylamine. Metabolic breakdown of these aromatic amines results in the production of the orthoaminophenol that is excreted in the urine. Epidemiologic studies have shown that 2 years of exposure to orthoaminophenol is necessary for the development of carcinoma that may develop after a variable latent period up to 40 years.

Other exogenous factors shown to produce increased risk for bladder cancer include pelvic irradiation, cyclophosphamide treatment, and phenacetin abuse. Women who received pelvic irradiation for gynecologic abnormalities have been shown to have a risk ratio of 2–3 times the nonirradiated female population. Several renal transplant patients with a history of cyclophosphamide cystitis have been reported to have developed transitional cell carcinoma of the bladder. Five percent of patients with a history of phenacetin abuse and renal papillary necrosis are said to develop urothelial tumors due to an orthoaminophenol resulting from the metabolism of phenacetin.

Other substances have been suspected of an association with increased risk for bladder cancer, such as coffee and artificial sweeteners, but this association has not been proven in humans.

ENDOGENOUS CAUSES.   Cigarette smoking is an exogenous cause of bladder cancer by interfering with the metabolism of an endogenous substance, the essential amino acid tryptophan. Normal tryptophan metabolism produces serotonin (5-hydroxytryptamine), which is further metabolized to 5-hydroxyindolacetic acid that is excreted from the bowel. Tryptophan may also be metabolized in the urine via the nicotinic acid pathway. This pathway results in the formation of two orthoaminophenol carcinogens (3-hydroxykinurenine and 3-hydroxyanthranilic acid) that are normally metabolized by pyridoxine (vitamin B_6) to harmless nicotinic acid. Cigarette smoking interferes with the converting action of pyridoxine. The resulting orthoaminophenol carcinogens are in high concentration in the urine and have a direct action on bladder transitional epithelium resulting in malignant change. It has also been found that α- and β-naphthaline (an aromatic amine) are products in cigarette smoke suggesting a direct exogenous etiology. This may be a factor in the production of urothelial tumors in heavy smokers. Pyridoxine deficiency also results in high levels of orthoaminophenol carcinogens in the urine.

Squamous Cell Carcinoma

Squamous cell carcinoma results in patients with long-standing mucosal irritation or bladder infection. Patients with low-grade outlet obstruction have a tendency to form bladder stones and to be subject to cystitis. Stone formation from chronic outlet obstruction occurs in elderly men and in neurogenic bladder patients. Chronic urinary tract infection is more common in females. Consequently, the incidence in males is not as high as is seen in transitional cell carcinoma. The most predominant group of patients developing squamous cell carcinoma are patients with bilharziasis, a condition endemic in the Nile Valley and Egypt. In Egypt 10% of bilharziasis patients develop squamous cell carcinoma, and squamous cell carcinoma is as common as transitional cell carcinoma.

Adenocarcinoma

Patients with bladder extrophy are at risk of developing adenocarcinoma. Chronic infection and bacterial toxins are implicated, but patients with bladder extrophy have an increase in the number of glandular elements trapped in the bladder mucosa during embryonal development. These are subject to malignant degeneration. In the nonextrophy patient, adenocarcinoma may occur after transitional cell metaplasia resulting in cystitis glandularis and cystitis cystica that may progress to adenocarcinoma. In the normal bladder, glandular rests are present within the transitional epithelium. Malignant degeneration in these glandular rests and metaplasia from transitional cell epithelium account for most bladder adenocarcinomas found in the trigone area, which is the most common site.

Pathology

Staging of bladder carcinoma is an attempted assessment of the extent of tumor spread, in particular the degree of bladder wall penetration. Consequently, Jewett and Strong's classification is based on the makeup of the bladder wall consisting of a mucosa, a submucosa, muscle layers, and perivesicle fat.

Stage 0 —mucosa only

Stage A —mucosal lesion extending into submucosa

Stage B_1—stage A with extension into muscle but less than halfway through muscle layer

Stage B_2—stage A with extension into muscle more than halfway through muscle layer

Stage C —tumor extending through muscle layer into perivesicle fat

Stage D —tumor through muscle and perivesicle fat with distant metastasis

The obvious difficulty with this classification is in the clinical assessment of Stage B_1 and B_2 carcinoma. The increase in the degree of bladder wall penetration from Stage B_1 to B_2 results in a decline of accurate staging. This classification does not take into consideration carcinoma in situ nor does it differentiate between local pelvic node invasion and distant metastasis. The tumor, nodes, and metastases (TNM) classification has been applied to bladder cancer but is felt by many to be overcomplicated and does not specifically clarify the difficulty in the staging of bladder cancer invading muscle. However, the TNM classification includes carcinoma in situ and differentiates Stage D into three stages.

Cellular grading of bladder cancer is a histologic assessment of cellular change and emphasizes the number of mitotic nuclei and the degree of differentiation. Broder's histologic classification was accepted for many years, and it described four grades of bladder carcinoma by the degree of differentiation.

Grade 1—75% of cells are well differentiated
Grade 2—50–75% of cells are well differentiated
Grade 3—25–50% of cells are well differentiated
Grade 4—0–25% of cells are well differentiated

Because of the difficulty the pathologist experiences with the differentiation of anaplasia as in Grade 4 from poorly differentiated cells in Grade 3, there is a recent emphasis on simplification of tumor grading into well, (Grade 1), moderately (Grade 2), and poorly differentiated (Grade 3). Grading of bladder carcinoma usually correlates well with staging or the degree of invasion. Therefore 80% of Grade 3 lesions are invasive, 50% of Grade 2 lesions are invasive, and 10% of Grade 1 lesions are invasive. Generally the higher the grade, the higher the probability of muscle and perivesicle fat invasion.

Both staging and grading should be considered in the management of bladder carcinoma. A high-grade, Stage A bladder cancer may occur, but careful frequent follow-up biopsies are necessary since high-grade tumors tend to be invasive. Grades 1 and 2, Stage 0, A, or B_1 are usually managed by local resection. Higher grades and stages require consideration of partial or total cystectomy.

Bladder papilloma is commonly considered a Stage 0 bladder cancer since the recurrence rate is approximately 50% and 10% will recur as bladder cancer.

Carcinoma in situ, although fitting into the staging classification as Stage 0, commonly has histologic evidence of a higher grade. Approximately 12% of patients with carcinoma in situ develop invasive carcinoma. It is not uncommon to find carcinoma in situ adjacent to an overt bladder tumor or in patients with a past history of resectable bladder cancer. Recurrence of multifocal areas of carcinoma in situ occur in approximately 75% of patients and 50% of these patients will be shown to have an increase in grade and stage. Carcinoma in situ has a high incidence among cigarette smokers.

Approximately 75% of patients with bladder cancer present with painless hematuria, sometimes also presenting with frequency, urgency, and dysuria. The remaining 25% may present without hematuria but with signs of bladder irritability. Occasionally flank pain may be the presenting symptom when the bladder cancer has invaded and obstructed a ureter.

Radiology

The plain film is usually normal. Approximately 0.3% of bladder tumors calcify (Fig. 15.24). These are epithelial in origin and are due to dystrophic calcification within tumor necrosis. This calcification is usually stippled or

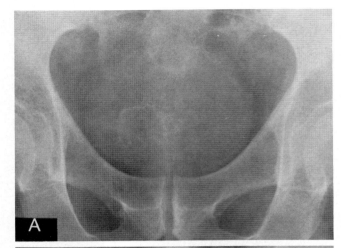

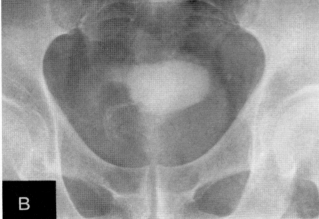

Figure 15.24.   A, Plain film demonstrating irregular crescentic calcification. (**B**), Excretory urogram showing some contrast medium within the bladder. The calcification on the plain film is seen to be part of a lobulated filling defect which proved to be transitional cell carcinoma.

floccular. Sessile carcinoma may cause curvilinear calcification at the base and should therefore be considered in the diagnosis of localized intramural calcification. Calcification may also occur at the tips of papillary villus tumors, which do not exhibit necrosis. Tumor calcification has also been reported in bladder hemangioma, neuroblastoma, and leiomyosarcoma.

Excretory urography should be performed in all cases of suspected or proven bladder cancer to exclude urothelial lesions in the collecting system and ureters, since multicentricity is common. Obstructive uropathy may be the result of bladder tumor obstructing the ureteric orifice (Fig. 15.25). Bladder cancers more than 1.5 cm in size are usually seen within the bladder filled with contrast medium. Occasionally bladder cancer is found within a bladder diverticulum (Fig. 15.20), and oblique views are commonly necessary for better visualization.

Overlying bowel gas is commonly difficult to distinguish from an intraluminal bladder filling defect. Overly-

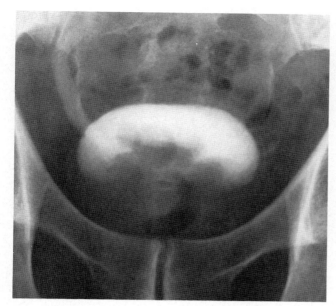

Figure 15.25.   Excretory urogram showing dilated right ureter due to irregular transitional cell carcinoma. The bladder base is elevated by enlarged prostate.

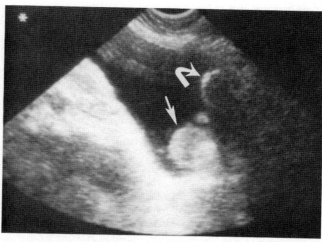

Figure 15.26.   Suprapubic ultrasound showing a filling defect of irregular echogenicity (*straight arrow*) in the bladder producing thickening of the adjacent bladder wall. Proven transitional cell carcinoma. The curvilinear echogenic area (*curved arrow*) is a bladder catheter.

ing bowel gas may sometimes be distinguished from a filling defect by the presence of Simpson's white line representing bowel wall. Oblique and upright views may also be helpful in this regard. Approximately 25% of bladder cancers are not recognized on excretory urography.

Cystography does not add significantly to the information obtained from urography, and it is rarely requested. Approximately 20% of bladder cancers are not visible on cystography even on retrospective studies.

Suprapubic ultrasound is an effective method of visualizing bladder cancer. The filled bladder and bladder wall are well visualized in the normal patient. Bladder cancer is seen as a filling defect within the bladder (Fig. 15.26). Stage 0 or Stage A bladder cancers are demonstrated as a filling defect arising from the bladder wall but do not alter the normal echogenicity of the bladder muscle. Tumor invasion of bladder muscle interrupts the normal regular echogenicity of bladder muscle resulting in an ill-defined area with abnormal echogenicity, usually an area of muscle wall thickening. Ultrasound can assess these tumors invading through the bladder wall into perivesicle fat but is not helpful in assessing the degree of penetration through bladder muscle, i.e., ultrasound cannot distinguish Stage B_1 and B_2. Bladder tumors causing ureteric obstruction or invasion into the ureter are well assessed. Although ultrasound can recognize a mass within the bladder, it cannot distinguish a primary bladder tumor from metastatic tumor without clinical history. It is doubtful that transrectal or transvaginal ultrasound will be an improvement over transabdominal ultrasound in the staging of bladder cancer. Transurethral bladder scanning may be a more helpful method.

The main advantage of CT over ultrasound is better definition of pelvic structures for staging. In addition, CT of the abdomen can delineate paraaortic lymph node enlargement (Fig. 15.27**A**) and can be used for guided biopsy of these nodes. Paraaortic node enlargement due to cancer of the bladder places the cancer in an advanced Stage D, which alters management. As with transabdominal ultrasound a filling defect within the bladder is readily visualized and involvement of the bladder wall can also be assessed (Fig. 15.27**B**).

Tumor invading through the wall into perivesical fat and surrounding structures (Fig. 15.28) is better assessed by CT than with ultrasound. Anatomic detail of tumor involving pelvic muscles, vessels, and adjacent viscera is better seen with CT. When enlarged nodes are identified, confirmation of the metastatic disease can be obtained from CT-guided thin-needle biopsy. Dynamic scanning can identify tumor capillary enhancement, which may help detect tumors invading the bladder musculature or extending into perivesicle fat.

Arteriography has been used in the staging of bladder cancer by the demonstration of abnormal vascularity. Malignant tumor vessels such as corkscrew vessels, abrupt changes in vessel caliber, abrupt vessel ending, and persistent capillary staining may be seen. Neovascularity in the muscularis or perivesicle fat requires numerous views including tangential views. Two major problems associated with arteriography in bladder cancer are that Stages B_1 and B_2 can seldom be differentiated and inflammatory vessels may also produce capillary staining. Coexistent tumor and inflammatory vessels are often indistinguishable and cause overstaging. In bladder

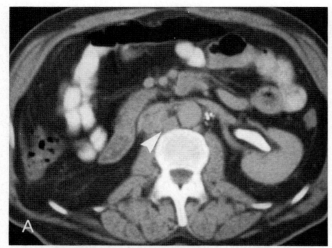

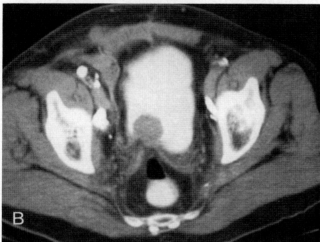

Figure 15.27. **A,** The right kidney has been removed for transitional cell carcinoma 1 year previously. Enlarged right paraaortic nodes are present (*arrowhead*). **B,** Same patient. The filling defect in the bladder is a second transitional cell carcinoma which has invaded through the bladder wall.

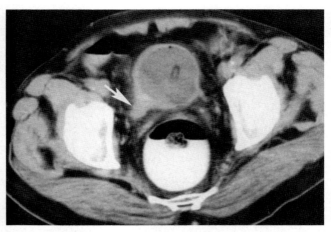

Figure 15.28. CT scan of pelvis in a patient with hematuria. The bladder wall is irregularly thickened and a mass is present at the UVJ (*arrow*) with invasion into the ureter. There is also early invasion of perivesicle fat.

joint conditions. Nuclear medicine scans are therefore highly sensitive but lack specificity, often requiring bone biopsy for definitive diagnosis.

MRI is a very promising method of examination in bladder cancer. T1-weighted images provide excellent anatomic detail. The fact that malignant tumors contain more water than normal tissue allows excellent tumor visualization on T2-weighted images (Fig. 15.29). Views can be obtained in the transverse, sagittal, and coronal planes, which may be a decided aid in the staging of bladder cancer. Muscle wall invasion may be clearly seen with MRI possibly solving the diagnostic problem of accurate differentiation of B_1 and B_2 tumors. The bladder should be filled with urine for this examination. MRI is also more useful in the examination of the postoperative patient and in the assessment of tumor spread. Nodes and

arteriography the bladder requires distention by the insertion of gas. Arteriography is seldom used for staging of bladder cancer.

Pedal lymphangiography opacifies the external iliac, common iliac, and paraaortic lymph nodes. Internal iliac nodes, obturator, presacral, and presciatic nodes are seldom visualized. The obturator, presacral, and presciatic nodes are the nodes initially affected by bladder cancer. Metastases within nodes may totally replace the node or produce a filling defect within the node. Suspected node involvement in partly opacified nodes aids localization for fluoroscopic guidance of needle biopsy of the node.

Technetium 99-labeled polyphosphate scans and technetium 99-sulfur colloid scans are used, respectively, for bone scanning and liver scanning for metastatic disease. However, bladder cancer rarely metastasizes to bone, and a positive scan may be due to a variety of bone and

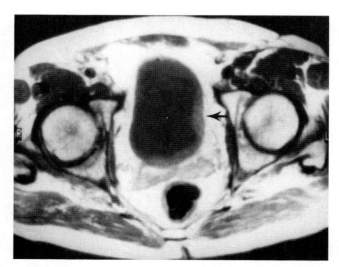

Figure 15.29. MRI examination showing a left bladder wall mass (*arrow*) extending to the posterior bladder wall on T2-weighted imaging.

vessels are clearly differentiated. The patient must be well enough to remain stationary within the magnet since movement deteriorates the images significantly. Contrast resolution is superior to CT and ultrasound. The normal low signal intensity of the bladder wall is increased in an area of tumor invasion. Perivesicle fat invasion by tumor decreases signal intensity of the perivesicle fat on T2-weighted images.

Urachal Carcinoma

In adults the urachus is a musculofibrous band 5–6 cm long extending from the umbilicus to the anterior superior surface of the bladder. It lies in the extraperitoneal space of Retzius, between the transversalis fascia anteriorly and the peritoneum posteriorly. The urachus represents a vestigial remnant of the obliterated umbilical arteries and the allantois. It retains a minute lumen lined by transitional epithelium in 70% of adults. Lumenal continuity between the adult urachus and the bladder is present in approximately 30% of adults. The bladder attachment of the urachus therefore consists of supravesical, intramuscular, and intramucosal segments.

Numerous anomalies of urachal closure may occur. *Patent urachus* is failure of closure along the entire length of the urachus resulting in excretion of urine from the umbilicus. *Urachal cyst* generally indicates cystic dilatation of the distal urachus proximal to the closed supravesical segment. *Urachal sinus* is a blind-end dilatation of the urachus at the umbilical end. *Vesicourachal diverticulum* is failure of closure and dilatation of the urachus in its distal half forming a diverticulum of the anterior superior aspect of the bladder. Patent urachus is rare and presents in infancy. Urachal cyst and sinus usually present in adults and not until infection occurs in the cyst or sinus. Vesicourachal diverticulum more commonly presents in adults and rarely calculi have been reported.

The transitional epithelium lining the urachus may undergo metaplasia to glandular epithelium that may be mucin producing. Consequently, malignant change in urachal epithelium includes mucin-producing adenocarcinoma that accounts for 69% of urachal cancers. Non-mucin-producing adenocarcinomas account for 15%. The remainder of urachal malignancies are transitional cell carcinoma, squamous cell carcinoma, or sarcoma. Squamous cell carcinomas are occasionally associated with urachal cysts and calculi in vesicourachal diverticulae. Urachal sarcomas occur in the young, and almost 70% occur before the age of 20 years. Urachal carcinoma may occur at any age but almost 70% occur between 40 and 70 years. Sixty-five percent of urachal carcinomas occur in males. Ninety percent are juxtavesicle. Three hundred and seventeen cases have been reported in the English and Japanese literature.

Clinical Presentation

Hematuria is the presenting symptom in 71% of patients. Mucus is found in the urine in 25% of patients and is an almost pathognomonic finding. Abdominal pain, a lower abdominal palpable mass, and dysuria are also presenting symptoms. Umbilical discharge is rare.

Urachal carcinoma may invade the bladder and is visible cystoscopically in 88% of cases.

Radiology

In less than 4% of urachal carcinomas, calcification is seen on the plain radiograph. The calcification may be stippled, granular, or curvilinear. Stippled calcification in the supravesicleal region on the filled bladder films, and deformity of the bladder dome, are virtually pathognomonic of urachal carcinoma. The ureters may be displaced laterally. However, 18% of excretory urograms are normal in urachal carcinoma. Ultrasound examination may show a supravesicle complex mass in the region of the palpable mass. Computed tomography offers the most hope for a definite preoperative diagnosis, as CT is capable of demonstrating calcification not seen on radiography or ultrasound. Computed tomography demonstration of a calcified mass above or anterior to the bladder is highly suggestive of urachal carcinoma. (Fig. 15.30). The mass may invade the bladder on CT examination, and calcification may be absent.

Computed tomography is also useful in assessing tumor spread and in assessing recurrence. Radionuclide imaging with technetium diphosphonate has been described in assessing metastases.

The prognosis of urachal carcinoma is poor—the 5-year survival rate is less than 10%. The poor prognosis is likely the result of late presentation of symptoms after the

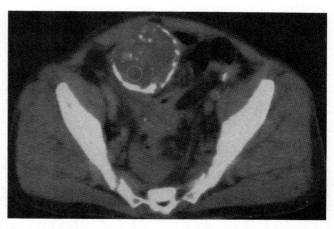

Figure 15.30. Computed tomography demonstrating an anterior abdominal mass with a thick rim of irregular calcification and invasion of the right anterior abdominal wall musculature. Proven urachal carcinoma. (Courtesy E. Fitzgerald, M.D.)

tumor is well established, an early tendency of local infiltration and the early development of lung and bone metastases.

The differential diagnosis includes primary carcinoma of the bladder (14% occur in the bladder dome) and a bladder metastasis from adenocarcinoma of the rectum, stomach, ovary, uterus, cervix, and prostate.

BLADDER CALCULI

Secondary Bladder Calculi

Secondary bladder calculi occur in the bladder of patients with chronic bladder infection or some form of urinary outlet obstruction such as prostatic hypertrophy, neurogenic bladder, urethral stricture, urethral or bladder diverticulum, cystocele, and bladder foreign bodies. They are more common in males and are the result of urinary solutes, supersaturation, crystalluria, clumping, and nidus formation.

A probable, or possible, cause and effect relationship can be demonstrated in 98% of secondary bladder stone formers. A definite cause and effect relationship can be demonstrated in struvite and carbonate apatite stones, which have been shown to be the result of urea-splitting bacteria. Cystine stones are found only in cystinuria. A presumptive cause and effect for bladder stone formation can be inferred by assessing risk factors, such as prostatic hypertrophy, neurogenic bladder, and urethral stricture.

Stones Resulting from Infection

Approximately 33% of bladder stones are associated with infection. The most common organisms are *E. coli* and *Proteus mirabilis,* accounting for approximately 80% of bladder stone formation in the infection group, *Proteus* being twice as common in Western countries. Other organisms involved are Pseudomonas, Klebsiella, and *Streptococcus faecalis.*

Attempts have been made to correlate the cause and composition of secondary bladder stones. It is generally accepted that struvite (magnesium ammonium phosphate) and carbonate apatite (calcium phosphate carbonate) stones are the result of supersaturation of these elements, and release of ammonium in hydrolysis of urea by the bacterial enzyme urease. All strains of Proteus that generally proliferate in urine where the pH is greater than 6.5 produce urease, and a high percentage of Pseudomonas and Klebsiella also produce urease. *E. coli,* which generally proliferates in urine where the pH is lower than 6.5, seldom if ever produces urease, and therefore would not be a causative effect of the formation of struvite or carbonate apatite stones. Both calcium oxalate and calcium phosphate crystalluria are common in urinary infection. Phosphate crystalluria is said to be more common with Proteus infection. Oxalate and urate crystalluria are said to be more common in *E. coli* infection. Struvite and carbonate apatite stones (urease stones) are pathognomonic of infection. Infection may also produce stones that are composed of calcium oxalate, calcium phosphate, or a mixture of both. Urease stones contain organic material (matrix). This is the result of proteinaceous and mucopolysaccharide debris from the inflamed urothelial lining of the ureter or bladder. Urease stones are poorly mineralized and therefore poorly visualized radiographically. If the infection is not eradicated, a urease stone may recur. Eradication of infection is difficult and requires long-term antimicrobial therapy and high fluid intake. Urease-inhibiting drugs such as hydroxyurea or acetohydroxamic acid (AHA) may be required. Urease-inhibiting drugs prevent urea splitting by urease. Some precautions are necessary in the administration of urease-inhibiting drugs, since they may depress bone marrow function.

Alkaline-encrusting cystitis may occur with the development of urease stones. Urea-splitting bacteria may cause a virulent cystitis resulting in areas of necrosis and sloughing in the mucosa and a severe inflammatory reaction in the muscularis and adventitia. An alkaline urine is produced by the release of ammonia from urea, which leads to calcium salt deposition in the necrotic areas of the mucosa, and calcification may then be seen in the bladder wall.

The recent literature suggests that *E. coli* is the organism most commonly associated with bladder stones in the Middle East, Turkey, and the Far East, and that *B. proteus* species are more commonly associated with bladder stones in Western Europe and the United States. Although bladder infection can be the sole cause of bladder stone formation giving rise to stones composed of calcium oxalate, calcium phosphate (or a mixture of these), and urease, infectious stones may also occur in the bladder of patients with some form of outlet obstruction, such as neurogenic bladder, prostatic hypertrophy, or urethral stricture. A significant number of neurogenic bladder patients with unacceptable residual urine and urine stagnation develop bladder infection that may result in stone formation. In addition, infectious bladder stones may form around foreign bodies such as sutures, pubic hairs, and catheters.

Stones Associated with Bladder Catheterization

An indwelling bladder catheter, although fulfilling its function of bladder drainage, will lead to bladder infection if left in position long enough. Strict aseptic technique of catheterization does not preclude stone formation. Struvite stones therefore account for approximately 50% of catheter-associated stones, the remainder are a mixture of calcium oxalate and phosphate or pure calcium phosphate. Catheter-associated stones are most frequently found in the neurogenic bladder and after surgical stone removal followed by catheterization.

Neurogenic bladder may result from congenital spinal defects, spinal cord trauma, or neuropathic disease. Neurogenic bladder patients may be treated with continual or preferably intermittent bladder catheterization or they may attain a catheter-free state by bladder training. Bladder catheterization and bladder training is necessary because patients with neurogenic bladder have outlet obstruction, usually at the bladder neck in lower motor neuron lesions, and at the distal sphincters in upper motor neuron lesions due to sphincter dyssynergia. Approximately 70% of neurogenic bladders after spinal cord trauma attain a catheter-free state after intermittent catheterization and bladder training. The remainder require continuous bladder catheterization. Bladder stones in neurogenic bladder patients are mostly associated with catheterization. Encrustations form around the balloon of the catheter. Disintegration of these crusts act as a nidus for the formation of characteristic neurogenic bladder calculi, which are crescentic in shape.

In addition, it has been demonstrated that intermittent clean catheterization in neurogenic bladder patients may introduce pubic hairs into the bladder that act as a nidus for calcareous deposits resulting in stone formation.

Transurethral stone crushing or electrohydraulic lithotripsy followed by catheter drainage have a stone recurrence rate of 44% and 50%. After suprapubic vesicolithotomy and catheterization, the recurrence rate is 7%. In transurethral procedures, small residual stone fragments remaining within the bladder form a nidus for stone formation, but the fact that stones occur with all three procedures implicates the bladder catheter.

Stones in Bilharziasis

Bilharziasis results in bladder stone formation in approximately 40% of patients. Bladder stone formation is not the direct result of the parasitic worm but rather the result of the fibrosis that occurs at the bladder neck in bilharziasis causing some degree of outlet obstruction. Superimposed bacterial infection results in supersaturation, crystalluria, clumping, and stone formation (Fig. 15.12).

Stones Resulting from Outlet Obstruction

In adult patients, outlet obstruction accounts for 70% of bladder stones. Outlet obstruction is most commonly the result of prostatic hypertrophy and hyperplasia. Urethral stricture, bladder neck hypertrophy, or neurogenic bladder dysfunction may also produce outlet obstruction. Thirty-eight percent of obstructive stones are mixtures of calcium oxalate and calcium phosphate and are the most common type. Pure calcium oxalate stones account for 18% of bladder stones and pure calcium phosphate stones (including brushite which is calcium phosphate dihydrate) account for approximately 13% of obstructive bladder stones. Infectious stones account for approximately 18% of bladder stones in association with outlet obstruction. Most of the remaining 13% of bladder stones are uric acid, cystine, or calcium carbonate. Xanthine stones have also been reported but are rare. The vast majority of these bladder stones have a presumptive cause, namely, obstruction, but no definite correlation between the composition of the stone and obstruction has been identified. Why obstruction produces a mixture of calcium oxalate and phosphate more commonly than pure calcium oxalate or pure calcium phosphate has yet to be clarified.

Miscellaneous Stone Formation

A rare complication of pelvic surgery is migrating sutures placed in the bladder wall extraluminally. These may migrate through the bladder wall into the bladder mucosa and act as a foreign body on which a stone may form. Such stones may be described as hanging stones as they hang from a suture attached to the bladder wall. They are usually small, less than 1 cm, and both stone and suture are readily removed cystoscopically. Foreign bodies introduced either surgically or self-induced transurethrally may form a nidus for stone formation. A variety of foreign bodies including pencils, pens, paperclips, hairpins, etc. introduced into the bladder per urethra have been shown with calcium encrustation (Fig. 15.3).

Migrant Calculi

A migrant bladder calculus is one that is produced in the kidney, migrates down the ureter, and is retained in the bladder. Most of these are usually passed per urethra. Consequently, migrant bladder calculi only remain in the bladder when there is some degree of outlet obstruction. Such calculi may increase in size and over a period of years may become large. Among the writings of Samuel Pepys is his own medical history in which he describes his painful affliction of kidney stones, resulting in a severe attack of ureteric colic. However, the sudden relief of ureteric colic was not followed by the passage of the stone per urethra. Some years later he suffered from severe bladder pain, dysuria, and a poor stream resulting in his consent to operation. A stone the size of a tennis ball and weighing 2 ounces was successfully removed.

Primary Idiopathic Endemic Calculi

These calculi occur in infants and young children. Documentation of idiopathic stone disease first occurred in the Norwich City Hospital, in Norfolk County on the

East Coast of England where bladder stones were endemic in children in the nineteenth century. Excellent hospital records from 1871 through 1947 indicate that the incidence of idiopathic stone disease in children under 10 years was high (44% of bladder stone patients) from 1871 to 1910, became markedly reduced between World Wars I and II, and by 1947 had been completely eradicated. Western European countries and the United States had a similar incidence of idiopathic bladder stone disease during these years. In 1874, Cadge suggested a dietary cause for primary bladder stone in children and noted an inadequate milk supply in the Norfolk area. The Norfolk and Norwich Hospital data also indicated a male : female ratio of approximately 10 : 1. Although idiopathic stone disease has been eradicated in developed countries, it still occurs in undeveloped countries. Bladder stones occur in North Africa, the Middle East, West India, Pakistan, Thailand, and in Australian aboriginal children.

There is general agreement that primary bladder stones are not related to congenital defects, infection, or bladder outlet obstruction. Idiopathic bladder stones differ from secondary stones in that once removed the recurrence rate is almost nil. Since 1963, studies of the natural history of idiopathic stone disease have been ongoing in endemic areas, in particular in Ubol Province, an endemic stone area on the eastern border of Thailand. Stones occur in the very young (the average age of stone passing episodes was 3 years) and symptoms, i.e., hematuria, dysuria, stream interruption, difficulty in micturition, and gravel in the urine were present as early as 18 months of age. It is suggested that bladder stone formation was closely associated with the practice of feeding glutinous and ordinary rice instead of milk to infants immediately or soon after birth. In such infants the incidence of bladder stone formation was twice as high as in those who were started on rice later in life. This suggests that primary idiopathic bladder stone formation is the result of milk replacement by carbohydrate food in the first few weeks of life, leading to phosphate deficiency and therefore low urinary phosphate excretion, and the formation of insoluble salts in the urine. It is suggested that although the above infant feeding practice is the same for male and females, a stone nidus in the bladder may be readily passed in females due to their short, straight urethra, thus accounting for the primary idiopathic bladder stone male : female ratio of 10 : 1. It is also suggested that besides low dietary phosphate intake and urinary excretion, other factors are implicated. These include high oxalate intake and perhaps high endogenous oxalate production, leading to oxalate crystalluria, crystal clumping, and nidus formation. Dehydration due to diarrhea and vomiting is also significant. Crystalluria was markedly reduced by the administration of milk in place of rice. Studies in endemic bladder stone areas agreed that affected children are from the lower socioeconomic

class and that renal stones in conjunction with bladder stones are rare. Such primary bladder stones usually consist of a combination of ammonium acid urate and calcium oxalate, and many contain calcium phosphate, but the composition of bladder stones varies from one endemic area to another.

Although there is now much information available on primary idiopathic bladder stone formation, all children with low phosphate urinary excretion do not form stones.

CLINICAL PRESENTATION OF BLADDER STONE

A significant number of bladder stones are asymptomatic and are only discovered on investigation for upper urinary tract disease, or on routine excretory urography and cystoscopy in the assessment of prostatic hypertrophy or other causes of outlet obstruction. Symptomatic patients present with bladder pain, which may be a dull ache suprapubically. Referred pain to the penis, buttock, perineum, or scrotum may also occur. The pain may be sudden, sharp, severe, or excruciating with the same referred areas. Fifty percent of patients present with intermittent obstruction. Microscopic hematuria in bladder stone disease may occur as a result of chronic irritation of bladder mucosa, but gross hematuria is rare. Foul-smelling urine in the presence of bladder stones strongly suggests infectious stones.

Investigation of Bladder Stone

Although extensive investigation of primary bladder stone disease is ongoing and important in endemic areas, a cost-effective investigative approach to migrant and secondary bladder stone disease is mandatory in Western countries. An initial plain film and excretory urogram may provide much useful information and guide further investigation. Such a study may show nephrocalcinosis suggesting hypercalcemia, hyperparathyroidism, medullary sponge kidney, or renal tubular acidosis. The visualization of a faintly radiopaque or ring calcification in the bladder would direct further investigation to urease stones, cystine stones, or uric acid stones. Urinary bacteriology, urinary cystine, and uric acid estimation may lead to the correct underlying diagnosis and the establishment of a definite cause and effect relationship. However, since 75% of stones are due to a mixture of calcium oxalate and calcium phosphate or pure calcium oxalate or pure calcium phosphate, and only a presumptive cause can be demonstrated in these cases, investigation can generally be limited to excretory urography and bacterial assessment of the urine. Recurrent stone formers deserve a complete blood and urine examination. This would include the assessment of serum electrolytes including Na^+, K^+, Ca^{++}, Cl^-, glucose, uric acid, total protein, albumin, creatinine, bilirubin, and alkaline phosphatase, in addition to the assessment of parathyroid hormone. Serum electrolyte studies repeated at least 3 times and preferrably 6 times are recommended. Urinary studies in this group of patients include estimation of urinary calcium, phosphate, oxalate, uric acid, and exact urinary pH. In addition to cystine estimation, urinary pH estimation should be repeated if the pH is over 5.5 after ammonium chloride challenge. In addition, crystallography studies including microscopic zone assay, x-ray diffractometry, chemical spot tests, and spectroscopy may be helpful. All of these investigations may lead to the establishment of a definite cause in patients in whom recurrent bladder stone may be the presenting symptom of a stone forming tendency. However, these extensive investigations are more commonly used in patients with upper urinary tract stones in which a probable or possible cause of stone formation is established in only 27% of cases.

Radiology

Studies in which bladder stones are visualized include plain radiography, excretory urography, ultrasound, and CT. Pure uric acid and urease stones will not be visualized on the plain film but may be seen as negative filling defects in the bladder on the urogram (Fig. 15.31). However, a significant number of bladder stones, less than 1 cm in diameter, both radiolucent and radiopaque, may not be seen on excretory urography.

Bladder stones vary from very dense to radiolucent. The best radiographic technique is essential for stone visualization. A low kilovoltage of between 60 and 70 kV to increase image contrast is generally best for plain film and excretory urography studies. A casual glance at the pelvic area on the plain film is insufficient. Careful scrutiny is required.

Bladder stones vary in size from a few millimeters to large stones filling the bladder (Fig. 15.32). Well-calcified stones over a few millimeters in size are usually apparent on the plain film. They may be obscured by overlying fecal material in the rectosigmoid colon, or they may overly the sacrum and coccyx where they are difficult to definitely identify. Consequently, any suspected calcification seen on the plain film should be pursued before the injection of contrast medium. Oblique views of the pelvis are often helpful in separating a calcified stone from the sacrum and coccyx and colonic or rectal fecal material. This also applies to suspicious faint ring calcification that may be a bladder or distal ureteric stone, difficult to differentiate from vascular calcification. Bladder stones should lie in the midline with the patient supine. Bladder stones identified on the plain film not lying in the midline may lie within a bladder diverticulum or be displaced to one side by a large prostatic adenoma, or they may be fixed in position as a hanging stone from a suture. However, large off-center stones may indicate an associ-

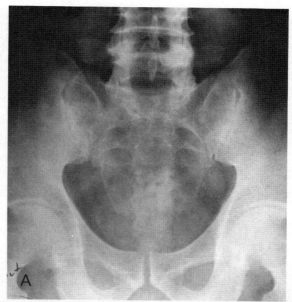
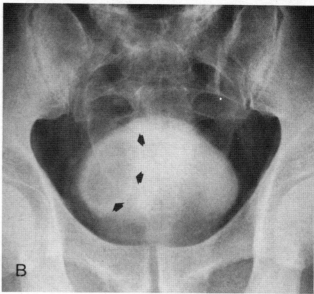

Figure 15.31. A, Plain film of the pelvis. No radiopaque calculus is visualized. **B,** Excretory urogram on the same patient showing the contrast-filled bladder with an oval filling defect (*arrowheads*) in the right side of the bladder which proved to be a uric acid stone.

ated intraluminal bladder carcinoma resulting from long-standing chronic irritation (Fig. 15.33).

Pure uric acid stones and urease stones are radiolucent and not seen on the plain film. Occasionally bladder calculi mainly composed of uric acid or struvite are faintly calcified producing a shadow of low density. Even after careful scrutiny and oblique views, it may be impossible to be certain that a bladder stone is present. Cystine stones contain no calcium but do contain sulfur, and they are generally round, less dense than calcium, and if over

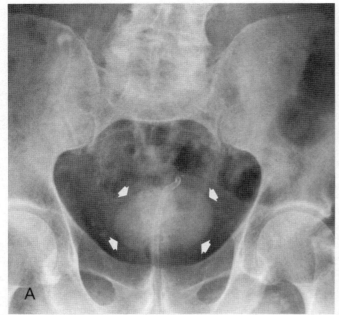

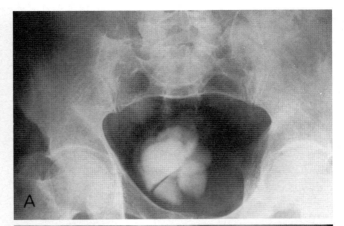

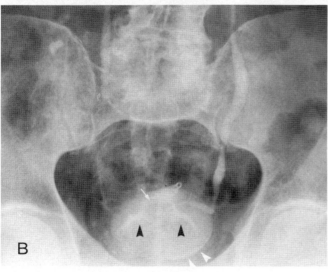

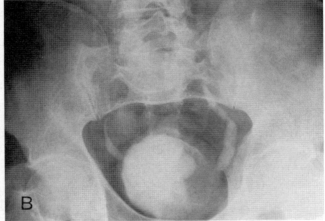

Figure 15.33.   A, Plain film of the pelvis showing multiple multifaceted stones lying to the right of midline. **B,** Same patient. Excretory urogram showing large filling defect in the left side of the bladder due to transitional cell carcinoma which is causing mild left ureteric dilatation. (From McCallum RW, Colapinto V: *Urological Radiology of the Adult Male Lower Urinary Tract.* Springfield, IL, Charles C Thomas, 1976.)

Figure 15.32.   A, Plain film of the pelvis showing a huge bladder calculus (*arrowheads*). There is also a catheter in the bladder because the patient has outlet obstruction. **B,** Same patient. Excretory urogram showing the stone almost completely fills the bladder. The ureters are **J**-shaped due to prostatic adenomata (*black arrowheads*) indenting the bladder base. Contrast medium outlines the balloon of the catheter (*white arrow*). A thin rim of contrast medium is seen between the stone and the bladder wall (*white arrowheads*). (Modified from McCallum RW, Colapinto V: *Urological Radiology of the Adult Male Lower Urinary Tract.* Springfield, IL, Charles C Thomas, 1976.)

1 cm in diameter should at least be suspected on the plain film by the addition of oblique pelvic views. On the plain film, a visible migrant stone in the distal ureter will not be midline. The migrant stone may be held up in the intramural ureter and lie low in the pelvis and close to midline.

Intraluminal bladder calculi are commonly solitary but there may be many bladder calculi visualized at the time of presentation. Bladder calculi vary in shape from round, oval, square, or multifaceted, and many calculi present a laminated appearance.

Well-calcified bladder calculi seen on the plain film may be completely obscured by contrast medium in the bladder. Consequently, small dense calcifications in the pelvis raising the suspicion of a bladder stone on the plain film may require oblique views of the contrast-filled bladder to prove they are intravesicle and do not lie outside the filled bladder. Many calcified bladder stones are less dense than contrast medium and therefore cast a negative shadow within the bladder on the contrast-filled films (Fig. 15.34**A**). However, oblique films may be necessary to distinguish bowel gas overlying the bladder from an intraluminal filling defect. A Simpson's "white line" can be identified around bowel gas (Fig. 15.34**B**). It represents the bowel wall seen between intraluminal gas

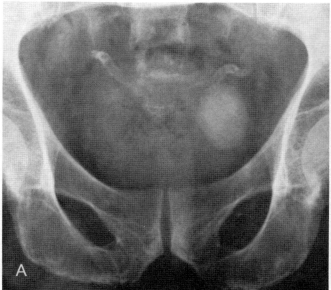
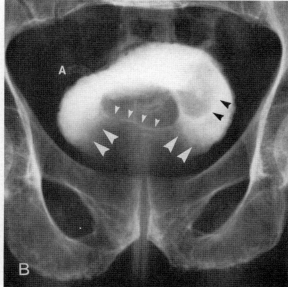

Figure 15.34. **A,** Plain film of the pelvis in a diabetic male patient showing calcification in the vas deferens due to diabetes mellitus and an oval, faintly calcified stone on the left side of the bladder. **B,** Excretory urogram showing the stone as a filling defect (*black arrowheads*) surrounded by denser contrast me- dium. The stone is pushed to the left of the bladder by an enlarged prostate (*large white arrowheads*). The radiolucent area in the center of the bladder outline is gas in the bowel emphasized by Simpson's white line (*small white arrowheads*). The ampulla of the vas deferens is again seen (A).

and paracolic fat. Radiolucent stones cast negative shadows within the contrast-filled bladder. Single radiolucent stones less than 1 cm may not be identified on intravenous urography. Single radiolucent stones over 1 cm in size should be seen to move within the bladder on oblique views unlike negative defects due to bladder tumor that do not move. The bladder base is often distorted and indented by prostatic adenomata so that the bladder base is well above the symphysis pubis. Stones in a bladder diverticulum may appear to be outside the bladder on excretory urography if the diverticulum neck is small and the stone obstructs the neck of the diverticulum. Varying the patient position usually allows contrast to fill the diverticulum.

On ultrasound study of the normal fluid-filled bladder, the fluid in the bladder is echo-free, the bladder wall is echogenic, and brighter echoes are seen projecting from the bladder wall posteriorly due to echo enhancement. When a calcified stone lies on the posterior wall of the bladder in a supine patient, the stone reflects the sound waves producing a bright echo that indicates the stone, and it interrupts the sound transmission through the bladder resulting in acoustic shadowing (Figs. 15.35 and 15.36). By rotating the patient into the high oblique position the stone can be seen to move freely within the bladder on real time ultrasonography. Radiolucent or poorly calcified stones on radiography are well seen on ultrasound and are not significantly different from well-calcified stones. Mobility of a stone within the bladder distinguishes stone from calcified bladder tumor. The

degree of ureteric obstruction and pelvicaliectasis can also be assessed when large bladder stones are present during the same examination.

Computed tomography demonstrates bladder stones well and demonstrates stones of high density. There may be associated transitional or squamous cell carcinoma that is well visualized on CT (Fig. 15.37).

Bladder stones that are radiolucent on the plain film can be seen well on CT as well-defined mobile high densities. A plain CT scan without contrast medium will clearly show a uric acid stone as a bright, well-defined

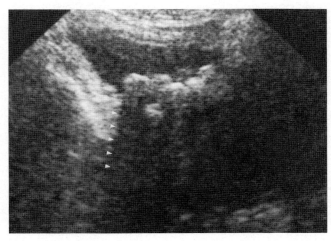

Figure 15.35. Transabdominal ultrasound in a patient with multiple bladder stones seen as bright echos with acoustic shadowing (*arrows*).

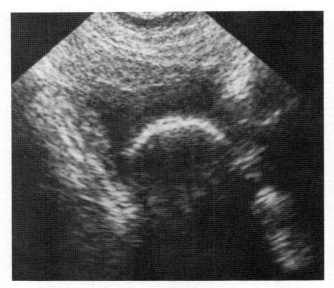

Figure 15.36.   Transabdominal ultrasound. A single large bladder stone is present producing acoustic shadowing.

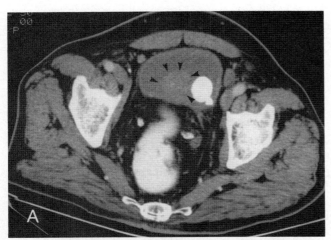

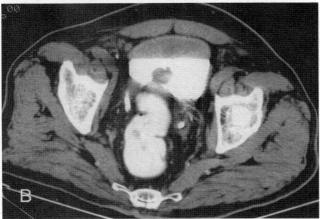

Figure 15.37.   A, Computed tomography of the pelvis before contrast medium enters the bladder. Two dense stones are well seen. In addition, there is a faintly seen mass centrally (*arrows*). **B,** The bladder contains contrast medium which obliterates the stones. The faintly seen mass is now obvious as a soft tissue mass arising from the posterior bladder wall. Proven transitional cell carcinoma.

area of high density with a CT number in excess of 150 HU. This is compared with transitional cell carcinoma in the renal pelvis or ureter, which presents as a soft tissue density with a low CT number in the range of 30–60 HU. Computed tomography scanning is probably more valuable in identifying the organ of origin of small calcific densities such as uterine or prostatic calcifications when the organ of origin is difficult to place on excretory urography. Extravesicle densities are readily identified in the organ of origin on CT, and intravesicle radiolucent stones are well visualized.

Management

The common approach to bladder stone removal is transurethral. Small bladder stones may be seen at cystoscopy and are readily removed using a basket, through the cystoscope. Larger stones must be broken. Large stones may be crushed (litholapaxy) using a lithotrite, or stones may be disintegrated to small fragments using electrohydraulic lithotripsy (EHL). Fragments are washed out per urethra by continuous irrigation throughout the procedure. Very large stones are usually removed by suprapubic vesicolithotomy, which is an extraperitoneal approach.

Pure uric acid stones too large for simple cystoscope removal may be dissolved by urinary alkalinization with oral sodium bicarbonate, hydration, and oral administration of allopurinol. This procedure may eliminate bladder uric acid stones or they may be sufficiently reduced in size for cystoscopic removal. Urease stones may be dissolved by bladder infusion of renacidin (hemiacidrin) or the instillation of Suby and Albright's solution G or M, G having a pH of 4.0, M having a pH of 4.5.

EXTRAVESICLE LESIONS
Benign Intestinal Lesions
Diverticulitis of the Sigmoid Colon Leading to Colovesical Fistula

Diverticulosis of the sigmoid colon is common. Diverticulitis of the sigmoid colon is relatively uncommon. When present a diverticular abscess may extend along the paracolic gutter and enlarge to distort the bladder shape, particularly superiorly and on the left side. Adhesions to the bladder wall may result in bladder mucosal edema and erosion through the bladder wall resulting in colovesicle fistula (Fig. 15.11). Up to 10% of patients with sigmoid diverticulitis develop a colovesicle fistula, and up to 60% of all vesicle fistulas are due to sigmoid diverticulitis. Most patients with colovesicle fistula present with colonic symptoms such as diarrhea, bleeding, and pain.

Such patients may present initially with urinary symptoms such as pneumaturia, cystitis, hematuria, or fecaluria. Colovesicle fistula is more common in males. Any nondiabetic patient presenting with pneumaturia should be considered to have a colovesicle fistula until proven otherwise. Clinically a tender mass in the pelvis may be palpable either in the suprapubic region or on rectal examination, but the clinical examination is occasionally negative. Cystoscopy commonly demonstrates the vesicle orifice of the fistula with a hemorrhagic edematous mucosa in the fistula region. Rarely the cystoscopic examination is negative, but this should not be considered as definite evidence that a colovesical fistula is absent. The administration of oral charcoal and recovery from the urine may be the only evidence that a colovesical fistula is present and the cause of the patient's pneumaturia.

Crohn's Disease

Crohn's disease may affect the terminal ileum and sigmoid colon. In either region the inflammatory change in the bowel may lead to pelvic abscess that may affect the bladder morphology and may lead to vesicoenteric or vesicocolic fistula. These complications of Crohn's disease usually follow long-standing severe granulomatous change in the ileum. Approximately 2% of ileal Crohn's granulomatous changes result in vesicoenteric fistula. The urinary tract may be affected by granulomatous abscess or fistula elsewhere resulting in ureteroenteric or pyeloenteric fistula.

Tuberculous Ileitis

Tuberculous ileitis is extremely rare and may simulate the effects of Crohn's disease on the urinary tract.

Radiation Ileitis or Colitis

Radiation therapy for the treatment of uterine or cervical carcinoma may result in radiation inflammatory changes in the distal small bowel, colon, or bladder. The mucosa in these regions affected by radiation becomes edematous and hemorrhagic and is susceptible to superimposed infection. In such circumstances abscess and fistula may develop between bowel and bladder.

Appendiceal Abscess

Occasionally the cecum and appendix abut the bladder. In these circumstances inflammatory disease of the appendix or cecum may result in associated extensive inflammatory process of the bladder wall resulting in vesicle mucosal edema hemorrhage and cystitis. The development of an appendiceal abscess may distort the bladder morphology and rarely may produce a vesicoappendiceal fistula resulting in cystitis, pyuria, and bladder pain.

Malignant Intestinal Lesions

Carcinoma of the sigmoid colon may result in invasion of the bladder and cause a colovesicle fistula. Rarely cecal carcinoma results in cecovesicle fistula when the cecum abuts the bladder. Lymphoma of the ileum is an exceedingly rare cause of vesicoenteric fistula.

Diagnosis of Intestinal Disease Affecting the Bladder

The diagnosis of the majority of intestinal diseases affecting the bladder can be made on clinical grounds. Colovesicle fistula can usually be seen on cystoscopy. In these cases, radiologic confirmation is helpful and provides visual proof of the intestinal lesion as well as the effects on the bladder. Occasionally the diagnosis can only be made radiologically. Rarely it may be almost impossible to elicit radiologically the presence of a sigmoid carcinoma in the presence of sigmoid diverticulitis as the cause of a colovesical fistula, when the patient's initial presentation is with urologic symptoms.

Plain Film

The plain film may contribute useful clues to the presence of an extravesicle mass or a colovesicle or enterovesicle fistula. The presence of a pelvic mass on the plain film distorting the bladder outline may be apparent when the bladder contains a significant amount of urine. Gas within the bladder resulting in an air fluid level on upright plain film is indicative of a fistula between bowel and bladder if the iatrogenic introduction of air into the bladder and acute infection are excluded. When gas is present in the bladder on the plain film, care must be taken to examine the bladder wall for streaky radiolucencies, which usually indicate diabetic emphysematosis. Gas in the bladder wall is not usually present in colovesicle fistula.

The plain film may suggest a pelvic mass on the right and the presence of dilated loops of small bowel may indicate complete or incomplete distal small bowel obstruction due to Crohn's disease. Fixed gas-filled small bowel loops may be seen, unchanged in position on supine, upright, and decubitus films. Acute Crohn's disease may show an adynamic ileus appearance that may be localized to the right side of the abdomen. Up to 10% of patients with long-standing Crohn's disease develop oxalate calculi in the urinary tract. When present they are obvious on the plain film. The sacroiliac joints may also provide a clue to Crohn's disease since unilateral sacroiliitis with sacroiliac sclerosis and ankylosis may be apparent.

Calcification in uterine fibromyomata may be seen on the plain film, and although the floccular nature of the calcification of fibromyomata is commonly seen, occasionally there may be difficulty in excluding bladder calcification (Fig. 15.38).

Excretory Urography

Excretory urography rarely provides significant information for bladder effects of bowel disease. A pelvic mass distorting the bladder outline on the filled bladder film

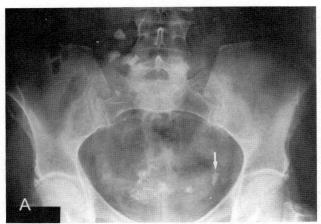

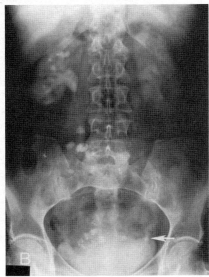

Figure 15.38.   A, Plain film of the pelvis showing irregular calcification in the bladder region. A calcific density (*arrow*) is seen in the left ureteric line. **B,** Excretory urogram showing the irregular calcification is above the bladder representing fibroid calcification. The linear calcific density is seen to be a stone in the distal left ureter (*arrow*).

may be apparent, or bladder mucosal edema may be seen as irregular filling defects in the dome and lateral wall adjacent to the pelvic mass. Colovesicle fistula is an extremely rare diagnosis on excretory urography.

Cystography

Although static cystography is commonly performed to demonstrate colovesicle fistula, voiding cystography is recommended, since only 35% of colovesicle fistulas are demonstrated by static cystography. Voiding cystography results in a marked increase in the intravesicle pressure. When the intravesicle pressure exceeds the intracolonic pressure as it may do in voiding cystography, the fistula may be demonstrated. On cystography bladder filling may demonstrate alteration in bladder morphology due to a pelvic mass. Paracolic abscess usually indents the

bladder dome and left side of the bladder. Pelvic mass resulting from ileal Crohn's disease or appendiceal abscess usually affects the right side of the bladder and bladder dome. Bladder mucosal edema occurs at the site of bladder contact with the pelvic abscess. Therefore edematous filling defects on the right side of the bladder result from Crohn's disease or appendiceal abscess. Paracolic abscess from sigmoid diverticulitis produces edema on the left side of the bladder mucosa. The presence of a colovesicle or vesicoenteric fistula may be shown on bladder filling, but the yield is usually low and bladder capacity must be obtained. If a fistula is clinically suspected and not demonstrated on bladder filling, a voiding cystogram must be obtained. Contrast medium outlining the bowel lumen is positive proof of fistula. It may be necessary to obtain oblique views in order to delineate the fistulous tract. On cystography visualization of contrast medium within bowel proves the presence of colovesicle or enterovesicle fistula.

Barium Enema

The barium enema diagnosis of diverticulitis and paracolic abscess depends on the demonstration of diverticula, circular muscle hypertrophy, barium outside the lumen, tracking along the paracolic gutter, and narrowing and irregularity of the sigmoid colon. If a colovesicle fistula is present, barium may be seen within the bladder (Fig. 15.8). Oblique, decubitus, and upright views may be necessary to delineate the actual fistulous tract. Air contrast barium enema is more likely to demonstrate the presence of a colovesicle fistula than barium enema without air. Insufflation of air per rectum will usually enter the bladder if colovesicle fistula is present. However, it may be difficult to demonstrate the fistulous tract. Diverticulitis of the colon and paracolic abscess generally affects a long segment of the sigmoid colon, with irregularity and narrowing. Carcinoma of the sigmoid colon affects a short segment with typical shoulder formation at each end of the lesion. Either may result in colovesicle fistula. Difficulty arises when both sigmoid carcinoma and diverticulitis are present together. Rarely a carcinoma of the cecum alters bladder morphology and may produce bladder mucosal edema or cecovesicle fistula. Air contrast barium enema is the best method of demonstrating carcinoma of the cecum. When the cecum abuts the bladder, air contrast enema may delineate a cecovesicle fistula with air and barium entering the bladder.

Ultrasound in an Extravesicle Inflammatory Pelvic Mass

Transabdominal ultrasound will clearly show a pelvic abscess adjacent to the filled bladder (Fig. 15.39). The pelvic abscess is mainly hypoechoic, but mixed echogenicity is usually present. The pelvic mass is well delineated. Abutment of a pelvic abscess on the bladder shows

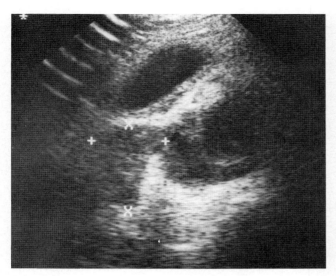

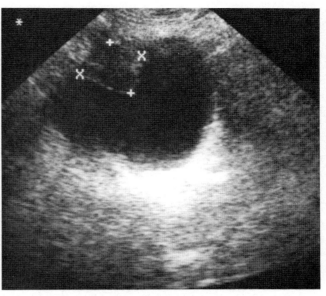

Figure 15.39.   Transabdominal ultrasound showing a pelvic abscess of mixed echogenicity adjacent to the bladder (*markers*). This abscess developed following hysterectomy.

Figure 15.41.   Transabdominal ultrasound scan in a patient with Crohn's disease. The inflammatory bowel process abuts the bladder causing localized bladder wall edema (*markers*). Proven at cystoscopy.

displacement of the fluid-filled bladder (Fig. 15.40). If the bladder wall is involved by the inflammatory process, irregularity of the bladder wall due to edematous blebs and bladder wall thickening is evident (Fig. 15.40). Pelvic abscess due to diverticulitis is present at the bladder dome and left side of the bladder. When due to Crohn's disease the abscess is seen more to the right side (Fig. 15.41). Interruption of the bladder wall outline is indicative of vesicle fistula. Carcinoma of the sigmoid colon

may invade the bladder and produce vesicocolic fistula. Carcinoma of the colon invading the bladder is seen as an echogenic mass projecting into the bladder on the left side (Fig. 15.42) and cannot be distinguished from primary carcinoma of the bladder. A lymphomatous pelvic mass may be seen as hypoechoic areas with through transmission adjacent to the bladder, giving the impression of a fluid-filled mass. However, the through transmission and acoustic enhancement are not as prevalent as that of the bladder. Gain alteration may define some echoes within a lymphomatous hypoechoic mass, but it

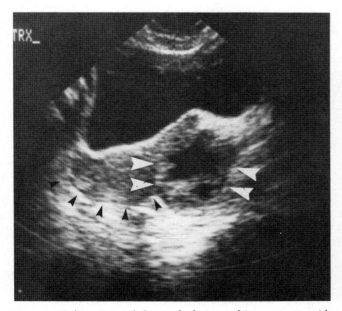

Figure 15.40.   Transabdominal ultrasound in a woman with pelvic inflammatory disease. A tuboovarian abscess is seen (*white arrows*) adjacent to the uterus (*black arrows*). The abscess distorts the bladder outline.

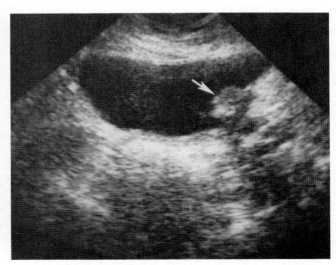

Figure 15.42.   Transabdominal ultrasound showing a soft tissue mass projecting into the left side of the bladder (*arrow*). Proven carcinoma of sigmoid colon.

may be difficult to distinguish a lymphomatous mass from a fluid filled cystic mass such as a lymphocyst.

Computed Tomography

Computed tomographic scans of the pelvis are an excellent method of assessing pelvic pathology affecting the bladder. As in ultrasound the bladder should be urine filled. The bladder wall is seen because of the difference in attenuation coefficient in urine, bladder detrusor muscle, and perivesicle fat. Adjacent pelvic abscesses from diverticulitis (Fig. 15.9), Crohn's disease, or appendicitis (Fig. 15.43) are readily diagnosed if oral contrast medium is administered 1–2 hours before the examination. The oral contrast medium fills the pelvic small bowel loops and colon. Water-soluble contrast medium may be inserted into the rectum and sigmoid colon so that bowel loops can be distinguished from enlarged nodes and abscess formation. The density of a pelvic abscess may be uniform and equivalent to soft tissue density but usually contains areas of gas and varying density. Abutment of a pelvic mass on the bladder may distort the bladder morphology producing indentations posteriorly or laterally. Hypoechoic lymphomatous masses seen on ultrasound are shown to be of soft tissue density on CT scanning. The presence of a vesicle fistula due to inflammatory bowel disease can be discerned as interruption of the bladder wall with contrast and air entering the bladder (Fig. 15.9).

Genital Lesions

Prostatic hypertrophy is the most common cause of alteration in bladder outline in males. Prostatic adenomas initially originate close to the bladder base and urethra. The bladder base is indented by median and lateral lobe hypertrophy. Median lobe hypertrophy indents the base centrally and may narrow the vesicourethral orifice. Lat-

eral lobe hypertrophy indents the lateral aspect of the base. Lateral lobe hypertrophy usually must attain a large size before producing urinary symptoms. Median lobe hypertrophy may be predominantly behind the bladder neck and cause minimal symptoms. Multiple small adenomata close to the bladder neck form an obstructing bar and cause symptoms early. Occasionally a large median lobe adenoma projecting into the bladder, termed "the lobe of Albarran," may appear as an intravesicle mass. An enlarged prostate may cause significant residual urine leading to a secondary bladder stone (Fig. 15.44).

Carcinoma of the prostate originates in the peripheral zone of the prostate and is initially distant from the bladder base and urethra. Local spread of carcinoma is initially to the seminal vesicles via the ejaculatory duct. Local invasion of the central and transitional zones of the prostate allows carcinoma to affect the bladder neck and

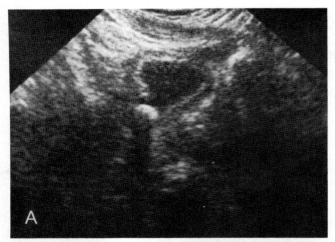

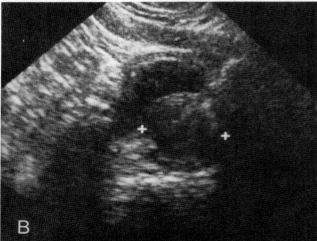

Figure 15.44. **A,** Transabdominal ultrasound showing a thick-walled bladder containing a stone which is seen as a bright echo-producing acoustic shadowing. **B,** A large prostate (*markers*) is demonstrated indenting the posterior bladder base resulting in stone formation.

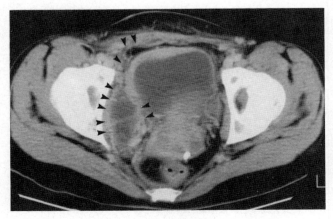

Figure 15.43. Computed tomography of the pelvis in a patient with an extensive thick-walled appendiceal abscess (*arrows*). Note the marked adjacent bladder wall thickening.

bladder base. Bladder neck invasion leads to outlet obstruction. Bladder base invasion usually affects the interureteric ridge causing unilateral or bilateral hydronephrosis. Unlike prostatic hypertrophy, which causes smooth indentation in the bladder base, prostatic carcinoma may cause irregular indentations.

Prostatic utricle cyst is a cystic dilatation of the prostatic utricle in the midline and may become large enough to indent the bladder base behind the bladder neck. It rarely causes urinary symptoms unless large.

Seminal vesicle cyst is commonly associated with urologic anomalies such as renal agenesis, ectopic kidney, and ectopic ureterocele. Cysts are usually unilateral and may be large enough to indent the bladder base posteriorly and laterally. Seminal vesicle carcinoma is rare. It may spread into the ejaculatory duct and prostatic urethra causing obstructive symptoms hematuria and hematospermia. It is an exceedingly rare cause of bladder indentation.

Uterine fibroids (fibroma, myoma, myofibroma, adenofibroma) are considered as submucosal, intramucosal, or subserosal. Submucosal and intramural fibroids cause enlargement of the uterine body. Intramural fibroids cause an irregular enlarged lumpy outline of the uterus. Subserosal fibroids may be pedunculated and may undergo torsion. Fibroids develop after puberty and tend to regress after menopause. They may undergo necrosis and calcify centrally (Fig. 15.37), or the periphery may calcify. Uterine retroversion with fibroid enlargement may displace the cervix anteriorly to the bladder neck causing some degree of outlet obstruction.

Endometriosis is ectopic endometrial tissue, the pathogenesis of which is poorly understood but may be of embryologic origin. The condition is invasive but does not normally exhibit histologic evidence of malignancy, although the rare case of malignant degeneration has been reported. Approximately 1% of patients with endometriosis have bladder involvement. The bladder may be affected by an extravesicle mass or the bladder wall may be invaded. The latter produces bladder pain, dysuria, frequency, and urgency. Cyclic hematuria may occur. Vesicle endometriosis is more common in patients who have had pelvic surgery.

Uterine malignancy affecting the bladder is either carcinoma of the cervix (Fig. 15.45) or less commonly carcinoma of the uterine body. In carcinoma of the cervix the close proximity of the uterine cervix to the bladder base and ureteric orifices results in the most frequent urinary effect of cervical carcinoma, which is ureteral obstruction. Less commonly the carcinoma invades the anterior vaginal wall, which may lead to invasion of the musculature of the posterior bladder wall and trigone and eventually to vesicovaginal fistula. Bladder wall invasion results in urinary symptoms of dysuria, frequency, and hematuria. Symptoms of outlet obstruction are rare.

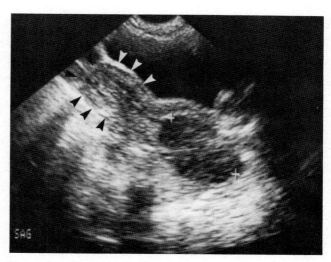

Figure 15.45. Transabdominal ultrasound showing the uterine body (*arrows*) and a large mass of mixed echogenicity arising from the cervix (*markers*). Proven carcinoma of the cervix.

Carcinoma of the uterine body is unlikely to affect the bladder other than the uterus being enlarged and indenting the bladder superiorly and posteriorly.

Ovarian cystadenomas and cystadenocarcinomas may reach a large size and affect bladder morphology. They are classified into pseudomucinous cystadenoma and serous or papilliferous cyst. Pseudomucinous cystadenoma are usually benign and may be large enough to rise out of the pelvis. Papilliferous cysts have a higher incidence of malignancy and commonly do not reach such a large size as pseudomucinous cysts. Ovarian cystadenoma or carcinoma are usually unilateral. Rupture of a pseudomucinous cystadenoma may lead to pseudomyxoma peritonei. This results in gelatinous cystic masses in the peritoneum. Pseudomyxoma peritonei may occur after surgical removal of a pseudomucinous cystadenoma, and a peritoneal mass may indent the bladder, usually near the dome. Ovarian cystadenocarcinoma may invade the bladder (Fig. 15.46) or displace the bladder (Fig. 15.47).

Ovarian dermoid cyst is ectodermal in origin. They may be unilateral or bilateral. The epithelial lining produces a thick oily secretion and may produce ectodermal derivatives such as hair and teeth (Fig. 15.48). There may be calcification in the cyst wall.

Pelvic inflammatory disease may produce pyosalpinx or hydrosalpinx, which rarely become large enough to affect bladder contour (Fig. 15.40).

Urethral diverticulum in females rarely becomes large enough to affect the bladder base. When sufficiently large it may indent the base, usually in the midline, and may contain stones simulating prostatic enlargement, hence the nomenclature "the female prostate."

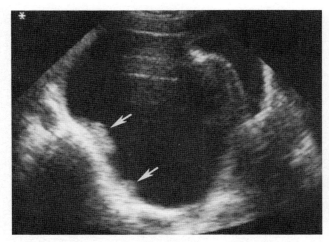

Figure 15.46.   Transabdominal ultrasound scan showing nodular lesions (*arrows*) in a thickened bladder wall, due to invasion of the bladder wall by ovarian cystadenocarcinoma.

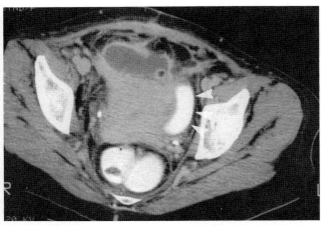

Figure 15.47.   Enhanced pelvic CT scan of a female with a pelvic mass. The bladder (*arrows*) is compressed and poorly filled due to a large mass with cystic and solid components. Proven ovarian cystadenocarcinoma.

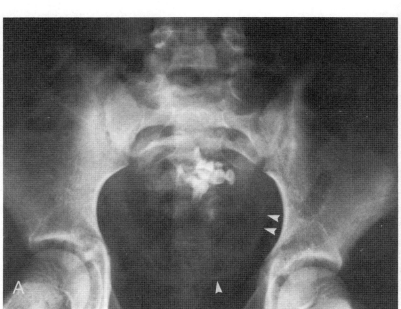

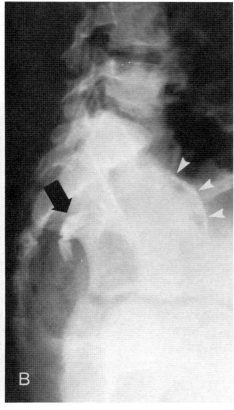

Figure 15.48.   A, A plain film of the pelvis in a young female. Multiple teeth are seen in a pelvic mass with faint irregular calcification (*arrowheads*). B, Lateral pelvic film. A pelvic mass containing teeth (*arrow*) and a partly calcified rim (*arrowheads*) is well visualized.

Sacral Lesions

Benign and malignant schwannoma arising from a sacral nerve may grow large enough to indent the posterior bladder. Lesions arising within the sacrum erode and destroy the anterior sacral bone, and growth progresses into the pelvis. It commonly presents between the third and fifth decades. There may be associated neurofibromatosis (Fig. 15.49).

Sacrococcygeal teratoma is the most common sacrococcygeal germ cell tumor. Four types are described. Type 1 is external to the sacrum and coccyx. Types 2 and 3 have both external and intrapelvic components. Type 4 is totally intrapelvic. Female : male ratio is 4 : 1. Both solid and cystic components are common. Over 80% are benign, but the incidence of malignancy increases with delayed presentation. Thus 70% are malignant after the age of 4 months. Eight percent of the Type 4 tumors have distal metastases on initial diagnosis. These lesions can attain a large size, up to 10 cm in diameter.

Chordoma is a lobular tumor of notochord origin. It commonly presents in the fifth and sixth decade but may occur at any age. It is rare before the age of 20 years. Over 50% of chordomas arise in the sacrococcygeal region. In this region they cause sacral bone destruction, and a mass projecting into the pelvis, reaching as far anterior as the bladder and producing bladder indentation posteriorly. Up to 20% of these tumors metastasize. Sacral neurofibroma may present a similar appearance (Fig. 15.49).

PELVIC LIPOMATOSIS AND DISPLACEMENT OF THE BLADDER

Pelvic Lipomatosis

Pelvic lipomatosis is a benign condition of unknown etiology characterized by an accumulation of histologically normal fat deep within the bony pelvis. Although considered relatively rare, as only 125 cases have been reported in the literature, most observers consider this to be related to underreporting because the disease is most commonly asymptomatic and is discovered incidentally upon radiologic studies performed for other reasons.

The process most commonly affects men in the fourth decade of life, although rare cases have been described in women and children. More than two-thirds of the reported cases are in black males. Hypertension is the most commonly reported associated finding. Cases of pelvic lipomatosis have been reported in association with cystitis glandularis and cystitis cystica. The most common presenting complaints are lower urinary tract symptoms including frequency, dysuria, nocturia, and hesitancy. Hematuria and urinary tract infection may also be present. Ureteral obstruction, which may result in renal failure in severe cases, is reported in 20–40% of the cases. In other advanced cases, rectal obstruction and occlusion of the inferior vena cava have been reported.

There has been considerable speculation about the etiology of pelvic lipomatosis, although no definite cause has ever been established. It has been postulated that the fat accumulation in the pelvis is a response to chronic perivesicle or pelvic inflammation owing to urinary tract infection. Others have suggested that the condition is a response to a hormonally induced metabolic process that results in fat deposition. Still other cases have been attributed to venous stasis, a local manifestation of obesity, a variant of Dercum's disease, or a type of lipodystrophy.

The diagnosis of pelvic lipomatosis is usually established on radiologic studies. Plain films of the pelvis typically reveal a pronounced radiolucency surrounding the bladder secondary to the fatty deposits. On contrast studies, the bladder is elongated with elevation of the bladder base (Fig. 15.50**A**). The abnormal configuration of the bladder has been variously described as teardrop-shaped, pear-shaped, gourd-shaped, or banana-shaped. There may be medial deviation of the distal ureters and a variable degree of hydronephrosis may be demonstrated on urography. The rectosigmoid colon characteristically is straightened and elevated from the pelvis on barium enema (Fig. 15.51). On ultrasound, the abnormal configuration of the bladder surrounded by variably echogenic pelvic fat is demonstrated. Pelvic venography may show venous compression that in severe cases may progress to frank venous occlusion. On MRI, an accumulation of fat within the pelvis with signal characteristics either identical to or of slightly lower intensity to those produced by subcutaneous fat on both T1- and T2-weighted images is present.

Although the characteristic radiologic triad of a lucent pelvis on plain films, a tear-drop bladder, and an elevated rectosigmoid colon are considered diagnostic, in recent years CT has been considered to be the most definitive diagnostic procedure. Characteristic CT findings include

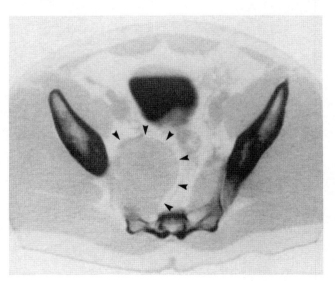

Figure 15.49.   Computed tomography scan in a patient with a large sacral neurofibroma (*arrows*) destroying part of the right ileum and extending into the pelvis approaching the bladder.

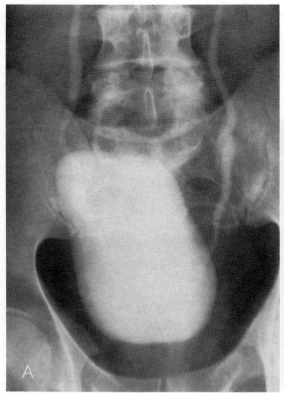

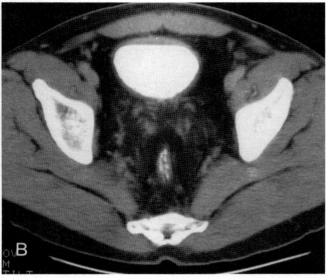

Figure 15.50. Pelvic lipomatosis. **A,** On an excretory urogram the bladder is vertically oriented and the base is elevated. Both ureters are deviated medially. **B,** Computed tomography demonstrates excess pelvic fat and the absence of soft tissue masses to explain the bladder deformity.

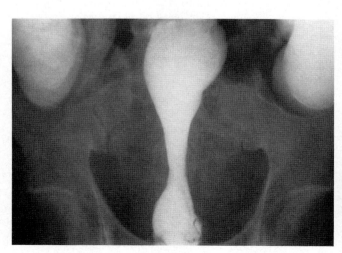

Figure 15.51. Pelvic lipomatosis. A barium enema demonstrates elevation of the rectosigmoid colon from the pelvis.

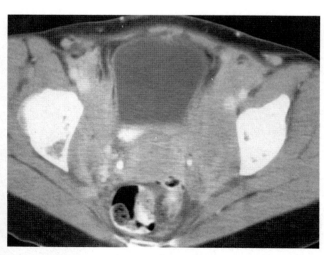

Figure 15.52. Lymphoma. Bilateral external iliac lymph node enlargement compresses the bladder resulting in a vertical orientation. This is easily distinguished from pelvic lipomatosis by CT.

excess pelvic fat, the absence of a soft tissue mass to explain the bladder deformity, an increased distance between the seminal vesicles and the posterior bladder wall, and elongation of the rectum (Fig. 15.50**B**).

A number of other conditions may result in a teardrop-shaped or pear-shaped bladder (Table 15.1). The most common of these, *iliopsoas hypertrophy,* is also common in black males. In contrast to the findings in pelvic lipomatosis, the bladder indentation in this condition is maximal in the upper portion of the organ and the other findings associated with pelvic lipomatosis will not be present. Wechsler and Brennan considered both iliopsoas hypertrophy and a narrow pelvis to be factors that predispose such patients to a teardrop bladder. An abnormal configuration of the bladder may be present in black patients in the absence of any demonstrable pathology. Indeed, Desai et al. found a pear-shaped bladder to be common among black patients and considered it to be a normal anatomic variation. In patients with *inferior vena cava obstruction,* the abnormal bladder configuration has been attributed to swelling of the pelvic muscles as a result of tissue edema and enlargement of pelvic venous collaterals. Any condition that results in *bilateral pelvic lymph node enlargement,* including lymphoma. (Fig. 15.52), prostatic carcinoma, or uterine or cervical carcinoma, may result in a teardrop bladder. Lipoplastic lymphadenopathy is an extremely rare condition that results in lymph node enlargement secondary to an accumulation of mature fat and has been associated with teardrop bladder. *Pelvic hematomas* secondary to bilateral pubic rami fractures frequently indent the bladder symmetrically (Fig. 15.53).

Table 15.1.
Causes of Teardrop Bladder

Perivesicle fluid (hematoma, urinoma, abscess)
Iliopsoas hypertrophy
Anatomic variant
Pelvic lymphadenopathy (lymphoma, etc.)
Pelvic tumor
Pelvic fibrosis
Pancreatic pseudocyst
Inferior vena cava obstruction
Retroperitoneal fibrosis
Pelvic lipomatosis

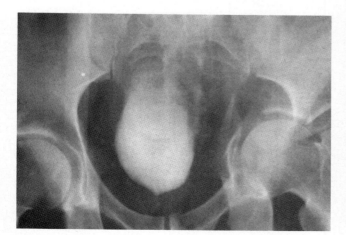

Figure 15.53. Pelvic fracture. Hematomas from pelvic fracture create bilateral pelvic masses and a teardrop configuration of the bladder.

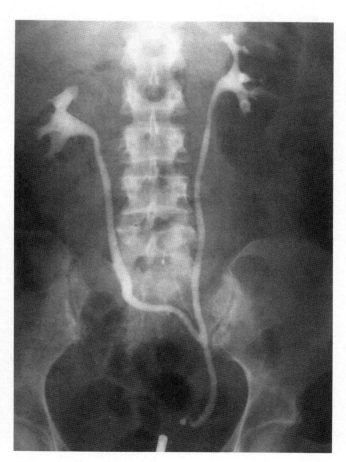

Figure 15.54. Transureteroureterostomy. The right ureter has been anastomosed to the left ureter.

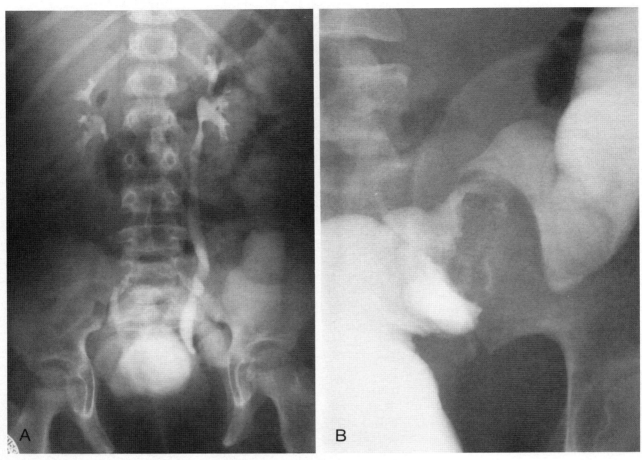

Figure 15.55. Ureterosigmoidostomy. **A,** Diastasis of the symphysis pubis is seen in this patient with bladder extrophy. A ureterosigmoidostomy was performed and contrast can be seen in the sigmoid colon during urography. **B,** Barium enema demonstrates development of colon cancer.

Other Causes of Bladder Displacement

A variety of conditions may result in unilateral asymmetric external compression of the bladder; such a finding implies the presence of a mass or mass effect. Among the conditions associated with such a finding include an aneurysm of the external iliac artery, unilateral pelvic hematoma, unilateral lymphadenopathy, lymphocele, bladder diverticulum, primary pelvic tumor, pelvic abscess, metastatic disease involving the bony pelvis, and fecal impaction.

Impressions on the base of the bladder are common in elderly males secondary to prostatic hypertrophy. In females, an impression on the base of the bladder simulating prostatic enlargement may be found after bladder suspension surgery or as the result of urethral diverticula, hypertrophy of the levator ani muscles, and from postpartum irregularity of the symphysis pubis.

Table 15.2.
Ureteral Urinary Diversion

Cutaneous ureterostomy
Transureteroureterostomy
Ureterosigmoidostomy
Ileal or ileocecal conduit
Kock pouch

URINARY DIVERSION

Urinary diversion may be performed at any level from the renal pelvis to the bladder. (Table 15.2) The indications for urinary diversion are widely varied, and the procedure used depends on the specific clinical problem. This section discusses diversion of urine flow at the level of the ureter and bladder.

Cutaneous Ureterostomy

In this procedure the ureter is brought out to the skin for direct external urine drainage. The incidence of stricture is small if the preoperative ureter was dilated. However, an external prosthesis is required to collect the urine.

Transureteroureterostomy

This technique is most often selected when the middle portions of the ureters are suitable for anastomosis (Fig. 15.54). It is contraindicated in patients with urolithiasis as both collecting systems could be obstructed by a single distal ureteral stone.

Ureterosigmoidostomy

Anastomosis of the ureters into the sigmoid colon (Fig. 15.55) avoids the need for an external urine collection prosthesis. Continence is preserved if there is normal rectal function. With antireflux techniques the incidence of pyelonephritis is low. The most serious long-term complication is the development of adenocarcinoma of the colon at the site of the ureteral anastomosis. However, the latent period required for an individual to develop these carcinomas is 15–20 years. These patients should be followed at regular intervals with sigmoidoscopy to detect the tumor.

Ileal Loop

Bricker described the construction of an ileal conduit as a form of urinary diversion in 1950. Both ureters are anastomosed to an isolated segment of ileum. The proximal end of the ileal conduit is closed, and the distal end is anastomosed to the skin in the right lower quadrant. An external prosthesis is required to collect urine drainage. This procedure has been used for many years and complications are relatively few.

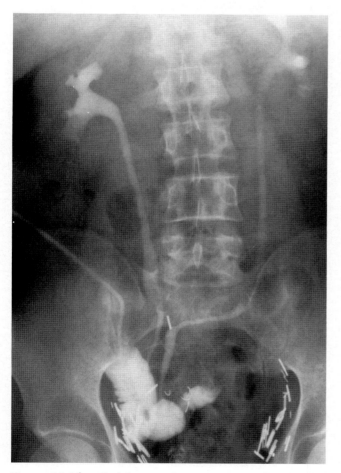

Figure 15.56.   Ileal loop. A loopogram opacifies the ileal loop and contrast refluxes into both upper tracts.

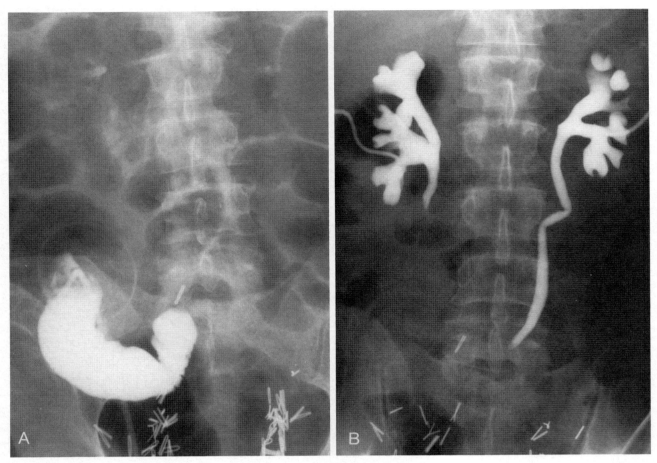

Figure 15.57.   Ureteral obstruction. **A,** The absence of reflux on a loopogram implies ureteral obstruction. **B,** Bilateral ante-grade pyelograms after percutaneous nephrostomies confirm bilateral ureteral obstruction.

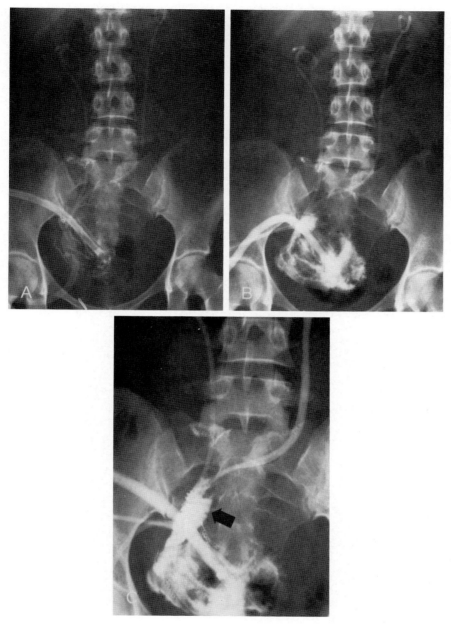

Figure 15.58. Kock pouch. **A,** Preliminary film demonstrates bilateral ureteral stents and a Malecot catheter in the pouch. **B,** No reflux or extravasation is seen after infusion of contrast material into the Malecot catheter. **C,** Injection of contrast into the ureteral stent catheters opacifies the upper tracts and the afferent loop (*arrow*).

Because the ureteroileal anastomosis usually refluxes, the collecting system can be evaluated radiographically by instilling dilute (30%) contrast material through a Foley catheter into the ileal loop (Fig. 15.56). Mild ureteropelvicaliectasis is expected, and gas may also be seen within the collecting system.

The absence of reflux implies obstruction (Fig. 15.57), and additional studies may be needed to exclude it. Thus, it is critical to use oblique positioning to try to demonstrate reflux. The loop should not be overdistended, however, as this may cause bacteremia or autonomic dysreflexia in patients with spinal cord injuries.

Ultrasound is often used to follow these patients, but mild degrees of dilation of the calyces is expected. A baseline examination 3 months after surgery is most helpful in interpreting subsequent examinations.

Kock Pouch

Modifications of Kock's continent ileostomy have resulted in a low-pressure, high-capacity urine reservoir. The intussuscepted ureteral nipples prevent reflux. Because it is a continent pouch, an external prosthesis is unnecessary. Urine is removed by intermittent self-catheterization.

The Kock pouch is constructed from an isolated segment of terminal ileum much longer (75 cm) than that used for an ileal loop (15–25 cm). A central reservoir is constructed in an antiperistaltic fashion so that a low pressure is maintained. Two ileal segments are intussuscepted into the pouch to create an antirefluxing anastomosis for the ureters. The second ileal segment serves as the efferent limb of the reservoir. The one-way nipple valve provides continence but can be easily catheterized by the patient for urine drainage.

Many modifications of the Kock pouch have been adapted for specific uses. In the hemi-Kock pouch, the efferent ileal limb is anastomosed to the urethra rather than the anterior abdominal wall.

The Mainz pouch uses the cecum and two ileal loops for greater reservoir capacity. The ureters are tunneled in the submucosa of the posterior cecum to prevent reflux.

Antirefluxing ureteroileal anastomoses are created at either end of a 40-cm segment of isolated ileum in the Camey procedure. The midportion of the antimesenteric border of this loop is anastomosed to the urethra. Continence depends upon an intact external sphincter.

The King pouch is similar to the Mainz pouch in that the ureters are tunneled in the posterior tenia of the cecal reservoir to prevent reflux. Continence is obtained by intussuscepting the terminal ileum deep into the cecal pouch through the ileocecal valve.

The radiographic evaluation is similar regardless of the specific surgical technique used. Initial evaluation is usually done with bilateral stents extending from both renal pelves through the pouch to drain into separate bags (Fig. 15.58). An additional large-bore catheter is used to drain the pouch and stent the efferent ileal limb.

The first radiographic evaluation of the Koch pouch is usually done 3 weeks after the operation. Instillation of 100–300 ml of contrast material into the Kock pouch is performed to look for reflux or extravasation. If no complications are seen, the stenting catheters are removed. Follow-up studies performed after 6 months require 500–1000 ml of contrast material as the mature pouch has a much larger capacity. Careful examination of the preliminary film is required as stone formation may occur on exposed surgical staples.

Contrast is passively instilled through the stent catheters by raising the contrast media bottle 36 inches above the patient. After evaluating the collecting systems, a postdrainage film is obtained to look for extravasation (Fig. 15.59). Excretory urography may be performed to detect ureteral obstruction after the stents have been removed.

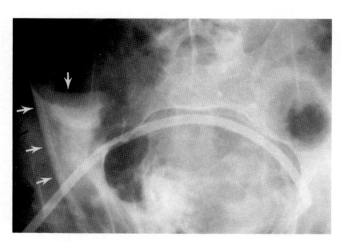

Figure 15.59. Extravasation from Kock pouch. After draining the contrast from the pouch, contrast is seen in the peritoneal cavity (*arrows*).

SUGGESTED READINGS

Benign Bladder Lesions

Bidwell JK, Dunne MG. Computed tomography of bladder malakoplakia. *J Comput Assist Tomogr* 11(5):909, 1987.

Das S, Bulusu NV, Lowe P: Primary vesical pheochromocytoma. *Urology* 21(1):20, 1983.

Frances RS, Shackleford GD: Cyclophosphamide cystitis with bladder wall calcification: report of a case. *J Can Assoc Radiol* 25:324, 1974.

Goldman IL, Caldamone AA, Gauderer M, et al: Infected urachal cysts: a review of 10 cases. *J Urol* 140:375, 1988.

Goldman SM, Salik JD: Benign mass lesions of the bladder wall. *Contemp Diagn Radiol* 12:1, 1978.

Harrison RB, Steir FM, Cochrane JA: Alkaline encrusting cystitis. *AJR* 130:575, 1978.

Joffe N: Roentgenologic abnormalities of the urinary bladder secondary to Crohn's disease. *Am J Roentgenol* 127:297, 1976.

Jorulf H, Lindstedt E: Urogenital schistosomiasis: CT evaluation. *Radiology* 157:745, 1985.

Murphy WD, Rovner AJ, Nazinitsky KJ: Condylomata acuminata of the bladder: a rare cause of intraluminal-filling defects. *Urol Radiol* 12:34, 1990.

Patel PS, Wilbur AC: Nephrogenic adenoma presenting as a calcified mass. *AJR* 150:1071, 1988.

Pollack HM, Banner MD, Martinez LO, Hodson CJ: Diagnostic considerations in urinary bladder wall calcification. *AJR* 136:791, 1981.

Pope TL, Harrison RB, Clark RL, Cuttino JT: Bladder base impressions in women: "female prostate." *Am J Roentgenol* 136:1105, 1981

Sandler, CM: *The Bladder in Text Book of Diagnostic Imaging.* Putman CE, Ravin CE (eds), Philadelphia, WB Saunders, 1988.

Warshawsky R, Bow SN, Waldbaum RS, et al: Bladder pheochromocytoma with MR correlation. *J Comput Assist Tomogr* 13(4):714, 1989.

Zilberman M, Loar E, Moriel E, et al: Paravesical granulomas masquerading as bladder neoplasma: late complications of inguinal hernia repair. *J Urol* 143:489, 1990.

Zimmermann K, Amis ES Jr, Newhouse JH: Nephrogenic adenoma of the bladder: urographic spectrum. *Urol Radiol* 11;123, 1989.

Malignant Bladder Lesions

Affre J, Michel JR, de Peyronnet R, et al: Secondary foci of primary tumors of the bladder in the upper urinary tract. *Urol Radiol* 3:7, 1981.

Amendola MA, Glazer GM, Grossman HB, et al: Staging of bladder carcinoma: MRI-CT-surgical correlation. *Am J Roentgenol* 146:1179, 1986.

Brick SH, Friedman AC, Pollack HM, et al: Urachal carcinoma: CT findings. *Radiology* 169:377, 1988.

Filmer RB, Spencer JR: Malignancies in bladder augmentations and intestinal conduits. *J Urol* 143:671, 1990.

Hillman BJ, Silvert M, Cook G, et al: Recognition of bladder tumors by excretory urography. *Radiology* 138:319, 1981.

Jewett HJ, Strong GH: Infiltrating carcinoma of the bladder: relation of depth of penetration of the bladder wall to the incidence of local extension and metastases. *J Urol* 55:366, 1946.

Johnson DE, Kaesler KE, Kaminsky S, et al: Lymphangiography as an aid in staging bladder carcinoma. *South Med J* 69(1):28, 1976

Korobkin M, Cambier L, Drake J: Computed tomography of urachal carcinoma. *J Comput Assist Tomogr* 12(6):981, 1988.

Lang EK: The roentgenographic assessment of bladder tumors. *Cancer* (Phila) 23:717, 1969.

Lee SH, Kitchens HH, Kim BS: Adenocarcinoma of the urachus: CT features. *J Comput Asst Tomogr* 14(2):232, 1990.

Miller SW, Pfister R: Calcification in uroepithelial tumors of the bladder. *AJR* 121(4):827, 1974.

Narumi Y, Sato T, Kuriyama K, et al: Vesical dome tumors: significance of extravesical extension on CT. *Radiology* 169:383, 1988.

Prout GR. Classification and staging of bladder carcinoma. *Cancer* (Phila) 45(8):1932, 1980.

Rholl KS, Lee JKT, Heiken JP, et al: Primary bladder carcinoma: evaluation with MR imaging. *Radiology* 163:117, 1987

Simpson W, Duncan AW, Clayton CB: A useful sign in the diagnosis of bladder tumors on intravenous urography. *Br J Radiol* 47:272, 1974.

Spataro RF, Davis RS, McLachlan MSF, et al: Urachal abnormalities in the adult. *Radiology* 149:659, 1983.

Strijk SP, Debruyne FMJ, Herman CJ: Lymphography in the management of urologic tumors. *Radiology* 146:39, 1983.

Tavares NJ, Demas BE, Hricak H: MR imaging of bladder neoplasms: correlation with pathologic staging. *Urol Radiol* 12:27, 1990.

Teefey SA, Baron RL, Schulte SJ, Shuman WP: Abdominal and gastrointestinal radiology. differentiating pelvic veins and enlarged lymph nodes: optimal CT techniques. *Radiology* 175:683, 1990.

Winterberger AR, Wajsman Z, Merrin C, Murphy GP: Eight years of experience with preoperative angiographic and lymphographic staging of bladder cancer. *J Urol* 119:208, 1978.

Bladder Calculi

Griffith DP, Musher DM, Itin C: Urease: the primary cause of infection-induced stones. *Invest Urol* 13:346, 1976.

McCallum RW, Banner MP: Lower urinary tract calculi and calcifications. In *Clinical Urography*. Polack HM (ed), Philadelphia, WB Saunders, 1990.

Otnes B: Correlation between causes and composition of urinary stones. *Scand J Urol Nephrol* 17:93, 1983.

Pelvic Lipomatosis

Allen FJ, De Kock MLS: Pelvic lipomatosis: the nuclear magnetic resonance appearance and associated vesicoureteral reflux. *J. Urol* 138:1228, 1987.

Ambos MA, Bosniak MA, Lefleur RS, et al: The pear-shaped bladder. *Radiology* 122:85, 1977.

Baath L, Nyman U, Aspelin P, et al: Computed tomography of pelvic lipomatosis. *Acta Radiol* 3:311, 1986.

Crane DB, Smith MJV: Pelvic lipomatosis: 5-year followup. *J Urol* 118:547, 1977.

Demas BE, Avallon A, Hricak H: Pelvic lipomatosis: diagnosis and characterization by magnetic resonance imaging. *Urol Radiol* 10:198, 1988.

Desai SC, Eliot CS, Lawton G: Bladder shape and racial origin. *Clin Radiol* 36:377, 1985.

Klein FA, Smith MJV, Kasenetz I: Pelvic lipomatosis: 35 year experience. *J Urol* 139:998, 1988.

Moss AA, Clark RE, Goldberg HI, et al: Pelvic lipomatosis: a roentgenographic diagnosis. *AJR* 115:411, 1972.

Pope TL, Harrison RB, Clark R, et al: Bladder base impression in women: "female prostate." *AJR* 136:1105, 1981.

Wechsler RJ, Brennan RE: Teardrop bladder: additional considerations. *Radiology* 144:281, 1982.

Urinary Diversion

Amis ES Jr, Cronan JJ, Pfister RC: Filling defects in small bowel urinary conduits. *AJR* 137:787, 1981.

Amis ES Jr, Newhouse JH, Olsson CA: Continent urinary diversions: review of current surgical procedures and radiologic imaging. *Radiology* 168:395, 1988.

Banner MP, Pollack HM, Bonavita JA, et al: The radiology of urinary diversions. *RadioGraphics* 4(6):885, 1984.

Bricker EM: Bladder substitution after pelvic evisceration. *Surg Clin North Am* 30:1511, 1950.

Camey M: Bladder replacement by ileocystoplasty following radical cystectomy. World *J Urol* 3:161, 1985.

Filmer RB, Spencer JR: Malignancies in bladder augmentations and intestinal conduits. *J Urol* 143:671, 1990.

Kenney PJ, Hamrick KM, Samuels LJ, et al: Radiologic evaluation of continent urinary reservoirs. *RadioGraphics* 10:455, 1990.

King LR, Stone AR, Webster GD: *Bladder Reconstruction and Continent Urinary Diversion.* Chicago, Year Book Medical, 1987, pp 209–251.

Kock NG, Nilson AE, Nilsson LO, et al: Urinary diversion via a continent ileal reservoir: clinical results in 12 patients. *J Urol* 128:469, 1982.

Lilien OM, Camey M: 25-year experience with replacement of the human bladder (Camey procedure). *J Urol* 132:886, 1984.

Princenthal RA, Lowman R, Zeman RK, et al: Ureterosigmoidostomy: the development of tumors, diagnosis, and pitfalls. *AJR* 141:77, 1983.

Ralls PW, Barakos JA, Skinner DG, et al: Imaging of the Kock continent ileal urinary reservoir. *Radiology* 161:477, 1986.

Rowland RG, Mitchell ME, Bihrle R, et al: Indiana continent urinary reservoir. *J Urol* 137:1136, 1987.

Skinner DG, Lieskovsky G, Boyd SD: Continuing experience with the continent ileal reservoir (Kock pouch) as an alternative to cutaneous urinary diversion: an update after 250 cases. *J Urol* 137:1140, 1987

Stockle M, Becht E, Voges G, et al: Ureterosigmoidostomy: an outdated approach to bladder exstrophy? *J Urol* 143:770, 1990.

NEUROGENIC BLADDER

Neurogenic bladder refers to neuromuscular dysfunction of the detrusor muscle and the urethral sphincter. Normal reciprocal parasympathetic and sympathetic activity is inhibited, causing voiding difficulties. Although there are numerous classifications of neurogenic bladder, the most useful for radiologists is based on the response of the bladder to the neurologic insult as described by McLellan in 1939 (Table 16.1).

NORMAL NEUROMUSCULAR ANATOMY OF THE BLADDER AND URETHRA

The neuroanatomy involved in micturition and in the maintenance of continence includes (*a*) the sympathetic (hypogastric) nerves, (*b*) the parasympathetic (pelvic) nerves, and (*c*) the somatic (pudendal) nerves. Passive continence is governed by the autonomic system. Active continence is governed by somatic nerves.

Sympathetic (Hypogastric) Nerves

Adrenergic α- and β-receptors within smooth muscle of the lower urinary tract have been mapped. Stimulation of α-receptors contracts smooth muscle. Stimulation of β-receptors relaxes smooth muscle. The fundus and body of the detrusor muscle is scant in α-receptors and rich in β-receptors. The bladder neck, internal sphincter, and intrinsic sphincter are rich in adrenergic receptors, with α-receptors predominating. Motor sympathetic activity relaxes the bladder and contracts the bladder neck while smooth muscle sphincters maintain passive continence. Sensory afferent fibers from the mucosa of the bladder body and fundus convey mucosal pain along the sympathetic "hypogastric" nerves. Both sympathetic hypogastric and parasympathetic pelvic nerves convey mucosal pain from the trigone area to the spinal cord. Sensory afferent impulses are stimulated when the detrusor is distended. Afferent sympathetic stimulation reduces sympathetic motor activity to the trigone and urethral sphincters causing relaxation. When done in reciprocity, with stimulation of the motor activity of the parasympathetic micturition reflex arc, voiding results. The sympathetic "hypogastric" nerves originate from the anterior horn cells from T11 to L2.

Parasympathetic Pelvic Nerves

The parasympathetic "pelvic" nerves are motor and sensory to the detrusor muscle. A reflex micturition arc is created through sacral segments S2–S4. Stretch receptors within the detrusor muscle are stimulated by a filled bladder causing sensory impulses to pass along a short postganglionic segment to the vesicle plexus where there is a synapse. The impulse passes along the preganglionic

Table 16.1.
Neurogenic Bladder

Upper motor neuron lesion
  Uninhibited
    Central nervous system lesions
    Demyelinating disease
    Multiple sclerosis
    Pernicious anemia
  Reflex
    Spinal cord lesions above L2
Lower motor neuron lesion
  Autonomous
    Spinal cord lesions below L2
  Motor paralytic
    Lesions affecting the motor limb of the
      micturition reflex arc, e.g.,
      poliomyelitis, pelvic or disc surgery
  Sensory paralytic
    Lesions affecting the sensory limb of the
      micturition reflex arc, e.g., diabetic
      mellitus and tabes dorsales
Mixed (features of both upper and lower
  motor neuron lesions)
    Trauma causing incomplete neurologic
      insult above and below L2

segment to the posterior root ganglion and the posterior horn of sacral segments S2–S4. Via an interneuronal synapse the sensory impulse passes to the anterior horn to stimulate a motor impulse. The motor impulse passes along the pelvic nerve to the detrusor muscle where the nerve ending produces acetylcholine, which causes detrusor contraction, resulting in voiding. Thus the micturition reflex arc is entirely autonomic for the first 18 months to 2 years of life. During this time micturition centers are developing in the brain. Several inhibitory centers have been described in the pons, hypothalamus, superior colliculus, and cerebellum. Centers in the cerebral cortex also develop that can both stimulate and inhibit micturition. Consequently, in infancy the bladder is uninhibited until the brain centers are sufficiently developed to control micturition. Passive continence control and normal voiding result from reciprocal activity of the sympathetic and parasympathetic nerve. Awareness of bladder filling after the development of brain centers occurs after 150-200 ml of urine is in the bladder. The centers learn to ignore these early stimuli and the brain centers do not release voiding until massive impulses pass through the micturition reflex arc and it is convenient to micturate. If it is not convenient to micturate, the brain centers can still inhibit voiding by stimulation of the voluntary striated muscles of the pelvic floor and external sphincter through the somatic pudendal nerves.

Somatic Pudendal Nerves

Striated muscles have both tone and active contraction. Striated fibers of the external sphincter intermingle with smooth muscle fibers of the intrinsic sphincter. Ac-

tive contraction of the external sphincter can only be maintained for a few minutes, which is sufficient time for the transference of impulses from the external sphincter striated fibers to the smooth muscle fibers of the intrinsic sphincter and internal sphincter thus converting active continence to passive continence and inhibition of the urge to void. The pudendal nerves originate in sacral segments S2–S4.

Patients with conditions leading to neuromuscular dysfunction of the bladder and urethra do not exhibit the normal neurologic functions. This results in uncoordinated detrusor contraction. Lesions arising from the cerebral cortex to the peripheral pelvic nerves interrupt normal neurologic function and precipitate neurogenic bladder.

CLASSIFICATIONS OF NEUROGENIC BLADDER

Lesions affecting the brain or spinal cord above the level of L2 result in upper motor neuron lesions or contractile bladder neuromuscular dysfunction. The micturition reflex arc is intact. Patients with upper motor neuron lesions whose lesion is above the level of T5 also exhibit detrusor sphincter dyssynergia. This results in nonrelaxation of the urinary sphincters when the detrusor contracts, resulting in outlet obstruction and increased residual urine. Sphincter dyssynergia may involve the bladder neck and internal sphincter or more commonly the distal sphincter. In patients with lesions below L2 the micturition reflex arc is compromised or obliterated. When the micturition reflex arc is obliterated the detrusor cannot contract. This results in a lower motor neuron lesion.

Patients with an acute upper motor neuron lesion such as trauma to the cord above L2 are initially in spinal shock. This is the autonomous neurogenic bladder that presents as a lower motor neuron lesion. In such patients, the autonomous neurogenic bladder is temporary, usually lasting less than 3 months. With the passage of spinal shock, the micturition reflex arc returns and the patient then presents as a reflex upper motor neuron lesion.

ETIOLOGY

The most common cause of neurogenic bladder in males is spinal cord injury. Other cord lesions include myelomeningocele, disc protrusion, tumor, syringomyelia, multiple sclerosis, spinal abscess, vascular insufficiency, transverse myelitis, diabetic myelitis, tabes dorsalis, and arachnoiditis. Brain lesions include cerebral atherosclerosis, multiple sclerosis, brain tumor, and brain injury.

INCIDENCE

There are 1–1.5 million North Americans with spinal cord injuries and this figure is increased by 20,000 new cases each year. When all of the lesions that contribute to neurogenic bladder are considered, the number of patients in North America suffering from neuromuscular dysfunction of the lower urinary tract is an astonishing 25 million. Several of the more common causes of neurogenic bladder require further discussion.

SPINAL CORD TRAUMA

Acute spinal cord trauma occurs almost exclusively in young men below the age of 30 years, the mean age being 19 years. Less than 0.5% of cases occur in females. The injury results from automobile or motorcycle accidents, diving accidents, and gunshot wounds. Most of these injuries are upper motor neuron lesions. Cervical spine and high thoracic lesions result in quadriplegia. Lower thoracic and lumbar lesions result in paraplegia. The cord trauma may result in complete or incomplete cord injury. The immediate result is spinal shock, in which the bladder is noncontractile, i.e., autonomous neurogenic bladder. Spinal shock may persist from a few weeks to 3 months. If trauma has occurred above L2, the micturition reflex arc returns to function after spinal shock subsides and the patient presents with findings indicative of reflex neurogenic bladder. These clinical findings include inability to initiate or inhibit voiding, increased residual urine, uninhibited bladder contractions causing urge incontinence, reduced bladder capacity, hyperactive bulbocavernous reflex, and in patients whose lesion is above T5, the manifestations of autonomic dysreflexia. If trauma has occurred at the level of L2 or below, the passage of spinal shock results in the persistence of the clinical findings of autonomous neurogenic bladder. These are a flaccid bladder that is unable to contract, increased residual urine, inability to initiate voiding, and an absent bulbocavernous reflex. These patients do not exhibit findings of autonomic dysreflexia.

AUTONOMIC DYSREFLEXIA

Autonomic dysreflexia is a serious complication of cord lesions above the T5 level, which is the level of the greater splanchnic nerves. It is said to occur in 70–90% of these patients.

Autonomic dysreflexia is the result of an α-adrenergic response resulting in peripheral vascular contraction below the cord lesion that is uncontrolled by central centers, and results in a rapid rise in blood pressure. The normal human experiences a small elevation in blood pressure during micturition due to this viscerovascular response but the peripheral vascular contraction is normally controlled by central centers. Consequently peripheral vascular contraction below the cord lesion is uncontrolled resulting in skin pallor below the lesion, flushing and sweating of the face and neck above the lesion, and nondilatation of the splanchnic veins resulting in a rapid rise in blood pressure. The blood pressure

may increase from normal to 250/110–120 mm Hg, within a few minutes of a bladder stimulation such as bladder filling with contrast medium or the initiation of voiding. The rapid rise in blood pressure may result in severe headache, coma, convulsions, and even death. In addition, baroreceptors in the carotid sinus are stimulated causing bradycardia.

In patients whose lesion is above T5, autonomic dysreflexia is to be anticipated during lower urinary tract examination. Blood pressure monitoring after the injection of every 50 ml of contrast medium during cystourethrography is recommended and particularly at the initiation of voiding. Blood pressure monitoring generally gives an early indication of pressure increase. Any indication of blood pressure increase is an indication for delay or termination of the procedure if the blood pressure rise is significant on bladder filling. A short-acting ganglion blocker (such as Regitine) should be readily available to control an excessive rise in blood pressure. It is to be emphasized that cystourethrography should be performed with the catheter balloon in the fossa navicularis and not in the bladder, which may cause involuntary hyperreflexic bladder contractions.

Patients with cord lesions above L2 and particularly those with lesions above T5 may exhibit detrusor sphincter dyssynergia. Detrusor sphincter dyssynergia may occur at the bladder neck, due to nonrelaxation of the internal sphincter during detrusor contraction, but in the author's experience, detrusor sphincter dyssynergia more commonly affects the distal sphincter mechanism. There is a reported association of sphincter dyssynergia with autonomic dysreflexia. Detrusor distal sphincter dyssynergia is common in upper motor neuron lesions since the micturition reflex is intact and therefore the detrusor muscle can be stimulated to contract. However, since the sympathetic hypogastric nerves and the somatic pudendal nerves control the distal intrinsic and external sphincters, the normal reciprocal activity between the parasympathetic, sympathetic, and somatic (pudendal) nerves is inhibited resulting in nonrelaxation of the distal sphincters during detrusor contraction. This results in some degree of outlet obstruction and increased residual urine. Both bladder neck dyssynergia and distal sphincter dyssynergia may arise in upper motor neuron lesions. Autonomic dysreflexia is said to be initiated by overdistention of the α-adrenergic fibers at the bladder neck and internal sphincter, resulting in the release of excess noradrenalin secretions. The excess noradrenalin causes peripheral vascular constriction leading to increased blood pressure. Perkash has indicated that a deep bladder neck sphincterotomy blocks the α-adrenergic response almost completely, reducing the incidence of autonomic dysreflexia. It has also been suggested that patients who are subject to autonomic dysreflexia should receive an α-adrenergic blocker before performing voiding cystourethrography. A modified sphincterotomy from the bladder neck to the distal sphincters may reduce the incidence of autonomic dysreflexia.

MULTIPLE SCLEROSIS

Over 50% of patients with multiple sclerosis have urinary symptoms, the most common being incontinence and urgency.

Cystourethrography has shown that 67–78% of multiple sclerosis patients with urinary symptoms have a hyperreflexic bladder. It has not yet been shown what percentage of these patients who have a dysreflexic bladder are due to bladder catheterization or to upper motor neuron lesions. Fifty percent of these patients had sphincter dyssynergia. Approximately 21% of patients presented with an areflexic bladder (lower motor neuron lesion) and 12% had normal detrusor function. The duration and mean age of multiple sclerosis patients is longer and higher in patients presenting with urinary symptoms, i.e., less severe early multiple sclerosis is less likely to produce urinary symptoms. Urodynamic studies correlate well with the severity of pyramidal and sensory lesions. Demyelinating lesions in the deep white matter of the lateral columns may result in interruption of the descending inhibitory pathways to the bladder resulting in detrusor hyperreflexia. Demyelination plaques in the white matter of the sacral cord affecting the reflex arc may result in detrusor areflexia. Detrusor sphincter dyssynergia is associated with detrusor hyperreflexia and demyelinating lesions of the pyramidal tracts. It is unusual for suprapontine demyelinating lesions to produce dyssynergia.

URINARY INCONTINENCE IN THE ELDERLY

Urinary incontinence in the elderly is becoming a more common problem since longevity in the Western world is increasing. It is therefore imperative that the distinction between neurogenic causes and nonneurogenic causes in elderly patients is made. Neurogenic bladder in the elderly may arise from a variety of geriatric causes. Advanced cerebral atherosclerosis, brain infarction, brain tumor, metastasis, vertebral body collapse, degenerative or arthritic changes in the spine, spinal metastasis, and diabetes mellitus are some causes giving rise to true neurogenic bladder incontinence.

Nonneurogenic causes include psychogenic polydipsia, neural insufficiency, chronic outlet obstruction, cystitis, bladder tumor, bladder stone, radiation cystitis, stress incontinence, urethral diverticulum in women, and postprostatectomy in men. Numerous drug therapies such as reserpine, furosemide, diazepam, phenothiazine, and phenytoin sodium may also contribute to urinary incontinence in the elderly. Naturally the management of many of the nonneurogenic causes differs significantly from that of a true neurogenic cause.

UROLOGIC INVESTIGATIONS IN NEUROGENIC BLADDER

Urologic investigations are aimed at assessing the degree of outlet obstruction, the site of obstruction, and the type of neurogenic bladder. The cystometrogram consists of the instillation of water, air, or carbon dioxide into the bladder and assessing intravesicle pressure during filling and voiding. Water instillation with manometric pressure measurement is the most commonly used. The method distinguishes reflexic from areflexic bladder, i.e., upper motor neuron lesion from lower motor neuron lesion. In normal voiding the intravesicle bladder pressure does not usually exceed 60 cm H_2O. If the intravesicle bladder pressure is higher than 60 cm H_2O some degree of bladder outlet obstruction exists, due either to sphincter dyssynergia, prostatic hypertrophy, or urethral stricture. A sustained intravesicle pressure of over 70 cm H_2O during voiding may result in vesicoureteral reflux.

Urodynamic Studies

The use of microtransducers has simplified the urodynamic assessment of the lower urinary tract. Dual-microtipped pressure transducer catheters enable measurement of intravesicle and urethral pressure simultaneously. Recently the dual-microtipped catheter transducer has progressed to five microtransducer catheters interfaced with a multichannel recorder in the assessment of neurogenic bladder. This enables simultaneous pressure recordings within the bladder, at the bladder neck, at the distal sphincters, and at the bulbous urethra during resting and voiding. Sphincter dyssynergia at the internal sphincter or the distal sphincters or both, can be clearly demonstrated. Intravenous injection of phentolamine during urethral pressure assessment may produce a dramatic fall in urethral pressure indicating bladder neck dyssynergia. Uroflow meter studies can be monitored. In normal males under 40 years the flow rate should be 22 ml/sec. This rate is reduced to 13 ml/sec in normal men over 60 years. In females under 50 years the flow rate is 25 ml/sec, diminishing to 18 ml/sec over the age of 50 years.

Electromyography

Striated muscle activity can be assessed by inserting a needle into the external sphincter. In normal humans moderate electrical activity is present in the external sphincter at rest. Electrical activity increases on increased intraabdominal pressure. Electrical activity ceases on voiding. In reflexic bladder, or upper motor neuron lesions, no increase in electrical activity on increased intraabdominal pressure indicates a lack of continuity of the neural pathways from the brain centers to the pudendal nerves and therefore neuromuscular dysfunction. During voiding, lack of cessation of electrical activity or increase in the electrical activity in the external sphincter indicates sphincter dyssynergia. In areflexic bladder or lower motor neuron lesions no electrical activity in the external sphincter is recorded at any time. Simultaneous urodynamic studies and radiologic studies are ideal.

RADIOLOGY

Upper motor neuron paraplegics have normal use of their hands and arms, and are therefore capable of bladder training. This involves the measurement of fluid intake, the stimulation of voiding at set intervals, and self-catheterization if necessary. Self-suprapubic tapping to stimulate detrusor contraction has long been known in the management of paraplegic patients and is part of bladder training. Many such individuals are also able to do sterile self-catheterization. The aim of bladder training and self-catheterization is to have an acceptable residual urine. This regimen is successful in 60–70% of upper motor neuron paraplegics. However, the remainder have an unacceptable residual urine in spite of this regimen. These patients require radiologic investigation, to pinpoint the site of outlet obstruction. In these patients outlet obstruction occurs due to sphincter dyssynergia, prostatic infection or hypertrophy, or urethral stricture, which is usually the result of catheterization (Fig. 16.1). Most paraplegics are young and unlikely to have developed prostatic hypertrophy, but they may be subject to pros-

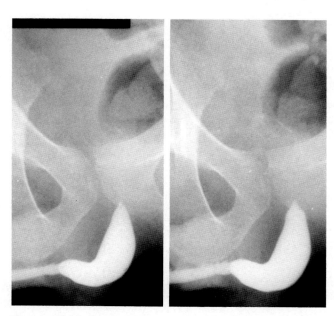

Figure 16.1. Dynamic retrograde urethrogram in a patient with upper motor neuron lesion. The study shows severe scarring in the distal bulbous urethra and penile urethra. The glands of Littre are also visualized. This scarring is due to catheterization causing pressure necrosis at the penoscrotal junction with superimposed infection spreading distally to the penile urethra and proximally along the bulbous urethra. *Note:* There is spasm of the distal sphincters obstructing the retrograde flow of contrast medium into the posterior urethra and bladder.

tatitis if obstruction is distal to the prostate, i.e., due to distal sphincter dyssynergia or urethral stricture. The site of obstruction cannot properly be assessed without obtaining a voiding study. Thus, the radiologist is asked to obtain a voiding study in a patient whose main complaint is that he cannot void properly. Although this appears to be paradoxical, it is not difficult to make an upper motor neuron paraplegic void. Two methods of assessing the site of outlet obstruction are described. The first is dynamic retrograde and voiding cystourethrography; the second is transrectal sonographic voiding cystourethrography.

Dynamic Retrograde and Voiding Cystourethrography

The method is as described for the assessment of urethral stricture with the exception that the catheter and syringe are left in place (with the balloon of the catheter in the fossa navicularis) during voiding. The catheter should not be inserted into the bladder. The dynamic retrograde urethrogram outlines the urethra from the fossa navicularis to the bladder neck. The presence or absence of urethral stricture can be assessed. During the retrograde urethrogram there may be a temporary holdup to the flow of contrast medium into the posterior urethra due to spasm of the distal sphincter (Fig. 16.2). Steady, gentle pressure on the syringe barrel and patience of the radiologist overcomes the spasm and contrast medium will flow into the bladder (Fig. 16.3). Iodine concentration of contrast medium is approximately 30%. In outlet obstruction there is usually some urine in the bladder, which mixes with the contrast medium. However, the 30% contrast medium mixed with this residual urine is sufficient to provide good visualization of the urethra during voiding. Retrograde injection of contrast medium into the bladder via the catheter in the fossa navicularis is continued until the micturition reflex arc is stimulated, either by bladder distention, which is common, or by suprapubic tapping after the insertion of 300–350 ml contrast medium. During bladder filling the possibility of low-pressure vesicoureteral reflux should be considered and the bladder intermittently fluoroscoped to assess this. If low-pressure reflux is demonstrated (which is rare) the examination can be continued after the application of a compression band (commonly used for compression in excretory urography) and elevation of the head of the table to 30°. The compression band serves two purposes. It stops the low-pressure reflux from reaching the kidneys, and it keeps the paraplegic patient in position on the table.

Cystourethrography in Upper Motor Neuron Paraplegics

In patients with upper motor neuron paraplegia, the voiding study demonstrates the site of outlet obstruction,

Figure 16.2. Dynamic retrograde urethrogram in a patient with a traumatic cord lesion at T6. The balloon of the Foley catheter is in the fossa navicularis. No urethral stricture is present in the anterior urethra but there is spasm of the distal sphincters and bulbocavernosus muscle restricting the flow of contrast medium into the posterior urethra.

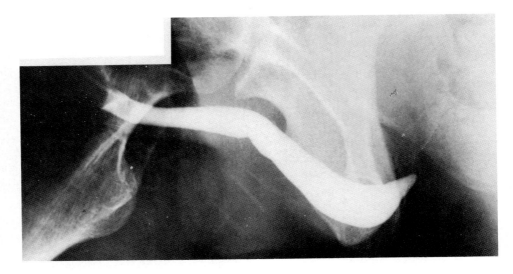

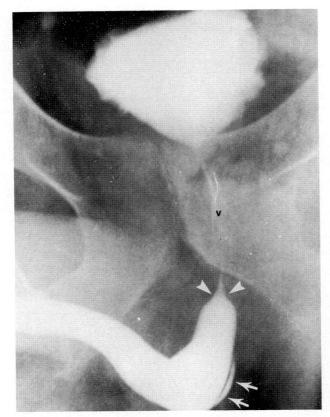

Figure 16.3. Dynamic retrograde urethrogram in upper motor neuron lesion patient with marked distal sphincter dyssynergia. Initially injection of contrast medium did not show contrast medium in the posterior urethra. Steady gentle pressure on the barrel of the syringe over a 3-minute period allowed visualization of the posterior urethra, verumontanum (v), and bladder neck. *Note:* unlike the situation in the normal human (convex cone) the cone of the proximal bulbous urethra is symmetric but concave (*arrowheads*). This is commonly seen in the retrograde study in patients with sphincter dyssynergia. Some reflux has occurred into the duct of the gland of Cowper (*arrows*) due to the spasm of the distal sphincters.

which is usually at the distal sphincters. The bladder neck opens normally to approximately 1 cm in diameter, contrast medium fills the prostatic urethra, but little or no contrast passes through the membranous urethra to the anterior urethra (Fig. 16.4). This is distal sphincter dyssynergia (Fig. 16.5). It is commonly intermittent and may

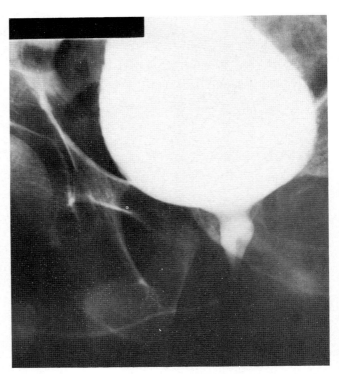

Figure 16.4. Upper motor neuron lesion voiding study after retrograde bladder filling and suprapubic tapping. The bladder neck opens and contrast medium fills the prostatic urethra. The verumontanum is visualized but detrusor distal sphincter dyssynergia allows only a trickle of contrast medium to pass into the anterior urethra.

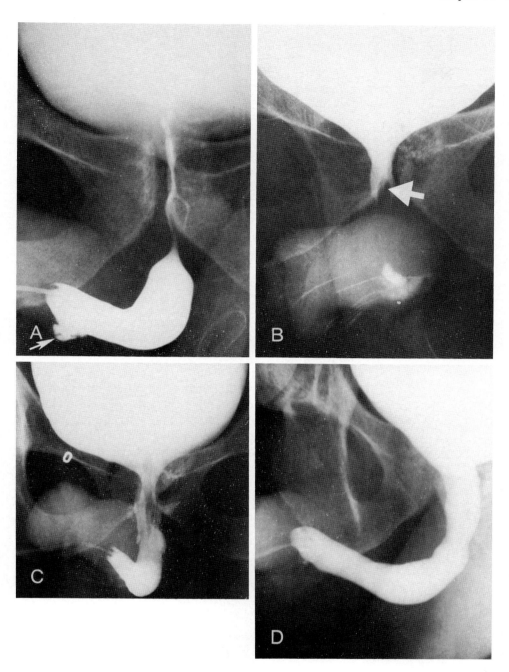

Figure 16.5.   A, Dynamic retrograde urethrogram in a patient with cord trauma at T7 causing neurogenic bladder. The retrograde study shows a small pseudodiverticulum (*arrow*) inferiorly in the distal urethra. The cone is symmetrical but concave. The verumontanum is well visualized, and contrast medium fills the bladder. **B,** Voiding cystourethrogram. The bladder is filled and suprapubic tapping stimulates detrusor contraction. The bladder neck is open and the posterior urethra fills down to the verumontanum (*arrow*). No contrast medium flows through the membranous urethra due to distal sphincter dyssynergia. **C,** Voiding cystourethrogram 1 week after sphincterectomy. The patient is voiding into the catheter and syringe. The irregularity of bulbomembranous urethra is the result of sphincterectomy. **D,** Voiding cystourethrogram three months after successful sphincterectomy. The patient voids well into the catheter and syringe. There is no obstruction due to sphincter dyssynergia.

be seen to relax, so that micturition continues (Fig. 16.6). However, when present, the dyssynergic sphincter contraction persists after voiding 100–200 ml, resulting in a significant residual urine. When distal sphincter dyssynergia has been present for some months before the procedure, posterior bladder lip hypertrophy (Fig. 16.7) may be demonstrated. Care should be taken to obtain voiding films that include the bladder neck and the whole of the urethra. Care should also be exercised to assess high-pressure reflux during the voiding study.

Cystourethrography in Quadriplegics and Patients with Cord Lesions above T5

The method of examination in quadriplegics and patients with cord lesions above T5 is the same as for paraplegics, but extra care is required because of the possibility of autonomic dysreflexia (Fig. 16.8), which is unpredictable and should be expected in such patients but does not occur to a significant degree in the majority

Figure 16.6.   A, Voiding cystourethrogram showing distal sphincter dyssynergia with complete cutoff of flow of urine through membranous urethra. **B,** Further suprapubic tapping initiates continued voiding with the patient passing contrast medium into the catheter and syringe.

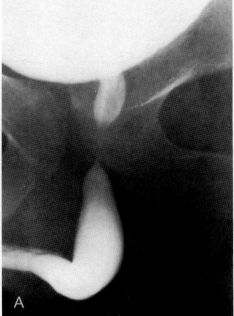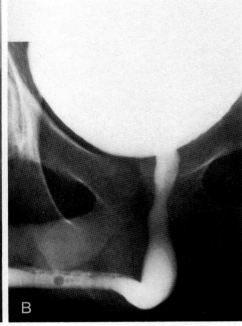

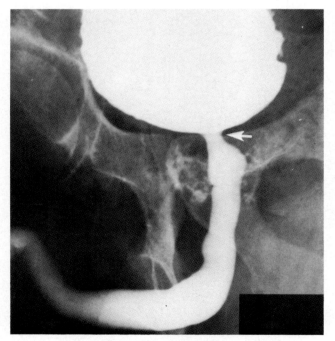

Figure 16.7.   Voiding cystourethrogram in a patient with a myelomatous mass at T7. The patient is voiding into the catheter and syringe. No sphincter dyssynergia is present during this examination. However, there is evidence of intermittent outlet obstruction as seen by the trabeculated bladder, the hypertrophied posterior bladder lip (*arrow*), and reflux into prostatic ducts. (From McCallum RW: Radiological assessment of the lower urinary tract in paraplegics—a new method. *J Can Assoc Radiol* 25:34, 1974.)

of patients having dynamic cystourethrography. Blood pressure monitoring with every 50 ml of contrast medium injected commonly elicits small blood pressure elevations, which is an indication to delay further injections for 5–15 minutes. Repeat blood pressure monitoring often results in the recording of more normal blood pressure during this delay and the examination can proceed (Fig. 16.9). If the blood pressure continues to rise the intravenous administration of a short-acting adrenergic blocker such as Regitine is usually sufficient to maintain relatively normal blood pressure, but is necessary in less than 5% of such patients. The incidence of distal sphincter dyssynergia that is sufficient to cause outlet obstruction in these patients is high and approaches 90%. It should be remembered that quadriplegic patients are managed by sterile intermittent catheterization.

Cystourethrography in Patients with Lower Motor Neuron Lesions

Patients with complete cord lesions below L2 have an interrupted micturition reflex arc and detrusor areflexia. Consequently detrusor contraction cannot be stimulated. Such patients produce voiding by increasing intraabdominal pressure or Crede's maneuver. The bladder neck and distal sphincters have to be forced open to obtain voiding, and voiding occurs only on continuous increase in the intraabdominal pressure.

Transrectal Sonographic Voiding Cystourethrography

Recent literature has emphasized the use of a linear array transducer inserted into the rectum to assess neuromuscular dysfunction in neurogenic bladder patients.

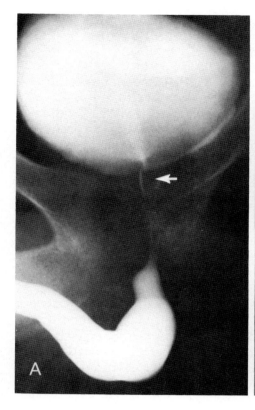

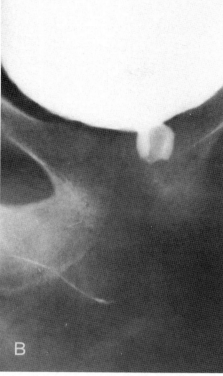

Figure 16.8. **A,** Dynamic retrograde urethrogram in a patient with cervical spine trauma. The study shows severe distal sphincter spasm sufficient to elevate the verumontanum (*arrow*) close to the bladder neck. **B,** Voiding cystourethrogram after bladder filling. Distal sphincter dyssynergia obstructs the flow of contrast medium through the membranous urethra. At the commencement of voiding the patient's face became sweaty and the blood pressure dramatically rose to 250/120 mm Hg. He complained of severe headache and required Regitine injection for blood pressure control. It was necessary to deflate the catheter balloon and advance the catheter into the bladder to drain the bladder. Repeat examination 1 week later did not produce autonomic dysreflexia.

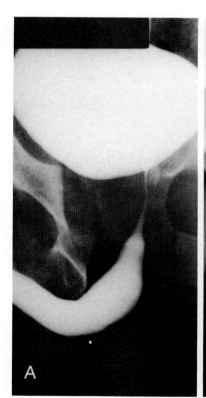

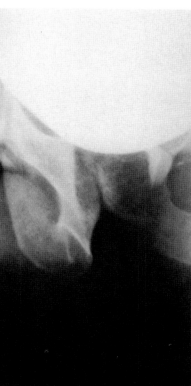

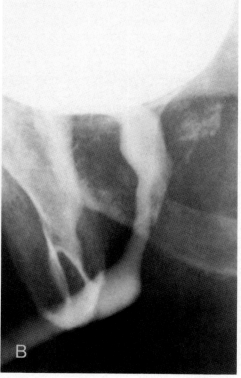

Figure 16.9. **A,** Dynamic retrograde urethrogram (on the *left*) in a patient with cervical spine trauma. Blood pressure monitoring with every 50 ml. of contrast medium injected showed blood pressure elevation from 115/76 to 120/90 mm Hg after 150 ml had been injected. The head of the table was elevated to 25° and the examination discontinued for 15 min. Blood pressure dropped to 115/80 mm Hg and the procedure continued. Voiding (on the right) occurred after the insertion of 400 ml of contrast medium with minimal blood pressure increase. **B,** Three months after successful sphincterectomy, voiding cystourethrogram shows no evidence of sphincter dyssynergia. The patient emptied his bladder completely into the catheter and syringe.

The procedure is performed at the same time as urodynamic studies. Claims that transrectal ultrasonography is more valuable than voiding cystourethrography are based on the cystourethrographic study being obtained with bladder filling via a catheter inserted into the bladder. However, no comparison has been made with transrectal ultrasonography and dynamic retrograde and voiding cystourethrography with the balloon of the catheter in the fossa navicularis. It is true that the examination obviates irradiation and that soft tissues adjacent to the urethra (prostate and seminal vesicles) can be better assessed with transrectal sonography, but it is controversial whether the information on neuromuscular dysfunction is better than dynamic retrograde and voiding cystourethrography. In addition, a bladder filling catheter and urodynamic transducers are present in the bladder and urethra during voiding if both studies are done simultaneously. The presence of the transrectal transducer and the urodynamic equipment are foreign objects in the area to be assessed and may affect the patient's pathophysiologic state. The transrectal sonographic study with combined urodynamic study is a time-consuming examination, unlike dynamic cystourethrography which usually takes only 15–20 minutes. The patient can be protected against irradiation with a lead testicular protector, which does not interfere with the retrograde and voiding films obtained. Bladder filling from a catheter inserted into the fossa navicularis and stimulation of the micturition reflex arc to produce voiding are more in keeping with the patient's pathophysiologic condition. A clear, concise radiographic record is obtained which can be compared with postoperative studies. In neurogenic bladder examination it should be emphasized that in dynamic retrograde and voiding cystourethrography the catheter and syringe are left in place during voiding and that the patient voids into the syringe in the operator's hand. When the syringe is filled by voiding the catheter is clamped and the syringe disconnected and emptied. Reconnection of the syringe to the catheter almost invariably shows continued voiding into the syringe.

The recent availability of linear array transducers for transurethral ultrasound (US) may indeed provide valuable information on neurovascular dysfunction (Figs. 16.10–16.12) but the equipment is expensive and may not readily be available in many centers providing radiologic assessment of lower urinary tract neuromuscular dysfunction.

Radionuclide studies in patients with neurogenic bladder are important in the assessment of renal damage due to reflux nephropathy or ureteric obstruction. Abnormal isotope renograms are not uncommon in patients with neurogenic bladder. Up to 70% of these patients have excretion delays within a few months after spinal cord injury. This situation has been shown to occur early, commonly due to obstruction at the ureterovesicle junction. Although excretory urography may show renal abnormalities as early as 5 months after spinal cord injury, the radionuclide study may show this abnormality sooner.

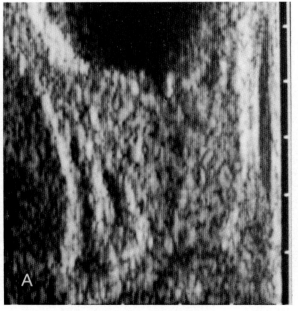
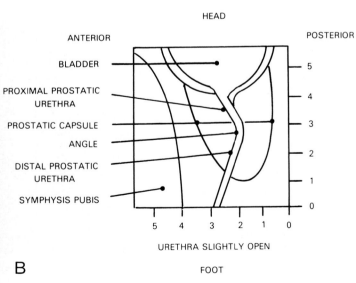

Figure 16.10.   A, Transrectal ultrasonography in a patient voiding normally. **B,** Diagrammatic representation of the visualized structures in (A). A small quantity of urine is seen in the prostatic and membranous urethra. The prostate and capsule are well visualized. (From Friedland GW, Perkash I. Neuromuscular dysfunction of the bladder and urethra. *Semin Roentgenol* 18:255, 1983.)

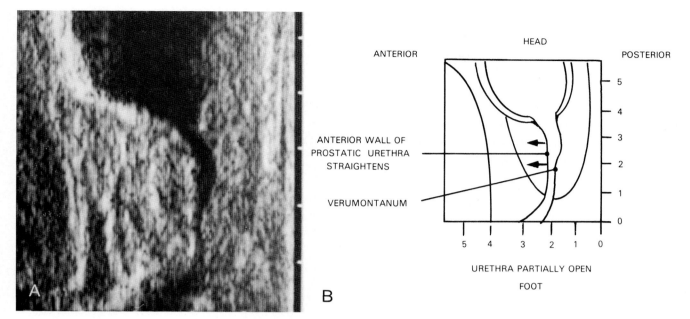

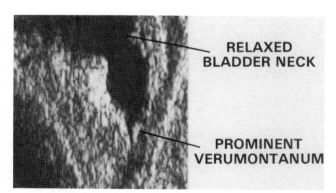

Figure 16.11.   A, Transrectal ultrasonography showing normal voiding. The posterior urethra, verumontanum, and proximal bulbous urethra are well visualized. **B,** Diagrammatic representation of the visualized structures in (A). (From Friedland GW, Perkash I. Neuromuscular dysfunction of the bladder and urethra. *Semin Roentgenol* 18:255, 1983.)

MANAGEMENT

The leading cause of death in patients with neurogenic bladder is urinary tract complications, mainly renal damage from outlet obstruction or vesicoureteral-renal reflux. The aim in management of these patients is to maintain normal renal function, an acceptable residual urine, and if possible urinary continence. Great progress in management has been made in the past decade and the incidence of the well-recognized Christmas tree bladder, vesicoureteral reflux, and renal damage has markedly reduced.

Figure 16.12. Transrectal ultrasonography in a patient with upper motor neuron lesion. The bladder neck is open. The prostatic urethra is visualized to the verumontanum. No urine is visualized distal to the verumontanum showing sphincter dyssynergia. (From Friedland GW, Perkash I. Neuromuscular dysfunction of the bladder and urethra. *Semin Roentgenol* 18:255, 1983.)

The initial reaction of spinal trauma patients with upper motor neuron lesions is spinal shock, in which the micturition reflex arc does not function although it is intact. Initial management therefore is to maintain bladder emptying. Since spinal shock may last up to 3 months, continuous catheter drainage is not recommended, since it may lead to bladder infection or urethral stricture. Sterile intermittent catheterization is used until the period of spinal shock subsides. Following this and the return of an active micturition reflex arc, the patient is bladder trained. Fluid intake is standardized and the patient is trained to stimulate detrusor contraction at timed intervals, by suprapubic tapping and increased intraabdominal pressure. It may be necessary to continue intermittent catheterization for some time, and this is used to estimate residual urine. The majority of upper motor neuron paraplegics are able to maintain an acceptable residual urine by this regimen. Approximately 30% of these patients have an unacceptable residual urine, either because they do not follow the regimen, they have sphincter dyssynergia, or they have developed a urethral stricture causing outlet obstruction. Further investigation of these patients is required, and includes full urodynamic and radiologic evaluation before the commencement of further treatment. Hyperreflexic bladder contractions alone may produce incontinence. These may be treated with anticholinergic drugs. Hyperreflexic bladder activity not controlled by anticholinergic drugs may require a surgical procedure to inhibit or obliterate the micturition reflex arc, such as dorsal root ganglionectomy. Sphincter dyssynergia may be treated with alpha-adrenergic blockers. However, the presence of persistent marked sphincter dyssynergia usually requires surgical intervention in the form of sphincterotomy (Figs. 16.5D, 16.9B), which more commonly is done at the distal sphincters but may include bladder neck sphincterotomy.

Clean intermittent catheterization is a safe and effective method of managing neurogenic bladder dysfunction. Urodynamic and radiologic evaluation in those patients not controlled by bladder training and considered for long-term intermittent catheterization is necessary to evaluate the need for adjunctive surgical therapy in patients with high intravesicle pressure. For intermittent catheterization the bladder capacity must be adequate. When the bladder capacity is considered inadequate it may be increased by anticholinergic drugs as well as cyclic bladder filling to increase the capacity. If this fails to increase bladder capacity to an acceptable level, dorsal root ganglionectomy or augmentation cystoplasty (usually using a loop of ileum) will increase the capacity. These patients are suitable for long-term intermittent catheterization, which has been shown to be safe and effective in maintaining normal renal function and obviating the need for sphincterotomy, which may contribute to incontinence. The regimen outlined is applicable to quadriplegics and upper motor neuron paraplegics. Patients with lower motor neuron lesions have an areflexic bladder and are best treated by intermittent catheterization.

Similarly, female patients with neurogenic bladder due to spinal cord trauma with hyperreflexic bladder and sphincter dyssynergia are best treated with anticholinergic drugs and intermittent catheterization. These patients cannot be treated by sphincterotomy as it may produce urinary incontinence.

NEUROMUSCULAR ACTIVITY IN FEMALE PATIENTS WITH NEUROGENIC BLADDER

Neuromuscular activity in female patients with neurogenic bladder is identical to that of male patients. Bladder training may be successful in maintaining an acceptable residual urine. Female patients with an unacceptable residual urine are more difficult to manage. Sphincterotomy is seldom performed in female patients with sphincter dyssynergia because incontinence may result and intermittent or continuous bladder catheterization is necessary. Consequently outlet obstruction in females with neurogenic bladder is managed by bladder catheterization without surgical intervention. After sphincterotomy, male patients with incontinence are able to wear a condom draining into a urine receptacle strapped to the patient's leg. This is not possible in females.

SUGGESTED READINGS

Amis ES Jr, Blaivas JG: The role of the radiologist in evaluating voiding dysfunction. *Radiology* 175:317, 1990.
Barbaric Z: Autonomic dysreflexia in patients with spinal cord lesions. Complication of voiding cystourethrography and ileal loopography. *AJR* 127:293, 1976.
Bors E, Comarr AE: *Neurologic Urology.* Baltimore, University Park Press, 1971.
Friedland GW, Perkash I: Neuromuscular dysfunction of the bladder and urethra. *Semin Roentgenol* 18:255, 1983.
McCallum RW: Radiological assessment of the lower urinary tract in paraplegics—a new method. *J Can Assoc Radiol* 25:34, 1974.
McLellan FC: *The Neurogenic Bladder* Springfield, IL, C C Thomas, 1939.
Perkash I: Detrusor—sphincter dyssynergia and dyssynergic responses: recognition and rationale for early modified transurethral sphincterotomy in complete spinal cord injury lesions. *J Urol* 120:778, 1978.
Rossier AB, Fam BA: 5-microtransducer catheter evaluation of neurogenic bladder function. *Urology* 27:371, 1986.
Tempkin A, Sullivan G, Paldi J, et al: Radioisotope renography in spinal cord injury. *J Urol* 133:228, 1985.

CHAPTER 17

PROSTATE AND SEMINAL VESICLES

PROSTATE

Prostatic Hypertrophy

The term *prostatic hypertrophy* describes hypertrophy and hyperplasia of inner periurethral glands (transitional zone of McNeal), which are only present above the verumontanum. The term *median lobe hypertrophy* refers to hypertrophy and hyperplasia of the inner periurethral glands posterior to the supracollicular prostatic urethra above the verumontanum, in the midline adjacent to the bladder neck. Similarly, lateral lobe hypertrophy arises from inner periurethral glands above the verumontanum adjacent to the supracollicular prostatic urethra extending laterally to indent the bladder base.

Etiology

Several factors influence the development of prostatic hypertrophy. Pituitary gonadotrophin stimulates the production of testosterone from the testes. Testosterone appears to stimulate prostatic growth, since eunuchs never develop prostatic hypertrophy and testosterone causes an increase in the size of the prostate of castrated patients. Estrogen administered to the uncastrated male causes prostatic atrophy. Outlet obstruction due to prostatic hypertrophy in poor risk operative patients, is improved in 50% of cases by the administration of progesterone. Against these recognized facts is the paradox that prostatic hypertrophy is associated with aging, gonadal involution, and consequently a reduction in the production of testosterone.

Incidence

The prostate usually maintains normal size and weight until the age of 40 years. Less than 10% of the male population between the ages of 30 and 40 years have clinical prostatic hypertrophy. After the age of 50 years, 50% of men have some degree of prostatic hypertrophy. The prostate may double in size before the age of 70 years. Up to 80% of men will have prostatic hypertrophy but only 10% require surgical intervention.

Pathology

Prostatic hypertrophy may be diffuse enlargement of the stromal and glandular elements in the transitional zone and periurethral glandular tissue but more commonly consists of nodular enlargement. Nodules may be stromal without glandular tissue. These nodules consist of vascular fibrous tissue and arise in the transitional zone. Similarly stromal nodules may consist of fibromuscular tissue and are prone to infarction and infiltration with plasma cells and histiocytes. Both types of stromal nodules may be incorporated in adenomatous hyperplasia. Fibroadenomas and myoadenomas are the most common and may attain a large size extending above the pubis causing interference with the function of the internal sphincter (Fig. 17.1), creating a large residual volume, and elevating the bladder base (Fig. 17.2). Such nodules commonly have areas of hemorrhage, infarction, and calcification.

Clinical Presentation

The clinical presentation depends on the site and size of the nodules. Even small nodules projecting into the prostatic urethra may cause stream reduction and eventual outlet obstruction. Nodules projecting into the bladder neck may interfere with the internal sphincter function resulting in mild dribbling at the end of micturition. Large nodules may reduce internal sphincter function and displace the verumontanum and distal sphincters dis-

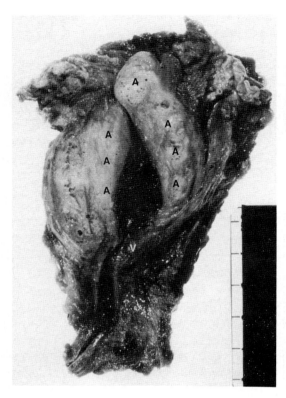

Figure 17.1. Gross specimen showing multiple adenomata (A). They project into the bladder neck and interfere with the normal function of the internal sphincter. In addition, the adenomata are all above the verumontanum (V), which is pushed inferiorly.

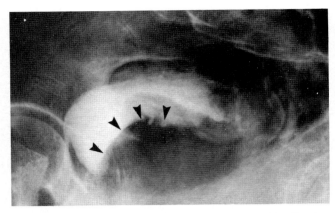

Figure 17.3. Oblique film from excretory urogram showing bladder base indentation (*arrowheads*) by prostatic adenoma.

tally so that stress incontinence occurs. Nodules arising laterally generally are asymptomatic until a large size is attained and difficulty in micturition occurs. The initial symptom is most commonly a reduction in force of the urine stream. Nocturia is common and is associated with a feeling of necessity to continue voiding even after void-

ing has ceased. Difficulty in initiating urination may have been present for some time before the patient seeks medical advice. Urinary retention may be of gradual onset or may occur suddenly. Although sudden acute retention is an indication for surgery, 50% of patients with acute retention are relieved by catheter drainage and may pass urine relatively well before requiring surgery.

Radiology

The plain film is commonly normal. Occasionally prostatic adenomata contain calculi, and these may be seen above and behind the symphysis pubis, most commonly in the midline. Excretory urography is a common method of assessing patients with prostatic hypertrophy. Films obtained after 15 minutes show the contrast-filled bladder. Supine, oblique (Fig. 17.3), and upright films identify the effects of prostatic hypertrophy on the bladder base (Fig. 17.4) and the postvoid film can give a

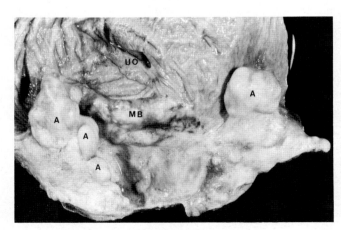

Figure 17.2. Gross specimen with the bladder open viewed from above. Multiple adenomata (A) are seen laterally. A hypertrophied ridge of prostatic tissue forms a median bar (MB) adjacent to the urethral orifice (UO).

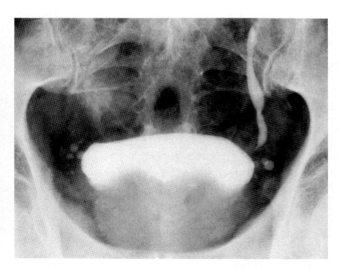

Figure 17.4. Excretory urogram showing bladder base elevation by large bilateral adenomata. The distal left ureter is slightly dilated.

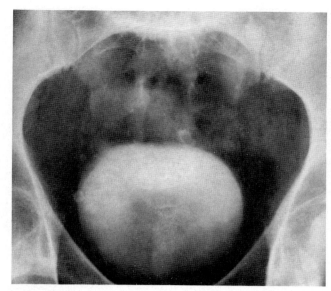

Figure 17.5.   Excretory urogram showing bladder base elevation by prostatic hypertrophy. Multiple discrete bladder stones are seen high in the bladder. These stones were only faintly visualized on the plain films.

rough estimate of residual urine. As the prostate enlarges, evidence of outlet obstruction increases. Bladder distention, distortion of the bladder base, and increased residual urine are apparent. The interureteric ridge is elevated producing the characteristic J-shaped ureters (See Chapter 15, Fig. 15.32). Ureteric dilatation may only be present

distally but commonly the pelvicalyceal system is also dilated with evidence of delayed excretion. Renal function may be impaired. The rate of contrast material excretion may be so low that the pelvicalyceal system and ureters do not become visible for 24 hours or more. In these cases, the bladder is usually markedly trabeculated, and the wall thickened due to detrusor hypertrophy. When detrusor hypertrophy cannot compensate any longer, the bladder dilates. The dilatation may be localized resulting in diverticulum formation. Large bladder diverticula result from long-standing outlet obstruction and may be larger than the bladder itself. It is occasionally difficult to say which is the bladder, and the insertion of a Foley catheter for cystography is required for clarification.

Excretory urography is frequently requested as a screening procedure in prostatic hypertrophy, mainly to exclude renal or ureteric lesions. It is questionable if this is justified since the yield for other lesions is low and the kidneys are well assessed by ultrasound. Unsuspected bladder stones resulting from long-standing, low-grade outlet obstruction by prostatic hypertrophy may be seen (Fig. 17.5). Urethrography and cystography may be helpful in a patient with some degree of outlet obstruction due to prostatic adenomata (Fig. 17.6**A,B**).

Transabdominal ultrasound of the filled bladder demonstrates indentation in the bladder contour by prostatic hypertrophy (see Chapter 15, Fig. 15.44**B**). Prostatic size, configuration, and the relationship to the bladder base

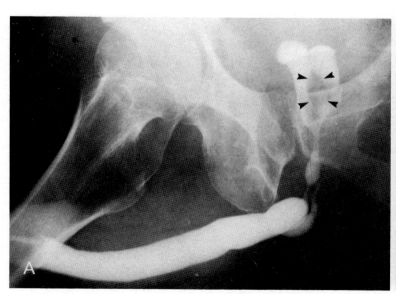

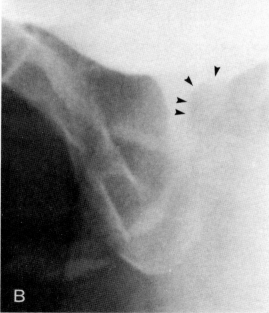

Figure 17.6.   **A,** Dynamic retrograde urethrogram in a patient with outlet obstruction. A proximal bulbous urethral stricture is present. Contrast medium flowing into the bladder passes around a filling defect close to the bladder orifice (*arrowheads*). (Modified from McCallum RW, Colapinto V: *Urological* *Radiology of the Adult Male Lower Urinary Tract.* Springfield, IL, Charles C. Thomas, 1976, p 202.) **B,** Voiding cystourethrogram showing the filling defect on the retrograde study represents a prostatic adenoma arising in the region of the median lobe (*arrowheads*).

can be assessed. Transverse and longitudinal scans are capable of delineating focal nodular bulging into the bladder base and bladder neck if the nodules are large enough. Small nodules capable of producing obstructive symptoms by projecting into the prostatic urethra may not be delineated. Prostatic calcifications may be identified as bright spots producing acoustic shadowing (Fig. 17.7). Although commonly associated with prostatic hypertrophy nodules, calcification may result from prostatitis or be idiopathic. Pelvicalyceal and ureteric dilatation are readily identified with ultrasound. Bladder diverticula, bladder trabeculation, and bladder wall thickening can also be assessed.

There has been a shift of emphasis to transrectal ultrasound because of better definition of prostatic lesions and the advent of transurethral balloon dilatation for prostatic hypertrophy. Transrectal ultrasound provides excellent definition of the internal glandular structure and prostatic adenomata arising in the transitional zone and periurethral glandular tissue are well visualized (Fig. 17.8). The transitional zone and periurethral glandular tissue is normally coarser and slightly less echogenic than the central and peripheral zones. Adenomata arising from the transitional zone vary in echogenicity but are more commonly hypoechoic or mixed echogenicity. Rarely they are isoechoic but the transitional zone usually shows clear demarcation from the central and peripheral zone. Transitional zone nodules commonly have a well-defined hypoechoic halo. Clear definition of the halo can be seen on both transverse (Fig. 17.9) and longitudinal views but is usually better seen on the transverse view. Longitudinal views give a better assessment of nodular

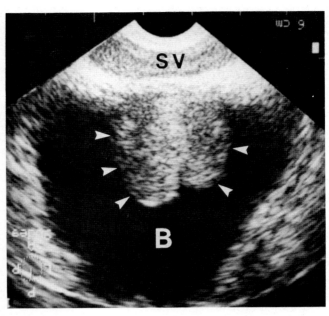

Figure 17.8. Transrectal ultrasound showing a urine-filled bladder (B) and a large bilobed adenoma (*arrowheads*) projecting into the bladder. The seminal vesicles (SV) are visualized posteriorly.

projection into the bladder base and bladder neck. Calcifications within adenomata produce acoustic shadowing (Fig. 17.9) and, if extensive, may make the appearance of the adenoma mainly hypoechoic. Digital rectal examination may reveal a stony hard nodule that suggests the possibility of carcinoma of the prostate. However, adeno-

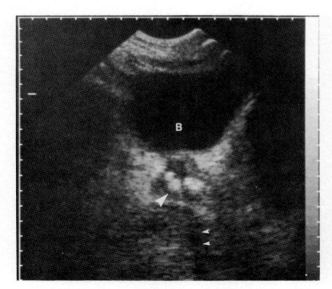

Figure 17.7. Transabdominal ultrasound showing the urine filled bladder (B) and the prostate posteriorly, containing several calcifications (*arrowhead*) producing acoustic shadowing (*small arrowheads*). (From Pollack HM (ed): *Clinical Urography*, Philadelphia, WB Saunders, 1989, p 1911.)

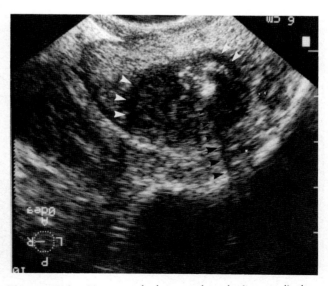

Figure 17.9. Transrectal ultrasound study (inverted) showing a mixed coarsely echogenic lesion clearly demarcated from the peripheral zone by a hypoechoic rim or halo (*arrowhead*) which usually indicates benign adenomatous formation. Acoustic shadowing (*black arrowheads*) is seen behind marked calcification.

mata containing calcification may be multiple and extend posteriorly and laterally compressing the central and peripheral zones. Transrectal ultrasound in such a case is likely to show the coarse echogenicity and halo appearance adjacent to the prostatic capsule or may even bulge the capsule, accounting for the hard palpable nodule felt digitally. Biopsy may be required to distinguish this from carcinoma. There may be only a generalized increase in size of the prostate without clearly defined nodules. The echogenicity is, however, coarser, and there may be areas of mixed, hypo-, and hyperechogenicity.

Computed tomography (CT) and magnetic resonance imaging (MRI) are both effective methods of assessing the effects of the hypertrophied prostate on the bladder but are not usually indicated. No assessment of the internal architecture can be made with CT, and to date no definite value of MRI over ultrasound has been clearly elicited in prostatic hypertrophy.

Prostatic Carcinoma

Incidence

Prostatic carcinoma is the second most common malignancy after bronchogenic carcinoma. The incidence is approximately 70 cases per 100,000 males per year. The disease is rare below the age of 40 years but increases with age. Prostatic carcinoma accounts for approximately 10% of cancer deaths in men. Significant geographic and racial differences in the incidence of prostatic carcinoma are reported. The incidence of clinical carcinoma is low in China, Japan, Hispanic areas, Israel, Latin and South America, and in American Indians. The incidence is high in North America and Northern Europe. North American blacks have an incidence approximately twice that of white Americans. However, the incidence of occult carcinoma is uniform throughout the world. The geographic incidence may be influenced by the lack of epidemiologic studies in low-incidence countries and by the lack of documentation of prostatic carcinoma.

Etiology

Etiologically, prostatic carcinoma, like prostatic hypertrophy, has been shown to be androgen dependent. Castrated males do not develop prostatic carcinoma. Marital status, sexual practices, occupation, dietary habits, socioeconomic status, tobacco consumption, and viral and bacterial infection have all been extensively investigated. No definite relationship has been shown to prostatic carcinoma by these investigations, but there appears to be a familial tendency.

Pathology

Pathologic investigation has shown that over 95% of prostatic carcinomas are adenocarcinomas, which originate in the epithelium of prostatic acini in the outer or peripheral zone of the prostate. Less commonly adenocarcinoma may arise from ductal epithelium, which may also undergo metaplasia to transitional cells and produce transitional cell carcinoma. Rarely mesenchymal tissue within the prostatic stroma become malignant producing rhabdomyosarcoma, leiomyosarcoma, or fibrosarcoma.

Grading of prostatic carcinoma is a histologic evaluation of tissue for glandular pattern, size, and distribution. The margins of tumor and stromal invasion are also evaluated. Gland pattern size and distribution involves an assessment of the definition of the cell border, the cell shape, smooth or ragged aggregates of cells, central necrosis, and the degree of cellular differentiation or dedifferentiation. The margins of tumor are examined for clearly or poorly defined edge of tumor cell aggregates, and stromal invasion is an assessment of tumor glandular cells between stromal planes or destruction of stromal tissue.

There are several grading systems in use. These are the Gleason, the M.D. Anderson, the Mostofi, the Gaeta, and the Mayo Clinic Systems. All systems vary slightly in grading numbers between 1 and 5. Grade 1 tumors in all systems are mild well-differentiated tumors, whereas Grades 3, 4 or 5 refer to anaplastic or severe lesions, depending on the grading system used. The lower the grade number the better differentiated is the tumor. The higher the grade, the less differentiation is present.

Staging

The Whitmore Jewett staging method is the most commonly used in North America. Stage A carcinoma has no clinical manifestations and is not suspected. It is incidentally found in pathology specimens of patients who have had prostatectomy for prostatic hypertrophy. Approximately 10% of all prostatic hypertrophy surgical specimens show the histologic presence of prostatic carcinoma. It is also found incidentally in autopsy specimens, with a frequency which increases with age. The natural history of stage A prostatic carcinoma is not clearly defined. It is generally accepted that well-differentiated carcinoma found in infrequent fields of surgical specimens is not a lethal disease. Most Stage A carcinomas fall into this category. Stage A_1 carcinoma is entirely within the substance on one side of the peripheral zone and does not bulge or break the capsule. Stage A_2 extensively involves the peripheral zone but does not invade through the capsule.

Stage B is a clinically palpable, stony hard nodule in the peripheral zone approximately 1 cm or less in size, without evidence of local or distant extension and without the development of urinary symptoms. Stage B_1 is palpable but has not invaded through the capsule. Stage B_2 is more extensive than Stage B_1 invading much of the prostate but does not invade through the capsule.

Stage C carcinomas invade the capsule and are usually

symptomatic. Digital rectal examination reveals a stony hard peripheral zone extending to the seminal vesicles. At least 50% of stage C carcinoma patients have metastases to the pelvic lymph nodes.

Stage D patients have urinary symptoms, soft tissue tumor extension, bony and lung metastasis, and hydronephrosis due to ureteric obstruction by carcinoma at the ureterovesical junction. Digital rectal examination usually reveals a diffusely hard nodular prostate, but occasionally only a single hard nodule is felt. Rarely the prostate feels entirely normal. The digital rectal examination may be initiated by evidence of bone or lung metastases.

The TNM staging method is more decisive and has been adopted by the American Joint Commission on Cancer, Staging, and End Results Reporting. T refers to tumor stage, N to node involvement, and M to distant metastases. A recently revised TNM staging system considers diagnostic imaging in the staging system. T categories are assessed by digital rectal examination, the N category is assessed by histology and or imaging studies, and the M category by imaging studies and several acid phosphatase studies. TA designates normal digital examination corresponding to Whitmore Jewett stage A. TA_1 is when less than 5% of the surgical specimen is histologically tumor and of low or medium grade. TA_2 is when more than 5% of the surgical specimen is tumor of high histologic grade. TB is a digitally palpable hard nodule not through the capsule. TB_1 is tumor less than one half of one lobe in size. TB_2 indicates tumor involving one lobe. TB_3 designates multiple tumors or tumor greater than one lobe. TC tumor is palpable and extends through the capsule. TC_1 indicates unilateral extension, while TC_2 indicates bilateral extension. TC_3 refers to extension involving the bladder base or rectum, or levator ani muscles or pelvic side walls.

The N category, i.e., the lymph node status, involves histologic (H) and imaging examinations (C). Thus NO (C&H) refers to no regional metastases. $N_1(H)$ indicates a microscopic regional node metastasis. N_2 (C&H) refers to gross regional node metastases and N_3 (C&H) refers to extraregional node metastases (inguinal, paraaortic, etc.).

The M category describes visceral (V) or bone (B) metastatic lesions. MO designates no evidence of metastases. M_1 designates at least three elevated acid phosphatase levels on separate occasions. M_2 (V&B) designates visceral or bone metastases.

Combined grading and staging assessment generally correlates well with the patient's risk of dying of prostatic cancer. Thus Grade 1 is commonly found in Stage A_1 carcinomas. Grades 3, 4, or 5 are commonly found in Stage C carcinomas. Undifferentiated carcinomas behave more aggressively than well-differentiated carcinomas and usually have a higher stage. However, there are exceptions to this. Stage B_1 lesions have a better prognosis than Stage A_2 lesions since only 25% of Stage A_2 lesions

are well differentiated whereas 85% of Stage B_1 lesions are well differentiated. Recent reports indicate that the incidence of diagnosis of Stage A carcinomas is increasing. In 1967, the Veterans Administration Cooperative Urological Research Group (VACURG) reported that only 6% of prostatic cancers were diagnosed as Stage A. Recent reports suggest that up to 50% of prostatic carcinomas are currently diagnosed as Stage A. In addition, only 2% of Stage A_1 carcinomas were found to have histologic evidence of regional node metastases and 23% of Stage A_2 carcinomas had similar histologic evidence. Such findings obviously alter the staging of prostatic carcinoma from Stage A to Stage C. Pathologically, carcinoma of the prostate is a combined report of stage and Gleason's grading.

Biochemical Studies

Biochemical studies may be helpful in assessing prostatic carcinoma. The serum acid phosphatase (SAP) is elevated in 60% of patients with Stage C and D carcinoma and in 80% of patients with bone metastases. Estimation of the prostatic fraction of SAP is more precise for prostatic carcinoma, since the SAP may be elevated in other conditions such as multiple myeloma, leukemia, and pancreatic carcinoma. Immunohistochemical techniques have been developed for detection of prostatic-specific antigen. It should be emphasized that although Paget's disease may slightly elevate the SAP, the serum alkaline phosphatase is significantly elevated in Paget's disease and not elevated in prostatic carcinoma.

Dissemination

Carcinoma of the prostate originates in the peripheral zone closer to the prostatic capsule than to the urethra. Capsular invasion opens a route to perineural lymphatics and to the periprostatic venous plexus allowing distant metastases to the lungs and axial skeleton. Spread of prostatic carcinoma occurs by three methods, local, lymphatic, and hematogenous.

Local spread is to the seminal vesicles, the urethra, the bladder neck, the bladder base, and the interureteric ridge, causing ureteric obstruction that occurs in over 10% of patients. Rarely prostatic carcinoma spreads posteriorly and superiorly to invade Denonvilliers' fascia. It then spreads between the two layers of this fascia and may encircle the rectosigmoid colon causing bowel obstruction. Rarely invasion occurs into the rectum producing an ulcerating lesion that is extremely difficult to distinguish clinically from rectal carcinoma. Late local spread to the corpus cavernosa, corpus spongiosum, and scrotum has been reported.

Lymphatic spread is initially from lymphatics within the prostate to the pelvic lymph nodes, which are usually dissected for histologic examination at the time of total prostatectomy. There is a high incidence of pelvic node metastases in carcinoma of the prostate. The pelvic lymph nodes include the obturator nodes, the hypogastric lymph nodes, and the presacral, presciatic, and external iliac lymph nodes. The obturator nodes are most commonly involved. Lymphatic spread beyond the pelvic nodes is rare, but the common iliac, inguinal, paraaortic, mediastinal, and supraclavicular nodes may be involved. Spread from the mediastinal nodes into lung lymphatics resulting in lymphangitic carcinomatosis has been reported. It is therefore important to include prostatic carcinoma in the differential diagnosis of lymphangitic carcinomatosis in males, since prostatic carcinoma may not be suspected clinically and it is the only lymphangitic carcinomatosis amenable to treatment with a hopeful prognosis, unlike other causes of lymphangitic carcinomatosis.

In autopsy cases up to 20% have pathologic evidence of pulmonary lymphangitic carcinomatosis, but only 5% of these cases were detected radiologically. Lymphangitic carcinomatosis results in progressive dyspnea and cor pulmonale and is commonly the result of carcinoma of the lung, stomach, breast, or pancreas. All have a very poor prognosis. It is to be emphasized that a male patient with this presentation should be investigated for carcinoma of the prostate since the condition and prognosis can be improved with estrogen therapy.

Hematogenous spread is to the axial skeleton or lungs. Eighty-five percent of patients dying of prostatic carcinoma exhibit bony metastases in the axial skeleton. Sites of skeletal metastases are the lumbar spine, proximal femur, bony pelvis, thoracic spine, ribs, sternum, skull, and proximal humerus in order of decreasing frequency. The route of hematogenous spread is via the intervertebral venous plexus (Batson's plexus), which is a low-pressure valveless venous system. Increasing intraabdominal pressure such as in coughing or straining increases the venous blood flow in the intervertebral venous plexus and may cause reversal of flow in ribs, pelvic girdle, and shoulder girdles. During increased intraabdominal pressure, tumor cells may be deposited in these regions due to reversal of flow. Over 90% of prostatic metastatic lesions to bone are blastic, and mixed osteolytic-osteoblastic lesions account for most of the remainder. Less than 1% of prostatic bone metastases are lytic alone.

Capsular invasion opens the hematogenous route for metastatic disease via the periprostatic venous plexus, which communicates with the pudendal and vesical venous plexuses. Drainage progresses through the veins to the lungs. Reduction of flow in the inferior vena cava, as occurs in increased intraabdominal pressure, produces increased flow to the intervertebral venous plexus resulting in reversal of flow and bony metastases to the axial skeleton. Metastases to bones below the level of the prostate, i.e., ischia and femora, likely result from malignant shunts with arterial metastases. Brain metastases from carcinoma of the prostate have been reported without lung metastases, which implies arterial embolization. This may occur in the presence of a cardiac right to left shunt. When lung metastases are present, it is possible that microscopic lesions may enter the pulmonary veins returning to the left heart and thus arterial embolization, but this is a rare form of tumor embolization.

Clinical Presentation

Prostatic carcinoma does not produce symptoms until significant local spread has occurred. Up to 25% of patients presenting with urinary retention have prostatic carcinoma, but the urinary retention may be solely the result of prostatic hypertrophy and the carcinoma is a histologic coincidental finding. When the carcinoma has attained sufficient bulk, dysuria, slow urinary stream, dribbling, and some degree of outlet obstruction are the presenting symptoms. Hematuria and rectal or perineal pain are less common symptoms. More commonly metastases cause bone pain, weight loss, and anemia. Digital rectal examination of the normal prostate reveals a consistency similar to the tip of the nose. Carcinoma of the prostate results in induration and the palpation of a stony hard nodule if localized, or if generalized, a uniform stony hardness. The normal seminal vesicles are soft and difficult to recognize with digital palpation. Palpation of firmness or hardness in the seminal vesicles are indicative of spread of carcinoma.

It is generally accepted that carcinoma of the prostate occurs most commonly in the posterior lobe. However, localized prostatic carcinoma has been reported in the lateral lobes in 50% of autopsy cases. Digital rectal examination can readily feel a hard nodule in the posterior lobe but palpation of a lateral lobe nodule may be more difficult. Digital rectal examination reveals only 60–80% of prostatic carcinomas.

Clinical Diagnosis

The preferred method of diagnosis of a suspicious nodule is by core needle biopsy. Using a Tru-cut or Vim-Silverman needle, biopsy routes include the transperineal or transrectal route. Recently the use of a mechanical, spring loaded, biopsy instrument has gained widespread popularity. Transperineal biopsy is more painful and cumbersome. Transrectal biopsy is associated with a higher incidence of sepsis and bleeding. After transrectal biopsy, blood cultures are positive in 85% of patients unless prophylactic antibiotics are administered. Less than 10% of transrectal biopsies result in urinary tract infection when prophylactic antibiotics are given. In transperineal biopsy the incidence of infection is almost negligible. Since the advent of transrectal ultrasound there has been a shift toward transrectal biopsy done with ultrasound guidance. Both techniques are falsely negative in approximately 10% of cases.

Fine-needle aspiration of the prostate may also be useful. A 20 or 22-gauge fine aspiration needle is inserted into the prostate substance and suction applied as the tip of the needle is moved back and forth. The smeared aspirate may be fixed in alcohol and Papanicolaou stained. False-negative results can be as high as 30% in patients with prostatic carcinoma proven by perineal biopsy.

Radiology

Plain film examination is not helpful unless metastatic lesions are present, but a radionuclide bone scan followed by plain film radiographs of suspicious areas should be obtained when carcinoma of the prostate is diagnosed. Most metastatic bone lesions are seen in the thoracolumbar spine, pelvis, and ribs, and the vast majority (90%) are blastic (Fig. 17.10). The remainder are mixed blastic and lytic. Approximately 1% are bone destructive and lytic, but may produce periosteal new bone. Metastatic bone lesions are discrete dense areas varying in size from a few millimeters to several centimeters. Solitary small discrete blastic lesions may represent bone islands, but in the presence of known prostatic carcinoma, follow-up examination is required. Metastatic lesions are commonly adjacent to joint surfaces such as the sacroiliac joints and hip joints but do not affect the joint space. Difficulty may be experienced when a metastatic lesion abuts a joint affected by degenerative or inflammatory change. Blastic lesions have a well-demarcated edge as opposed to degenerative sclerosis, which is more diffuse. Blastic metastases in pedicles may be obscured by

degenerative arthritic change in the apophyseal joints in the lumbar spine and extraoblique lumbar spine views may be necessary for clarification. Blastic metastatic lesions in the vertebral bodies typically lie adjacent to the vertebral body cortex but may increase in size to involve the complete vertebral body resulting in a sclerotic vertebra. Unlike Paget's disease, the sclerotic vertebra is not enlarged in carcinoma of the prostate. Bone biopsy may be required to distinguish prostatic carcinoma from lymphoma although lymphoma more commonly occurs in a younger age group. Multiple bone islands and osteopoikilosis are small discrete bone densities that never change in size or density, unlike blastic metastases, which are less discrete and increase in size without therapy.

Osteoblastic-osteolytic lesions may be produced by both carcinoma of the prostate and by Paget's disease. Paget's disease generally produces cortical thickening, coarse trabeculation, and an increase in the size of the affected bone. The lytic lesions in Paget's disease are well demarcated. Areas of reparation become blastic leading to the mixed blastic and lytic appearance. Although the appearance of metastases from carcinoma of the prostate and Paget's disease are similar, there are distinguishing features. Difficulty with this differentiation can be clarified by assessing the SAP and serum alkaline phosphatase. The latter is markedly elevated in Paget's disease, whereas the acid phosphatate is not. The reverse is true in carcinoma of the prostate with metastases.

Generalized increase in bone density may be due to carcinoma of the prostate. The spine, pelvis, ribs, and shoulders may show a generalized increase in bone density (Fig. 17.11). If a generalized increase in bone density is seen without a diagnosis of carcinoma of the prostate, a differential diagnosis of carcinoma of the prostate, myelosclerosis, urticaria pigmentosa, and fluorine poisoning must be entertained. Urticaria pigmentosa producing generalized increased bone density is associated with multiple pigmented skin nodules. Myelosclerosis invariably is associated with splenomegaly and cardiomegaly. Fluorine poisoning occurs in geographic areas where the water content of fluorine is high and in occupations producing fertilizer, or in the smelting of metals. Generalized increased bone density is present, but the trabeculae are coarsened, the cortex is thickened, and ligamentous calcification is common. None of these features of myelosclerosis, urticaria pigmentosa, or fluorine poisoning is seen in generalized increased bone density due to carcinoma of the prostate. The chest examination may be normal, but a careful search for small nodular lesions and increased interstitial lung markings is mandatory. Hematogenous nodules in the lungs may vary in size from a few millimeters to several centimeters. Lymphangitic spread may be recognized as hilar node enlargement and increased interstitial lung markings, particularly Kerley A and B lines. Kerley A lines are several

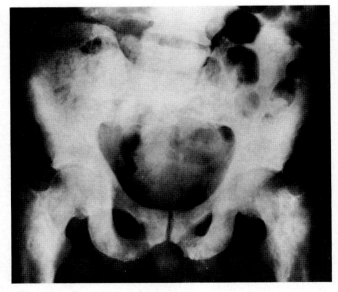

Figure 17.10.   Plain film of the pelvis in Stage D carcinoma of prostate. Multiple blastic lesions are present in the pelvis and femora.

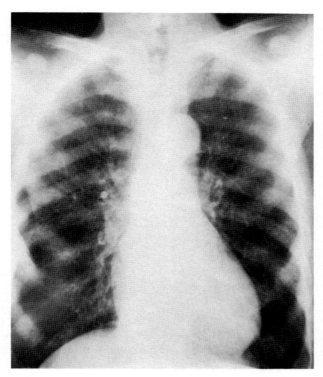

Figure 17.11. Generalized increased bone density in the ribs and shoulder girdle in carcinoma of the prostate. (From McCallum RW, Colapinto V: *Urological Radiology of the Adult Male Lower Urinary Tract.* Springfield, IL, Charles C. Thomas, 1976, p 236.)

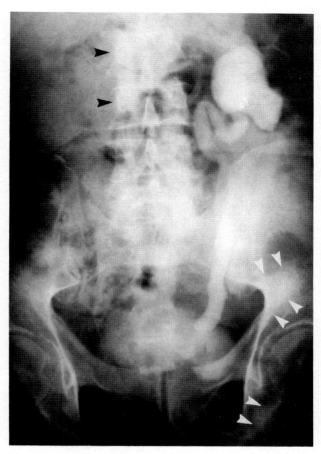

Figure 17.12. Excretory urogram in a patient with carcinoma of the prostate and well demarcated bone metastases (*white arrowheads*). Blastic pedicles are also seen (*black arrowheads*). Carcinoma of the prostate has spread locally to involve the interureteric ridge completely obstructing the right ureter and causing marked pelvicalyceal and ureteric dilatation on the left.

centimeters long extending from the hila into the lungs. Kerley B lines are short, extending to the lung periphery in the costophrenic angles. There may be small effusions obliterating the costophrenic angles.

Excretory urography may be performed as a screening procedure in carcinoma of the prostate but is more important in the assessment of the urinary tract in outlet obstruction (Fig. 17.12). Rarely carcinoma of the prostate is seen with a marked degree of outlet obstruction. More commonly there is clinical evidence of mild outlet obstruction, but if the carcinoma has locally invaded the seminal vesicles and bladder base, the degree of ureteric obstruction may be severe enough to cause pelvicalyceal dilatation and a significant delay in excretion. It may eventually progress to renal failure. This may require intervention with urinary diversion and the insertion of stents if possible, or percutaneous nephrostomy drainage. Bladder distention, trabeculation, and sacculation result from coexisting prostatic hypertrophy.

Cystourethrography is seldom necessary in carcinoma of the prostate. It may be indicated in outlet obstruction, to distinguish a possible urethral stricture causing obstruction, from carcinoma invading the bladder neck and prostatic urethra. If no stricture is present, the posterior urethra and bladder neck should be carefully assessed

for nodular projections in this region, but benign and malignant nodules cannot be distinguished.

When Stage C or D carcinoma of the prostate is present, the voiding study generally shows a fixed posterior urethra without the normal descent of the bladder orifice, posterior, and membranous urethra. Local spread of carcinoma of the prostate may involve the corpus spongiosum producing irregular urethral narrowing on the retrograde study, but insufficient narrowing to cause proximal urethral dilatation on voiding.

Nuclear medicine studies are valuable in the initial staging of prostatic cancer. A clinical Stage A_2 or Stage B may be restaged to Stage D when bone metastases are demonstrated by radioisotope bone scanning. It has been well demonstrated that radioisotope studies can detect bone metastases earlier than metastatic lesions are seen on skeletal surveys (Fig. 17.13). Metastatic bone lesions cause hypervascularity, and the radioisotope reveals an

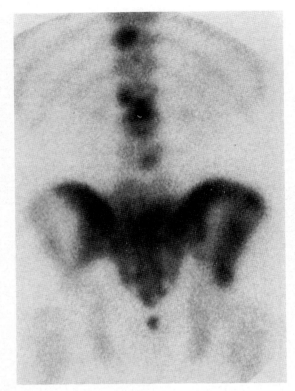

Figure 17.13. Bone metastases. A radionuclide bone scan with ^{99m}Tc-medronate demonstrates metastases to the pelvis and lumbar spine.

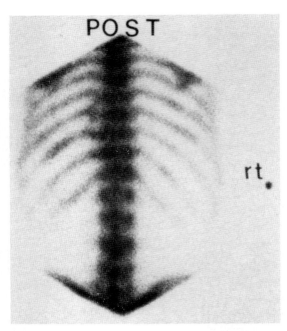

Figure 17.14. Bone metastases. Occasionally, diffuse blastic metastases have such avid radionuclide uptake that no tracer activity is seen in the kidneys.

area of increased activity before bone is replaced by the metastatic lesion. In some patients, blastic metastases take up so much of the radionuclide that no tracer activity is seen in the kidneys (Fig. 17.14). This is referred to as a "superscan." Areas of increased radionuclide uptake are seen in any condition producing hypervascularity, such as arthritis, osteomyelitis, fracture, and Paget's disease. Patients with carcinoma of the prostate are usually in a similar age group as those with arthritis and Paget's disease. Consequently the demonstration of increased uptake, particularly in the spine, may require further investigation such as CT to help differentiate these conditions. Hot spots in the ribs are diagnostic if no rib fracture is seen on the radiographs. In addition to initial staging, radioisotope studies are helpful in treatment evaluation. Metastatic bone lesions may be reduced or even obliterated by estrogen therapy. Serial technetium-99m diphosphonate studies may show alteration in the hypervascularity of the lesion and reduction or disappearance of the initial hot spot.

Lymphangiography is seldom used in the assessment of prostatic carcinoma. Bipedal lymphangiography is more commonly used in testicular malignancy and occasionally in bladder cancer. The normal pedal lymphangiogram is unlikely to show the obturator nodes that are most commonly involved in carcinoma of the prostate.

The external iliac, common iliac, and paraaortic lymph nodes are visualized in pedal lymphangiography, but involvement of these nodes is less common. Involved nodes are increased in size, with discrete filling defects (Fig. 17.15).

Barium enema is seldom indicated unless bowel obstructive symptoms are present in a case of known carcinoma of the prostate. More commonly the barium enema is performed because of rectal bleeding or if there are obstructive symptoms of unknown etiology. Carcinoma of the prostate affecting the rectum and sigmoid colon has been described. The most common effect is an annular constriction around the rectum leading to obstruction. Carcinoma of the prostate spreading into the space between the two layers of Denonvilliers' fascia provides an easy route for encircling the rectum, or it may extend proximally and encircle the rectosigmoid region or extend inferiorly to cause an anal stricture. Stricture extending inferiorly to involve the rectum may result in difficulty in the insertion of the barium enema tube and the performance of the study. More commonly the stricture involves only the rectum and the examination may be easily performed. The flow of barium into the bowel is slow and the rectal constriction may be so severe that only a thin narrow passage through the rectum is seen. The appearance is similar to advanced rectal carcinoma because of the apple core appearance but typical shoulder formation is absent. Rectal carcinoma is usually a rectal filling defect.

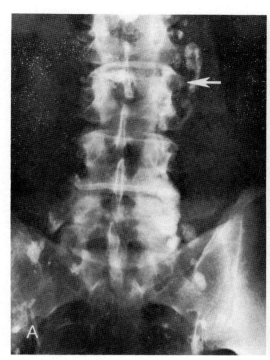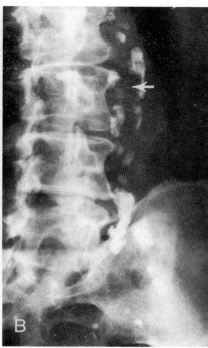

Figure 17.15. Paraaortic lymph node metastasis. Lymphography demonstrates a peripheral filling defect (*arrow*) seen on (**A**) anteroposterior (AP) and (**B**) left posterior oblique (LPO) radiographs indicating metastatic tumor.

Carcinoma of the prostate may also invade the anterior rectal wall (Fig. 17.16). Patients with this condition are more likely to present with rectal bleeding, tenesmus, and diarrhea. Urinary symptoms may be minimal. Digital rectal examination reveals the ulcerating mass on the anterior rectal wall. The barium enema outlines the ulcerating mass, which may have a very similar appearance to rectal carcinoma, although typically rectal carcinoma is more likely to produce a mass projecting into the rectum. Prostatic carcinoma ulcerating into the rectum is unlikely to produce a significant rectal mass. In ulcerating prostatic carcinoma the correct diagnosis is of prime impor-

tance since the management of rectal carcinoma is entirely different from that of prostatic carcinoma. Prostatic carcinoma may produce an anterior rectal indentation without encirclement or ulceration. This is seen on barium enema as an irregular indentation in the anterior rectal wall without mucosal involvement. This appearance is rarely produced by extensive prostatic hypertrophy and the barium enema is not helpful in distinguishing these indentations.

Computed tomography is of no help in the staging of Stage A or B carcinoma, but CT is useful in assessment of Stage C and D carcinoma. Contrast medium inserted into the colon by rectal tube or by large amounts of oral contrast opacifies these regions. Rapid infusion of intravenous contrast medium and dynamic scanning serve to differentiate nodes from blood vessels (Fig. 17.17).

Pelvic extension of prostatic carcinoma may be clearly delineated, and tumor extension into obturator and internal iliac nodes causing nodal enlargement over 1 cm may be identified. Although lymph nodes involved with metastases from prostate carcinoma are usually only mildly enlarged, occasionally bulky metastases are seen (Fig. 17.18).

Although nodal enlargement may be seen on CT, it should be remembered that all nodal enlargement is not due to metastatic carcinoma but may be inflammatory or reactive fibrosis. Consequently the visualization of enlarged obturator or internal iliac nodes requires thinneedle biopsy or aspiration of the node for the definitive diagnosis. This can be done with biplane fluoroscopy as in the case of opacified enlarged nodes on lymphangiog-

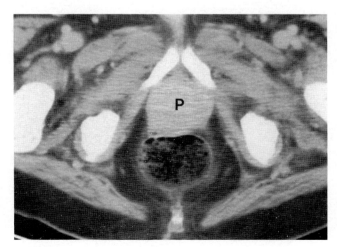

Figure 17.16. Prostate carcinoma. Tumor (P) invading the anterior rectal wall is well visualized on pelvic CT.

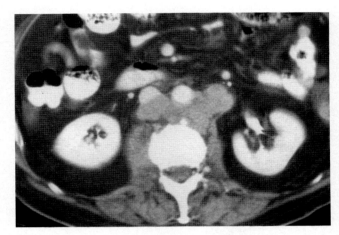

Figure 17.17. Prostate carcinoma. Paraaortic metastases are clearly distinguished from the opacified aorta and inferior vena cava on this enhanced CT scan.

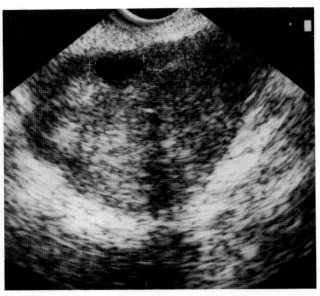

Figure 17.19. Prostate carcinoma. Digital rectal examination did not reveal a nodule in this asymptomatic 60-year-old man. The anechoic lesion (*markers*) was proven to be Stage A prostatic carcinoma.

raphy, or by CT localization and control of needle insertion into the enlarged node. This needle biopsy is usually performed by a transabdominal approach with the insertion of a 20- or 22-gauge needle.

Endorectal ultrasound studies have produced significant expectations in the diagnosis of Stage A and B disease. Transabdominal ultrasound is only able to detect prostatic carcinoma when the carcinoma is bulky, extensive, and invasive into surrounding periprostatic structures. Although early reports on transrectal ultrasound were confusing, the recent development of high-resolution 6- to 7.5-MHz transducers and improved near-field focus have improved results. The aim of these diagnostic procedures is to make a malignant diagnosis while the lesion is operable and has not spread. It is possible that the more often Stage A or Stage B carcinoma of the prostate can be diagnosed the better the prognosis is for the

patient. Small carcinomas (Stages A and B) are mostly hypoechoic, and the vast majority (80–90%) occur in the peripheral zone. Some carcinomas may be well defined without any internal echoes (Fig. 17.19), but unlike cysts there is no through-transmission. Others may be irregular and poorly defined (Fig. 17.20). However, most carcinomas of Stage A or B are hypoechoic in relation to the echogenicity of the remainder of the peripheral zone. When a small hypoechoic lesion is seen on the transverse

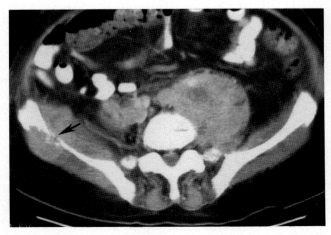

Figure 17.18. Prostate carcinoma. Bulky metastases to common iliac lymph nodes are seen. Metastatic tumor has also destroyed a portion of the right ilium (*arrow*).

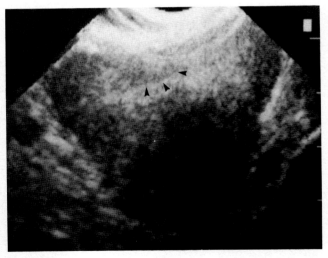

Figure 17.20. Transrectal ultrasound in a patient with a digitally palpable nodule in the left lobe of the prostate. The study shows an ill-defined hypoechoic area left of center in the peripheral zone (*arrowheads*). Transrectal ultrasound biopsy proven prostatic carcinoma.

view, every effort should be made to visualize the same lesion on longitudinal views (Fig. 17.21). The majority of carcinomas in the peripheral zone are adjacent to the apex of the prostate where the capsule is thin. Extension of carcinoma through the capsule is recognized as capsular bulging with interruption of the hyperechoic capsule and pericapsular fat. Such a finding indicates Stage C carcinoma. Lesions from 4 mm to 1 cm are now readily detectable with high-resolution equipment. Because most hypoechoic areas in the peripheral zone are not malignant, biopsy should be performed. Ultrasound guidance of transrectal biopsy is accurate and allows early diagnosis. At least three needle cores are often ob-

tained from the lesion, and random biopsy cores may be obtained from the opposite peripheral zone.

Santorini's venous plexus, which surrounds the anterolateral portion of the prostate, may be seen as longitudinal hypoechoic areas along the edge of the peripheral zone. This should not be taken for infiltrating carcinoma. Usually the venous plexus has a fairly characteristic curvilinear appearance. Rarely it is not well visualized and gives rise to concern and confusion with hypoechoic carcinoma. Carcinomas in the peripheral zone may extend through the capsule or extend anterosuperiorly into the central (Fig. 17.22) and transitional zone, resulting in varying degrees of echogenicity throughout

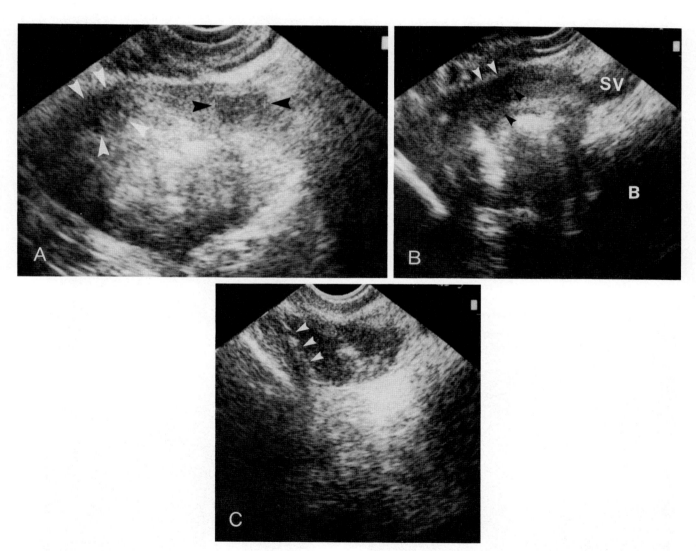

Figure 17.21. **A,** Transrectal ultrasound transverse view showing an irregular hypoechoic area in the left peripheral zone (*white arrows*) and a faintly seen hypoechoic area in the right peripheral zone (*black arrows*). R = right prostate. **B,** Longitudinal scan of the left lobe of prostate. The hypoechoic area in the left peripheral zone (*arrows*) is well seen. The faintly hypoechoic area in the right peripheral zone was not seen on longitudinal views of the right lobe. B = bladder, SV = seminal vesicles. **C,** Transrectal ultrasound biopsy of hypoechoic lesion in the left peripheral zone. The needle tract is well seen (*arrowheads*). Random biopsies were also obtained from the right peripheral zone. All cores obtained were adenocarcinoma Stage B.

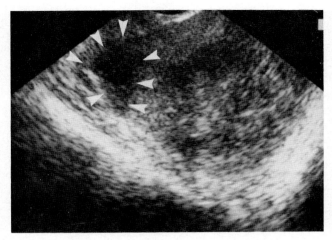

Figure 17.22. Transrectal ultrasound study in a 65-year-old man with a digitally hard palpable nodule in the left lobe. The study shows an irregular hypoechoic area in the left peripheral zone extending into the central zone. There was transrectal ultrasound biopsy proven carcinoma.

the prostate, producing some difficulty in distinguishing carcinoma from hypertrophy. However, since most carcinomas originate in the peripheral zone, hypoechogenicity in this region with varying echogenicity and loss of demarcation of the usually well-defined junction of the peripheral and central zone should suggest malignancy (Fig. 17.23).

Approximately 25% of prostatic carcinomas are iso-echoic or faintly hypoechoic in the peripheral zone and are therefore difficult to demonstrate by transrectal ultra-

sound. Isoechoic carcinomas can only be suspected when they bulge or invade the capsule. As carcinomas gain bulk and invade the central and peripheral zones, areas of hyperechogenicity may be seen (Fig. 17.24). This appearance simulates prostatic hypertrophy, and it is often difficult to definitely identify the lesion as malignant unless capsular invasion and partial or complete obliteration of the capsule and pericapsular fat echogenicity are present. Tumor extension into the seminal vesicles alters the normal sharp beak shape of the seminal vesicle on the longitudinal scan. The normal seminal vesicle is slightly less echogenic than the adjacent prostate (Fig. 17.21**B**) and provides a small beak or nipple that is sharply angled. Tumor extension into the seminal vesicle usually increases the seminal vesicle echogenicity and widens or obliterates the normal beak or nipple.

Transurethral prostatectomy for prostatic hypertrophy not uncommonly reveals malignant change on specimen pathologic examination. There is pathologic evidence that 10–20% of prostatic carcinomas arise in the transitional zone, and the peripheral zone is clear of carcinomas. Prostatic carcinomas arising in the transitional zone are almost impossible to diagnose with transrectal ultrasound since this is the area that results in prostatic hypertrophy, which may be hypoechoic. Few characteristic signs of malignancy are available using transrectal ultrasound. Capsular invasion (Fig. 17.24), loss of the seminal

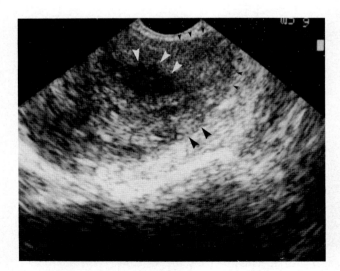

Figure 17.23. Transrectal ultrasound study showing an irregular hypoechoic area at the junction of the peripheral and central zones (*white arrowheads*). Note the coarser echogenicity of the central zone (*large black arrowheads*) when compared to the peripheral zone (*small black arrowheads*). There was transrectal ultrasound biopsy proven adenocarcinoma.

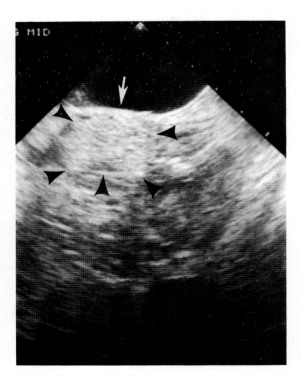

Figure 17.24. Transrectal ultrasound demonstrating a large hyperechoic mass (*black arrowheads*) and capsular bulging (*white arrow*). Biopsy proved this to be a large infiltrating carcinoma.

vesicle beak, or small hypoechoic areas with asymmetry of the peripheral zone are helpful. Any asymmetry of the peripheral zone echogenicity requires biopsy. It is to be emphasized that all hypoechoic lesions seen in the peripheral zone are not carcinomas. Only 25–50% of hypoechoic areas in the peripheral zone are proven carcinomas. The remainder include prostatitis, normal prostatic tissue, prostatic infarcts, and benign hypertrophy. However, any success in diagnosing Stage A or B prostatic carcinomas is an improvement on previous experience.

MRI provides clear visualization of the prostate in transverse, sagittal, and coronal planes. Although the prostate is well visualized on T1-weighted images (i.e., short repetition and echo time 500/28 msec), T2-weighted images (long TR and TE 2000/60 ms) are necessary for visualization of the internal architecture of the prostate. Spin echo technique with a long TR and TE is able to differentiate the peripheral from the central zone in young men, but this differentiation may be less apparent in elderly men (Fig. 17.25). The transitional zone has the same signal intensity as the peripheral zone since both are histologically similar but may be recognized by position on sagittal and coronal views. Pathologic states within the prostate can be identified by varying areas of signal intensity. However, MRI examination of the prostate is promising in staging prostate carcinoma although Stage A cannot be distinguished from Stage B. Coronal views of the prostate with spin echo technique and long TR and TE (2000/60) have been used to identify the periprostatic venous plexus, which appears as a bright rim around the prostate due to the slow blood flow. It has been proven that this bright rim and high signal intensity is not fat since it is not visualized when the TE is reduced

to 30 msec. The visualization of the periprostatic venous plexus is valuable in the assessment of carcinoma that has spread through the capsule. Using this technique on coronal views, a complete uninterrupted bright rim of high signal intensity should indicate that if a known prostate carcinoma is present, it remains within the prostatic capsule and is therefore Stage B. When the bright rim is interrupted (Fig. 17.26), this would indicate Stage C or D.

Both T1- and T2-weighted images are necessary to assess local spread of prostatic carcinoma. T1-weighted images provide excellent contrast between the prostate, fat, and urine. T2-weighted images provide the best contrast between muscle, the prostate, fascial planes such as Denonvilliers' fascia, and the membranous urethra. Volumetric assessment of the prostate can be done using all three planes. The multiplane imaging allows the assessment of spread of prostatic carcinoma to the seminal vesicles, rectum, bladder neck, and base, and to the levator ani muscles. On T2-weighted images increased signal intensity in the seminal vesicles and levator ani muscles, or interruption of the low signal intensity of Denonvilliers' fascia are indications of Stage C disease in a patient with known prostatic carcinoma. Abnormally large pelvic lymph nodes are best seen on T1-weighted images and indicate Stage D_1 carcinoma. Much of recent MRI investigation has been performed using resistive low field strength units. Equipment of 1.5 Tesla and above is more likely to provide better resolution, and it is to be hoped that future studies will show differentiation of Stage A and Stage B prostatic carcinoma. Although a transrectal MRI coil has been demonstrated, transrectal ultrasound re-

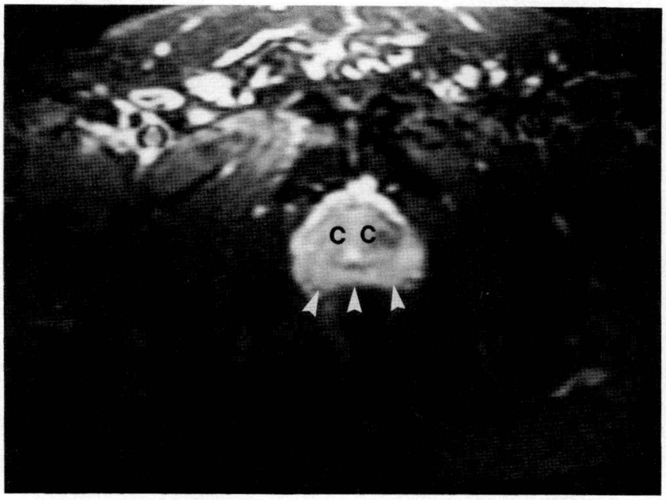

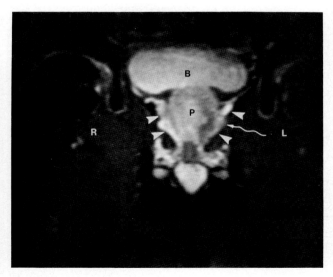

Figure 17.26. MRI examination of the prostate (P) coronal view. The periprostatic venous plexus is clearly seen as a high signal intensity around the prostate (*arrowheads*). The low signal intensity area in the left prostate is proven carcinoma invading and interrupting the periprostatic venous plexus (*curved arrow*). R = right side; L = left side; B = bladder.

Figure 17.25. MRI examination of the prostate, transverse view, showing clear differentiation of the peripheral (*arrowheads*) and central zone (C).

mains the only radiologic method of obtaining prostatic biopsy.

Prostatitis

Inflammatory conditions of the prostate arise from a variety of causes. The clinical presentation includes frequency, urgency, nocturia, dysuria, perineal pain, and frequently urethral discharge. In acute prostatitis, digital rectal examination reveals a "boggy" tender prostate. In chronic prostatitis the prostate may be normal to the examining finger, stony, asymmetrically hard, or diffusely enlarged and slightly tender.

The etiology of acute prostatitis is bacterial infection. The etiology of chronic prostatitis, which commonly occurs without any acute episode, varies between bacterial, nonbacterial, and no pathologic lesion found, i.e., the patient is symptomatic but all investigations are normal. Bacterial prostatitis is more commonly a retrograde infection. Literature reports vary in their demonstration of the most common organism, either Gram-positive or Gram-negative organisms. *Staphylococcus epidermis* and alpha Streptococcus have been found to be the most common organisms in some series whereas much of the literature implicates Gram-negative organisms, the most common being *Escherichia coli*. It is said that *E. coli* accounts for over 80% of bacterial prostatitis, with an additional 15% being composed of either *Klebsiella, Proteus, Pseudomonas,* and *Enterobacter* or *Gonococcus.* Any of these bacterial organisms may produce acute prostatitis or may present as chronic prostatitis.

Granulomatous prostatitis may result from nonbacterial agents such as tuberculosis, coccidioidomycosis, histoplasmosis, blastomycosis, and fungal infections. The third group of patients with a clinical diagnosis of chronic prostatitis without evidence of bacterial or nonbacterial infection and with normal digital rectal examination and normal prostatic secretion remain controversial, but the possibility that *Mycoplasma, Chlamydia,* and viruses are responsible should be considered.

The clinical diagnosis rests on digital examination, bacterial examination of prostate secretions expressed by digital prostatic massage, and prostatic biopsy of suspected areas. Bacterial and nonbacterial prostatitis are usually diagnosable. When all clinical examinations are negative but the patient has chronic prostatitis, clinically, controversy occurs. Anatomic controversy as to the common sites of prostatitis still prevails, although there is a shift of emphasis from the periurethral glands to the peripheral zone that is now mainly accepted as the most common site of prostatic infection and inflammation. In those patients without abnormal clinical signs, autoimmune or localized allergic phenomenon have been implicated in chronic granulomatous prostatitis.

Radiology

Neither the plain film nor the excretory urogram provides pathognomonic findings to suggest prostatitis. Prostatic calcification and an enlarged prostate indenting the bladder base are more common in prostatic hypertrophy than in prostatitis. Transabdominal ultrasound and CT are likewise nondiagnostic. In chronic prostatitis, transrectal ultrasound may demonstrate varying areas of altered echogenicity in the bulk of the prostate similar to the findings in prostatic hypertrophy. Areas of low echogenicity are seen in the peripheral zone similar to that seen in prostatic carcinoma (Fig. 17.27). Such areas may be the result of chronic prostatitis or infarction, which is the result of infection. Up to 20% of transrectal biopsies in such cases represent chronic prostatitis.

Prostatic abscesses generally demonstrate decreased echogenicity. Combined with the clinical presentation, a prostatic abscess may be suspected and proven by transrectal ultrasound-guided aspiration. Computed tomography and MRI, while incapable of diagnosing acute or chronic prostatitis, may be extremely helpful in the diagnosis of a prostatic abscess. On CT they are seen as irregular areas of low density. With MRI, fluid collections within the prostate can be identified on T1- and T2-weighted images. Evidence of an old prostatic abscess that has sloughed into the urethra (Fig. 17.28) or rectum may be demonstrated on cystourethrography. Rarely prostatic cavities are found to contain stones (Fig. 17.29).

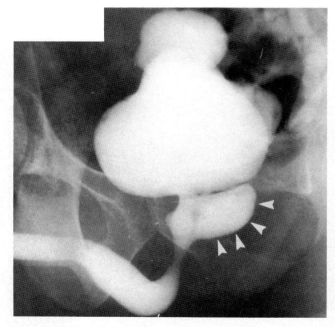

Figure 17.27. Retrograde urethrocystogram in a patient with known tuberculosis. He had a right autonephrectomy and was treated for tuberculous prostatitis and abscess. The abscess sloughed into the urethra leaving a cavity (*arrowheads*).

Prostatic Calcification

Primary Calcification

The peripheral zone of the prostate is the seat of the corpora amylacea where calcification may occur. The etiology is unknown and these calcifications have no known pathologic effects. Up to 30% of men over 50 years may show corpora amylaceous calcification on plain films. These calcifications are discrete, vary in size from 1 to 5 mm, and are usually multiple. Rarely these calcifications move into a prostatic duct and may be passed per urethra. If maintained in the ductal orifice for some time, they are exposed to urine flow. Corpora amylaceous calcifications are calcium phosphate (apatite). When exposed to urine flow they may contain oxalate, cystine, uric acid, or struvite.

Secondary prostatic calculi occur in areas of necrosis that may occur in adenomata, carcinoma, granulomatous prostatitis, or after radiation therapy. Calcification occurs in 7–10% of patients with prostatic adenomata. In prostatic adenomatous calcification, the only distinguishing feature from corpora amylaceous calcification is the position, seen on plain film. Adenomatous calcification is commonly seen above the symphysis pubis. Corpora amylaceous calcification is seen in the normal prostate position, i.e., below or behind the symphysis pubis. Calcification is rare in prostatic carcinoma but may occur in approximately 5% of patients. Most of the calcifications seen in the prostate in patients with carcinoma were in corpora amylacea. In a small number of carcinomas there is necrotic calcification. Calcification in prostatic carcinoma becomes more common as the carcinoma becomes more invasive.

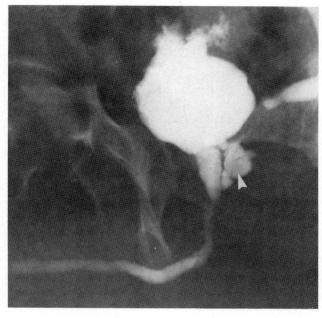

Figure 17.29. Retrograde urethrocystogram showing a prostatic cavity containing a filling defect (*arrowhead*) which proved to be calcium encrusted debris.

Granulomatous prostatitis resulting from tuberculosis causes significant calcification. Calcifications may be small, or the whole prostate may be calcified and separated from the prostatic capsule. Bilharziasis calcification is extremely rare although bilharziasis is a very destructive lesion in the prostate and urethra. Granulomatous prostatitis without evidence of bacterial or nonbacterial infection is thought to be a severe histiocytic granulomatous reaction. Up to 15% of this type of granulomatous

Figure 17.28. Prostatitis. **A,** Transrectal ultrasound demonstrated a hypoechoic region (*arrowheads*) in the peripheral zone. **B,** Transrectal biopsy with an 18-gauge needle (*arrow*) demonstrated prostatitis.

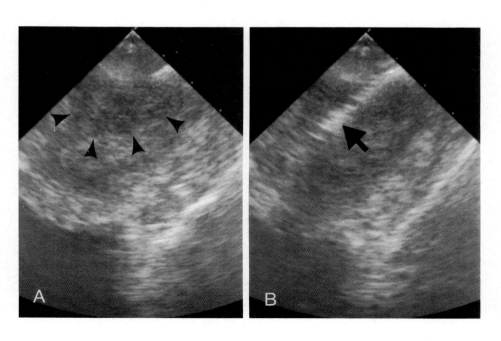

prostatitis show dystrophic prostatic calcification. Prostatic cancer treated by radiation may produce symptomatic prostatic calcification, resulting in dysuria and hematuria. Transurethral resection with removal of the prostatic calculi relieves the condition.

Prostatic calcification is detected on 15–30% of plain films of men over the age of 50 years. It is most commonly seen about the age of 65 years. Sixty percent of patients between the ages of 50 and 70 years will show prostatic calcification on CT as it is more sensitive than plain radiography.

Radiology

Plain film examination is essential in assessing prostatic calcification. Care must be observed to obtain as much of the prostate area on the film so that calcification in the prostate is visualized. Prostate calcification may be difficult to see since primary calcification (i.e., amylaceous body calcification) with a relatively normal-sized prostate may overlie the symphysis pubis. Secondary or dystrophic calcification such as tuberculous granulomatous calcification is usually well visualized on plain film since it is commonly extensive (Fig. 17.30). Dystrophic

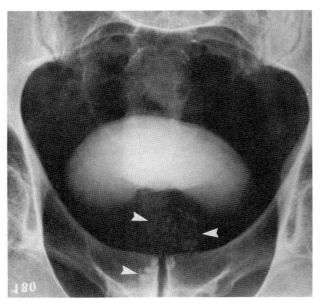

Figure 17.31. Excretory urogram in a patient with a large median lobe adenoma contains dystrophic calcification. (From Pollack HM (ed): *Clinical Urography.* Philadelphia, WB Saunders, 1990, p 1906.)

calcification within the prostate may occur in chronic prostatitis resulting from outlet obstruction. This is rarely seen in young patients. Excretory urography is useful in assessing bladder indentation by calcified prostatic adenomata (Fig. 17.31). Transabdominal ultrasound readily shows calcification within the prostate as bright echoes producing acoustic shadowing (Fig. 17.7). Computed tomography is more accurate in showing faint calcification (Fig. 17.32) not apparent on plain film or transabdominal ultrasound.

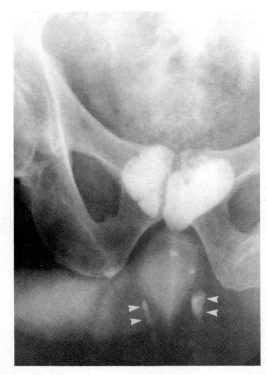

Figure 17.30. Plain film in a patient with known pulmonary and renal tuberculosis. The prostate is almost completely calcified due to tuberculous granulomatous prostatitis. Calcification is also seen in the epydidimii bilaterally (*arrows*) from tuberculous epydidimitis. (From McCallum RW, Colapinto V: *Urological Radiology of the Adult Male Lower Urinary Tract.* Springfield, IL, Charles C Thomas, 1976, p 80.)

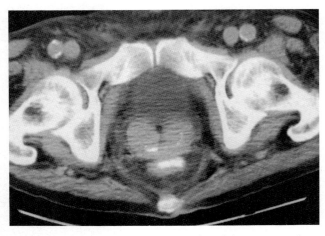

Figure 17.32. Computed tomography of the prostate showing faint calcification within the prostate. This calcification was not visualized on plain film.

SEMINAL VESICLES

Until the advent of cross-sectional imaging, the seminal vesicles could only be visualized by seminal vesiculography. This required opening the scrotum, cannulating the vas deferens, and injecting contrast medium into the vas deferens. The seminal vesicles were visualized by contrast medium refluxing into the seminal vesicles from the junction of the ducts of the seminal vesicle and the ampulla of the vas deferens or by direct reflux from the ejaculatory ducts. The clinical indications for the procedure included persistent perineal pain, suprapubic pain, pain on ejaculation, hematospermia, and infertility. The pain described by patients has often been attributed to chronic prostatitis, but the persistence of pain in spite of adequate antibiotic therapy should raise the possibility of a seminal vesicle disorder. Patients with hematospermia should be considered to have a seminal vesicle lesion. Seminal vesicle and ejaculatory duct calculi should be excluded.

Patients with postgerminal hypofertility are candidates for seminal vesiculography. These patients are oligospermic or azoospermic and have normal follicle stimulating hormone (FSH) serum levels. In these patients seminal vesiculography is diagnostic of postgerminal lesions in 15–40% of patients. These lesions include obstruction of the vas deferens or obstruction of the ejaculatory duct or verumontanum. Relief of the obstruction surgically usually results in an increase in the patient's sperm count and semen volume.

The results of seminal vesiculography are disappointing when the procedure is performed to assess seminal vesiculitis. Although over 70% of these patients had abnormal vesiculograms, less than 20% had abnormal histology in those patients who had seminal vesiculectomies. Seminal vesiculitis may be an extension from acute or chronic prostatitis. Untreated seminal vesiculitis may result in extension of the inflammatory process to the ampulla of the vas deferens resulting in asymmetry, fibrosis, and contraction of the seminal vesicle and narrowing and diverticular formation of the ampulla of the vas deferens.

Fifty-five percent of patients with hematospermia have seminal vesicle or ejaculatory duct calculi. Seminal vesicle cysts may also produce hematospermia. The pain due to calculi commonly occurs during ejaculation. Seminal vesicle cyst more commonly produces perineal pain or low-grade perineal ache. Seminal vesicle cysts occasionally contain calculi. Dilated seminal vesicles may be present without any obvious cause for the dilatation being found.

Radiology

The plain film and excretory urogram are seldom helpful in assessing seminal vesicle disease. Seminal vesicle cysts rarely calcify and are seldom large enough to displace the bladder, usually being less than 5 cm.

Giant seminal vesicle cysts associated with renal agenesis have been reported. These giant cysts may be 12 cm or more in diameter and displace the bladder. Calcification in the rim has been recorded. It is to be emphasized that seminal vesicle calcification is extremely rare but that calcification of the ampulla of the vas deferens is relatively common, especially in patients with diabetes mellitus in whom it is virtually pathognomic (Fig. 17.33).

In a normal patient, contrast material injected into the vas deferens opacifies the vas, the ampulla of the vas deferens, the seminal vesicle, and the ejaculatory duct. Contrast in the bladder or urethra indicates patency (Fig. 17.34). In patients with postgerminal infertility the vaso-

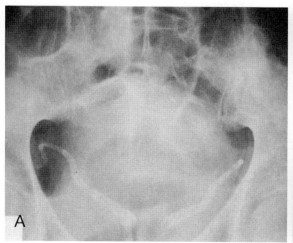
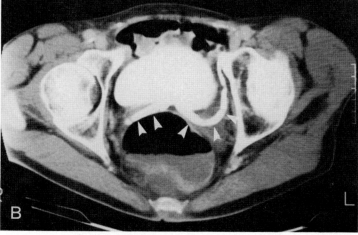

Figure 17.33. **A,** Plain film of the pelvis showing characteristic appearance of calcified ampulla of the vas deferens bilaterally in a patient with diabetes mellitus. **B,** Computed tomography scan in a diabetic patient showing calcified ampullae of the vas deferens (*arrows*).

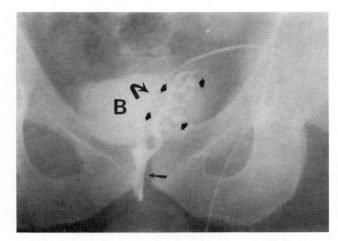

Figure 17.34. Normal seminal vesiculogram. Contrast injected into the left vas as deferens opacifies the vas, the ampulla of the vas deferens (*curved arrow*), the seminal vesicle (*arrowheads*), and the ejaculatory duct (*arrow*). Contrast material in the bladder (B) indicates patency.

gram may demonstrate obstruction either along the vas deferens (Fig. 17.35) or at the verumontanum. In seminal vesiculitis, the seminal vesicle may be displaced or poorly filled (Fig. 17.36). The ampulla of the vas may also present a feathery appearance with narrowing, loss of the normal convoluted (string of beads) appearance, and multiple small diverticulae. The normal separation of the seminal vesicle and ampulla of the vas is commonly obliterated. All of these findings may be indicative of chronic inflammatory change in the seminal vesicles. Rarely tuberculosis affects the seminal vesicles and ampulla resulting in contraction and narrowing of the seminal vesicle with loss of the normal convoluted appearance (Fig. 17.37**A**). If too much contrast medium is injected via the vas deferens, reflux occurs into the bladder and this may obscure the seminal vesicles (Fig. 17.37**B**).

Retrograde and voiding cystourothrography is seldom helpful in assessing the seminal vesicles. Rarely either study may show reflux of contrast medium in the ejaculatory duct and seminal vesicle. This condition may occur in postprostatectomy patients or in patients who have severe urethral stricture causing hydrostatic backpressure. In the latter case reflux into the ejaculatory duct may persist long after the distal urethral obstruction has been surgically corrected (Fig. 17.38).

Computed tomography is a useful method of assessing pathology in the seminal vesicles since they are well visualized. A benign cyst of the seminal vesicle is the most common abnormality and is well visualized on CT (Fig. 17.39). Primary carcinoma of the seminal vesicle is rare. More commonly the seminal vesicle is invaded by carcinoma of the prostate (Fig. 17.40), bladder, or rectum.

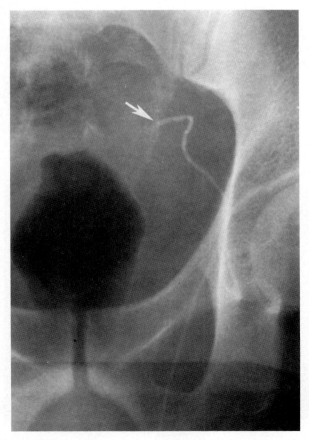

Figure 17.35. Obstructed vas deferens. A left vasogram demonstrates complete obstruction (*arrow*) of the vas deferens.

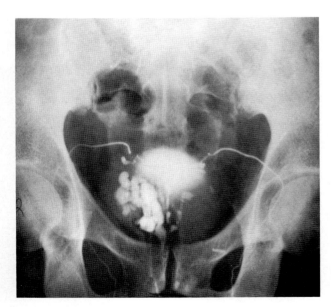

Figure 17.36. Seminal vesiculitis. A bilateral vasogram demonstrates marked asymmetry with poor filling of the left seminal vesicle.

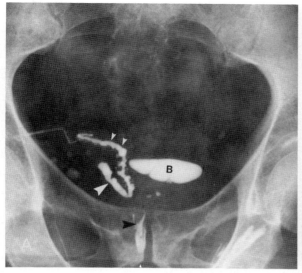

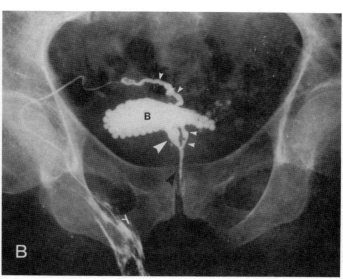

Figure 17.37. **A,** Right seminal vesiculogram in a patient with tuberculosis. The ampulla of the vas deferens shows a beaded appearance (*small white arrowheads*) and the seminal vesicle is contracted and small (*large white arrowheads*) with loss of the normal convoluted appearance. The ejaculatory duct (*black arrow*) is visualized. B = bladder. (From Putman CE, Ravin CE (eds): *Textbook of Diagnostic Imaging*. Philadelphia, WB Saunders, 1988, p 1359.) **B,** Seminal vesiculogram with the injection of too much contrast medium, much of which has refluxed into the bladder (B) obscuring the seminal vesicle (*large white arrowheads*). The ampulla of the vas deferens is also partly obscured (*small white arrowheads*). The ejaculatory duct (*black arrowhead*) is visualized.

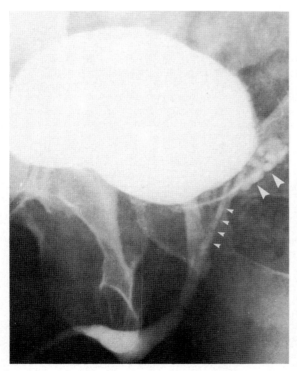

Figure 17.38. Voiding cystourethrogram in a patient with a previous history of bulbous urethral stricture which was surgically corrected by urethroplasty. The voiding study shows reflux into the ejaculatory duct (*small arrowheads*) and seminal vesicle (*large arrowheads*).

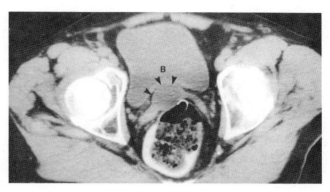

Figure 17.39. Computed tomography scan of the pelvis showing a full bladder (B) and a cyst of the right seminal vesicle (*arrowheads*) lying centrally and indenting the bladder base.

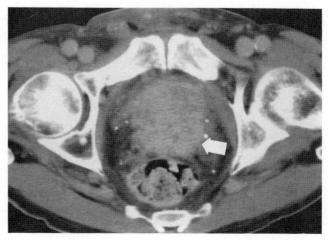

Figure 17.40. Direct extension of prostate carcinoma into the seminal vesicles (*arrow*) is demonstrated by CT.

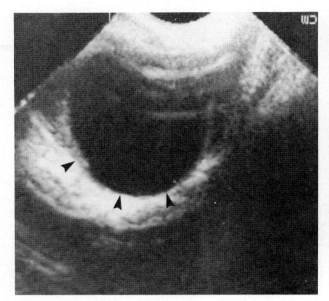

Figure 17.41. Seminal vesicle cyst. The transverse image from a transrectal ultrasound examination shows a large left echo-free seminal vesicle cyst (*arrowheads*).

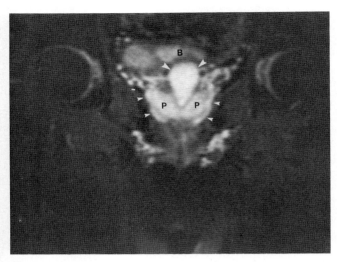

Figure 17.43. MRI examination performed for prostatic carcinoma demonstrates clear definition of a seminal vesicle cyst lying in the midline (*large arrowheads*). The periprostatic venous plexus is also well seen (*small arrowheads*). P = prostate; B = bladder.

Transrectal ultrasound of the seminal vesicles is the most promising method of assessment and may be extremely helpful in differentiating seminal vesicle disease from prostatis. Seminal vesicle cysts are readily seen (Fig. 17.41) and seminal vesicle abscesses are well demonstrated (Fig. 17.42). Seminal vesicle abscess may be a complication of seminal vesiculography and of vasectomy or may occur as an extension of infection from prostatitis. MRI examination is usually not required in the assessment of the seminal vesicles, but they are well visualized

on MRI examination. Occasionally a seminal vesicle abnormality is demonstrated during MRI study of the prostate (Fig. 17.43).

SUGGESTED READINGS

Prostatic Hypertrophy

Haylen BT, Parys BT, West CR: Transrectal ultrasound to measure bladder volumes in men. *J Urol* 143:687, 1990.

Pope TL Jr, Harrison RB, Clark RL, et al: Bladder base impressions in women: "female prostate." *AJR* 136:1105, 1981.

Villers A, Terris MK, McNeal JE, Stamey TA: Ultrasound anatomy of the prostate: the normal gland and anatomical variations. *J Urol* 143:732, 1990

Wasserman NF, Lapointe S, Eckmann DR, et al: Assessment of prostatism: role of intravenous urography. *Radiology* 165:831, 1987.

Prostate Cancer

Ajzen SA, Goldenberg SL, Allen GJ, et al: Palpable prostatic nodules: comparison of US and digital guidance for fine-needle aspiration biopsy. *Radiology* 171:521, 1989.

Andriole GL, Kavoussi LR, Torrence RJ, et al: Transrectal ultrasonography in the diagnosis and staging of carcinoma of the prostate. *J Urol* 140:758, 1988.

Benson CB, Doubilet PM, Richie JP: Sonography of the male gential tract. *AJR* 153:705, 1989.

Catalana WJ: *Prostate Cancer.* Orlando, Grune & Stratton, 1984, pp 1–84.

Chang P, Friedland GW: Hypoechoic lesions of the prostate: Clinical relevance of tumor size, digital rectal examination, and prostate specific antigen. *Radiology* 175:581, 1990.

Chang P, Friedland GW: The role of imaging in screening of prostate cancer: a decision analysis perspective. *Invest Radiol* 25(5):591, 1990.

Connolly JG. Surgery of the prostate gland. In Tannenbaum M (ed): *Urologic Pathology: The Prostate.* Philadelphia, Lea & Febiger, 1977, p 283.

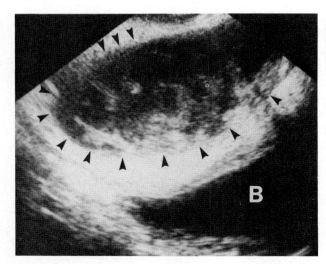

Figure 17.42. Seminal vesicle abscess. The transverse image from a transrectal ultrasound examination demonstrates a large mixed echogenic seminal vesicle abscess (*arrowheads*). B = bladder.

Cooner WH, Mosley BR, Rutherford CL, et al: Prostate cancer detection in a clinical urological practice by ultrasonography, digital rectal examination and prostate specific antigen. *J Urol* 143:1146, 1990.

Devonec M, Fendler JP, Monsallier M, et al: The significance of the prostatic hypoechoic area: results in 226 ultrasonically guided prostatic biopsies. *J Urol* 143:316, 1990.

Donohue RE, Fauver HE, Whitesel JA, et al: Prostatic carcinoma. Influence of tumor grade on results of pelvic lymphadenectomy. *Urology* 17:435, 1981.

Donohue RE, Fauver HE, Whitesel JA, et al: Staging prostatic cancer. A different distribution. *J Urol* 122:327, 1979.

Fritzsche PJ, Axford PD, Ching VC, et al: Correlation of transrectal sonographic findings in patients with suspected and unsuspected prostatic disease. *J Urol* 130:272, 1983.

Gleason DF: Histologic grading and clinical staging of prostatic carcinoma. In Tannenbaum M (ed): *Urologic Pathology: The Prostate*. Philadelphia, Lea & Febiger, 1977, p 171.

Hricak H, Dooms GC, Jeffrey RB, Availlone A, et al: Prostatic carcinoma: staging by clinical assessment, CT, and MR imaging. *Radiology* 162:331, 1987.

Hodge KK, McNeal JE, Stamey T: Ultrasound guided transrectal core biopsies of the palpably abnormal prostate. *J Urol* 142:66, 1989.

Kahn T, Burrig K, Schmitz-Drager B, et al: Prostatic carcinoma and benign prostatic hyperplasia: MR imaging with histopathologic correlation. *Radiology* 173:847, 1989.

Kidd R, Crane RD, Dail DH: Lymphangiography and fine-needle aspiration biopsy: ineffective for staging early prostate cancer. *AJR* 141:1007, 1984.

Lee F, Littrup PJ, Torp-Pedersen ST, et al: Prostate cancer: comparison of transrectal US and digital rectal examination for screening. *Radiology* 168:389, 1988.

McMillen SM, Wettlaufer JN: The role of repeat transurethral biopsy in stage A carcinoma of the prostate. *J Urol* 116:759, 1976.

Platt JF, Bree RL, Schwab RE: The accuracy of CT in the staging of carcinoma of the prostate. *AJR* 149:315, 1987.

Poon PY, McCallum RW, Henkelman MM, et al: Magnetic resonance imaging of the prostate. *Radiology* 154:143, 1985.

Rifkin MD: Prostate sonography: clinical indications and implications. *Urol Radiol* 11:238, 1989.

Rifkin MD, McGlynn ET, Choi H: Echogenicity of prostate cancer correlated with histologic grade and stromal fibrosis: endorectal US studies. *Radiology* 170:549, 1989.

Spellman MC, Castellino RA, Ray GR, et al: An evaluation of lymphography in localized carcinoma of the prostate. *Radiology* 125:637, 1977.

Seminal Vesicles

Banner MP, Hassler R: The normal seminal vesiculogram. *Radiology* 128:339, 1978.

Dunnick NR, Ford K, Osborne D, et al: Seminal vesiculography: limited value in vesiculitis. *Urology* 20(4):454.

Ford K, Carson CC, Dunnick NR, et al: The role of seminal vesiculography in the evaluation of male infertility. *Fertility & Sterility* 37(4):552, 1982.

Heaney JA, Pfister RC, Meares EM Jr: Giant cyst of the seminal vesicle with renal agenesis. *AJR* 149:139, 1987.

Kenney PJ, Leeson MD: Congenital anomalies of the seminal vesicles: spectrum of computed tomographic findings. *Radiology* 149:247, 1983.

King BF, Hattery RR, Lieber MM, et al: Seminal vesicle imaging. *RadioGraphics* 9(4):653, 1989.

Littrup PJ, Lee F, McLeary RD, et al: Transrectal US of the seminal vesicles and ejaculatory ducts: clinical correlation. *Radiology* 168:625, 1988.

Premkumar A, Newhouse JH: Seminal vesicle tuberculosis: CT appearance. *J Comput Assist Tomogr* 12(4):676, 1988.

Schabsigh R, Lerner S, Fishman IJ, et al: The role of transrectal ultrasonography in the diagnosis and management of prostatic and seminal vesicle cysts. *J Urol* 141:1206, 1989.

Schwartz JM, Bosniak MA, Hulnick DH, et al: Computed tomography of midline cysts of the prostate. *J Comput Assist Tomogr* 12(2):215, 1988.

Silverman PM, Dunnick NR, Ford KK: Computed tomography of the normal seminal vesicles. *Comput Radiol* 9(6):379, 1985.

CHAPTER **18**

URETHRA AND PENIS

ACQUIRED URETHRAL LESIONS

Gonorrhea

Gonorrhea is a sexually transmitted disease more prevalent in underdeveloped countries where low hygenic standards prevail. Sexual promiscuity is a major contributing factor. The estimated number of cases of gonorrhea in North America in 1974 reached 2.7 million. Since the early 1980s, sexual promiscuity has decreased due to the fear of acquired immunodeficiency syndrome (AIDS), and thus the incidence of gonorrhea has decreased. The estimated number of cases of gonorrhea in North America in 1985 was 1.8 million. Adequate early antibiotic treatment of gonorrhea eradicates the disease without sequelae. No treatment or inadequate treatment results in a chronic inflammatory reaction resulting in urethral stricture.

Although the incidence of gonorrhea in North America is relatively high, the incidence of urethral stricture resulting from gonorrhea is low. Approximately 40% of urethral strictures in North America are due to gonorrhea, while the remainder are due to trauma iatrogenic injury or other inflammatory etiologies.

The gonococcus ascends the anterior urethra affecting the columnar epithelial cells which become congested. The submucosal glands of Littre that are predominant in the bulbous urethra become infected and produce a copious, thick, purulent, urethral discharge within 48 hours. Adequate treatment at this stage should eradicate the disease. Without treatment, the infection extends into the corpus spongiosum causing venous thrombosis and necrosis. A mild watery chronic discharge results and granulation develops where columnar cells have desquamated and sloughed. Necrosis and granulation tissue in the submucosa develops into fibrous scarring that is more prominent in the bulbar sump, due to less effective flushing by urination and the preponderance of glands of Littre in this area. Over a period of months or years the scarring becomes irregular. Some scarring is hard fibrous tissue, which is difficult to dilate whereas other scarring is softer and more easily dilated. Gonococcal scarring or stricture is usually several centimeters long and 70% of the hard fibrous scars are present in the sump of the bulbous urethra. Months or years after the initial infection, the hard fibrous scar or stricture results in a gradual reduction of the urinary stream. Surgical or radiologic intervention is usually required to alleviate obstructive symptoms.

Effects of Stricture

PROXIMAL DILATATION. Infection spreads for several centimeters both proximal and distal to the hard fibrous scar, producing further scarring that is not as advanced as the initial site and is consequently softer. The proximal spread of the infection may extend as far as the membranous urethra, but the patient's presenting symptoms of stream reduction or outlet obstruction are due to the hard scarring in the sump of the bulbous urethra. This is the primary stricture, and the adjacent softer scars are secondary strictures. As the scarring in the bulbous urethral sump gradually hardens, the urethra proximal to this hard scar becomes dilated. The hydrostatic pressure on voiding in the urethra proximal to hard scarring is sufficient to dilate softer proximal scarring. Consequently, scarred tissue dilates; this is known as *paradoxical dilatation* (Fig. 18.1**A** and **B**).

PSEUDODIVERTICULUM. Pseudodiverticulum formation results from a gonococcal periurethral abscess that eventually sloughs into the urethra leaving a cavity. The vast majority of pseudodiverticula affect the inferior aspect of the urethra but rarely they occur anteriorly in the region of the penoscrotal junction. They vary in size from small (about 1 cm) to huge (up to 10 cm) (Fig. 18.2**A** and **B**).

URETHRAL FISTULA. Occasionally a periurethral abscess is large enough to extend to the perineum and penetrate both into the urethra and through the perineum creating a urethrocutaneous fistula. Consequently, urination usually occurs through the perineal fistula creating a "watering pot perineum." The cavity generally contracts by fibrosis leaving only a fistulous tract from the urethra to the perineum (Fig. 18.3).

URETHRAL STONE. Most urethral stones are migrant, either from the kidney or bladder. A native urethral stone, which is rare, forms proximal to a stricture. Proximal dilatation in which eddying may occur results in supersaturation and crystallization of calcium salts and the formation of calculi (Fig. 18.4**A** and **B**, Fig. 18.5**A** and **B**).

URETHRAL CARCINOMA. Approximately 70% of cases of urethral carcinoma occur in patients who have had previous urethral infection and most are squamous cell carcinomas (Fig. 18.6**A** and **B**).

EFFECTS ON THE PROSTATE AND BLADDER. Urethral gonorrhea resulting in stricture produces a high hydrostatic pressure proximal to the stricture. This may force open the prostatic ducts that empty into the prostatic sulcus, allowing infection to enter the prostate (Fig. 18.7**A** and **B**). Similarly, the pressure necessary to urinate through a hard stricture is increased by a gradual increase in hypertrophy of the detrusor muscle, resulting in bladder trabeculation and diverticulum formation. If the urine in the bladder is infected, ureterovesical junction dysfunction may occur resulting in vesicoureteral reflux. Long-standing partial outlet obstruction due to gonococcal stricture can result in supersaturation and crystallization of calcium salts producing bladder stones.

Urethrography in Gonococcal Infection

The main impact of untreated or poorly treated gonococcal infection is in the sump of the bulbous urethra, and results in bulbous urethral scarring. Dynamic retrograde urethrography commonly shows several centimeters of irregular urethra, of varying caliber, and there is generally a hard scar in the sump of the bulbous urethra. Irregularity of the urethra may extend for 2–3 cm toward the penoscrotal junction and 1–2 cm proximally. If the disease has spread proximally to involve the membranous urethra, the normal cone shape of the proximal bulbous urethra becomes asymmetric and narrowed, giving an elongated appearance to the membranous urethra (Fig. 18.8). Abnormality of the normal convex cone shape of the proximal bulbous urethra almost invariably indicates scarring involving the membranous urethra. This radiologic finding is of prime importance to the urologist, since surgical intervention in this region involves cutting the scar tissue and consequently the distal sphinc-

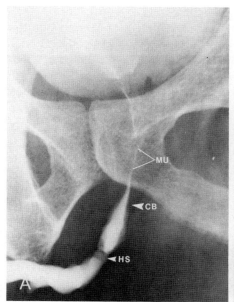
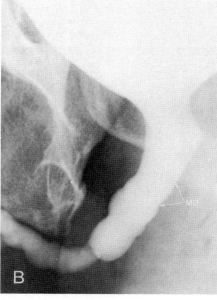

Figure 18.1.   A, Dynamic retrograde urethrogram in a patient who had a previous anterior urethroplasty for gonococcal stricture and developed outlet obstruction 2 years after urethroplasty. Note recurrent hard scar (HS) in the proximal bulbous urethra. Abnormal irregular narrowed cone to the proximal bulbous urethra (CB) indicates scarring extends into the membranous urethra (MU). **B,** Same patient voiding. Note marked dilatation of urethra from bladder neck to hard scar. The soft scarring in the membranous urethra (MU) is markedly dilated due to the high hydrostatic back-pressure produced by the hard scar in the proximal bulbous urethra.

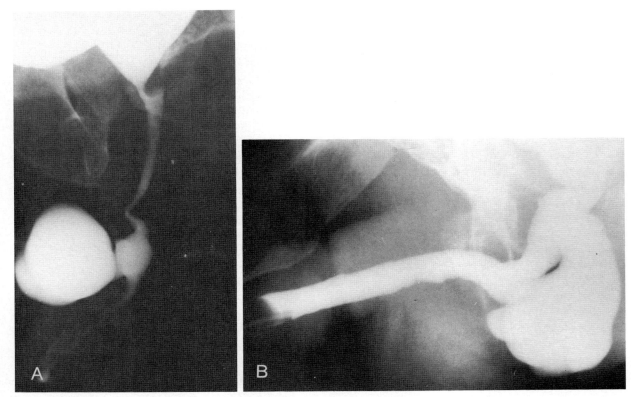

Figure 18.2. **A,** A voiding cystourethrogram in a patient with bulbous urethral scarring and old sloughed periurethral abscess at the penoscrotal junction producing an anterior divertic-ulum. **B,** Dynamic retrograde urethrogram in a patient with two diverticula (one large) extending posteroinferiorly from the bulbomembranous urethra.

ter mechanism, which may result in iatrogenic incontinence.

The verumontanum must always be seen on the dynamic retrograde examination. If the normal cone of the bulbous urethra is distorted, the membranous urethra can be localized 1–1.5 cm below the bulk of the verumontanum. Above the verumontanum, the supracollicular part of the prostatic urethra is visualized as contrast

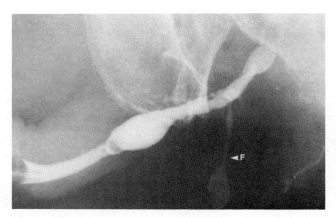

Figure 18.3. Dynamic retrograde urethrogram showing irregular scarring in the bulbous urethra with a fistula extending from the bulbous urethra to the perineum.

medium enters the bladder. On dynamic retrograde urethrography, the bladder neck cannot accurately be localized in the supine patient until the bladder is almost full of contrast medium. Occasionally the bladder neck is localized early in the procedure as a jet of contrast medium is seen entering the bladder (Fig. 18.9). When the bladder is almost full, the bladder neck is readily identified and is seen to be closed (Fig. 18.10).

The voiding cystourethrogram is obtained when the bladder is absolutely full. It is sometimes difficult to assess when the bladder is really full and voiding is imminent. The presence of a urethral stricture may alter the bladder capacity. In normal man, voiding usually occurs after the insertion of 300–400 ml of contrast medium. In men with urethral stricture the bladder capacity may increase to 1000 ml before the urge to void is felt. It is usually a mistake to remove the catheter for voiding when the patient first indicates he is ready to void. He may not void after catheter removal, resulting in lost time and reinsertion of the catheter. We recommend inserting a further 100 ml of contrast medium into the bladder after the patient indicates he is ready to void. This usually results in an immediate and good voiding study, and the bladder neck will open to 1 cm in diameter (Fig. 18.11**B**).

In the presence of a gonococcal bulbar stricture, the voiding study usually shows dilatation of the proximal

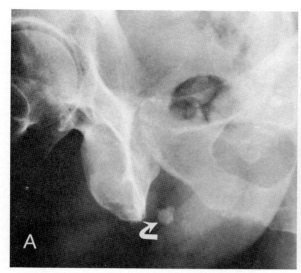

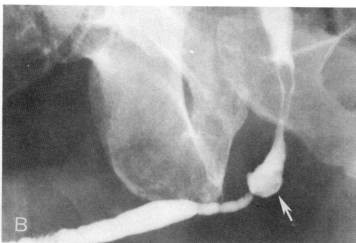

Figure 18.4.   A, Plain film showing a stone (*curved arrow*) in the expected position of the urethra. **B,** Dynamic retrograde urethrogram showing severe scarring in the bulbous urethra.

The filling defect (*arrow*) in the dilated urethra proximal to the scarring is a urethral stone.

urethra down to the scarring in the bulbous urethra (Fig. 18.11**A** and **B**). The dilatation may include the membranous urethra even when the dynamic retrograde study indicates bulbous scarring extending into the membranous urethra. Dilatation of a scarred membranous urethra indicates softer scarring in the membranous urethra than the hard scarring in the bulbous urethra and is known as *paradoxical* dilatation. Consequently, voiding cystourethrography alone, without dynamic retrograde urethrography, may erroneously indicate bulbar scarring alone without involvement of the membranous urethra (Fig. 18.7**B**). The voiding study almost invariably shows

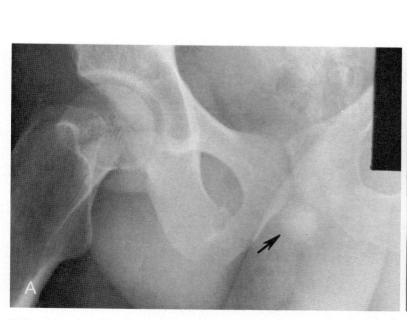

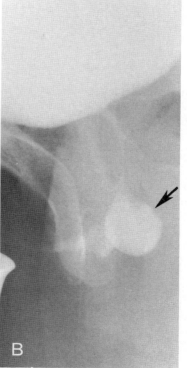

Figure 18.5.   A, A plain film showing a round stone (*arrow*) in the urethral area. **B,** Voiding cystourethrogram showing urethral stone (*arrow*) is present in a diverticulum proximal to a urethral stricture.

Figure 18.6. **A,** Voiding cystourethrogram in a patient who had previous urethroplasty for proximal bulbous urethral stricture. The stricture has recurred and proximal dilatation is present. No biopsy was performed at this time. **B,** The same patient 1 year later. The patient had a perineal mass and fistula. The retrograde urethrogram shows the perineal fistula with a fixed mass producing a scalloped appearance in the bulbous urethra at the site of origin of the fistula. Proven urethral carcinoma. (From McCallum RW, Colapinto V: *Urological Radiology of the Adult Lower Urinary Tract.* Springfield, IL, Charles C Thomas, 1976, p 111.)

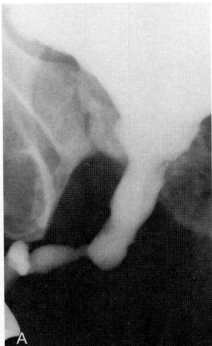
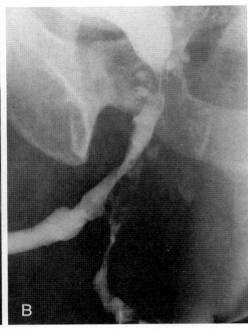

Figure 18.7. **A,** Dynamic retrograde urethrogram showing grossly abnormal cone to proximal bulbous urethra indicating scarring extends into the membranous urethra. Marked reflux of contrast medium into dilated open prostatic ducts indicating previous prostatitis and outlet obstruction. **B,** The same patient voiding. There is marked paradoxical dilatation with increased reflux into the prostatic ducts.

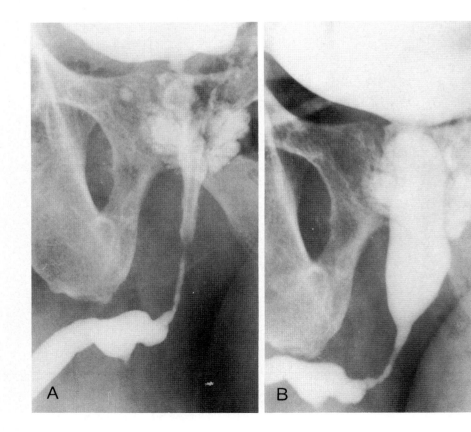

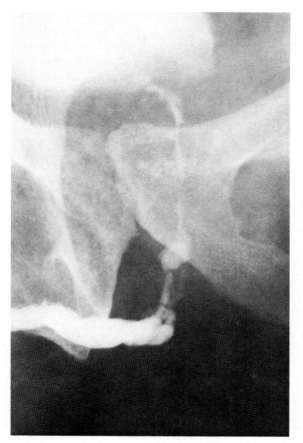

Figure 18.8. Dynamic retrograde urethrogram showing infectious scarring in the bulbous urethra, marked hard scarring in the proximal bulbous urethra, abnormal cone of the proximal bulbous urethra indicating scarring extends into the membranous urethra. By permission. (From Putnam, Putman CE, Ravin CE: *Textbook of Diagnostic Imaging.* Philadelphia, WB Saunders, 1989.)

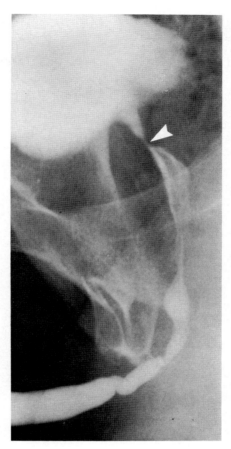

Figure 18.9. Dynamic retrograde urethrogram showing jet of contrast medium (*arrow*) passing into the bladder at the internal sphincter.

contrast medium outlining the hard bulbous scar and the urethral irregularity distal to the hard scar. The contrast medium stream is reduced distal to the scarring. In addition to proximal dilatation, the dynamic retrograde and voiding examination may also indicate other complications of gonococcal urethral stricture. Reflux into prostatic ducts (Fig. 18.7**B**), or Cowper's duct, as well as the development of bladder and urethral diverticula are not uncommon findings. Reflux into the ejaculatory duct, seminal vesicle, and vas deferens is uncommon (Fig. 18.13) as is reflux into a dilated prostatic utricle (Fig. 18.14).

Recent literature has emphasized the use of ultrasound in the assessment of urethral disease. There is no doubt that ultrasound can give adequate information on scarring in the anterior urethra. This procedure is unlikely to indicate bulbous urethral scarring extending into the membranous urethra. The assessment of bulbous urethral scarring extending into the membranous urethra is essential for the urologist in the decision re-

garding operative procedure. Consequently, it would appear that dynamic retrograde urethrography is of more value than ultrasound since the urologist has an excellent indication of the necessity for trans-sphincter urethroplasty.

Tuberculosis

Tuberculous stricture of the urethra is rare without evidence of tuberculous involvement of the prostate. Usually genital tuberculosis is a descending infection and renal tuberculosis is evident, but cases of genital tuberculosis are reported in which the kidneys are normal. These cases are presumed to be blood-borne infection. The prostate is involved in genital tuberculosis in 70% of cases. Prostatic abscess, prostatorectal fistula, and prostatoperineal fistula are all clinical findings in genital tuberculosis. Tuberculous epididymitis, scrotal abscess, fistula, and induration may also be seen with genital tuberculosis, but less than 4% of cases have urethral involvement. Tuberculous prostatic abscess may rupture into the urethra, posteriorly into the rectum, inferiorly into the perineum, or both, producing numerous fistulae and water-

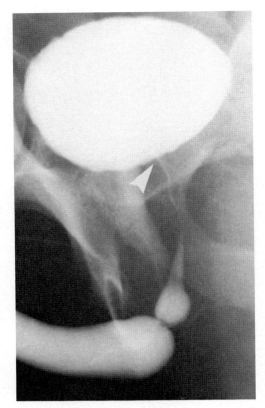

Figure 18.10. The bladder is almost filled by retrograde urethrography. The verumontanum is well visualized and the bladder neck (*arrow*) is closed.

ing can-perineum. Urine examination for *Mycobacterium tuberculosis* may be negative until the discharge from the prostatic abscess ruptures into the urethra. Granulation tissue may affect a localized area of the anterior urethra but may also cause stricturing along the whole of the anterior urethra. Urethral stricture due to unsuspected urethral tuberculosis tends to recur after urethroplasty. *M. tuberculosis* may not be found at stricture biopsy but evidence of old inactive tuberculosis in the lungs should raise the possibility of tuberculous urethral stricture and triple antibiotic therapy should be considered.

Radiology

Dynamic retrograde and voiding cystourethrography may outline an anterior urethral stricture and commonly demonstrates perineal and occasionaly rectourethral fistulae. The retrograde injection of contrast medium may not show the posterior urethra since most of the contrast medium exits via the perineal fistulae. It is then necessary to insert catheters into the perineal fistulae and inject the fistulous catheters and the penile catheter at the same time thus filling the posterior urethra, and bladder (Fig. 18.15). During bladder filling there may be evidence of bladder trabeculation and low-pressure vesicourethral

reflux. Four percent of cases of bladder and ureteric tuberculosis demonstrate reflux. When the bladder is filled, a voiding study can be obtained. Fistulous tracts not seen on the dynamic retrograde urethrogram may be demonstrated. If scrotal abscess or fistula is present, scrotal ultrasound may reveal fluid collections within the tunica vaginalis or epididymal collections of fluid, within a thick-walled cavity. Generally there are echoes within the fluid collections if the abscess contains thick pus.

Schistosomiasis (Bilharziasis)

Schistosomiasis haematobium is the parasite that involves the urinary tract. Bilharziomas form in the bladder and prostate, destroying tissue, and allowing secondary infection, cavitation, and fistulous tract formation. Marked fibrosis occurs and dead ova calcify. This calcification can be seen on plain radiography, particularly in the bladder wall (Fig. 18.16). Urethral stricture is secondary to fistulous tract formation. Strictures most commonly occur in the bulbous urethra. In patients with a fistula lasting more than 4 years, 100% develop urethral stricture.

Iatrogenic Injury

Instrument Strictures in Males

The initial insult to the urethra is pressure necrosis. Pressure necrosis results from the passage of a straight metallic instrument along an S-shaped urethra that is fixed at two points. Fixation points are the penoscrotal junction fixed by the suspensory ligament, and the membranous urethra fixed by the urogenital diaphragm. When a straight metallic instrument is passed along the S-shaped urethra, a fulcrum is created at the inferior aspect of the penoscrotal junction. A second fulcrum is present at the anterior aspect of the bulbomembranous urethra. If the instrument is too large in diameter, pressure necrosis occurs at these fixed points. If the instrument is the correct size, prolonged use of the instrument may cause similar site pressure necrosis. Pressure necrosis involves tissue destruction resulting in scar formation. The anterior urethra is fragile, the mucous membrane consisting of stratified columnar epithelium surrounded by a loose connective tissue stroma. The corpus spongiosum surrounds most of the anterior urethra except the proximal 1.5 cm of the bulbous urethra, the pars nuda, which has only loose connective and fatty tissue anteriorly. Stratified columnar epithelium is also present in the membranous urethra, but the membranous urethra is supported by the intrinsic and external sphincter within the urogenital diaphragm. Consequently, it does not require much pressure to produce necrosis at the fixed points.

The most common instrument producing urethral scarring or stricture is a resectoscope used in trans-

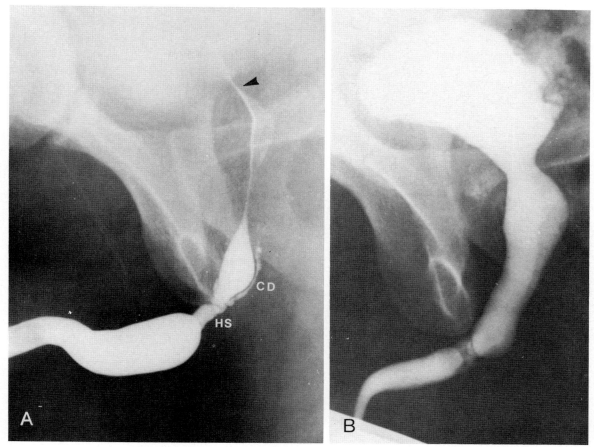

Figure 18.11.   A, Dynamic retrograde urethrogram showing hard scar in mid-bulbous urethra (HS). Contrast medium also outlines Cowper's duct (CD). *Black arrow* indicates closed bladder neck. **B,** The same patient voiding. Note that the bladder neck is open. The urethra is dilated down to the hard scar in the mid bulbous urethra.

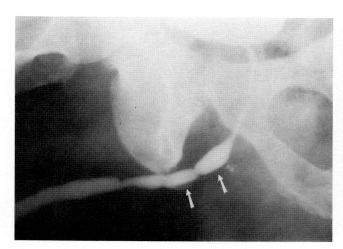

Figure 18.12. Cowper's duct. Multiple strictures indicate previous inflammatory disease. Filling of Cowper's duct (*arrows*) is seen during retrograde urethrography.

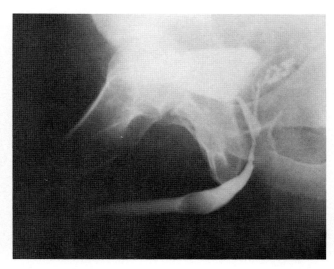

Figure 18.13. Dynamic retrograde urethrogram showing bulbomembranous stricture and reflux into ejaculatory duct, seminal vesicle, and vas deferens.

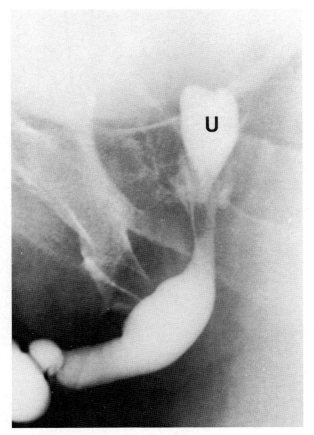

Figure 18.14. Dynamic retrograde urethrogram in a patient with multiple anterior urethral strictures. A dilated prostatic utricle (U) is arising from the verumontanum.

urethral resection for prostatic hypertrophy. The incidence of urethra stricture after transurethral resection of the prostate (TURP) is approximately 4%. Urology centers specializing in urethral disease or trauma to which cases are referred by other centers can have a much higher incidence of postprostatectomy stricture in their published series. Only from such centers with large series can the etiology be suspected by evaluation of the stricture site and length of the stricture. Urethrography has demonstrated that strictures arising from instrumentation are short and well defined and that the vast majority occur in the bulbomembranous region (Fig. 18.17). Less than 20% of instrument strictures occur at the penoscrotal junction (Fig. 18.18).

Catheter Strictures

Indwelling transurethral bladder catheters may cause pressure necrosis at the fixed points of the urethra and almost invariably cause infection if the catheter is left in position for more than a few days. The catheter causes pressure necrosis if it is too large for the urethra or if the catheter is allowed to dangle from the penis, such as drainage into a bag strapped to the lower thigh. Penoscrotal junction pressure necrosis due to catheterization can usually be avoided if the catheter is strapped up the anterior abdominal wall, thus removing the bend at the penoscrotal junction.

Occasionally catheter material (rubber, latex, plastic, Teflon, silicone) may evoke an inflammatory response and superimposed infection, which leads to urethral scarring involving the whole of the urethra.

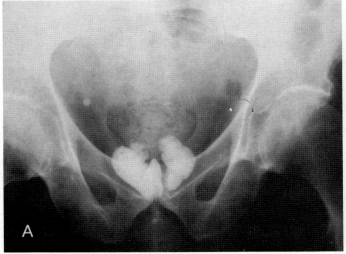

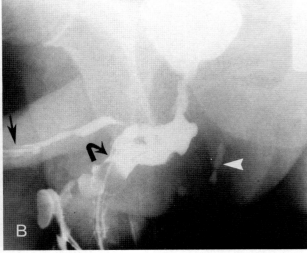

Figure 18.15. **A,** A plain film in a patient with known pulmonary and renal tuberculosis. The prostate gland is almost completely calcified. **B,** Same patient. Dynamic retrograde urethrogram with injection of contrast medium into the catheter (*arrow*) in the fossa navicularis shows a perineal fistula. A second catheter (*curved arrow*) is inserted into the perineal fistula orifice. Injection of both catheters simultaneously outlines a urethro-perineal abscess cavity and scarred urethra. Calcification is seen in the epididymis (*arrowhead*).

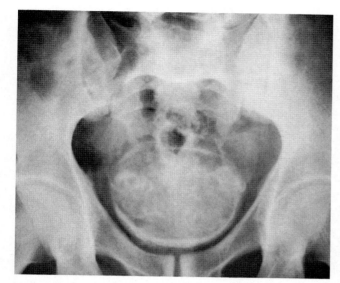

Figure 18.16. Bilharziasis. The bladder wall is markedly calcified. The convoluted calcification seen through the bladder is in the seminal vesicles. There is also faint calcification of a dilated left distal ureter.

Although the primary origin of the catheter stricture is pressure necrosis at the fixed points, superimposed infection spreads along the urethra involving the glands of Littre, and can cause an almost continuous inflammatory reaction in the submucosa for several centimeters on both sides of the original area of pressure necrosis. On

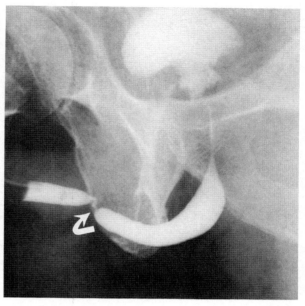

Figure 18.18. Instrument stricture: post-TURP. Dynamic retrograde urethrogram shows a short tight instrument stricture (*arrow*) at the penoscrotal junction. Note resected prostatic bed. The cone of the bulbous urethra is elongated and narrowed suggesting bulbomembranous urethral scarring.

urethrography, catheter strictures are therefore usually long and irregular, often with visualization of the glands of Littre (Figs. 18.19 and 18.20). Seventy to 80% of catheter strictures affect the penoscrotal junction alone, and 95% of catheter strictures are several centimeters long and irregular in outline. Catheter strictures affecting the bulbomembranous urethra cause distortion, irregularity,

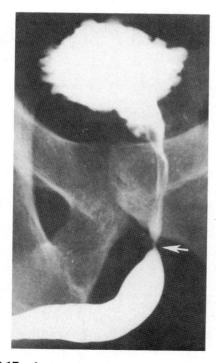

Figure 18.17. Instrument stricture: post-TURP. Dynamic retrograde urethrogram shows a short tight instrument stricture (*arrow*) in the bulbous urethra.

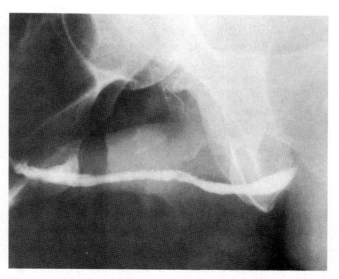

Figure 18.19. Catheter stricture: dynamic retrograde urethrogram 1 year following abdominal operation requiring 7 days of bladder catheterization. The penile and distal bulbous urethra is markedly narrowed and irregular—most marked at the penoscrotal junction. Glands of Littre are visualized.

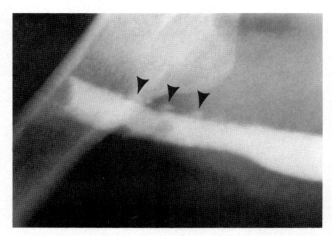

Figure 18.20.   Glands of Littre. A retrograde urethrogram was performed for evaluation of strictures. Glands of Littre are opacified (*arrowheads*) in the anterior urethra.

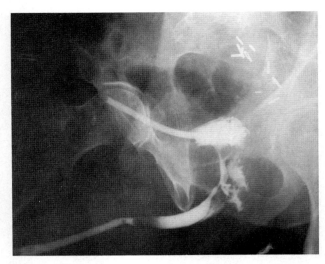

Figure 18.21.   Post-abdominoperineal resection for carcinoma of the rectum. The patient had severe pain on micturition and retention. A suprapubic catheter was inserted. Dynamic retrograde urethrogram shows extravasation of contrast medium due to a tear in the membranous urethra which occurred at the pull-through part of the abdomino-perineal resection. (From McCallum RW, Rogers JM, Alexander MW: The radiologic assessment of iatrogenic urethral injury. *J Can Assoc Radiol* 36:122, 1985.)

elongation, and asymmetry of the cone of the proximal bulbous urethra. The glands of Littre are not visualized since they are sparse proximal to the sump of the bulbous urethra. In approximately 10% of patients with catheter strictures, combined penoscrotal and bulbomembranous strictures are present. Approximately 12% of patients who have had coronary artery bypass surgery develop urethral strictures from bladder catheterization.

Abdominoperineal Resection

Abdominoperineal resection may result in a bulbomembranous urethral tear at the time of the perineal or pull-through part of the operation (Fig. 18.21). The close proximity of the anterior rectal wall and the membranous urethra contributes to this complication. This complication is unusual. It begins as a bulbomembranous urethral tear that creates a urethral fistula. Suprapubic drainage is required for closing of the fistula, which results in a bulbomembranous urethral stricture.

Special Considerations in Bulbomembranous Urethral Stricture

Pressure necrosis in the bulbomembranous urethra usually affects the mucosa and submucosa resulting in stricture. If the pressure necrosis is prolonged, necrosis may extend deeper than the submucosa and may compromise the passive function of the intrinsic sphincter. If the internal sphincter has been ablated, as occurs in prostatectomy, impairment of the function of the intrinsic sphincter by pressure necrosis may result in some degree of urinary incontinence. Urinary incontinence after transurethral prostatectomy occurs in less than 4% of prostatectomy patients and is the result of ablation of the internal sphincter at the bladder neck and damage to the distal sphincter mechanism. A second important consid-

eration in postprostatectomy bulbomembranous strictures is the possibility of producing incontinence when an attempt is made to surgically correct the bulbomembranous stricture. Ten to 12% of continent postprostatectomy patients with bulbomembranous urethral stricture are incontinent as a result of surgery to correct the bulbomembranous stricture.

Management of Urethral Stricture

All urethral stricture patients are assessed by dynamic retrograde and voiding urethrography and urethroscopy. Anterior urethral strictures that are present 1.5 cm or more below the urogenital diaphragm do not require surgical intervention involving the distal sphincters. Urethral stricture repair may be managed by internal visual urethrotomy, which consists of incising the stricture with a urethrotome under direct visualization or urethroplasty. Anterior urethroplasty is used to repair a stricture that is distal to 1.5 cm below the urogenital diaphragm. A patch or pedicle penile skin graft is the usual method. Posterior or transphincter urethroplasty is used to repair a bulbomembranous urethral stricture and is a surgical procedure not to be taken lightly since it involves cutting the distal sphincters at the site of the stricture. A scrotal skin flap to make a new urethra from the verumontanum to 2 cm into healthy urethra distal to the stricture is required. Both anterior and posterior urethroplasty may be done as a one- or two-stage procedure. Posturethroplasty urethrography follow-up for 1 year delineates the success of the operative procedure.

Urethral stricture may also be treated by balloon dilatation. Three methods are described.

1. Direct passage of the balloon catheter through the stricture with dilatation of the balloon in the stricture area. This can only be done in soft strictures or hard strictures that are not too tight to allow passage of the balloon (Fig. 18.22**A**–**C**).
2. More commonly a guidewire has to be passed through the stricture into the bladder. Over the guide-wire the balloon catheter is passed through the stricture and the balloon dilated in the stricture area.

3. Impassable strictures causing almost total obstruction are initially treated by a suprapubic cystostomy tube. The urethral stricture is approached suprapubically. A guidewire is passed through the suprapubic orifice into the bladder neck and down through the urethral stricture and out the external meatus. With the guide wire fixed at both ends, the balloon catheter is passed per urethra over the guide wire to the strictured area and the balloon is dilated (Fig. 18.23**A**–**D**).

Balloon dilatation in all three approaches may require several attempts. The balloon should be dilated and held in position for several minutes until the "waist defect" in the balloon produced by the stricture is obliterated.

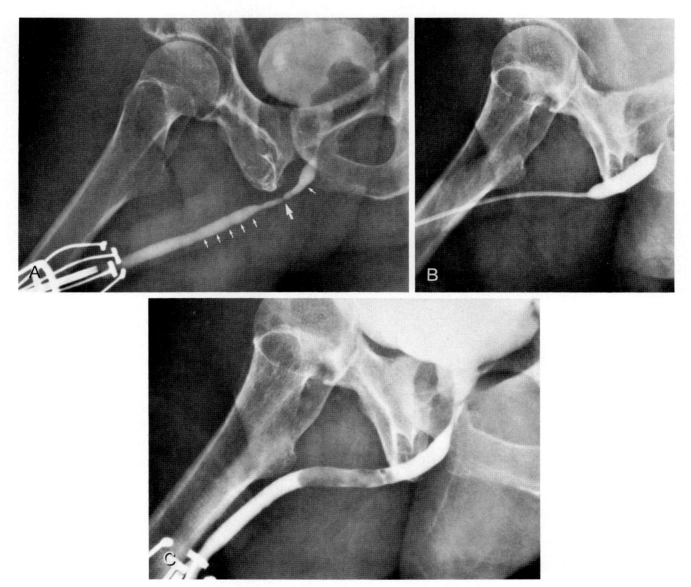

Figure 18.22.   **A,** Dynamic retrograde urethrogram done using a Brodny clamp. Severe scarring is seen in the bulbous urethra (*big arrow*). Lesser softer scarring is present both proximal and distal to the hard scar. **B,** A balloon catheter has been inserted into the stricture area, and the balloon inflated with dilute contrast medium. **C,** Postdilatation urethrogram showing stricture is dilated to a normal urethral caliber. (From Russinovich NAE, Lloyd LK, Griggs WP, et al: Impassable urethral strictures: Percutaneous transvesical catheterization and balloon dilatation. *Radiology* 2:33, 1980.)

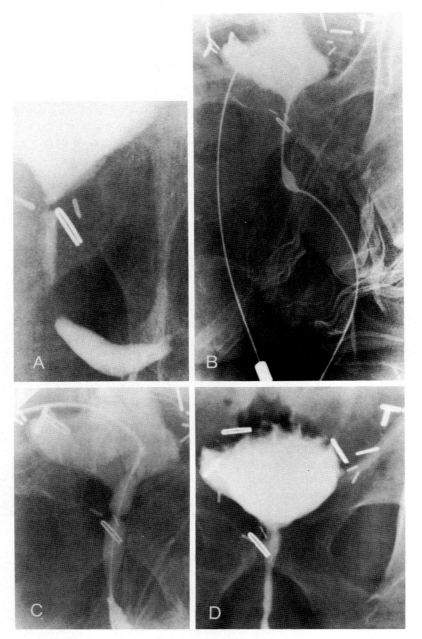

Figure 18.23. **A,** A voiding cystourethrogram in a patient after total suprapubic prostatectomy. A tight stricture has developed at the anastomosis of the cut bladder ends and the membranous urethra. This stricture is impassable from below. **B,** Via a suprapubic cystostomy tube a guidewire is passed through the stricture and extends from the external urethral orifice. **C,** The balloon catheter is then passed over the guidewire to the strictured area, and the balloon is inflated with contrast medium.

Note the waist in the balloon at the stricture site. The balloon may require several deflations and inflations until the waist disappears. (From Scales FE, Katzen BT, van Breda A, et al: Impassable urethral strictures: Percutaneous transvesical catheterization and balloon dilatation. *Radiology* 157:59, 1985.) **D,** Postdilatation voiding cystourethrogram showing marked improvement in the caliber of the urethra at the stricture site.

URETHRAL TUMORS

Benign Tumors

Benign tumors of the urethra are rare. They may have a mesenchymal or epithelial origin.

Epithelial Origin

Three types of epithelial cells make up the mucosa of the urethra. Transitional cell epithelium lines the prostatic urethra to the membranous urethra where it changes to pseudostratified tall columnar epithelium. This type continues from the membranous throughout the bulbous and penile urethra to the fossa navicularis where it becomes stratified squamous epithelium. However, there may be rests of squamous or transitional epithelium throughout the bulbous and penile urethra.

Transitional cell papilloma (papillary adenoma) is the most common benign tumor in the prostatic urethra. It arises from the transitional cell epithelium, has a vascular stroma, and is difficult to identify radiographically at the time of presentation. Clinically it presents with hematuria, nocturia, and stream reduction in elderly males and is diagnosed by urethroscopy. It is seen as a sessile polyp with multiple papillary outgrowths. The lesion is not associated with multifocal origin or malignant change, and recurrence is unlikely after urethroscopic resection.

Adenomatous tumors in the prostatic urethra arise from the prostatic epithelium and project into the prostatic urethra. They commonly have a sessile base but may be polypoid or papillary. There is a covering of transitional cell epithelium, but this benign tumor consists mainly of tall columnar epithelium with a fibromuscular stroma. Immunohistologic techniques are positive for prostatic acid phosphatase and specific prostatic epithelial antigen. This lesion usually presents with hematuria or hematospermia and may be identified on cystourethrography. The lesion occurs below the verumontanum and consequently is not associated with prostatic hyperplasia. Recurrence is rare after resection. Although considered a benign lesion, adenocarcinoma within an adenomatous polyp has been reported.

Adenomatoid metaplasia (nephrogenic adenoma, nephrogenic metaplasia) is rare and is more common in the bladder than in the urethra. It may be present only in the prostatic urethra and is found in elderly men who have had a previous history of bladder or urethral trauma or previous bladder, prostatic, or urethral surgery. Lesions are small, 5 mm or less, and may be multiple. Histologically there is metaplastic urothelium and the presence of metaplastic tubules that resemble renal tubules accounting for the inclusion of "nephrogenic" in the variety of names given to this lesion. These small lesions are friable and present with gross hematuria. Diagnosis is by urethroscopy, although a slightly irregular appearance to the prostatic urethra may be seen on cystourethrography.

Papillary urethritis (polypoid urethritis) in the prostatic urethra is an inflammatory reaction resulting in transitional cell proliferation, ectatic capillaries, and edema, producing multiple small cystic strictures similar to ureteritis cystica. Clinically the ectatic capillaries bleed, producing hematuria, which is the most common presentation. There may be a reduction in the urinary stream. Urethroscopy may show an irregular appearance to the prostatic urethra similar to the appearance of adenomatoid metaplasia and inflammatory polyps.

Inflammatory polyps in the anterior urethra are the result of previous urethral infection or previous urethral

surgery for stricture. They are usually symptomless but may increase in size to over 1 cm, when they may produce stream reduction. They may be diagnosed by urethrography (Fig. 18.24) or urethroscopy.

Squamous cell papillomas occur in younger men and present at the urethral meatus. These lesions recur after surgical excision and malignant change has been reported. Squamous cell papillomas arising elsewhere in the urethra arise from squamous cell rests amid the columnar epithelium.

Transitional cell papillomas are extremely rare in the anterior urethra and arise either due to metaplasia of the columnar epithelium due to chronic infection, or they may arise within rests of transitional cells amid the columnar epithelium.

Mesenchymal Tumors

Fibrous polyps are congenital lesions arising in the prostatic urethra. The polyp may protrude into the bladder when resting and may prolapse as far as the membranous or bulbous urethra on voiding (Fig. 18.25). The growth of fibrous polyps commonly gives rise to intermittent obstructive symptoms and is found in the male pediatric age group; it has not been reported in females. There may be frequency and dysuria and occasional mi-

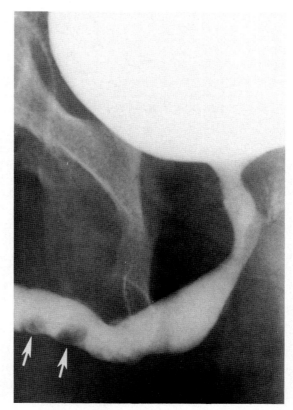

Figure 18.24.   Voiding cystourethrogram showing inflammatory polyps (*arrows*) in the anterior urethra following urethroplasty for gonococcal stricture.

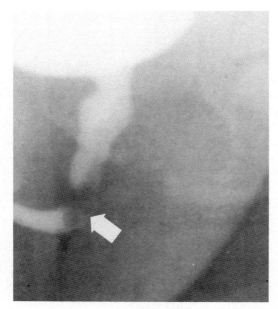

Figure 18.25. Voiding cystourethrogram in a child with difficulty in micturition. The filling defect in the bulbomembranous urethra is a fibrous polyp (*arrow*) on a stalk arising from the verumontanum. (Courtesy of Dr. R. Lebowitz. From Pollack HM ed: *Clinical Urography.* vol 2 Philadelphia, WB Saunders, 1990, p. 1404.

crohematuria accompanying intermittent obstructive symptoms. The lesion is easily demonstrated by dynamic retrograde and voiding cystourethrography. Transurethral resection is the treatment. Lesions do not recur.

Hemangioma and myoblastoma are exceedingly rare but have been reported.

Tumor-like Lesions

Amyloidosis of the urethra is characterized by penile bleeding and a palpable hard mass along the ventral surface of the penile or bulbous urethra and consequently may be confused clinically with carcinoma of the urethra. Fewer than 25 cases have been reported and most have occurred in men under 50 years of age. Amyloidosis should always be considered in any young male presenting with penile bleeding and a palpable mass without previous urethral disease or trauma. Urethrography shows an irregular narrowed anterior urethra that may be indistinguishable from infective urethral stricture, but glands of Littre are not visualized in amyloidosis. On urethrography it cannot be distinguished from a metastasis to the corpus spongiosum.

Condylomata acuminata (venereal warts) is a viral infection that usually produces sessile squamous papillomas on the glans penis and prepuce that may extend to the perineum. Occasionally these warts spread along the urethra (Fig. 18.26) and even reach the bladder. Urethral involvement is a serious complication and may require numerous treatment sessions with the instillation of po-

dophyllin, thiotepa, or 5-fluorouracil into the urethra. If urethral involvement is suspected clinically, the patient should not have any urethral instrumentation or catheterization because of the possibility of retrograde seeding. Retrograde urethrography should not be done for the same reason. The diagnostic procedure of choice is voiding cystourethrography at the end of excretory urography (excretory voiding urethrography). The urethrographic study shows a characteristic appearance of multiple frond-like papillary filling defects if the whole urethra is involved. Occasionally only isolated filling defects are seen in the penile urethra.

Sarcoidosis rarely affects the lower urinary tract. It has been reported in the female urethra and simulates urethral carcinoma. Biopsy is diagnostic.

Balanitis xerotica obliterans (BXO) is rare and affects the glans penis, prepuce, and urethral meatus. The lesion is seen as white, dry, hyperkeratotic plaques. Rarely BXO extends into the anterior urethra and may cause pain on micturition. It may be premalignant and associated with squamous cell carcinoma.

Malignant Tumors

Malignant tumors of the urethra are rare and are almost all of epithelial origin. Leiomyosarcoma, malignant melanoma, and urethral metastases have been reported but are exceedingly rare. Malignant urethral tumors are twice as common in the female urethra than in the male urethra. The most common urethral carcinomas are squamous cell carcinoma and transitional cell carcinoma. Adenocarcinoma is rare and arises from Skene's glands in the female and from Cowper's gland or ducts or glands of Littre in the male. In both men and women, carcinoma of the urethra usually occurs over the age of 50 years.

Carcinoma of the Male Urethra

Almost 80% of male urethral carcinomas are squamous cell and 60% occur in the bulbomembranous region. Fifteen percent are transitional cell carcinoma. The remainder are adenocarcinoma or undifferentiated carcinoma. Approximately 6% occur in the prostatic urethra, and the remainder occur in the anterior urethra or bulbomembranous region. Fewer than 500 cases of urethral carcinoma in males have been reported.

Squamous Cell Carcinoma

Squamous cell carcinoma is associated with previous urethral stricture in between 35 and 76% of cases. Chronic irritation producing squamous metaplasia adjacent to a urethral stricture is common and therefore the tumor is seen most often in the bulbomembranous region. Approximately 50% are associated with urethral stricture due to previous external or iatrogenic trauma.

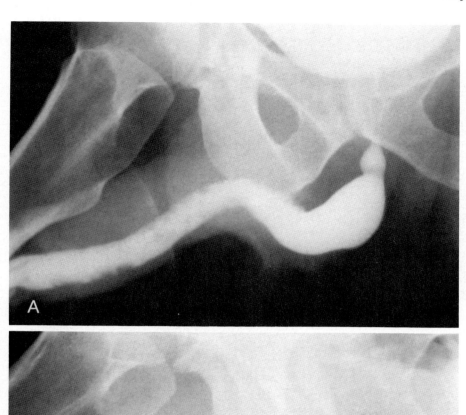

Figure 18.26. Condylomata acuminata. **A,** Multiple filling defects are seen in the anterior urethra. **B,** After treatment with podophyllin, there is complete clearing of the urethra.

Consequently, any condition that may result in urethral stricture should be considered a predisposing factor to squamous cell carcinoma. These include gonococcal urethritis, bladder catheterization, and urethral trauma. The diagnosis is often difficult and unsuspected. Recurrent stricture after urethroplasty, excess bleeding after stricture dilatation, or the development of perineal fistula or a palpable hard mass in the bulbar region are all clues to the development of squamous cell carcinoma (Fig. 18.27). The incidence of squamous cell carcinoma after successful urethroplasty for stricture is low. Only five such cases have been reported. Successful urethroplasty appears to reduce the incidence of squamous cell carci-

noma of the urethra. However, urethroplasty with recurrent stricture should invoke biopsy of the recurrent strictured area to exclude carcinoma.

Spontaneous squamous cell carcinoma occurs in patients without previous history of urethral disease or trauma and is thought to arise in rests of squamous cell epithelium within the normal stratified columnar epithelium. Columnar epithelium changes to stratified squamous epithelium in the glans penis and spontaneous squamous cell carcinoma may also occur in this site and usually protrudes from the external meatus. Spontaneous squamous cell carcinoma accounts for approximately 20% of male urethral squamous cell carcinomas.

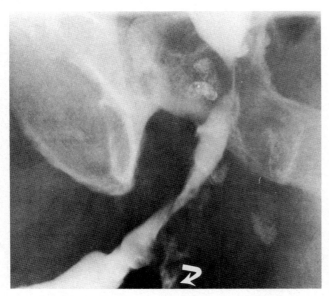

Figure 18.27. Biopsy-proven squamous cell carcinoma of the bulbous urethra, which developed after urethroplasty for recurrent bulbous urethral stricture. A mass effect is seen in the bulbous urethra and contrast medium is seen in a perineal fistula (*arrow*). Numerous opacified lymph nodes are seen due to previous lymphography. (Adapted from McCallum RW, Colapinto V: *Urological Radiology of the Adult Male Lower Urinary Tract.* Springfield, IL, Charles C Thomas, 1976.)

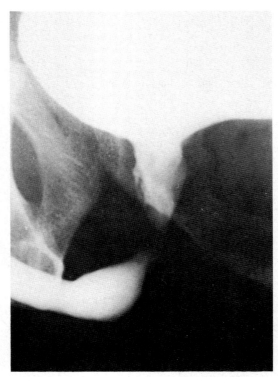

Figure 18.28. Spontaneous transitional cell carcinoma in the prostatic urethra causing gross hematuria in a 55-year-old man. The remainder of the urinary tract was free of transitional cell carcinoma. (From Pollack HM (ed): *Clinical Urography,* Philadelphia, WB Saunders, 1990, Vol 2, p 1408.)

Spontaneous transitional cell carcinoma is found in the prostatic urethra where over 60% of transitional cell carcinomas of the urethra occur (Fig. 18.28). The multicentric origin of transitional cell carcinoma in the urinary tract may account for some prostatic urethral transitional cell carcinomas. Seeding of malignant transitional cells from elsewhere in the urinary tract to the prostatic urethra, especially by instrumentation, may be an etiologic factor. Radiation therapy for carcinoma of the prostate has been noted as an etiologic factor in transitional cell carcinoma of the proximal bulbous urethra.

Transitional cell carcinoma of the anterior urethra has been associated with carcinoma of the bladder (Fig. 18.29). Patients having cystectomy for carcinoma of the bladder may develop transitional cell carcinoma of the anterior urethra. Total cystectomy involves removal of the bladder, prostate, and prostatic urethra. Urethral carcinomas may present with obstructive symptoms, serosanguineous discharge, perineal fistula, periurethral abscess, or palpable mass in the perineum or along the shaft of the urethra. Obstructive symptoms are the commonest presentation, occurring in approximately 60% of patients.

Based on prognosis and treatment, carcinoma of the urethra can be classified into two groups. Group 1 is carcinoma involving most of the anterior urethra up to the distal bulbous urethra. Group 2 patients have carcinoma of the posterior urethra and proximal bulbous urethra. Patients with group 1 lesions present earlier, within 1 year, and seldom present with the complications of periurethral abscess or perineal fistula. Treatment with penectomy and radiotherapy results in a 5-year survival

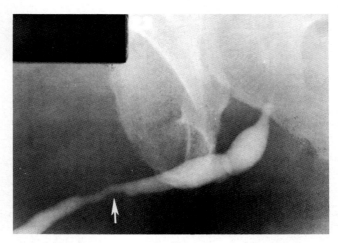

Figure 18.29. Transitional cell carcinoma of the anterior urethra producing irregular narrowing (*arrow*). This patient had cystectomy 1 year previously for transitional cell carcinoma of the bladder. (From Pollack HM (ed): *Clinical Urography.* Philadelphia, WB Saunders, 1990, Vol 2, p 1409.)

rate of 43%. Group 2 patients present later, approximately 18 months after the onset of symptoms, and have a poor prognosis. The 5-year survival rate of group 2 lesions is 14%. Untreated patients with carcinoma of the urethra survive only 3 months after presentation.

Adenocarcinoma of the midurethra is rare. It may arise from the ducts or glands of Littre or Cowper's glands. Adenocarcinoma presents with hematuria, partial outlet obstruction, penile or perineal mass, and filling defects or scar in the urethra on urethrography.

Metastatic Tumors to the Male Urethra

Bladder transitional cell carcinoma may be spread to the anterior urethra by seeding in patients having urethral instrumentation or at the time of cystectomy. Contiguous spread of carcinoma of the prostate (Fig. 18.30), rectum, spermatic cord, and testes may involve the corpus spongiosum causing extensive urethral narrowing and filling defects. Erosion into the urethra from metastases to the corpus spongiosum (Fig. 18.31) may produce some degree of obstruction or urethral bleeding. Blood-

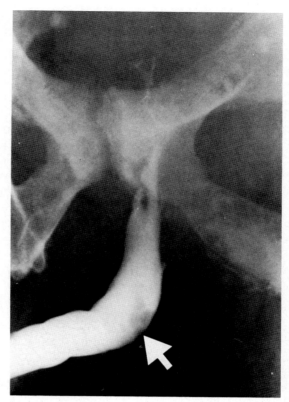

Figure 18.31. Carcinoma of the prostate metastasizing to bones and corpus spongiosum producing an irregular filling defect (*arrow*) in the bulbous urethra.

borne metastases to the corpora cavernosa and corpus spongiosum are exceedingly rare, but a metastasis to the corpus spongiosum from renal cell carcinoma has been reported.

Malignant Tumors of the Female Urethra

Although twice as common as male urethral carcinoma, carcinoma of the female urethra is still a rare condition and accounts for less than 1% of genitoururinary malignancies. Ninety-two percent of female malignant urethral tumors are carcinomas, of which 74% are squamous cell carcinoma and 16% are adenocarcinoma. The remainder are transitional cell carcinomas or undifferentiated carcinoma. Mucinous adenocarcinoma has been reported. Eight percent of female urethral malignant tumors are sarcomas or malignant melanomas. Carcinoma of the female urethra has been recorded in patients between 30 and 90 years of age and 75% of patients come for treatment after 50 years of age.

The etiology of female urethral carcinomas remains controversial, but previous urethral infection, urethral trauma, and urethral caruncle may be predisposing factors. Approximately 2.5% of patients with urethral caruncle have an associated carcinoma. Female urethral diver-

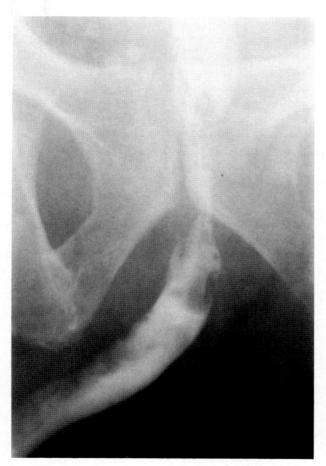

Figure 18.30. Contiguous spread of carcinoma of prostate into urethra. Multiple filling defects are appreciated in the bulbous and membranous portions of the urethra.

ticula may contain carcinoma as well as stones. The female urethral mucosa consists of transitional cells in the proximal third of the urethra. Squamous epithelium is present in the distal two-thirds. Carcinomas presenting in the distal one-third of the urethra are classified as "anterior" urethral tumors and are usually low-grade tumors with early presentation and good prognosis. Tumors involving the proximal two-thirds of the urethra are classified as "entire" urethral tumors and are of more advanced grade, become apparent later, and have a less favorable prognosis (Fig. 18.32). Clinically "anterior" urethral tumors present with a mass projecting from the urethral orifice, urethral bleeding, dysuria, and frequency. "Entire" urethral tumors may have a similar presentation early in the course of the disease but may not present until urinary retention, urethral abscess, or urethrovaginal fistula have developed. Urethral and pelvic pain are late and uncommon presentations.

URINARY INCONTINENCE

Urinary continence is passive or active. Passive continence is the maintenance of urine within the bladder without conscious effort and is controlled by the two smooth muscle sphincters—the internal sphincter at the bladder neck and the intrinsic sphincter around the distal prostatic and membranous urethra. Active continence is a conscious effort to interrupt or inhibit micturition and is

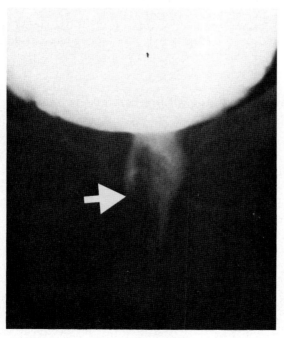

Figure 18.32. A voiding cystourethrogram in a female complaining of dysuria and poor urinary stream. The filling defect in the proximal urethra (*arrow*) represents transitional cell carcinoma. (From Pollack HM (ed): *Clinical Urography.* Philadelphia, WB Saunders, 1990, Vol 2, p 1411.)

controlled by the external (striated muscle) sphincter and by the levator ani and pelvic floor muscles. Active continence can only be maintained for a few minutes at a time. Under certain circumstances the urge to void can be inhibited by an active effort lasting seconds or minutes. It is assumed that electrical impulses pass from the external sphincter to the intrinsic and internal sphincters so that inhibition becomes passive after a few minutes. The internal sphincter at the bladder neck is the primary muscle of passive continence. When damage occurs to the internal sphincter, such as may occur in external trauma or in transurethral prostatectomy (which ablates the internal sphincter), urinary continence is passively maintained by the intrinsic sphincter. Damage to both the internal and intrinsic sphincters will result in urinary incontinence.

Males

The clinical assessment of male urinary incontinence is classified into three grades. In grade 1 or stress incontinence, the patient is continent in the upright or supine position but dribbling incontinence occurs on increased intraabdominal pressure. There are several degrees of stress incontinence from a few drops of urine to a significant stream on increased intraabdominal pressure. Grade 2 or moderate incontinence occurs when there is persistent dribbling in the upright position but no dribbling in the supine position. This is usually accompanied by stress incontinence when the persistent dribbling stream is increased by increased intraabdominal pressure such as straining or coughing. Grade 3 or total incontinence occurs when there is complete loss of function of the smooth muscle sphincters resulting in a continual flow of urine in any position.

In normal man the detrusor muscle is activated by the parasympathetic (pelvic) nerves and the smooth muscle sphincters are activated by the sympathetic (hypogastric) nerves. The external striated muscle sphincter, levator ani, and pelvic floor muscles are controlled by somatic (pudendal) nerves. Reciprocity occurs between the parasympathetic and sympathetic activity so that with detrusor contraction the sphincters relax reciprocally, and the reverse reciprocity occurs at the end of micturition, with contraction of the sphincters and relaxation of the detrusor. Passive continence is therefore controlled by the autonomic sympathetic system. Active continence is controlled by the somatic voluntary nerves.

Incontinence Due to Urethral Injury in Pelvic Fracture

The urethral injury in pelvic fracture commonly occurs in the bulbomembranous region and may disrupt the intrinsic and external sphincters. In these patients the internal sphincter is usually undamaged and passive continence can be maintained. The incidence of incontinence after primary repair for urethral injury in pelvic fracture approximates 30% although the internal sphincter is not damaged by the pelvic fracture. This incidence is reduced to 2% if delayed repair is the elected treatment. Occasionally the pelvic fracture injury is severe enough to damage both the bladder neck and the bulbomembranous region in which case both smooth muscle sphincters are damaged and urinary incontinence will result. However, this is a rare injury. More commonly the bladder neck is not injured and therefore the internal sphincter is intact.

After successful primary or delayed repair of Type II or III urethral injury the patient remains continent because of an intact undamaged internal sphincter. However, if in later years the patient requires prostatectomy, the possibility of urinary incontinence is high since the intrinsic sphincter has been damaged by the pelvic fracture injury or cut intraoperatively at urethroplasty, and the internal sphincter is ablated by the prostatectomy.

Urinary Incontinence After Prostatectomy

Suprapubic, retropubic, and transurethral prostatectomy all ablate the internal sphincter at the bladder neck. If the suprapubic or retropubic prostatectomy is total, the distal sphincters may also be damaged resulting in incontinence. After transurethral prostatectomy, urinary incontinence is uncommon. It occurs when the internal sphincter is ablated by the prostatectomy and the distal sphincters are damaged. Damage to the intrinsic sphincter occurs by pressure necrosis either due to the resectoscope being too large or the resection taking a long time. If pressure necrosis is slight and only affects the mucosa, bulbomembranous urethral stricture will occur. If pressure necrosis is more severe and deeper than the mucosa the intrinsic sphincter may suffer varying degrees of damage. The external sphincter is rarely damaged, but the nerve supply to the external sphincter and pelvic floor muscles may be damaged resulting in some degree of loss of function of these muscles and consequently loss of reflex inhibition of stress incontinence on suddenly increased intraabdominal pressure.

Urinary Incontinence in Neurogenic Bladder

Lower motor neuron lesions producing neurogenic bladder have an interrupted micturition reflex arc. Without bladder training and good management, the bladder becomes dilated and flaccid. Overflow incontinence is common in these patients but is usually intermittent since there is still intact sympathetic activity affecting the smooth muscle sphincters. In upper motor neuron lesions the micturition reflex arc is intact and detrusor activity is still present. The normal recriprocity between parasympathetic and sympathetic nerves is absent and sphincter dyssynergia is present. Detrusor contraction is readily stimulated by touching or pressure on the lower abdomen or penis and urine flow may be produced. Overflow incontinence in upper motor neuron lesions is therefore uncommon.

Radiology

A radiologic method of assessing male urinary incontinence has been described as an adjunct to the clinical assessment and to provide a visual record of the dynamics of urinary incontinence. The method uses the Foley catheter for dynamic retrograde urethrography and bladder filling through the same catheter. On removal of the catheter a sequence of four antegrade films are obtained in clinical grade 1 or 2 incontinence. The dynamic retrograde study is obtained to assess the urethra for diverticulum and urethral stricture. Anterior urethral diverticulum may be a cause of postmicturition incontinence. Postprostatectomy incontinence shows an abnormal cone to the proximal bulbous urethra indicating stricture in the bulbomembranous region. After bladder filling, films are obtained upright, "resting," "coughing," "voiding," and stop voiding.

In stress incontinence no contrast medium passes through the membranous urethra until the coughing film. In moderate grade 2 incontinence there is a continual trickle of contrast medium through the membranous urethra at rest. This trickle is increased by coughing. The voiding study shows an increased stream and the stop voiding study delineates interruption of micturition.

In total grade 3 incontinence only three antegrade films are required. At rest the patient with total incontinence shows a voiding stream throughout the whole urethra. Asking the patient to void may show slight increase in the stream but this may not be significant. A stop voiding film demonstrates the ability to interrupt micturition.

Almost all men with postprostatectomy incontinence are able to interrupt micturition voluntarily. However, there is some damage to the somatic nerve supply since the reflex contraction of the external sphincter and pelvic floor muscles on increased intraabdominal pressure is inhibited allowing stress incontinence.

Management of Urinary Incontinence

The fact that there are so many operative procedures available for male urinary incontinence is evidence that none is totally satisfactory. Tendinous and Marlix slings, the Kaufman balloon, and numerous artificial sphincters all have been used and each has shown success in some cases. However, there is no definitive mechanism for urinary incontinence that is trouble free and effective.

Females

Stress incontinence in females is not uncommon and is usually the result of difficult childbirth or aging. It is commonly associated with a cystocele. Stress incontinence must be distinguished from urge incontinence clinically. The intrinsic bladder pressure in the normal woman does not increase significantly during bladder filling, coughing, or change of posture. Bladder intrinsic pressure only increases during voiding. In stress incontinence, bladder pressure readings are similar to normal on bladder filling, but coughing or the erect position produce urine leakage. Urge incontinence is the result of an unstable bladder of non-neurogenic origin when the urge to void is felt strongly on bladder filling, change of posture, or the erect position.

The best method of assessing stress incontinence in females is a urodynamic study. However, the bead chain method is still of value to prove a tendency to stress incontinence, and according to Green's classification, it indicates the type of operative procedure that is necessary. The bead chain method consists of the insertion of a metal bead chain into the bladder via a metal adaptor, leaving much of the bead chain within the urethra. The posterior vesicourethral angle and the anterior angle of inclination (angle between the urethra and the vertical) can be measured at rest and on straining. A Green Type 1 deformity is a posterior vesicourethral angle of over 100° with a normal (less than 30°) anterior angle of inclination. Green Type 2 deformity occurs when both angles are abnormally increased. Green Type 1 deformities are usually repaired per vagina. Green Type 2 deformities usually require a suprapubic approach and a Marshall-Marchetti type of sling to lengthen the urethra and elevate the bladder base.

Urethral Diverticulum

Urethral diverticulum in females may be more common than has been suspected. It should be excluded in patients with a diagnosis of urethral syndrome. At present it is considered acquired and originates in periurethral glands. Mild urinary incontinence, frequency dysuria, and dyspareunia are presenting symptoms. Urethral diverticulum is best demonstrated by the double-balloon catheter method (Figs. 18.33 and 18.34). A diverticulum may also be visualized on a voiding cystourethrogram (Fig. 18.35). This method may require cine or video recording for accurate assessment.

PENIS

Benign and malignant lesions of the penis are readily visible and may be diagnosed clinically. These include adenomas, polyps, condylomata acuminata, chancres, melanomas, basal cell carcinomas, and squamous cell carcinomas. Radiology makes little or no contribution to the diagnosis of these lesions. However, radiology procedures in the form of radiography, penile arteriography, cavernosography, and Doppler examinations are useful in the investigation of organic impotence, Peyronie's disease, and trauma.

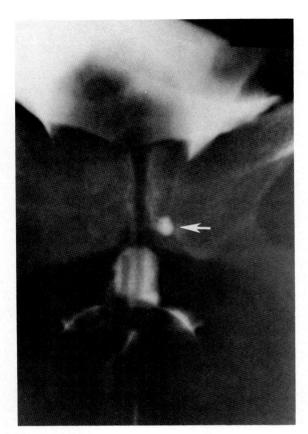

Figure 18.33.   Double-balloon catheter method for visualization of a female urethral diverticulum. There is no opening in the distal end of the catheter. The hole in the catheter is between the balloons. The inner balloon is pulled against the bladder neck and the outer balloon is against the urethral orifice. Injection of contrast medium shows a small diverticulum (*arrow*) on the left of the urethra.

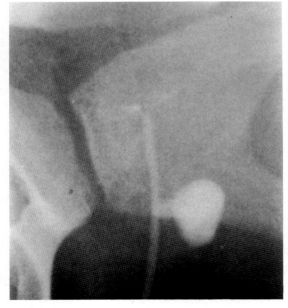

Figure 18.34.   Urethral diverticulum. Contrast is opacifying the lumen of a double-balloon catheter. The diverticulum is clearly seen in this oblique projection.

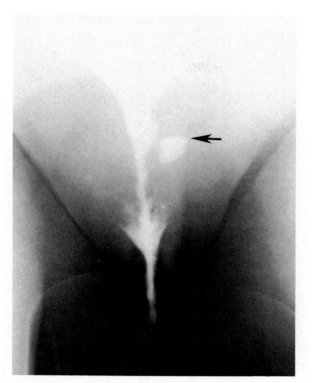

Figure 18.35. A voiding cystourethrogram showing a fluid level (*arrow*) in a diverticulum to the left of the urethra.

forators and transverse root communicators were the most common variations and unilateral or bilateral accessory cavernosal branches were also common. Numerous intrapenile arterial communications are also demonstrated that may act as collateral pathways in patients with intrapenile arterial obstructive disease.

Cavernosography and cavernosometry have recently been shown to be of value in the evaluation of impotence. The method involves the injection of contrast material directly into the corpus cavernosum (Chapter 3). Only one side is injected as the septum between the corpora is fenestrated and both corpora will fill (Fig. 18.36). If pressures are measured, a second needle is used to infuse saline after the injection of papaverine.

Duplex sonography has also been employed in the diagnosis of vasculogenic impotence. A penile-brachial index, the ratio of systolic penile and brachial pressures, can be measured by Doppler techniques and is used to screen for arteriogenic impotence. However, this index does not appear to be as accurate as the intracorporeal injection of papaverine. Evaluation of the diastolic waveform may prove to be useful as an indicator of the veno-occlusive mechanism within the penis. However, more work is needed to define the role of these techniques in the evaluation of the impotent patient.

Organic Impotence

Organic impotence may be due to arteriogenic or veno-occlusive insufficiency. Arteriogenic impotence has recently been clarified by advances in contrast medium, selective pudendal catheterization, vasodilation, and magnification. Intrapenile arterial anatomy is best shown by penile magnification pharmacoarteriography. This method has shown a high degree of variability of penile arteries, often differing from the classic arterial descriptions found in anatomy textbooks. The method consists of the use of a low-osmolar, high-concentration contrast medium, the intrapudendal arterial injection of nitroglycerin and papaverine, or the intracavernosal injection of papaverine alone to achieve vasodilation and obviate arterial small vessel spasm. In experienced hands internal pudendal artery catheterization can be achieved in 95% of cases. Direct magnification is necessary to visualize intrapenile arteries.

Clinical anatomy textbooks describe each penile artery branching from the internal pudendal artery. The penile artery gives rise to a dorsal penile artery, a cavernous artery, an artery to the bulbous spongiosum, and a urethral artery. The bulbous spongiosum artery forms small anastomoses with the urethral arteries. However, penile magnification pharmacoangiography demonstrates variable branching patterns to the dorsal penile and cavernosal artery. The classic description above is seen in a minority of cases. Dorsal penile cavernosal per-

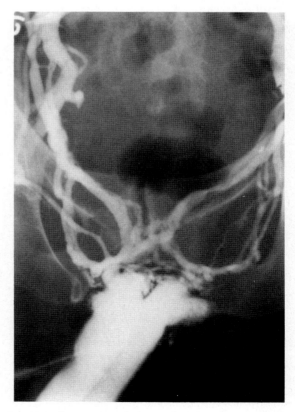

Figure 18.36. Venous leak. Both corpora cavernosa are filled, but the erection is not maintained. Rapid filling of large veins indicates a venous leak.

Penile Prostheses

In recent years impotence has been the subject of intense study. Better understanding of the etiologies has allowed more physiologic treatment to minimize the problem of erectile dysfunction. Failure to initiate an erection can be treated with intracorporeal injections of papaverine. Selected patients with arteriogenic impotence may be treated with large vessel angioplasty or microvascular bypass techniques. Patients who are unable to maintain erection may suffer from a venous leak that can be treated with ligation or transvascular occlusion of the draining veins. However, many patients have an organic cause of impotence that is not amenable to these treatment options. Implantable penile prostheses have become an attractive alternative treatment, and in many cases a prosthesis is the preferred option.

Types of Penile Prostheses

The first successful penile prostheses were semirigid or malleable rods designed for placement into each corpus cavernosum. The Small-Carion prosthesis (Heyer-Schulte Corp., Minneapolis, MN) consists of a silicone sponge interior surrounded by a medical grade silicone exterior. This prosthesis is only faintly radioopaque (Fig. 18.37).

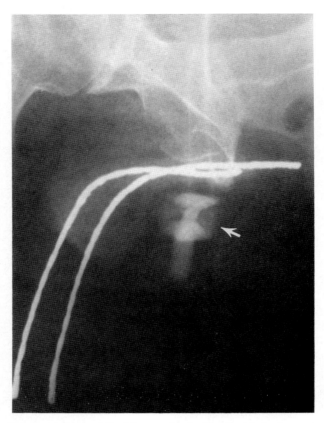

Figure 18.38. Malleable prosthesis. The braided wire cores are readily visualized but the silicone shell can only barely be appreciated. An artificial urethral sphincter (*arrow*) is also present. (From Cohan RH: Radiology of penile prostheses: Normal appearance and evaluation of malfunctions. In *Uroradiology Syllabus—American Roentgen Ray Society:* 1989, pp 167.)

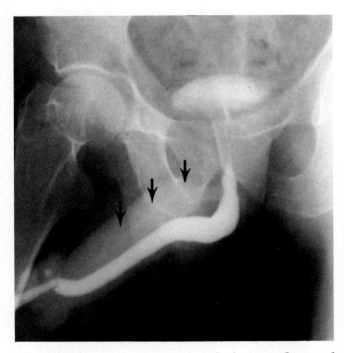

Figure 18.37. Semirigid prosthesis. The faint opacification of a Small-Carion prosthesis (*arrows*) is appreciated during retrograde urethrography. (From Cohan RH: Radiology of penile prostheses: Normal appearance and evaluation of malfunctions. In *Uroradiology Syllabus—American Roentgen Ray Society:* 1989, pp 167.)

Malleable prostheses consist of braided stainless steel or silver wire cores surrounded by Teflon (Fig. 18.38). Although less rigid than the solid silicone prostheses, they are more malleable and concealable.

These prostheses come in many sizes and widths or can be tailored to an individual patient. However, rigidity, length, and width cannot be altered once a particular device has been inserted. Patient satisfaction has been high, greater than 80%. Complications including pain, infection, perforation, and erosion have been observed in 7–16% of patients.

The development of an inflatable penile prosthesis provided significant improvement as both erect and flaccid states could be achieved. Concealment was no longer a problem and the quality of the erection was superior to that obtained with the noninflatable devices. Early versions suffered from a high mechanical failure rate due to the increased number of components. However, revised versions have significantly reduced the incidence of malfunction.

Two of the newer multicomponent inflatable prostheses have a 97% likelihood of remaining functional 3–4 years after implantation. The AMS 700 (American Medical Systems) and Mentor IPP (Mentor Corp. Goleta, CA) consist of four components interconnected by kink-resistant plastic tubing (Fig. 18.39). A spherical reservoir comprised of a single piece of silicone rubber is implanted immediately beneath the rectus abdominus muscle in the pelvis. It is filled with isoosmolar contrast media so that the status of the fluid can be followed with plain film radiographs. Two inflatable penile cylinders are made of expansile silicone rubber that widens and stiffens when inflated. These are inserted into the corpora cavernosa. The pump mechanism is placed in the scrotum where it is easily accessible for activation. Recent modifications have eliminated the reservoir by using a larger, more capacious pump so the reservoir is not needed (Fig. 18.40). Patient satisfaction of greater than 90% is improved over the noninflatable devices.

A self-contained mechanical prosthesis has been developed by Dacomed (Minneapolis, MN). It consists of an outer core of silicone covering a series of articulating plastic segments. The Omni Phase prosthesis uses an interconnecting spring cable (Fig. 18.41). The prosthesis is activated into an erect state by an abrupt flicking motion that shortens the cable and forces all of the segments to tighten against each other. The Dura Phase prosthesis (Dacomed) is similar to the malleable prosthesis but uses articulating plastic segments rather than the braided wire. A central cable connects both ends of the prosthesis and it retains the position in which it has been placed. Clinical

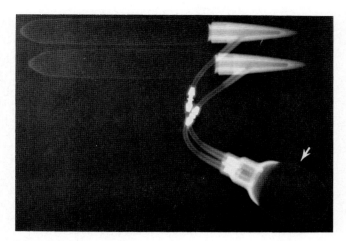

Figure 18.40.   Multicomponent inflatable penile prosthesis. This newer version has the reservoir (*arrow*) contained in the valve mechanism. (From Cohan RH: Radiology of penile prostheses: Normal appearance and evaluation of malfunctions. In *Uroradiology Syllabus—American Roentgen Ray Society*: 1989, pp. 167.)

experience has not yet been sufficient for proper evaluation of these newer devices.

Radiology

Plain films are usually sufficient for radiographic evaluation of the malfunctioning prosthesis. Fracture or erosion may be seen with semirigid or malleable prostheses. These are usually obvious on physical examination and radiographic confirmation is not necessary. The silver

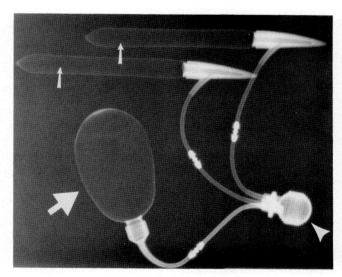

Figure 18.39.   Multicomponent inflatable penile prosthesis (IPP). This specimen radiograph of a Mentor IPP demonstrates the reservoir (*large arrow*), valve mechanism (*arrowhead*), and penile cylinders (*small arrows*). (From Cohan RH: Radiology of penile prostheses: Normal appearance and evaluation of malfunctions. In *Uroradiology Syllabus—American Roentgen Ray Society*: 1989, pp. 167.)

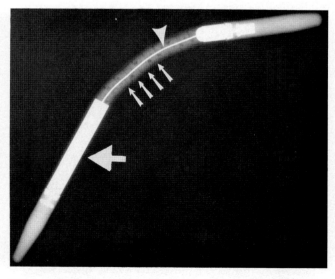

Figure 18.41.   Omni Phase prosthesis. The spring action cable (*arrowhead*) and interconnecting plastic segments (*small arrows*) are well seen. The spring action assembly is housed in the radioopaque metallic segment (*large arrow*). (From Cohan RH: Radiology of penile prostheses: Normal appearance and evaluation of malfunctions. In *Uroradiology Syllabus—American Roentgen Ray Society*: 1989, pp. 167.)

braided core of the older Jonas prosthesis may break or fray. Patients may complain of loss of rigidity or audible crackling on movement. Although these breaks may be detected radiographically, their severity is often underestimated due to breaks or fraying of individual wire braids that comprise the core.

Radiography plays a much more important role in identifying the cause of mechanical malfunction of inflatable penile prostheses. A single AP or oblique pelvic radiograph with the prosthesis inflated is often diagnostic.

Fluid may leak from an inflatable prosthesis due to erosion of the tubing against the cylinders or kinks in the tubing or deflated cylinder fabric. This complication has been seen in as many as 50% of patients with older models but is less commonly encountered with newer devices. Cohan et al. reported that 20% of 179 patients with a variety of inflatable penile prostheses had leaks from the cylinders, connectors, or tubing.

If there has been a leak of fluid, the prosthesis will not inflate adequately and the patient is unable to achieve erection. A pelvic radiograph reveals a decrease or complete absence of fluid in the reservoir and the penile cylinders are underinflated (Fig. 18.42). Once a leak is detected the defective component can be identified at surgery using an ohmmeter and is then replaced.

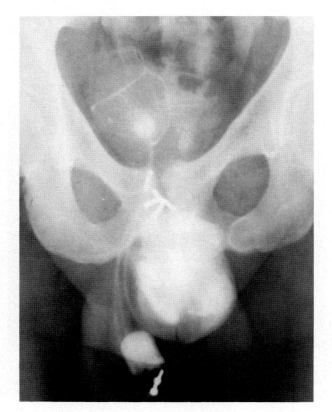

Figure 18.42.   Fluid leak from an inflatable penile prosthesis. Only a minimal amount of fluid remains within the reservoir and penile cylinders, indicating fluid leak.

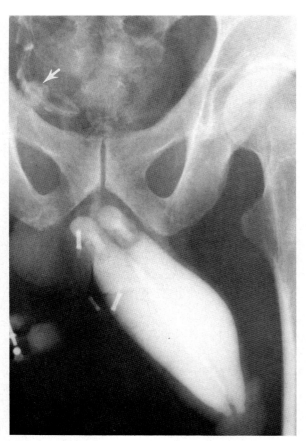

Figure 18.43.   Aneurysmal ballooning of inflatable penile cylinders. The reservoir (*arrow*) is empty. (From Cohan RH, Dunnick NR, Carson CC: Radiology of penile prostheses. *AJR* 152:925, 1989.)

Structural weakness may develop in the cylinders themselves after multiple inflations and deflations. These weaknesses may be apparent as buckling of the prostheses, cylinders, or even aneurysmal dilatation. (Fig. 18.43). Weakness of the tunica albuginea may predispose to the development of these problems. They have been reported in 1.6–8% of patients and were seen in 1.7% of patients in the series reported by Cohan et al. These problems can frequently be detected on physical examination and confirmed with a pelvic radiograph. The defective cylinders must be replaced, and because the surrounding tunica albuginea has been expanded it must be reinforced or resected.

Kinks in the tubing connecting the reservoir and pump were reported in approximately 5% of cases. They usually develop within the first few months of surgery. They cannot be detected on physical examination but may be identified on abdominal radiography (Fig. 18.44). This problem is seen less frequently with the introduction of "kinkproof" tubing.

Separation of the tubing from the reservoir pump or connector is rare but can easily be detected on a plain radiograph.

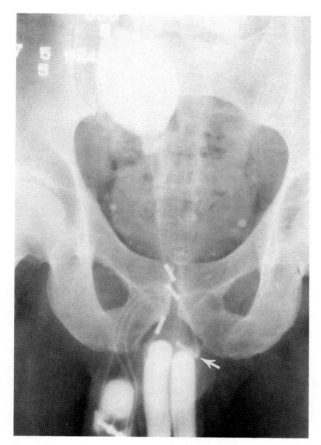

Figure 18.44. Kink in connecting tubing. The abrupt angulation (*arrow*) indicates a kink in the connecting tubing. (From Cohan RH: Radiology of penile prostheses: Normal appearance and evaluation of malfunctions. In: *Uroradiology Syllabus—American Roentgen Ray Society*: 1989, pp 167.)

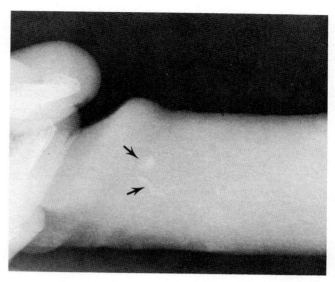

Figure 18.45. A plain film of the penis showing several calcified plaques (*arrows*) in the distal penis. (From Gray R, Grosman H, St. Louis EL, et al: The use of corpus cavernosography: a review. *J Can Assoc Radiol* 35:338, 1987.)

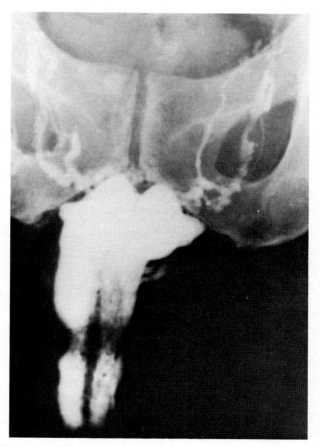

Figure 18.46. Cavernosogram in a patient with Peyronie's disease. Filling defects are present in both corpora cavernosa due to fibrous plaques. Excess venous drainage is also present contributing to the patient's impotence. (From Gray R, Grosman H, St. Louis EL, et al: The use of corpus cavernosography: a review. *J Can Assoc Radiol* 35:338, 1984.)

Erosions, encountered in 1–3% of patients, probably result from local tissue ischemia. Most erosions involve the pump or reservoir, which most commonly erodes into the bladder. Cylinder and pump erosions are detected on physical examination. A reservoir erosion can be suggested on the plain radiograph by identifying an unusual position of the reservoir or change in position since the previous film. Confirmation may require endoscopy or surgery.

Peyronie's Disease

Peyronie's disease is the development of fibrous plaques in the corpora cavernosa, which may contribute to painful erection and erect penile deviation. Plain film radiography may show calcification (Fig. 18.45) in these plaques, but this is uncommon. Computed tomography of the penis has been reported as showing faint calcifications in penile plaques that cannot be demonstrated on plain radiography. Cavernosography shows fibrous plaque defects in the contrast media–filled corpora (Fig. 18.46). Most plaques are peripheral and produce a filling defect in the outline of the corpus. The septum between the corpora may be significantly thickened. In severe Peyronie's disease cavernosography may show areas of fibrous obliteration of the corpora.

SUGGESTED READINGS

Urethra

Al-Ghorab NM: Radiological manifestations of genitourinary bilharziasis. *Clin Radiol* 10:100, 1968.

Amis ES Jr, Newhouse JH, Cronan JJ: Radiology of male periurethral strictures. *AJR* 151:321, 1988.

Bolduan JP, Farah RN: Primary urethral neoplasms: review of 30 cases. *J Urol* 125:198, 1981.

Campbell JE, Sniderman KW: Urethral diverticula in the adult female. *J Can Assoc Radiol* 27:232, 1976.

Colodny AH, Lebowitz RL: Lesions of Cowper's ducts and glands in infants and children. *Urology* 9:321, 1978.

DiSantis DJ: Urethral inflammation. In Pollack HM (ed): *Clin Urography,* Philadelphia, WB Saunders, 1990, pp. 925.

Fitts FB Jr, Herbert SG, Mellins HZ: Criteria for examination of the urethra during excretory urography. *Radiology* 125:47, 1977.

Gluck CD, Bundy AL, Fine C, et al: Sonographic urethrogram: comparison to roentgenographic techniques in 22 patients. *J Urol* 140:1404, 1988.

Levine RL: Urethral cancer. *Cancer* (Phila) 45(8):1965, 1980.

Macpherson RI, Leithiser RE, Gordon L, et al: Posterior urethral valves: an update and review. *RadioGraphics* 6:753, 1986.

McCallum RW: Urethral disease and interventional cystourethrography. *Radiol Clin North Am* 24:651, 1986.

McCallum RW: Urethral neoplasms. In Pollack HM (ed): *Clinical Urography,* Philadelphia, WB Saunders, 1990, pp. 1404.

McCallum RW, Alexander MWT, Rogers JM: Etiology and method of radiologic assessment of male urinary incontinence. *J Can Assoc Radiol* 36:4, 1985.

McCallum RW, Colapinto V: *Urological Radiology of the Adult Male Lower Urinary Tract.* Springfield, IL, Charles C Thomas, 1976.

McCallum RW, Rogers JM, Alexander MW: The radiologic assessment of iatrogenic urethral injury. *J Can Assoc Radiol* 36:122, 1985.

McGuire EJ: Urethral Sphincter Mechanisms and the Evaluation of Incontinence. In Pollack HM (ed): *Clinical Urography,* Philadelphia, WB Saunders, 1990, pp. 2045.

Mogg RA: Congenital anomalies of the urethra. *Br J Urol* 45:638, 1973.

Ortlip SA, Gonzalez R, Williams RD: Diverticula of the male urethra. *J Urol* 124:350, 1980.

Palmer PES, Reeder MM: Parasitic Disease of the Urinary Tract. In Pollack HM (ed): *Clinical Urography,* Philadelphia, WB Saunders, 1990, pp. 999.

Pollack HM, DeBenedictis TJ, Marmar JL, et al: Urethrographic manifestations of venereal warts (condyloma acuminata). *Radiology* 126:643, 1978.

Raz S: Pathophysiology of male incontinence. *Urol Clin North Am* 5:295, 1978.

Russinovich NAE, Lloyd LK, Griggs WP, et al: Balloon dilatation of urethral strictures. *Urol Radiol* 2:33, 1980.

Scales FE, Katzen BT, van Breda A, et al: Impassable urethral strictures: percutaneous transvesical catheterization and balloon dilatation. *Radiology* 157:59, 1985.

Stern AJ, Patel SK: Diverticulum of the female urethra. *Radiology* 121:222, 1976.

Symes JM, Blandy JP: Tuberculosis of the male urethra. *Br J Urol* 5:432, 1973.

Penis

Bookstein JJ, Lang EV: Penile magnification pharmacoarteriography: details of intrapenile arterial anatomy. *AJR* 148:883, 1987.

Bookstein JJ, Lurie AL: Selective penile venography: anatomical and hemodynamic observations. *J Urol* 140:55, 1988.

Cohan RH, Dunnick NR, Carson CC: Radiology of penile prostheses. *AJR* 152:925, 1989.

Delcour C, Wespes E, Vandenbosch G, et al: Impotence: evaluation with cavernosography. *Radiology* 161:803, 1986.

Frank RG, Gerard PS, Wise GJ: Human penile ossification: a case report and review of the literature. *Urol Radiol* 11:179, 1989.

Fuchs AM, Mehringer CM, Rajfer J: Anatomy of penile venous drainage in potent and impotent men during cavernosography. *J Urol* 141:1353, 1989.

Goldstein I, Krane RM, Greenfield AJ, et al: Vascular disease of the penis: impotence and priapism. In Pollack HM (ed): *Clinical Urography,* Philadelphia, WB Saunders, 1990, pp. 2231.

Gray R, Grosman H, St. Louis EL, et al: The uses of corpus cavernosography: a review. *J Can Assoc Radiol* 35:338, 1984.

Hovsepian DM, Amis ES: Penile prosthetic implants: a radiographic atlas. *RadioGraphics* 9(4):707, 1989.

Hricak H, Marotti M, Gilbert TJ, et al: Normal penile anatomy and abnormal penile conditions: evaluation with MR imaging. *Radiology* 169:683, 1988.

Krysiewicz S, Mellinger BC: The role of imaging in the diagnostic evaluation of impotence. *AJR* 153:1133, 1989.

Macpherson RI, Leithiser RE, Gordon L, et al: Posterior urethral valves: an update and review. *RadioGraphics* 6:753, 1986.

Malhotra CM, Balko A, Wincze JP, et al: Cavernosography in conjunction with artificial erection for evaluation of venous leakage in impotent men. *Radiology* 161:799, 1986.

Miller K, Kaplan L, Weitzman AF, et al: The radiology of male impotence. *RadioGraphics* 2(2):131, 1982.

Mulcahy JJ, Krane RJ, Lloyd LK, et al: DuraPhase penile prosthesis: results of clinical trials in 63 patients. *J Urol* 143:518, 1990.

Paushter DM: Role of duplex sonography in the evaluation of sexual impotence. *AJR* 153:1161, 1989.

Porst H, van Ahlen H, Vahlensieck W: Relevance of dynamic cavernosography to the diagnosis of venous incompetence in erectile dysfunction. *J Urol* 137:1163, 1987.

Quam JP, King BJ, James EM, et al: Duplex and color Doppler sonographic evaluation of vasculogenic impotence. *AJR* 153:1141, 1989.

Rajfer J, Canan V, Dorey FJ, Mehringer CM: Correlation between penile angiography and duplex scanning of cavernous arteries in impotent men. *J. Urol* 143:1128, 1990.

Rajfer J, Mehringer M: Cavernosography following clinical failure of penile vein ligation for erectile dysfunction. *J Urol* 143:514, 1990.

Rajfer J, Rosciszewski A, Mehringer M: Prevalence of corporeal venous leakage in impotent men. *J Urol* 140:69, 1988.

Schwartz AN, Lowe MA, Ireton R, et al: A comparison of penile brachial index and angiography: evaluation of corpora cavernosa arterial flow. *J Urol* 143:510, 1990.

St. Louis EL, Gray RR, Grosman H: Simplified technique of internal pudendal angiography in the investigation of impotence. *Cardiovasc Intervent Radiol* 9:22, 1986.

Velcek D, Evans JA: Cavernosography. *Radiology* 144:781, 1982.

Vickers MA, Benson CB, Richie JP: High resolution ultrasonography and pulsed wave Doppler for detection of corporovenous incompetence in erectile dysfunction. *J Urol* 143:125, 1990.

Wespes E, Schulman CC: Venous leakage: surgical treatment of a curable cause of impotence. *J Urol* 133:796, 1985.

CHAPTER **19**

SCROTUM AND CONTENTS

Until the advent of cross-sectional imaging, scrotal contents were examined only by palpation and transillumination. Even the best of clinical examinations often failed to differentiate intra- from extratesticular disease. Transillumination could define the presence of a hydrocele but could not detect the presence of associated testicular disease.

Cross-sectional imaging techniques now available for scrotal examination include scrotal ultrasound (US) and magnetic resonance imaging (MRI) examination, neither of which involves ionizing radiation.

Scrotal US is now widely accepted as the method of choice, and readily separates intra- from extratesticular lesions. Real-time high-resolution US can be obtained by 7.5- or 10-MHz transducers. A towel draped over the patient's thighs supporting the scrotum may be used, but the preferable technique is to support the scrotum in the examiner's gloved hand thereby allowing testicular and epididymal palpation to correlate with the US appearance.

In normal men uniform echogenicity of the testes is obtained by gain alteration. The normal testes demonstrate medium-level echogenicity which is uniform throughout and similar to thyroid echogenicity. A bright linear echogenicity in the longitudinal axis of the testes parallel to the epididymis represents the mediastinum testis (Fig. 19.1). The normal testis measures 3.5 cm in length and 2–3 cm in diameter. Along the posterolateral aspect of the testis lies the epididymis. The epididymis is of coarser echogenicity than the testis but of similar medium-level echoes. The head of the epididymis (globus major) is separate from the testis and lies lateral to the superior pole; it normally measures 7–8 mm. The body and tail of the epididymis pass inferiorly along the posterior wall of the tunica vaginalis and are seen separate from the testis as an isoechoic band 2 mm thick expanding slightly at the tail (globus minor). Cephalad to the testes, the pampiniform venous plexus and testicular and deferens arteries are seen within the spermatic cord extending into the inguinal canal within the two layers of the tunica vaginalis. These almost completely surround the testes and attach the testes to the posterior scrotal wall. A 2-mm layer of hypoechoic fluid is commonly seen and is normal. The eight layers of tissue forming the scrotum are not distinguishable except the tunica vaginalis because of the thin layer of fluid between the parietal and visceral layers. The scrotal layers together present as a hyperechoic band surrounding the scrotal contents. Distinction between intra- and extratesticular lesions by scrotal US is accurate in over 90% of cases.

INTRATESTICULAR LESIONS

Testicular Tumors

Testicular tumors may be classified as (a) germ cell tumors, (b) tumors arising from gonadal stroma, (c) metastases or (d) lymphoma.

Germ cell tumors include seminoma, embryonal cell carcinoma, choriocarcinoma, and teratoma. They may be of single or mixed cell type and constitute approximately 95% of testicular tumors and 5% of male genitourinary tumors.

423

Figure 19.1. Mediastinum testis. **A,** Sagittal section. **B,** Transverse section. The bright linear echo represents the mediastinum testis.

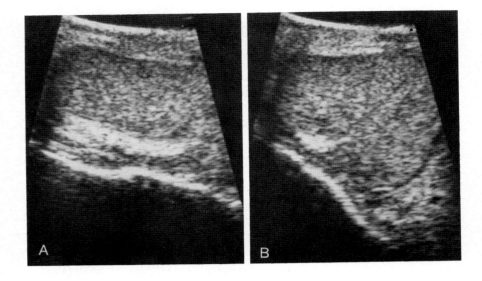

Seminomas are the most common testicular neoplasms, accounting for approximately 40% of all germ cell tumors. They occur in slightly older men, aged 30–45 years, than nonseminomatous germ cell tumors, which occur most commonly in men aged 17–32 years.

Ultrasound demonstrates uniform hypoechogenicity, usually in clinically enlarged but painless testes. Tumors may be seen as well-circumscribed, discrete, hypoechoic areas (Figs. 19.2, 19.3), or they may involve the entire testis, resulting in uniform hypoechogenicity. They rarely involve the tunica albuginea, become necrotic, or bleed (Fig. 19.4).

Seminomas are quite sensitive to radiation therapy and have a cure rate of over 95% when diagnosed before the advent of metastases (Fig. 19.5). However, distant me-

tastases occur in approximately 25% of cases by the time the patient presents.

Embryonal cell carcinoma occurs in younger men and accounts for approximately 30% of germ cell tumors. This aggressive tumor may invade the tunica albuginea and alter the testicular shape. Sonographically this lesion is a poorly circumscribed, hypoechoic mass of nonuniform echogenicity. It often contains focal areas of increased echogenicity due to areas of necrosis and hemorrhage, resulting in a coarse speckled echogenic pattern.

Choriocarcinoma is less common, accounting for only 2% of testicular tumors. This tumor is aggressive, metastasizes early, and the patient may seek treatment because of metastases. The primary lesion may be small and sonographically is mainly hypoechoic with mixed areas of

Figure 19.2. Seminoma. **A,** Sagittal and **B,** transverse scans demonstrate well-defined hypoechoic areas corresponding to a 1.5-cm seminoma.

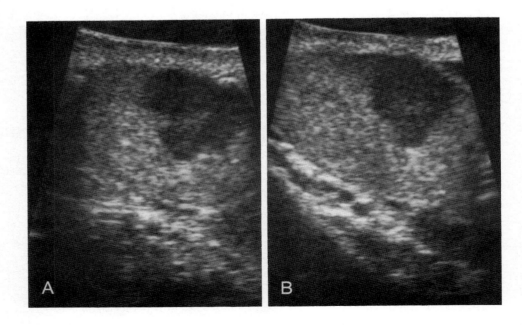

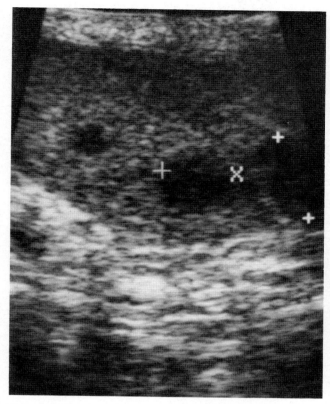

Figure 19.3. Seminoma. Several small hypoechoic foci are appreciated in this 32-year-old man with a testicular seminoma.

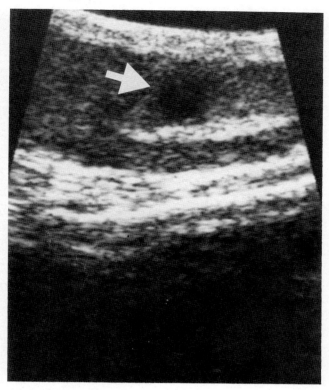

Figure 19.5. Recurrent seminoma. Five years after orchiectomy for left seminoma this recurrent seminoma (*arrow*) was found in the right testis.

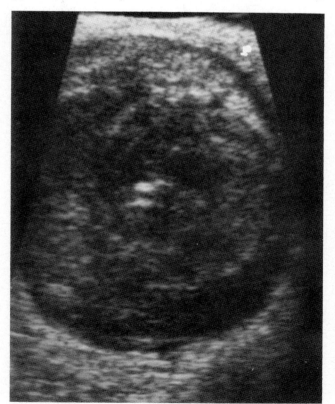

Figure 19.4. Seminoma. A large seminoma with bleeding was found in this 45-year-old man presenting with a swollen right testicle.

increased echogenicity due to necrosis, hemorrhage, and calcification.

Most of the remaining germ cell tumors are of mixed histologic pattern and show more than one germ layer. These include teratoma, teratocarcinoma, seminoteratoma, and seminoembryonal cell carcinoma. The most common of these tumors are teratoma and teratocarcinoma.

Testicular teratoma accounts for 10–20% of testicular tumors. Commonly they form a well-differentiated squamous cystic lesion containing keratinaceous fatty material, muscle, cartilage, bone, and mucous glandular tissue. Rarely these tissues are poorly differentiated. Although considered benign by many, there is a shift of emphasis to considering these tumors as malignant since over 30% of patients develop metastases within 5–10 years. The sonogram commonly shows cystic hypoechoic areas with areas of marked hyperechogenicity due to the mixed nature of the lesion.

Teratocarcinoma is a mixture of teratoma and embryonal cell carcinoma and is slightly less common than seminoma. Metastasis is an early occurrence of this very aggressive tumor which may break through the tunica albuginea, and is subject to necrosis and hemorrhage. The sonogram shows a mainly hypoechoic cystic lesion that is poorly demarcated and may contain areas of increased echogenicity due to necrosis and hemorrhage (Fig. 19.6).

Approximately 15% of testicular tumors present with evidence of distant metastatic disease without clinical suspicion of testicular tumor. Ultrasonography therefore is important in the detection of occult testicular tumor. The testis may be normal to palpation, but the occult tumor is usually visible as a hypoechoic area. Occasionally the primary tumor is "burned out" and is seen only as a hyperechoic focal area or a linear area of calcification. Although a focal hyperechoic lesion is not specific for primary burned-out testicular tumor, the presence of proven testicular metastasis strongly suggests burnout of the primary tumor.

Intratesticular papillary adenocarcinoma is a rare cystic malignancy. Less than 25 cases have been reported in the urologic and pathologic literature. The sonographic findings in one case has recently been reported in the radiologic literature. Papillary adenocarcinoma usually occurs in the superior pole of the testis arising in the rete testis, and is most common in the fourth and fifth decades. A well-defined echo-free multicystic septated intratesticular lesion is seen. Within the cysts are solid echogenic nodules, some arising from the septations. Other malignancies affecting the testis include metastatic disease, lymphoma, and leukemic infiltration.

Metastatic disease to the testes is more common than germ cell tumors in men over 50 years old. Although more commonly from the urinary tract (prostate and kidney), testicular metastases have been reported from almost any primary site. Testicular metastases are commonly bilateral and multiple and are usually hypoechoic, although hyperechoic metastases have been observed.

Testicular lymphoma may be primary in the testes without nodal or systemic involvement, or it may be associated as a complication of systemic lymphoma. Testicular lymphoma accounts for 25% of testicular tumor in men over 50 years old. Poorly differentiated lymphoma is more common bilaterally. Lymphoma and leukemic infiltrates are seen as either focal areas of hypoechogenicity (Fig. 19.7) or a diffusely enlarged hypoechoic testis. Although the sonographic appearance is nonspecific, such an appearance in a man over 50 years should raise the possibility of lymphoma.

Gonadal Stromal Tumors

Tumors arising from the gonadal stroma are either Leydig cell or Sertoli cell tumors. Leydig cell tumors arise from the interstitial cell of the fibrovascular stroma which produce testosterone, and therefore result in increased muscle weight in the patient. Leydig cell hyperplasia has been described in the presence of seminoma. Sertoli cell

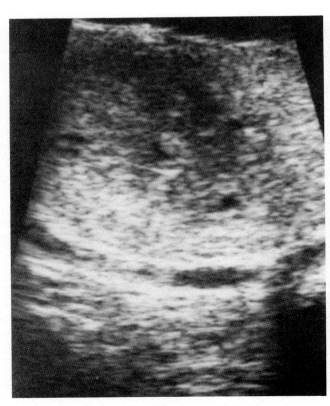

Figure 19.6. Teratocarcinoma. Cystic areas in a hyperechoic lesions are seen in this 32-year-old man with teratocarcinoma.

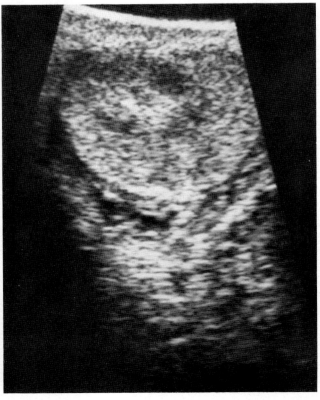

Figure 19.7. Lymphoma. Focal hypoechoic areas are seen within an enlarged testis.

tumors occur in the basement membrane of the seminiferous tubules and produce estrogen. These tumors are usually benign and are rare. The sonogram in these tumors usually shows spotty hypoechoic areas, with several associated cysts.

Benign Testicular Masses

Rarely, in patients with increased adrenocorticotropic hormone, adrenal rest tumors of the testis may develop. These tumors may occur in congenital adrenal hyperplasia or in primary adrenal insufficiency. The tumors most likely represent hypertrophy of ectopic adrenal rests that have migrated with the testis in fetal development. Adrenal rest tumors are usually multiple, producing testicular enlargement. Sonographically the lesions are eccentrically placed intratesticular hypoechoic nodules, some of which produce acoustic shadowing. In one case associated with Addison's disease, hyperechoic nodules that also produced acoustic shadowing were seen.

Other benign testicular lesions include testicular abscess, infarcts, and cysts.

Testicular abscess is most common in diabetic patients and results from epididymo-orchitis. Orchitis and testicular abscess have been reported as a complication of many bacterial and viral infections including tuberculosis, syphilis, and mumps. Both tuberculosis and syphilitic abscesses may break through the tunica albuginea and tunica vaginalis resulting in pyelocele and fistula to the scrotum. Up to 25% of patients with mumps develop orchitis, which may progress to abscess formation. Abscess formation in the testicle is seen sonographically as a hypoechoic area often with internal echoes and septations.

Testicular infarcts are seen in blood dyscrasia, testicular torsion, trauma, and bacterial endocarditis. Sonographically they are hypoechoic unless the infarct has fibrosed when they are hyperechoic.

Testicular Fluid Collections

Testicular cysts are rare. They are often idiopathic but may be postinflammatory or posttraumatic. They arise from efferent ductules or the rete testis and are located peripherally adjacent to the mediastinum testis. Their average size is 5–7 mm. Histologic examination demonstrates that the cyst is lined by cuboidal or low-columnar epithelium and some cases demonstrate cilia. Intratesticular cysts are not palpable. Ultrasound examination shows a peripheral, well-defined, hypoechoic lesion without internal echoes and with normal surrounding testicular echogenicity (Fig. 19.8). Ten to 20% of benign testicular cysts arise from the tunica albuginea. These cysts are palpable as a small 2- to 5-mm mass on the periphery of the testis. It should be emphasized that

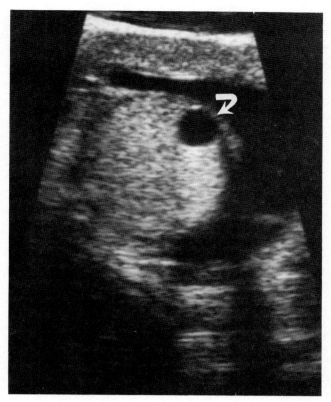

Figure 19.8. Cyst. A well-defined anechoic mass with increased through sound transmission in the testis indicates a cyst (*arrow*). A hydrocele is also present.

such a clinical finding cannot be distinguished from tumor. Ultrasound examination of this digitally localized lesion shows an echo-free cyst with acoustic enhancement and normal surrounding testicular echogenicity. When a cyst is positioned posteriorly against the epididymis, acoustic enhancement may not be apparent. Histologic examination is similar to that seen in an intratesticular benign cyst.

Epidermoid cysts of the testis are rare. These present as a palpable mass. On US examination they are seen as solitary cystic structures with an echogenic rim.

Since testicular tumors are also usually hypoechoic, the presence of a cystic lesion raises a diagnostic dilemma, as both benign and malignant lesions have to be considered. Benign cysts are usually well defined and peripheral, are completely anechoic, and usually show acoustic enhancement. Surrounding testicular echogenicity is normal. Malignant cysts are either primary with necrosis and liquification of the tumor or secondary to tumor occlusion of the ducts of the rete testis resulting in cystic dilatation. Seminomas are rarely cystic but may cause secondary cysts. Teratomatous cysts, on the other hand, are more commonly the result of necrotic liquification. Intratesticular hypoechoic lesions with or without cystic development should probably be considered malignant.

A *hydrocele* is an abnormal collection of fluid between the layers of the tunica vaginalis. Hydroceles may be congenital or acquired. A congenital hydrocele is usually due to a patent communication between the peritoneum and the vaginalis process. This is therefore not uncommon in premature infants, and may be demonstrated in the male fetus after 30 weeks' gestation. Normally, as the premature infant develops, the communication closes and the hydrocele is resolved. Nonresorption of the hydrocele indicates persistence of the communication. This condition is commonly associated with an inguinal hernia but may be the result of a defect in lymphatic drainage.

An acquired hydrocele may be primary or secondary. A primary hydrocele is idiopathic and more common than a secondary hydrocele. Small, presumably primary hydroceles may be present in over 60% of otherwise normal males (Fig. 19.9). When large, however, they may completely surround the testis (Fig. 19.10).

Secondary hydroceles result from trauma, infection, or tumor. They are seldom large. Secondary hydroceles due to trauma are usually the result of a hematocele. Orchitis and tumor hydroceles are usually filled with serous fluid but may also contain hemorrhage or purulent fluid.

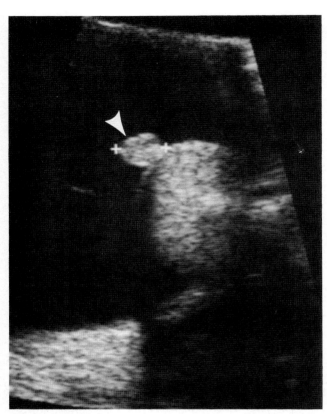

Figure 19.10. Hydrocele. A large hydrocele almost completely surrounds the testis. The appendix testis is seen (*arrowhead*) projecting off the testis.

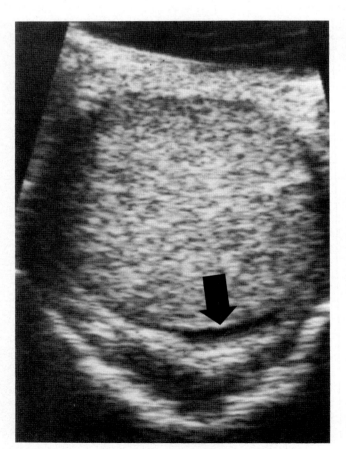

Figure 19.9. Hydrocele. Small hydroceles (*arrow*) are found in as many as 60% of normal males.

Hydroceles are usually anechoic, and the overlying normal scrotal skin has a normal thickness. Hematoceles and purulent hydroceles may be associated with thickened scrotal skin. They commonly contain internal echoes which may be due to septation or fibrous strand formation producing adhesions. However, it is emphasized that such internal echoes may occasionally be seen in a primary hydrocele; the explanation of this is obscure.

With the exception of primary hydrocele, it is apparent that almost all of these testicular lesions are hypoechoic and that the sonographic appearance is not specific for any one lesion. The clinical history and presentation are important in the differential diagnosis of a hypoechoic testicular lesion and frequently point the way to the diagnosis.

Testicular Blunt Trauma

Testicular trauma is rare but is an indication for emergency ultrasonographic examination. If rupture is diagnosed, emergency surgery is indicated. In approximately 90% of cases of testicular rupture the testis can be saved if surgical intervention occurs within 72 hours. When delay occurs beyond 72 hours the salvage rate drops to 55%. Ultrasonography allows the correct diagnosis in almost 100% of cases with virtually no false-positive or false-negative results.

Testicular rupture results most commonly from athletic injuries and occasionally from traffic accidents or violent attacks. Rupture is the result of compression of the testicle between the pubic or ischial bones and the offending object. The tunica albuginea ruptures and hemorrhage occurs into the scrotum. The sonographic appearance is that of an irregular change in the normal testicular echogenicity, with areas of hypo- and hyperechogenicity (Fig. 19.11). Normal testicular echogenicity and outline may not be visualized. The presence of a hydrocele or hematocele without the appearance of a normal testicular outline and echogenicity is an indication of testicular rupture (Fig. 19.12). It is rare to demonstrate rupture planes.

Testicular Torsion

Testicular torsion occurs when there is anomalous development of the epididymal attachment to the posterior scrotal wall by the processus vaginalis. Torsion may occur spontaneously in young males and adolescents but may also be a complication of scrotal trauma. In testicular torsion the testicle can be salvaged in the vast majority of cases if operation occurs within 24 hours. However, the

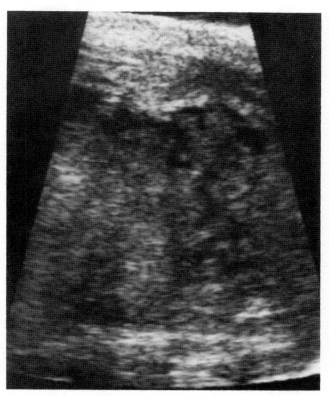

Figure 19.12.   Testicular rupture. The testis cannot be visualized, but a large hematoma of mixed echogenicity is seen.

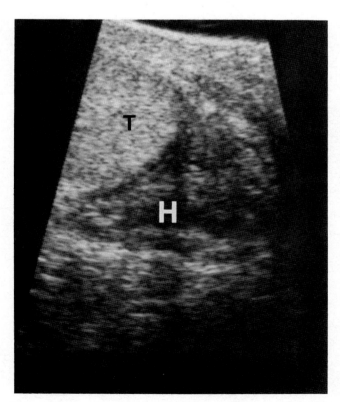

Figure 19.11.   Hematoma. A hematoma (H) is identified adjacent to the tesis (T).

salvage rate drops to 20% if operation is delayed more than 24 hours. Sonography is helpful in the early diagnosis when used in conjunction with Doppler US analysis of the spermatic cord and with radioisotope studies, although none of these studies done singly is diagnostic. The important differentiation is between torsion and epididymitis.

Sonographic abnormalities of the testicle are dependent on the duration of the torsion. Early sonographic findings include a decrease in testicular echogenicity, increase in size of the epididymis and testis, increase in size of the spermatic cord, and a reactive hydrocele. Doppler analysis of the spermatic cord indicates reduced or absent arterial flow. Radionuclide angiography usually indicates diminished perfusion on the affected side, with a "cold spot" replacing the epididymis and testis, unlike epididymitis which is indicated by increased perfusion and increased radionuclide activity within the affected scrotum. The radionuclide angiographic study alone is nonspecific since a similar "cold spot" may be produced by torsion, hydrocele, hematoma, or tumor while a "hot spot" may be produced by epididymitis, abscess, varicocele, or tumor. However, US, Doppler analysis, and radionuclide examination together may well point the way to the definitive diagnosis. In approximately 5% of cases only the appendix testis undergoes torsion.

Undescended Testicle

The embryonal gonad descends to the internal inguinal ring. Descent through the inguinal ring is guided by the gubernaculum which leads the testicle into the scrotum. This process occurs about the 34th–36th week of fetal life. Premature infants therefore have a relatively high incidence (30%) of undescended testicle at birth. By 4 months of age, the testicle usually descends into the scrotum with less than 1% remaining with undescended. Although 75% of undescended testicles are found in the inguinal canal, arrested descent may occur at any level and the testicle may be found within the abdominal cavity or pelvis.

Normal testicular development only occurs when the testicle is in the scrotum. A persistent undescended testicle is sterile and has a high incidence of malignant change, especially when intraabdominal. Consequently, localization of the testis and surgical intervention to bring the testis into the scrotum are essential to produce normal testicular development and to avoid malignant change. Approximately 10% of cases are bilateral.

Undescended testes may lie high in the scrotum, in the inguinal canal or anywhere along the line of testicular descent from the lower pole of the ipsilateral kidney to the internal ring. Testes that lie high in the scrotum are usually palpable. The most common location of an impalpable testis is the inguinal canal.

Ultrasound accurately localizes the undescended testis in over 90% of cases located in or near the inguinal canal. The US examination should begin with the scrotum to identify the normally descended testis. On the undescended side, the empty scrotum and inguinal canal are examined where the undescended testicle is commonly found. It is usually smaller and more elongated than the normal testis, but of similar echogenicity. It is important to identify the mediastinum testes in the undescended testis since the bulbous end of the gubernaculum, the pars infravaginalis gubernaculi, may be of similar size and echogenicity as the testis, and only the identification of the mediastinum testes within the undescended testis confirms the localization.

The reported sensitivity of CT in the detection of undescended testes in or near the inguinal canal is excellent. An ovoid mass of soft tissue density is seen along the line of testicular descent (Fig. 19.13). There have been too few cases of upper abdominal testes reported for evaluation.

MRI may also be used to localize undescended testes. The imaging sequences selected depend on the field strength of the magnet, but early reports have shown good results.

Gonadal venography is the oldest radiologic examination used to localize an undescended testis. It relies on identification of the pampiniform plexus which usually indicates the location of the testis. A blind-ending internal spermatic vein suggests that the testis is absent. However, these criteria not completely accurate. Furthermore, valves in the gonadal vein may prevent contrast from reaching the most terminal portion of the vein. Thus gonadal venography is seldom utilized for the detection or localization of an undescended testis.

EXTRATESTICULAR LESIONS

Extratesticular lesions are either epididymal or vascular, and most are benign. The most common abnormali-

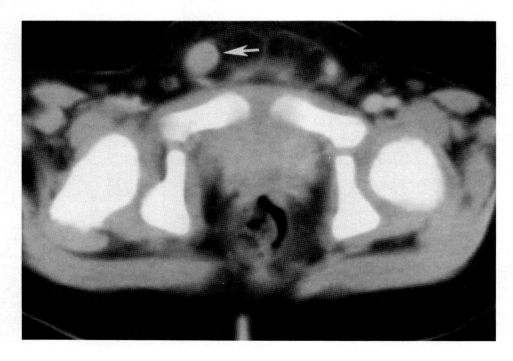

Figure 19.13. Undescended testis. The right testis is seen (*arrow*) in the inguinal canal.

ties are epididymal cysts and spermatoceles. Epididymal cysts are due to dilatation of tubules in the epididymis. They may be small and multiple but may be up to 2 cm in size. These cysts contain serous fluid as opposed to spermatoceles, which contain thick sperm-filled fluid. Epididymal cysts may occur anywhere within the epididymis.

Spermatoceles usually represent retention cysts of the small tubules in the epididymal head and may be loculated. Both epididymal cysts and spermatoceles may be unilateral or bilateral and are usually palpated as an extratesticular mass posterior to the testis. Cystic replacement of the epididymis is rare but has been reported following vasectomy.

Ultrasound studies show these lesions are well-defined anechoic cysts with through-transmission within the epididymis (Fig. 19.14). They are readily distinguished from hydrocele by position. Hydrocele is seen anteriorly surrounding the testis. Epididymal cyst and spermatocele are seen in the epididymis superior or posterior to the testis. Epididymal cysts and spermatoceles are usually echo free with the same acoustic characteristics and cannot be distinguished. Occasionally a spermatocele has a few internal echoes due to cellular debris.

Varicocele

Varicoceles may be primary or secondary and consist of dilated veins draining the testis, usually in the pampiniform plexus, the main venous drainage of the testis. They have also been reported to occur in the cremasteric plexus, which drains the epididymis and scrotal wall. Primary varicoceles are idiopathic and are most commonly seen in male children or adolescents. Secondary varicocele is more common in the left scrotum and usually results from incompetent valves in the left spermatic vein, resulting in stasis. Up to 15% of normal males have been shown to have a varicocele.

Varicocele is present in approximately 40% of infertile males. In these patients, the infertility is said to be due to venous stasis resulting in decreased sperm mortality. Venous drainage may be sluggish or intermittent or continuous reflux may be present. Large varicoceles may be palpated. Moderate and small varicoceles are commonly not palpable. Consequently the management of infertility must include the examination for small or moderate varicoceles.

High-resolution real-time US is a suitable method to demonstrate varicocele. The procedure is best performed in the upright position or with the patient supine performing a Valsalva maneuver. By these methods, small varicoceles may be demonstrated as serpiginous, tubular, elongated, anechoic fluid collections (Fig. 19.15). Varico-

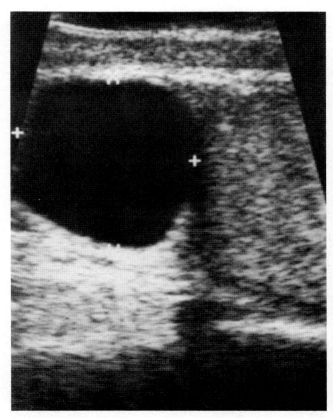

Figure 19.14. Spermatocele. A large cystic mass in the region of the epididymis is consistent with a spermatocele, but cannot be distinguished from an epididymal cyst.

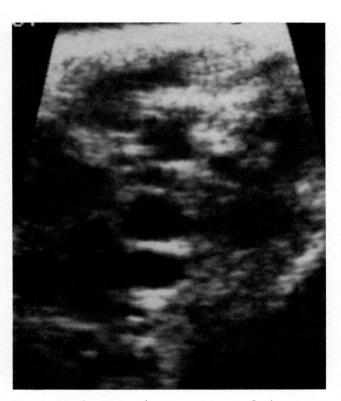

Figure 19.15. Varicocele. A serpiginous, fluid-containing structure is consistent with varicocele.

cele of the pampiniform plexus can be differentiated from cremasteric varicoceles since cremasteric varicoceles are posterior to pampiniform varicoceles. High-resolution 10-MHz transducers may allow assessment of antegrade or retrograde flow.

Continuous-wave Doppler US is an excellent method of varicocele assessment. Flow direction and rate can be recorded on a monitoring device to distinguish antegrade flow, stasis, or retrograde flow. Doppler auscultation is accurate in clinically palpable lesions, and slightly less accurate in small or moderate varicoceles.

Spermatic vein angiography is reserved for men who are symptomatic and require surgical intervention. Although this is the most invasive method of diagnosis, it supplies anatomic detail and demonstrates reflux of contrast medium from the renal vein (or IVC in right-sided varicoceles) into the internal spermatic vein. Collateral veins from the internal spermatic vein to the pampiniform plexus are also demonstrated. Interventional venous ablation may be performed by venous occlusion techniques including the insertion of detachable balloons or stainless steel coils for occlusion of the abnormal internal spermatic vein. However, the demonstration of multiple collateral veins may make embolization impractical. The recurrence rate of varicocele after balloon occlusion of approximately 10% is comparable with the recurrence rate of 10–20% following surgical ligation of the internal spermatic vein.

Radioisotope examination with ^{99m}Tc-pertechnetate demonstrates clinically palpable varicoceles. The dynamic study provides an isotope angiogram demonstrating increased uptake in the varicocele. Stasis is detected by increased uptake in late static images.

Epididymitis

Epididymitis is the most common inflammatory process in the scrotum. Middle-aged men who have undergone prostatectomy and adolescents are most commonly affected. It is rare in children.

The most common pathogens are *E. coli* and Pseudomonas. Tuberculous epididymitis is seen in tuberculous patients, and the epididymis may also be infected by bilharziasis (*Schistosoma hematobium*). Men who have had transurethral prostatectomy with resection involving the verumontanum may have reflux of infected urine into the vas deferens resulting in epididymitis. Occasionally epididymitis is idiopathic without demonstration of a pathogenic organism. Epididymitis is also commonly associated with prostatitis and associated orchitis is found in up to 20% of cases of epididymitis.

Clinically acute epididymitis presents as acute pain and tenderness in the scrotum making palpation difficult. Pain, tenderness, and pyrexia increase over the first 2 days followed by dysuria and pyuria. Urethral discharge is common. There may be initial difficulty in differentiat-

ing epididymitis from acute torsion of the cord in 50% of cases. Rarely hemorrhagic testicular tumor may have a similar initial presentation of pain and tenderness.

Ultrasound examination is extremely helpful in the differential diagnosis after initial clinical examination. The head and body of the epididymis are enlarged and of altered echogenicity. Although echogenicity is often decreased, acute epididymitis presents as a hyperechoic epididymal head. The entire body of the epididymis or only the head may be affected. There is commonly an associated reactive hydrocele (Fig. 19.16). Focal hypoechoic areas within the head or body of the epididymis suggest abscess formation.

When orchitis coexists (Fig. 19.17) the testicle is enlarged and of reduced echogenicity. Focal areas of markedly reduced echogenicity within the testis indicate abscess formation. The presence of suppuration within the epididymis or testis usually leads to infection within the reactive hydrocele resulting in pyelocele. Chronic epididymitis may present as a painless, nodular, palpable mass, difficult to clinically separate from the testis. Ultrasound examination reveals the epididymal site of the lesion; most of these sites are hyperechoic.

Inflammation

Scrotal inflammation, abscess, or gangrene may be a complication of an intrascrotal infectious process that

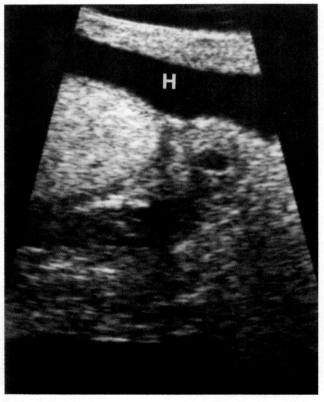

Figure 19.16. Epididymitis. The head of the epididymis is enlarged and there is an associated hydrocele (H).

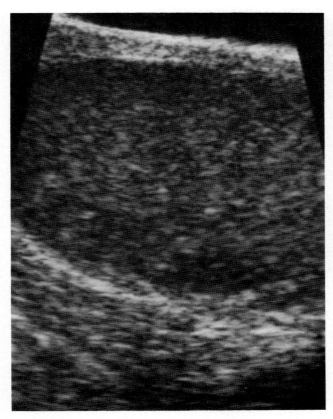

Figure 19.17. Orchitis. The testis is enlarged with decreased echogenicity.

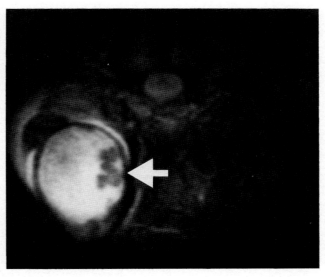

Figure 19.18. Scrotal MRI. A right testicular seminoma (*arrow*) is clearly seen as an intratesticular lesion on this T2-weighted (TR 2000, TE 80) coronal image.

may also result from trauma, surgery, or extension of an adjacent perineal infection.

A rare but fulminant necrotizing fasciitis of the penis and scrotum was described by Fournier in 1883. There is an abrupt onset and rapid progression to gangrene. Most of these patients have an underlying chronic urinary tract infection, recent urologic instrumentation, or perirectal or colonic disease. Many patients have a history of diabetes mellitus, paraplegia, or alcohol abuse.

The diagnosis can usually be made on physical examination. Gas can be detected on the plain radiograph in the scrotal wall and may spread anteriorly along the anterior abdominal wall or posteriorly into the perineum.

Treatment includes broad-spectrum intravenous antibiotics, as a wide variety of both aerobic and anaerobic bacteria have been found. Surgical management includes wide incision and drainage of involved areas with excision of necrotic tissue. Despite aggressive treatment, mortality remains as high as 50% in some series.

MAGNETIC RESONANCE IMAGING

Recently normal scrotal anatomy and scrotal pathology have been described using MRI. High-resolution MRI using a surface coil provides excellent spatial resolution and high contrast within a wide field of view. Signal intensities of the testis, epididymis, tunica albuginea, spermatic cord, fluid, and fat produce excellent detailed delineation of these structures. As with US, no radiation is involved, and the scrotal contents may be viewed in transverse, sagittal, or coronal planes.

All pathologic processes are best seen on T2-weighted images in the coronal plane (Fig. 19.18). On T2-weighted images, all pathologic testicular processes are less intense than the normal testicular intensity (except for old blood). Testicular lesions are readily separated from epididymal lesions. Varicocele is readily recognized. Excellent visualization of the tunica albuginea is a distinct advantage of MRI over US in the assessment of trauma or tumor invasion.

In patients with extremely painful scrotal lesions, MRI may have an advantage over US since US requires close contact of the transducer to the scrotal surface. In MRI the surface coil is not in contact with the scrotum, allowing for a less painful examination.

Magnetic resonance spectroscopy may produce specificity in identifying a scrotal mass, however, neither US nor MRI are specific at present. The disadvantages of MRI include the expense of the procedure, reduction in image quality by patient motion, and the length of the examination.

SUGGESTED READINGS

Baker LL, Hajek PC, Burkhard TK, et al: MR imaging of the scrotum: normal antomy. *Radiology* 163:89, 1987.

Baker LL, Hajek PC, Burkhard TK, et al: MR imaging of the scrotum: pathologic conditions. *Radiology* 163:93, 1987.

Benson CB, Doubilet PM, Richie JP: Sonography of the male genital tract. *AJR* 153:705, 1989.

Burks DD, Markey BJ, Burkhard TK, et al: Suspected testicular torsion and ischemia: evaluation with color Doppler sonography. *Radiology* 175:815, 1990.

Friedland GW, Chang P: The role of imaging in the management of the impalpable undescended testis. *AJR* 151:1107, 1988.

Gooding GAW: Sonography of the spermatic cord. *AJR* 151:721, 1988.

Grant RW, Mitchell-Heggs P: Radiological features of Fournier gangrene. *Radiology* 140:641, 1981.

Hricak H, Filly RA: Sonography of acute scrotal abnormalities. *Radiol Clin North Am* 21:595, 1983.

Hricak H, Jeffrey RB: Sonography of acute scrotal contents. *Urol Radiol* 4:147, 1982.

Krone KD, Carroll BA: Scrotal ultrasound. *Radiol Clin North Am* 23:121, 1985.

Panicek DM, Toner GC, Heelan RTT, Bosl GJ: Nonseminomatous germ cell tumors: enlarging masses despite chemotherapy. *Radiology* 175:499, 1990.

Rholl KS, Lee JKT, Heiken JP, et al: MR imaging of the scrotum with a high resolution surface coil. *Radiology* 163:99, 1987.

Rifkin MD: Inflammation of the lower urinary tract: the prostate, seminal vesicles and scrotum. in Pollack HM (ed): *Clinical Urography.* Philadelphia, WB Saunders, 1990.

Seidenwurm D, Smathers RL, Kan P, et al: Intratesticular adrenal rests diagnosed by ultrasound. *Radiology* 155:479, 1985.

Seidenwurm D, Smathers RL, Lo RK, et al: Testes and scrotum: MR imaging at 1.5 T. *Radiology* 164:393, 1987.

Smith SJ, Vogelzang RL, Smith WM, et al: Papillary adenocarcinoma of the rete testis: sonographic findings. *AJR* 148:1147, 1987.

Spirnak JP, Resnick MI, Hampel N, et al: Fournier's gangrene: report of 20 patients. *J Urol* 131:289, 1984.

Steinfeld AD: Testicular germ cell tumors: review of contemporary evaluation and management. *Radiology* 175:603, 1990.

Sussman EB, Hadju SI, Lieberman PH, et al: Malignant lymphoma of the testis: a clinicopathologic study of 37 cases. *J Urol* 118:1004, 1977.

CHAPTER 20

RENAL FAILURE AND MEDICAL RENAL DISEASE

Renal Failure
    Acute Renal Failure
    Chronic Renal Failure

Imaging Studies in Renal Failure
    Plain Film Radiography
    Excretory Urography
    Ultrasonography
    Computed Tomography
    Radionuclide Studies
    Other Imaging Studies

Medical Renal Disease
    Acute Tubular Necrosis
    Acute Cortical Necrosis
    Acute Interstitial Nephritis
    Hematologic Disorders
    Acute Urate Nephropathy
    AIDS Nephropathy
    Alport's Syndrome
    Miscellaneous Conditions

RENAL FAILURE

There is no clearly defined set of biochemical or clinical criteria that characterize the term "renal failure." Most authors use this term to describe a patient whose renal function is insufficient to maintain homeostasis. In this fashion, renal failure is distinguished from the term "renal insufficiency," which characterizes a patient whose renal function is abnormal but capable of sustaining essential bodily functions. Uremia, the clinical syndrome that results from renal dysfunction, may be present in untreated patients with both renal insufficiency and renal failure. Uremia may result in symptoms related to a number of different organ systems including the gastrointestinal tract (nausea, vomiting), the cardiovascular system (hypertension, cardiac arrhythmias, pericarditis), the nervous system (personality changes, seizures, somnolence),

and the hematopoietic system (anemia, bleeding diathesis), among others. The term "end-stage renal disease" is often used to describe a patient with chronic renal failure whose renal deterioration is irreversible and requires either dialysis or renal transplantation to sustain life.

Acute Renal Failure

Acute renal failure (ARF) is the sudden rapid deterioration in renal function. Classically, the causes of acute renal failure are divided into three broad categories, (*a*) *prerenal*, (*b*) *renal*, and (*c*) *postrenal*.

Prerenal causes are generally associated with volume depletion or renal hypoperfusion and are the most common causes of ARF. Such conditions include congestive heart failure, diuretic use, sepsis, dehydration, burns, hemorrhage, cirrhosis with ascites, and diabetic ketoacidosis.

Renal causes for ARF may result from damage to any portion of the kidney (i.e., the tubules, the glomerulus, the interstitium or the blood supply). *Acute tubular necrosis* (ATN) is among the most common of these. *Interstitial* causes for ARF include acute urate nephropathy, myeloma, and acute interstitial nephritis. *Glomerular* damage may cause ARF as a result of acute glomerulonephritis, drug toxicity, Goodpasture's syndrome, systemic lupus erythematosus, and others. *Vascular* causes for ARF include acute renal vein thrombosis, renal artery occlusion, and scleroderma.

Postrenal causes for ARF refer to the onset of renal failure secondary to acute obstruction. Although postrenal causes of ARF account for only 15% of the cases, this entity is the most commonly sought cause for ARF, since acute obstruction represents the most easily reversed cause of acute renal dysfunction.

Chronic Renal Failure

The gradual progressive loss of renal function characterizes chronic renal failure (CRF). The renal dysfunction is attributable to the loss of functioning renal parenchyma and as such is irreversible. The causes of CRF are protean, but may be related to vascular disease (i.e., generalized arteriosclerosis, arterial infarction), intrinsic renal disease (i.e., chronic glomerulonephritis, adult polycystic kidney disease), systemic disease (i.e., diabetes mellitus, hypertension), or as a result of long-standing obstruction (i.e., neurogenic bladder disease, posterior urethral valves). In most cases the process eventually results in the requirement for dialysis or renal transplantation.

IMAGING STUDIES IN RENAL FAILURE

Plain Film Radiography

A plain film of the abdomen offers much valuable information about the patient with renal failure. Although the older literature stressed the value of this study for determining renal size, such information is much more reliably obtained with ultrasound. However, the plain film should be used to detect the presence of renal calculi or abnormal gas collections in the patient with urosepsis, and gives valuable information about the bony pelvis, including the detection of unsuspected renal osteodystrophy or metastatic disease.

Excretory Urography

The role of excretory urography in the assessment of patients with renal failure has greatly declined since the advent of cross-sectional imaging techniques. High-dose urography with tomography became the accepted technique for the evaluation of the renal failure patient in the mid-1960s. When dose of contrast material in the range of 600 mg iodine/kg, careful radiographic technique, tomography, and delayed films were used, such studies were reported to have reliably demonstrated the renal outlines and the collecting system in over 90% of patients with renal failure. In this fashion it was possible to exclude obstruction as the cause of the renal failure and to make an assessment whether the renal failure was acute or chronic. However, the rapid development of cross-sectional imaging techniques coupled with the concern over the use of contrast material in patients with renal insufficiency have relegated this procedure to instances where high-quality ultrasonography or computed tomography (CT) is not available.

Fry and Cattell reported that analysis of the pattern of the nephrogram in such cases could sometimes yield information as to the cause of the renal dysfunction. They reported three distinct patterns: (a) the *immediate, faint, persistent nephrogram* associated with chronic glomeru-

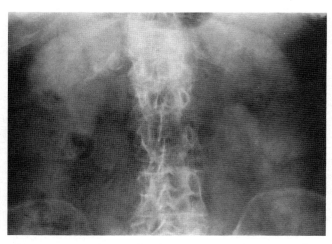

Figure 20.1. A 10-min film from an excretory urogram demonstrates an increasing dense nephrogram without a pyelogram in a patient who became hypotensive following contrast administration. After fluid resuscitation, the findings resolved.

lar disease; (b) the *increasing dense nephrogram*, usually present in acute extrarenal obstruction, but also present with hypotension (Fig. 20.1), renal ischemia, acute glomerular disease, intratubular obstruction, and acute renal vein thrombosis; and (c) the *immediate, dense, persistent nephrogram* which is characteristically present in acute tubular necrosis (Fig. 20.2) and occasionally in severe renal inflammatory disease.

The immediate faint, persistent nephrogram represents a decrease in the number of functioning nephrons, a decrease in the ability of the kidney to concentrate urine, and an increased diuresis secondary to azotemia. The pathogenesis of the obstructive nephrogram is poorly understood but probably represents a combination of increasing tubular distention and increased salt and water resorption in the tubule as the result of ob-

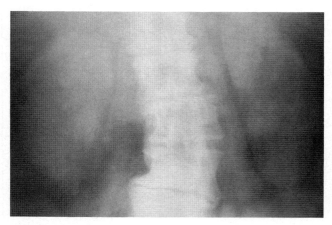

Figure 20.2. A 25-min film from an excretory urogram in a patient with drug-induced acute tubular necrosis. An unchanging dense nephrogram is present.

struction. In systemic hypotension, the increasingly dense nephrogram is thought to occur as a result of increased salt and water resorption from the tabules and a reduced rate of clearance of the contrast from the plasma. The precise pathophysiology responsible for the immediate dense persistent nephrogram is also poorly understood but may be related to recirculation of the contrast through the venous or lymphatic systems.

Subsequent authors have shown that while these patterns are not always specific, nephrogram analysis is nonetheless frequently helpful in differential diagnosis.

Ultrasound

Ultrasound represents the best available imaging study for the patient with renal failure. The obvious advantage of ultrasound is its lack of dependence on renal function for the demonstration of renal anatomy; this is in contrast to urography and to a lesser extent, computed tomography which depend on the kidney's ability to excrete contrast material. Therefore, in a patient with renal failure, sonography can easily distinguish a patient with normal sized kidneys (which generally indicates acute renal failure) from one with small kidneys (which generally indicates chronic renal failure) (Fig. 20.3). Ultrasound can also readily define the patient with adult polycystic kidney disease in whom the kidneys are large and display obvious morphologic abnormalities. Ultrasound accurately depicts the presence of renal calculi, either as a cause of or in association with renal failure.

Ultrasound can screen for renal failure caused by obstruction. Except for patients with bilateral iatrogenic postoperative obstruction, obstructive renal failure is usually chronic in nature and is associated with hydronephrosis; it is therefore readily detectable by ultrasound. Ritchie et al. retrospectively evaluated the diagnostic yield of sonography in 394 azotemic patients and found a 29% incidence of obstructive renal failure in a group of patients considered clinically to be at high risk for obstruction (i.e., known pelvic malignancy, known or suspected renal calculus disease, suspected urosepsis, a palpable mass, recent pelvic surgery, or bladder outlet obstruction). In patients without known risk factors, the incidence of obstructive renal failure was 1%. Similar conclusions were reached by Stuck et al. in a prospective study.

The accuracy of ultrasound in screening for chronic renal obstruction has been discussed in Chapter 14.

Ultrasound may also give limited information about the nature of the underlying renal disease. Normal kidneys have an echogenicity less than that of the liver or spleen, although with the use of newer ultrasound equipment it has been observed that in many normal patients the echogenicity of the renal cortex is equal to that of the liver. Most renal parenchymal diseases result in increased cortical echogenicity (Fig. 20.3), however, although such a finding has a high specificity, it has a relatively low sensitivity for detecting renal disease on screening sonography. A small number of renal diseases including lymphoma, acute pyelonephritis, and renal vein thrombosis characteristically result in decreased cortical echoes. Gouty nephropathy, medullary nephrocalcinosis, renal tubular acidosis, and medullary sponge kidney may result in increased medullary echogenicity. Hricak et al. compared the ultrasound appearance of the kidneys with the results of renal biopsy in 109 patients. Although there was no direct correlation between the ultrasound appearance and a specific disease process, there was a significant correlation between increased cortical echogenicity and a decreased level of renal function.

Computed Tomography

Computed tomography should be considered as an imaging study in patients with renal failure when the result of sonography is inconclusive. Even without intravenous contrast material, CT is often capable of detecting hydronephrosis, although in some cases differentiation from some forms of renal cystic disease may be difficult. CT may be useful in delineating the point and nature of an obstruction, as the dilated ureter may be imaged on sequential sections (Fig. 20.4). Computed tomography may be used to obtain an accurate assessment of renal size and the degree of cortical atrophy that may be present. In some forms of renal cystic disease, CT is the imaging study of choice to detect a complication of the disease process, i.e., hemorrhage complicating adult polycystic disease or the development of a solid renal tumor in patients with acquired cystic disease. Computed

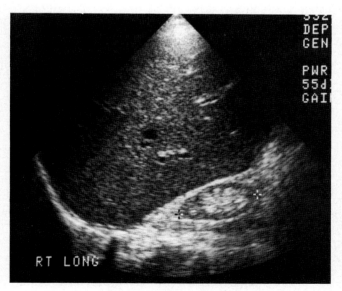

Figure 20.3. Longitudinal sonogram of the right kidney demonstrates a small echogenic kidney characteristic of chronic renal parenchymal disease.

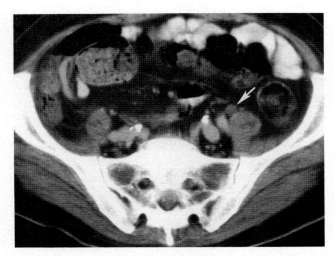

Figure 20.4. Noncontrast CT scan through the pelvis demonstrates a dilated ureter (arrow).

tomography detects the presence of renal calculi, even those not demonstrated on conventional radiography.

Radionuclide Studies

Because the excretion of radiopharmaceuticals depends on renal function, they cannot be used to evaluate all patients with renal failure. This is particularly the case with technetium-99m diethylenetriaminetetraacetic acid (^{99m}Tc-DTPA), as it is excreted primarily by glomerular filtration. ^{131}I-Hippuran, however, is excreted by tubular secretion and thus it may visualize the kidneys even when renal dysfunction is relatively advanced. Because this agent has relatively poor imaging characteristics, its primary use is to produce time-activity curves (radionuclide renogram—see Chapter 3) and to evaluate differential renal function when a unilateral process is present. If obstruction is present, a percutaneous nephrostomy tube or a double-J ureteral catheter should be placed prior to the performance of a radionuclide scan made to estimate residual renal function since potentially recoverable renal function will likely be overestimated if renography is performed while the kidney(s) are still obstructed.

Radionuclide determination of the glomerular filtration rate may also be of value in some forms of medical renal disease (see Chapter 3).

Other Imaging Studies

The role of *angiography* is extremely limited in the diagnostic evaluation of renal failure. Occasionally the angiographic features of end-stage renal disease will be encountered in patients being evaluated for another purpose. Such features include a pruned, tortuous appearance of the intrarenal vessels, thinning of the cortex, and a slowing of arterial flow within the kidneys. The angiographic nephrogram may have a mottled or lucent appearance. A number of systemic diseases associated with renal failure may demonstrate multiple microaneurysms, including Wegener's granulomatosis, polyarteritis nodosa, and systemic lupus erythematosus (see Chapter 8). *Renal venography* is frequently necessary to confirm the diagnosis of renal vein thrombosis.

MRI was initially thought to have great promise for the evaluation of chronic renal failure. This hope was based upon reports that loss of the corticomedullary distinction (CMD) was a relatively specific finding in some forms of medical renal disease. It has subsequently been shown, however, that the loss of the CMD is not specific and may be present in normal patients who are well hydrated. There is continued hope, however, that phosphorus-31 magnetic resonance spectroscopy may provide relatively disease specific patterns in some forms of renal failure.

Antegrade and *retrograde pyelography* are useful in establishing the diagnosis of ureteral obstruction as a cause for renal failure (see Chapter 14).

Small kidneys are found in many conditions that lead to chronic renal failure including chronic glomerulonephritis, diabetic nephrosclerosis, hypertensive nephropathy, generalized renal arteriosclerosis, and analgesic nephropathy (see Chapter 11).

MEDICAL RENAL DISEASE

Acute Tubular Necrosis

Acute tubular necrosis (ATN) is the most common form of acute reversible renal failure. ATN has a wide range of causes including hemolysis, dehydration, hypotension, drugs (contrast material, aminoglycosides, and other antibiotics), heavy metal, and solvent exposure. ATN is commonly seen after cadaveric renal transplantation (see Chapter 21). The exact pathogenesis of ATN is poorly understood, but some authorities believe that direct tubular damage is the initiating event and results in filling of the tubular lumen with cellular debris. Others believe that ATN is probably related to a disturbance in the renin-angiotensin axis that results in a global decrease in renal blood flow. Proponents of this theory prefer the term "acute vasomotor nephropathy," as they believe that there is little primary tubular damage and that the renal failure occurs because of a redistribution of blood flow within the kidney.

The renal failure may be oliguric or nonoliguric. During the acute phase, azotemia is present with blood urea nitrogen and creatinine levels peaking after 10–30 days. The return of renal function is typically heralded by the onset of a diuresis and a rapid return of renal function.

The kidneys in patients with ATN are enlarged bilaterally. Urography, although no longer recommended as a diagnostic procedure, characteristically demonstrates a dense persistent nephrogram as discussed above (Fig. 20.2). In a minority of patients, an increasingly dense nephrogram, more characteristic of acute extrarenal obstruction, may be found. The nephrogram may be present for as long as 24 hours after the contrast administration. There is typically no opacification of the collecting system.

A variety of sonographic appearances of ATN have been reported. Some authors report an increase in cortical echogenicity with preservation of corticomedullary definition. Others have noted an increase in the echogenicity of the pyramids with a normal cortical appearance while the completely opposite appearance, i.e., a decrease in the echogenicity and swelling of the pyramids, has been observed by still other authors. Rosenfield et al. have suggested, based on experimentally induced ATN in rats, that the sonographic appearance of ATN depends on its etiology thus accounting for the variable appearance reported among the various series.

Initial enthusiastic reports that MRI would be helpful in differentiating renal transplant rejection from ATN have not been borne out, however, a more recent report by Carvlin et al. demonstrated that gadolinium-enhanced MRI studies may show perfusion abnormalities in experimentally induced ATN. Additional work will be necessary to confirm the clinical utility of these observations.

Acute Cortical Necrosis

Acute cortical necrosis is a distinct form of ARF that results in ischemic necrosis of the renal cortex, including the columns of Bertin, while the medullary portions of the kidney are relatively spared. The process may occur diffusely throughout both kidneys and result in complete absence of renal function or may occur in a patchy distribution resulting in renal insufficiency. In both instances there is characteristically sparing of a thin rim of cortical tissue on the outer surface of the kidney because of preservation of the capsular blood supply. A large number of conditions are reported in association with cortical necrosis including burns, sepsis, toxins, transfusion of incompatible blood, dehydration, and peritonitis. More than two-thirds of the cases, however, are reported to be associated with pregnancy, especially those complicated by placental abruption, septic abortion, or placenta previa. The precise mechanism by which cortical necrosis occurs remains obscure, however, a transient episode of intrarenal vasospasm leading to cortical ischemia is regarded as the probable mechanism by most authors. Other possible explanations include intravascular thrombosis and damage to the glomerular capillary endothelium.

The radiographic findings depend on the stage of the illness. In the early stages of the disease, the kidneys are diffusely enlarged. On urography there may be faint opacification of the collecting system, particularly if patchy cortical involvement is present. Over the course of several months, there will be smooth renal shrinkage. Characteristically, this will be accompanied by a distinctive form of tram-like calcification throughout the cortex, including the septal cortex (Fig. 20.5). The appearance of this calcification has been reported as early as 24 days after the onset of the illness but more characteristically is reported at approximately 2 months. On sonography, the outer cortex is hypoechoic, a finding that has been reported soon after the onset of the disease. On contrast-enhanced CT scans, a radiolucent zone bordering the circumference of the kidneys has been reported.

Acute Interstitial Nephritis

Acute interstitial nephritis (AIN) is an acute hypersensitivity reaction in the kidney that may result in renal insufficiency or frank renal failure. Three forms of AIN have been described, (*a*) in association with a variety of drugs; (*b*) in association with a number of nonrenal infectious processes, e.g., infectious mononucleosis; and (*c*) in an idiopathic form. Drug-induced AIN is the most common of these. More than 40 compounds including penicillin and particularly methicillin, as well as rifampin, sulfonamide derivatives, nonsteroidal antiinflammatory agents, cimetidine, furosemide, and thiazide diuretics have been associated with AIN.

Cell-mediated immune mechanisms appear to be more important than humorally mediated mechanisms in the pathogenesis of AIN. Histologically, AIN is characterized by an interstitial infiltration of inflammatory cells including eosinophils and mononuclear cells without a significant component of arteritis or glomerulitis. In some forms of AIN, eosinophiluria may be found on clinical examination. Other common clinical signs and symp-

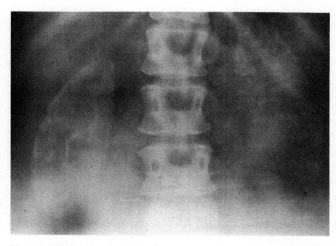

Figure 20.5. Acute cortical necrosis. Bilateral cortical calcifications characteristic of cortical necrosis are present. (From Pollack HM (ed): *Clinical Urography*. Philadelphia, WB Saunders, 1990, p. 1771.)

toms include macroscopic or microscopic hematuria, non-nephrotic range proteinuria, fever, eosinophilia, skin rash, and oliguria. Typically, there is recovery from the renal failure upon withdrawal of the drug.

On urography, bilateral nephromegaly with diminished opacification of the collecting system has been reported (Fig. 20.6). On ultrasound, increased cortical echogenicity and renal enlargement may be found. Increased accumulation of gallium-67 (^{67}Ga) citrate in the kidneys has also been reported.

Hematologic Disorders

Sickle Cell Anemia

A variety of morphologic abnormalities, including bilateral renal enlargement, lobar infarction, papillary necrosis (Fig. 20.7), and dilatation of the collecting system have been described in patients with both heterozygous and homozygous sickle cell disease. The later abnormality is thought to occur secondary to a decrease in the kidney's ability to concentrate urine. In addition to these structural defects, a number of functional abnormalities including hyposthenuria, hematuria, renal tubular acidosis, and progressive renal insufficiency have been described in sickle cell patients. This constellation of functional abnormalities is known as *sickle cell nephropathy*.

The older literature suggested that papillary necrosis is uncommon among homozygous patients while it is common in the heterozygous forms, particularly when hemoglobin S is combined with hemoglobin A (SA disease) or hemoglobin C (SC disease). The more recent literature, however, reports that changes of papillary necrosis are present in approximately 25–40% of homozygous patients. The appearance of the radiologic abnormalities, however, does not necessarily correlate with the

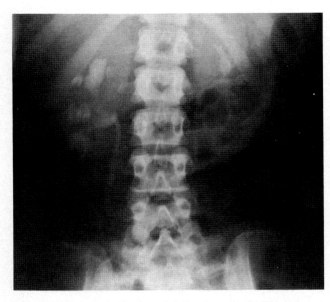

Figure 20.7. Marked calyceal deformity compatible with papillary necrosis is present bilaterally in this patient with known homozygous sickle cell anemia.

presence of renal functional abnormalities. Papillary necrosis is thought to occur as a result of low oxygen tension in the renal papilla which promotes sickling of the abnormal red blood cells. This, in turn, results in necrosis and ischemia of the papillary tips.

Lande et al. found that MRI in patients with sickle cell disease demonstrates decreased signal from the renal cortex which is especially apparent on T$_2$-weighted images. These authors speculated that the findings were secondary to iron deposition in the renal cortex. Similar findings, however, were not present in a group of patients suffering from β-thalassemia who were also clinically suffering from iron overload.

Hemophilia

A variety of urographic abnormalities including bilateral renal enlargement, retroperitoneal hemorrhage, and obstructive uropathy secondary to clots within the collecting system or ureter have been described in patients with hemophilia. The most striking feature, bilateral nephromegaly, is of uncertain etiology. Papillary necrosis, thought to be related to concomitant analgesic ingestion, has also been described.

Acute Leukemia

Leukemia is the most common malignant cause of bilateral nephromegaly in children (Fig. 20.8). The renal enlargement is commonly attributed to infiltration of the kidneys by leukemic cells, however, intrarenal hemorrhage and edema may also contribute to this appearance. The degree of renal enlargement may be striking, simulating the appearance of polycystic disease. In some

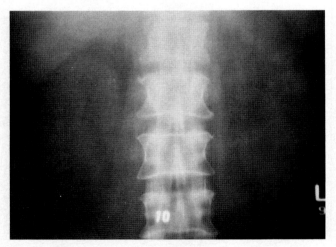

Figure 20.6. Acute interstitial nephritis. Bilateral nephromegaly, a diminished nephrogram, and a faintly opacified collecting system are demonstrated in this patient with drug-induced acute interstitial nephritis.

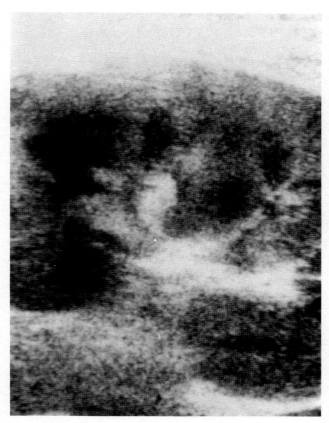

Figure 20.8. Marked nephromegaly is present in this child with proven leukemic infiltration of the kidneys.

cases, the renal enlargement may be asymmetric, and rarely may occur as a focal intrarenal mass (chloroma). The collecting system is generally attenuated and there may be filling defects in the renal pelvis or calyces secondary to blood clots or uric acid stones.

Multiple Myeloma

Multiple myeloma is one of a group of plasma cell dyscrasias which also includes Waldenström's macroglobulinemia, heavy- and light-chain disease, and benign monoclonal gammopathy. The disease results in the excess production of immunoglobulins and is characterized by the presence of Bence-Jones proteins in the urine. Renal failure occurs in 30–50% of such patients and has been attributed to the abnormal precipitation of myeloma proteins within the renal tubules. Hypercalcemia, as a result of the bone destruction that accompanies the myelomatous lesions in bone, may result in nephrocalcinosis. Because there is excess uric acid production, uric acid calculi may also be found. Amyloidosis develops in approximately 10% of the patients.

Radiologically, the kidneys are enlarged and there may be attenuation of the collecting system as the result of interstitial edema. Poor opacification on urography typically occurs because of the diminished renal function. On sonography, the kidneys are enlarged with decreased echogenicity which reflects the abnormal fluid accumulation within the kidney.

In the past, the administration of radiographic contrast material to patients with multiple myeloma was thought to be contraindicated because of reports that contrast material caused precipitation of the myeloma proteins within the renal tubules thereby hastening the onset of renal failure. More recent literature, however, suggests that the risks associated with contrast administration in patients with myeloma can be minimized as long as dehydration is avoided.

Amyloidosis

Amyloidosis is characterized by the extracellular deposition of an insoluble fibrillar proteinaceous material with a β-sheet configuration. Although the disease may be localized to one organ, in more than 85% of the cases a systemic multiorgan form of involvement is present. The disease is known to occur as an idiopathic systemic process (*primary amyloidosis*); in association with a variety of other chronic diseases including rheumatoid arthritis, tuberculosis, leprosy, chronic osteomyelitis, and some malignancies (*secondary amyloidosis*); in a familial form including that associated with familial Mediterranean fever; in a senile form; or in association with endocrine disorders including medullary carcinoma of the thyroid and diabetes. Each of these forms is associated with its own characteristic protein subunit. The protein found in patients with primary amyloidosis and those with amyloid disease associated with multiple myeloma are identical and resemble a portion of an immunoglobulin light chain. This fact suggests that the two diseases are different manifestations of a similar underlying blood dyscrasia and most authorities now classify amyloidosis as a blood dyscrasia.

Virtually every organ in the body may be involved; men are affected more commonly than women. The usual age of onset is 55–60 years. Most patients experience nonspecific symptoms including weight loss, weakness, and fatigue. Renal involvement occurs in 80% of patients with secondary amyloidosis and 35–40% of patients with primary disease. Fifty percent of patients with secondary amyloidosis die of renal failure. Although the kidneys are the most commonly involved organ in the urinary tract, isolated involvement of the renal pelvis, ureter, bladder, urethra, prostate, and seminal vesicles has been described. Amyloidosis of the renal pelvis, without renal parenchymal involvement, may be associated with a characteristic pattern of submucosal calcification visible on plain films. Renal vein thrombosis is a well-described complication of renal amyloidosis and may only affect the segmental or interlobar veins as a unique feature. The sudden onset of nephrotic syndrome in a patient with amyloidosis should suggest the development of this complication.

The radiologic findings in renal amyloidosis are non-specific. Although some patients have normally sized kidneys, the most consistently described feature is smooth bilateral renal enlargement (Fig. 20.9). As the disease progresses and renal failure ensues, the kidneys become shrunken while retaining their smooth contour. On urography, the nephrogram is typically diminished and there may be attenuation of the collecting system. On ultrasound examination, there is renal enlargement in the acute phase with an increase in cortical echogenicity, presumably related to the abnormal protein deposition. Angiographic features include tortuosity and irregularity of the interlobar arteries which may be localized to one portion of the kidney. An abnormal accumulation of ⁶⁷Ga citrate in the kidneys 48–72 hours after injection has been described on radionuclide examination.

Acute Urate Nephropathy

Increased nucleoprotein catabolism may occur as a complication of chemotherapy or radiation therapy in patients with leukemia, lymphoma, and other neoplastic disorders. As a consequence, there is a marked rise in plasma uric acid concentration, increased renal tubular secretion, and possibly decreased resorption of the filtered urate load. In such cases, precipitation of urate crystals within the tubules resulting in oliguric renal failure may occur. This form of acute renal failure is termed urate nephropathy.

An increasingly dense nephrogram with enlarged kidneys and an absent or markedly diminished pyelogram has been reported on urography (Fig. 20.10). As contrast material is a known uricosuric agent, precipitation of acute urate nephropathy in patients with high plasma uric

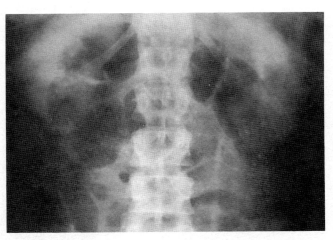

Figure 20.10. Bilateral renal enlargement and an increasing dense nephrogram are present in this patient with acute urate nephropathy.

acid concentrations may also theoretically occur after contrast administration.

Increased medullary echogenicity on sonography has been reported in patients with hyperuricemia and clinical evidence of gout.

AIDS Nephropathy

Azotemia, with moderate to severe proteinuria, occurs in approximately 10% of patients with acquired immunodeficiency syndrome (AIDS). A variety of glomerular lesions including focal and segmental glomerulosclerosis as well as tubular atrophy have been found on histologic examination. The combination of renal insufficiency, nephrotic syndrome, and glomerular changes has been called *AIDS nephropathy*.

On ultrasound, increased cortical echogenicity with normal-size kidneys has been observed. Hamper et al. found there was a correlation between the degree of increased cortical echogenicity and the severity of both the tubular and glomerular changes on histologic examination. A case of partial nephrocalcinosis secondary to *Mycobacterium avium intracellulare* renal infection associated with AIDS has also been reported.

Alports' Syndrome

The association of chronic hereditary renal disease, deafness, and ocular abnormalities is known as *Alport's syndrome*. Although both sexes are affected equally, males have a much worse prognosis and usually die of renal failure at an earlier age than do females. Clinically, symptoms begin in early childhood and include episodic hematuria, progressive renal failure, and a progressive high-frequency nerve deafness. Ocular abnormalities include congenital cataracts, nystagmus, and myopia. Although there is typically a strong familial history of renal

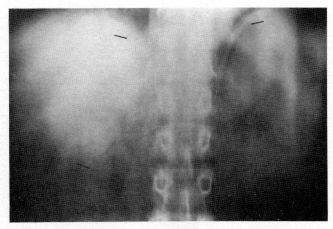

Figure 20.9. Renal amyloidosis. Bilaterally enlarged, poorly functioning kidneys are present on urography in this patient with proven renal amyloidosis. (Courtesy Marco A. Amendola, M.D.)

failure, the precise mode of transmission has not been established. On pathologic examination, the kidneys are small but smooth and exhibit a variety of histologic abnormalities including interstitial fibrosis with patchy glomerular involvement. A distinctive histologic feature is the presence of foam cells throughout the renal cortex, but most prominently near the corticomedullary junction.

Small smooth kidneys with impaired excretion of contrast material are found on radiologic examination. Pruning of the interlobar arteries with an indistinct corticomedullary junction has been reported on angiography.

Miscellaneous Conditions

Nephromegaly has been reported in a variety of other medical conditions including hepatic cirrhosis, diabetes mellitus, infectious mononucleosis, hyperalimentation, paroxysmal nocturnal hemoglobinuria, acute glomerulonephritis, heroin abuse, and Fabry's disease.

Diabetes, in patients with normal renal function, is the most common cause for bilateral nephromegaly. In some cases, the nephromegaly may be found before overt glycosuria develops. Although the exact etiology of the renal enlargement is not known, nephron hypertrophy is a possible explanation.

SUGGESTED READINGS

General References and Imaging Studies in Renal Failure

Davidson AJ: Radiology of the Kidney. Philadelphia, WB Saunders, 1985.

Evans C: Annotation: renal failure radiology—1987. *Clin Radiol* 38:457, 1987.

Fry IK, Cattell WR: The nephrographic pattern during excretion urography. *Br Med Bull* 28:227, 1972.

Hansen ME, Dunnick NR: Percutaneous intervention in renal failure. *Radiology Rep* 2:137, 1990.

Hricak H, Cruz C, Romanski R, et al: Renal parenchymal disease: Sonographic-histologic correlation. *Radiology* 144:141, 1982.

Keeton GR, Pillay GP: Diagnostic role of intravenous urography in acute and chronic renal failure. *Urol Radiol* 8:72, 1986.

Mena E, Bookstein JJ, Gikas PW: Angiographic diagnosis of renal parenchymal disease. *Radiology* 108:523, 1973.

Platt JF, Rubin JM, Bowerman RA, et al: The inability to detect kidney disease on the basis of echogenicity. *AJR* 151:317, 1988.

Ritchie WW, Vick CW, Glocheski SK, et al: Evaluation of azotemic patients: diagnostic yield of initial US examination. *Radiology* 167:245, 1988.

Schwartz WB, Hurwit A, Ettinger A: Intravenous urography in the patient with renal insufficiency. *New Engl J Med* 269:277, 1963.

Stuck KJ, White GM, Granke DS, et al: Urinary obstruction in azotemic patient: detection by sonography. *AJR* 149:1191, 1987.

Toyoda K, Miyamoto Y, Ida M, et al: Hyperechoic medulla of the kidneys. *Radiology* 173:431, 1989.

Acute Tubular Necrosis

Carvlin MJ, Arger PH, Kundel HL, et al: Acute tubular necrosis: use of gadolinium-DTPA and fast MR imaging to evaluate renal function in the rabbit. *J Comput Assist Tomogr* 11(3):488, 1987.

Love L, Lind JA Jr, Olson MC: Persistent CT nephrogram: significance in the diagnosis of contrast nephropathy. *Radiology* 172:125, 1989.

Nomura G, Kinoshita E, Yamagata Y, et al: Usefulness of renal ultrasonography for assessment of severity and course of acute tubular necrosis. *J Clin Ultrasound* 12:135, 1984.

Rosenfield AT, Zeman RK, Cicchetti DV, et al: Experimental acute tubular necrosis: US appearance. *Radiology* 157:771, 1985.

Acute Cortical Necrosis

Goergen TG, Lindstrom RR, Tan H, et al: CT appearance of acute renal cortical necrosis. *AJR* 137:176, 1981.

McAlister WH, Nedelman SH: The roentgen manifestations of bilateral renal cortical necrosis. *AJR* 86(1):129, 1961.

Sefczek RJ, Beckman I, Lupetin AR, et al: Sonography of acute renal cortical necrosis. *AJR* 142:553, 1984.

Acute Interstitial Nephritis

Adler SG, Cogen AH, Border WA: Hypersensitivity phenomena and the kidney: role of drugs and environmental agents. *Am J Kid Dis* 5(2):75, 1985.

Baldwin DS, Levine BB, McCluskey RT, et al: Renal failure and interstitial nephritis due to penicillin and methicillin. *New Engl J Med* 279(23):1245, 1968.

Ten RM, Torres VE, Milliner DS, et al: Acute interstitial nephritis: immunologic and clinical aspects. *Mayo Clin Proc* 63:921, 1988.

Hematologic Disorders

Dalinka MK, Lally JF, Rancier LF, et al: Nephromegaly in hemophilia. *Radiology* 115:337, 1975.

Ekelund L: Radiologic findings in renal amyloidosis. *AJR* 129:851, 1977.

Lande IM, Glazer GM, Sarnaik S, et al: Sickle-cell nephropathy: MR imaging. *Radiology* 158:379, 1986.

Lee VW, Skinner M, Cohen AS, et al: Renal amyloidosis: evaluation by gallium imaging. *Clin Nucl Med* 11(9):642, 1986.

Mapp E, Karasick S, Pollack H, et al: Uroradiological manifestations of S-hemoglobinopathy. *Semin Roentgenol* 22(3):186, 1987.

Marquis JR, Khazen B: Sickle-cell disease. *Radiology* 98:47, 1971.

McCall IW, Moule N, Desai P, et al: Urographic findings in homozygous sickle cell disease. *Radiology* 126:99, 1978.

Odita JC, Ugbodaga CI, Okafor LA, et al: Urographic changes in homozygous sickle cell disease. *Diagn Imaging* 52:259, 1983.

Pear BL: Other organs and other amyloids. *Semin Roentgenol* 21(2):150, 1986.

Scott PP, Scott WW Jr, Siegelman SS: Amyloidosis: an overview. *Semin Roentgenol* 21(2):103, 1986.

Acute Urate Nephropathy

Martin DJ, Jaffe N: Prolonged nephrogram due to hyperuricaemia. *Br J Radiol* 44:806, 1971.

Postlewaite AE, Kelley WM: Uricosuric effect of radiocontrast agents. A study in man of four commonly used preparations. *Ann Intern Med* 74:845, 1971.

AIDS Nephropathy

Bourgoignie JJ, Meneses R, Ortiz C, et al: The clinical spectrum of renal disease associated with human immunodeficiency virus. *Am J Kidney Dis* 12(2):131, 1988.

Falkof GE, Rigsby CM, Rosenfield AT: Partial, combined cortical and medullary nephrocalcinosis: US and CT patterns in AIDS-associated MAI infection. *Radiology* 162:343, 1987.

Hamper UM, Goldblum LE, Hutchins GM, et al: Renal involvement in AIDS: Sonographic-pathologic correlation. *AJR* 150:1321, 1988.

Alport's Syndrome

Chuang VP, Reuter SR: Angiographic features of Alport's syndrome. *AJR* 121(3):539, 1974.

RENAL TRANSPLANTATION

During the past 10 years renal allotransplantation has become the standard therapy for end-stage renal disease. The advent of the immunosuppressive drug cyclosporine has made successful allograft transplantation a clinical reality so that a 95% 1-year patient survival and an 80% 1-year graft survival, even after cadaver transplantation, can now be expected.

In 1988, 8932 renal transplants were performed in the United States of which 7116 were cadaver donors, 56 were living unrelated donors, and 1760 were living related donors. This represents an increase of approximately 30% when compared with the number of transplants performed in 1983.

Radiologic evaluation plays an important role in both the pretransplant evaluation of prospective kidney recipients and potential kidney donors as well as in the evaluation of posttransplant renal dysfunction.

PRETRANSPLANT EVALUATION

A voiding cystourethrogram is customarily performed on every prospective renal transplant recipient to determine whether vesicoureteral reflux is present. Pretransplant native kidney nephrectomy will usually be performed when significant vesicoureteral reflux is present

to minimize the possibility of posttransplant pyelonephritis in an immunosuppressed patient. The voiding cystourethrogram is also of value in ascertaining whether normal bladder function is present. If the patient has had a prolonged period of anuria prior to evaluation, the voiding cystourethrogram may well show a small capacity bladder because of disuse. Benign extravasation of the contrast material from the bladder in these patients has been described (Fig. 21.1). Such extravasation does not represent frank perforation of the bladder. Cystoscopy performed in such patients generally reveals no abnormality; it requires no specific therapy, and it is not a contraindication to subsequent transplantation. It has been speculated that such extravasation occurs through the fascial plane adjacent to the sheath of Waldeyer, a tube-like structure that extends from the trigone of the bladder through the ureteral orifices and merges with the wall of the ureter 2–3 cm outside the bladder.

The presence of significant uncorrectable bladder dysfunction, either as the cause of or in association with the patient's renal failure is not a contraindication to transplantation. In such patients, vesicle augmentation procedures, intermittent catheterization, or the construction of an ileal conduit prior to transplantation may be considered.

Ultrasonography of the potential recipient's native kidneys is performed to evaluate the size of the kidneys, the presence or absence of hydronephrosis, and the presence of renal calculi. Plain film tomography of the kidney may also be utilized for this purpose especially if there is a prior history of renal calculus disease.

Other radiologic studies commonly performed in the pretransplant period include chest radiography, a bone survey to determine the presence of renal osteodystrophy, ultrasonography of the gallbladder to detect the presence of cholelithiasis, and in patients with a history of prior gastrointestinal disease, an upper gastrointestinal series and barium enema.

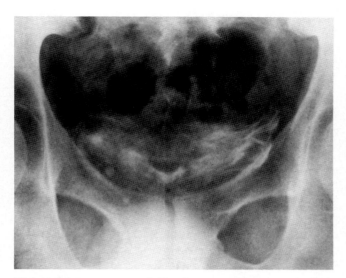

Figure 21.1. A postvoid film from a voiding cystourethrogram patient with an unused bladder demonstrates benign extraperitoneal extravasation.

In addition to radiologic evaluation, patients being prepared for renal transplant undergo a large number of laboratory studies including tissue typing, an extensive cardiovascular evaluation, and an extensive medical and psychological evaluation.

LIVING RELATED DONOR EVALUATION

Patients receiving living related donor kidneys have a 5-year graft survival that approaches 90%. For transplants involving human leukocyte antigen (HLA)-identical siblings, long-term graft survival approaches 95%. For haploidentical living related donors (parent or non-HLA-identical sibling), 1-year graft survival is somewhat lower, but still approaches 90%. Patients receiving HLA-identical kidneys have fewer instances of rejection and require less immunosuppression than do patients receiving cadaver kidneys or haploidentical kidneys.

Potential living related donors should be screened radiologically with an excretory urogram to determine the number and size of the kidneys, the presence of congenital anomalies, including duplication of the ureters, and the presence of unsuspected renal pathology. If the results of urography and screening laboratory studies are normal and histocompatability studies are compatible, angiography is then performed to evaluate the number of renal vessels that are present.

For the purpose of transplantation, a kidney having only a single artery is preferable to one having multiple arteries. It is generally preferable to use the left kidney as a donor, as its renal vein is longer, making the venous anastomosis technically easier to perform. Kidneys with three or more renal arteries are generally considered unsuitable for donation but may be used at a considerably higher risk for technical complications.

Evaluation of the number of renal vessels that are present is usually performed by standard catheter angiography. In some centers, however, a combined urogram and intravenous digital subtraction angiographic (DSA) study of the renal vessels (Fig. 21.2) is performed in one examination, eliminating the need for catheter angiography. In 100 consecutive such patients reported by Flechner et al., the intravenous DSA study satisfactorily imaged the renal arteries in 89% of the patients; 11% of the patients required further study with conventional catheter angiography because of inadequate intravenous DSA studies. Intravenous DSA was found to have an accuracy of 96% in identifying the number of renal vessels present. In a separate study, McElroy et al. found that a satisfactory intravenous DSA study was accurate in identifying the number of renal arteries in 21 out of 23 patients. This approach has a major advantage in that it can be performed completely on an outpatient basis and is less costly than conventional angiography by a factor of at least 50%.

TECHNIQUE OF RENAL TRANSPLANTATION

Patients undergoing renal allograft placement are generally considered to be at a higher risk for surgical complications than patients without renal failure. In addition, many of these patients suffer from a systemic disease that also adds to the risk of surgery. Therefore, careful surgical technique is even more important so that complications associated with graft placement can be minimized.

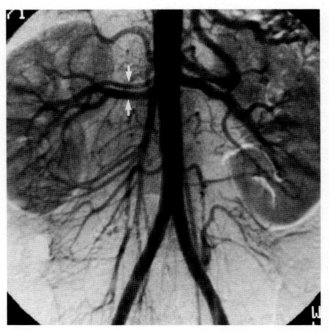

Figure 21.2. Intravenous digital subtraction angiogram of the abdominal aorta demonstrates two right renal arteries (*arrows*).

Renal allograft placement is generally accomplished in either the right or left iliac fossae through an extraperitoneal incision made above, but parallel to the inguinal ligament. The vascular dissection is somewhat technically easier on the right side and, therefore, this is the preferred site of graft placement. The lymphatics, especially, must be carefully dissected and ligated to avoid subsequent development of a lymphocele. In patients receiving a kidney containing a single renal artery, either an end-to-end renal artery to hypogastric artery anastomosis is performed with an end-to-side anastomosis between the renal vein and the external iliac vein or an end-to-side anastomosis between the renal artery and the external iliac artery with an end-to-side anastomosis between the renal vein and the external iliac vein can be performed. Normally the venous anastomosis is accomplished before the arterial anastomosis is made. If there are multiple renal vessels, a patch of the aorta or vena cava is utilized and generally end-to-side anastomoses are performed. Alternatively, side-to-side anastomoses between the renal vessels can be accomplished and a single anastomosis with the recipient vessel made.

There are many variations in surgical technique for dealing with donor kidneys containing multiple vessels which depend on the experience of the surgeon and the exact anatomy that must be reconstructed.

The ureter of the transplanted kidney is generally implanted into the bladder via a ureteroneocystostomy commonly using the Ledbetter-Politano or Litch technique. In this fashion, an antirefluxing anastomosis is accomplished. As with vascular anastomoses, there are many variations in technique that largely depend on the experience and preference of the surgeon. Ureteral stents are rarely utilized.

The transplanted kidney usually starts functioning almost immediately after the vascular anastomoses are completed, provided there has not been a prolonged period of warm or cold ischemia.

COMPLICATIONS OF RENAL TRANSPLANTATION

Complications of renal transplantation can generally be divided into three groups; those related to (*a*) malfunction of the renal parenchyma including acute tubular necrosis (ATN), graft rejection, cyclosporine nephrotoxicity, renal rupture, and renal infection; (*b*) technical complications involving the renal artery or vein, urologic complications, and the development of peritransplant fluid collections; and (*c*) long-term complications such as the subsequent development of malignancy.

Clinically it is convenient to classify the causes of transplant dysfunction by the time frame in which the dysfunction occurs. Early transplant dysfunction is usually caused by ATN, acute rejection, or cyclosporine nephrotoxicity or is related to a mechanical problem with the vascular anastomosis or the ureteroneocystostomy. Later causes of transplant dysfunction include rejection, nephrotoxicity, vascular stenoses, and the development of urologic complications, or peritransplant fluid collections.

RENAL COMPLICATIONS

Acute Tubular Necrosis

ATN occurs in the immediate posttransplant period as the result of ischemia of the transplant prior to revascularization. In patients receiving living related transplants, posttransplant renal dysfunction secondary to ATN is rarely found, however, in patients receiving cadaver kidneys, the incidence of ATN ranges from 5 to 80% and is directly related to the period of warm and cold ischemia, the method by which renal preservation was accomplished, and to the presence of such adverse conditions in the donor as preterminal hypotension. The present methods of renal preservation may allow storage for periods up to 48 hours, however, with longer times the rate of ATN is very high. As a general rule, however, the presence of ATN in the initial posttransplant period does not appear to have a major adverse effect on ultimate graft survival.

ATN may be manifest in the immediate posttransplant period or its onset may be delayed for up to 24–48 hours. It is generally self-limiting and renal function generally recovers within a few days to a few weeks. Persistence of ATN for periods up to 1 month with subsequent function, however, have been reported.

Radionuclide studies are the major method by which ATN is diagnosed radiologically. In patients studied using a combination of DTPA and Hippuran, those exhibiting ATN generally demonstrate a relative preservation of renal perfusion, however, while the Hippuran curve generally shows prompt uptake of the isotope, there is a prolonged excretion phase with the renogram curve demonstrating an ascending slope (Fig. 21.3). Static images demonstrate retention of the tracer in the transplant kidney.

Most studies indicate that sonography in patients with ATN is normal, however, sonographic abnormalities in ATN have occasionally been reported. Most authorities, however, feel that sonography is not a reliable way to distinguish ATN from other causes of early transplant dysfunction.

Nephrotoxicity

The introduction of the fungal metabolite, cyclosporine, has had a major effect on kidney transplantation in the United States. Multiple studies show an improvement in 1-year graft survival with cadaver kidneys that approaches 30% when immunosuppression with cyclosporine plus prednisone was compared with conven-

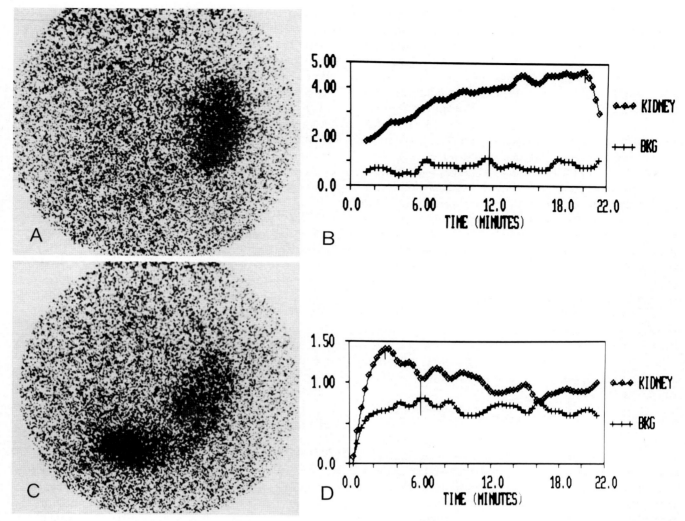

Figure 21.3. Acute tubular necrosis. A ^{131}I-Hippuran scan (**A**) in the immediate postoperative period in a patient who received a cadaver kidney demonstrates retention of the radiopharmaceutical within the kidney. The corresponding renogram curve (**B**) demonstrates an ascending slope. Five days later, a repeat study (**C**) demonstrates prompt excretion of the tracer into the bladder and the renogram curve (**D**) has normalized indicating resolution of the ATN.

tional therapy with azathioprine and prednisone. Cyclosporine also represents a major advance over conventional immunosuppressive therapy in that the incidence of opportunistic infection appears to be markedly reduced with this drug. This is particularly true for infections caused by bacterial pathogens. However, cyclosporine has both nephrotoxicity and hepatotoxicity as major side effects. In this setting of renal transplantation, nephrotoxicity is the major clinical concern.

The level of cyclosporine concentration in the blood is usually monitored utilizing one of two methods. The first method is a selective cyclosporine assay utilizing high-performance liquid chromatography or specific monoclonal antibodies by radioimmunoassay. The second method is a nonselective method that measures both the level of cyclosporine and its metabolites. The results of the two methods give differing results, and it is unclear which method more closely correlates with the clinical syndrome of nephrotoxicity. As a further complicating factor, individuals also appear to have varying sensitivity to a given drug level.

Cyclosporine nephrotoxicity may be acute, subacute, or chronic. Acute cyclosporine toxicity is dose related, appears to potentiate initial graft dysfunction related to ischemia, and in some cases is manifested by a prolonged period of ATN. Subacute toxicity also is dose related and is reversible by a reduction in the dose of immunosuppression given. Clinically, subacute cyclosporine nephrotoxicity occurs in the first 60 days following transplantation and is usually associated with elevated serum trough levels of the drug of greater than 250 mg/ml by radioimmunoassay. Chronic nephrotoxicity is usually seen following the 60th day of therapy with the drug and does not respond to a reduction in the dose of drug administered. On biopsy, patients suffering from cyclosporine nephrotoxicity have nonspecific findings such as interstitial fibrosis that may be difficult to reliably differentiate from rejection.

On radionuclide examination, cyclosporine toxicity has been shown to result in a disassociation between ^{99m}Tc-DTPA perfusion studies and ^{131}I-Hippuran studies. In such cases, the perfusion portion of the examination remains relatively intact while the Hippuran curve shows a prolonged rate of clearance of the tracer (Fig. 21.4). This is particularly the case in patients with subacute nephrotoxicity. Thus, the findings in cyclosporine toxicity are similar to the radionuclide findings produced by ATN or obstruction. The diagnosis of cyclosporine toxicity, therefore, can only be suggested when serial studies have demonstrated a resolution of the immediate posttransplant ATN; the reappearance of an ascending slope of the Hippuran curve without a new ischemic episode suggests the diagnosis of cyclosporine nephrotoxicity.

At present, no other imaging studies appear to be as reliable as the radionuclide studies in differentiating cyclosporine toxicity from other causes of transplant dysfunction. Early hopes that MRI would allow differentiation between nephrotoxicity and rejection have not been borne out.

Rejection

Graft rejection represents a significant source of morbidity in the transplant patient. Clinically, rejection is classified into four categories: (*a*) hyperacute rejection, (*b*) accelerated acute rejection, (*c*) acute rejection, and (*d*) chronic rejection. Virtually every patient receiving a renal transplant experiences some form of rejection in the posttransplant period and differentiation of rejection episodes from other causes of graft dysfunction continues to be a difficult and perplexing clinical problem. This difficulty has been compounded by the widespread use of cyclosporine as an immunosuppressive agent. The therapy of early graft dysfunction obviously depends on the diagnosis; if the cause is rejection, increased immunosuppression is indicated. If, on the other hand, the cause is cyclosporine toxicity, the opposite treatment should be instituted; that is, the dose of cyclosporine should be reduced. A further complicating issue is the fact that in many instances, the etiology of the graft dysfunction is multifactorial; for example, ATN may be superimposed on acute rejection.

Hyperacute Rejection

Hyperacute rejection is mediated by humoral antibodies originating from β-lymphocytes and is usually manifested at the operating table when the graft is revascularized. As soon as the vascular clamps are removed, a transplant exhibiting hyperacute rejection will become swollen and cyanotic. The antigen-antibody reaction results in complement activation that in turn damages the vascular endothelium, particularly involving the small vessels of the kidney. As a result, they become filled with fibrin thrombi and there is extensive cortical necrosis. An allograft exhibiting hyperacute rejection is usually considered unsalvageable, and transplant nephrectomy is usually performed. If nephrectomy is not immediately undertaken, renal perfusion studies using technetium-DTPA generally show a virtual absence of renal perfusion. Pretransplant screening of the recipient for antibodies cytotoxic to donor lymphocytes has reduced the incidence of this form of rejection.

Accelerated Acute Rejection

The mechanism for accelerated acute rejection is poorly understood. Some authors maintain that accelerated acute rejection is an antibody-mediated form of rejection that is mechanistically identical to hyperacute rejection, however, the onset of the rejection episode is delayed until the first 2–3 days after transplantation. Other authors believe that accelerated acute rejection is merely an anamnestic manifestation of cell-mediated immunity. Accelerated acute rejection is usually considered to be present when a rejection episode is documented within the first week following transplantation. Accelerated acute rejection is frequently, but not always, successfully treated with immunosuppressive drugs.

Acute Rejection

The term "acute rejection" is utilized to characterize a group of morphologic and pathologic changes that characterize a rapid course of renal allograft dysfunction. Clinically, acute rejection is characterized by a relatively rapid rise in serum creatinine (a rise of 25% or more above the baseline level occurring within 24–48 hours), graft swelling and tenderness on physical examination, and fever. Decreased urine output is usually present as well. Laboratory studies may demonstrate a decrease in active T rosette–forming cells and increased spontaneous lymphocyte blastogenesis.

Acute rejection is thought to occur because of a proliferation of T-lymphocytes and represents a cell-mediated form of immunity. Histologically, it is characterized by a proliferation of mononuclear cells, eosinophils, and plasma cells that infiltrate the interstitium of the kidney. A vascular component may also be present and biopsies showing acute rejection are sometimes classified as showing primarily interstitial rejection or a mixed pattern in which both an interstitial and vascular component are present. The degree of interstitial infiltration that is present determines whether mild, moderate, or severe rejection is present.

While clinical signs suggest the diagnosis of acute rejection, none of these signs is absolutely specific and there is a significant overlap with patients who are pri-

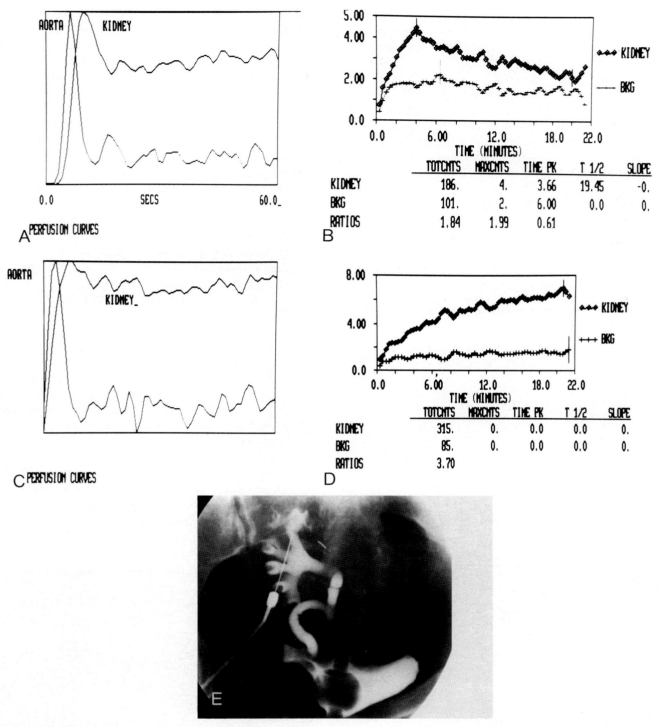

Figure 21.4. Cyclosporine nephrotoxicity. Immediate post-transplant ^{99m}Tc-DTPA perfusion (**A**) and ^{131}I-Hippuran renogram (**B**) curves in a patient who received a living related kidney show good perfusion and excretion. Three days later, the perfusion curve (**C**) remains relatively intact, however, the Hippuran curve (**D**) now demonstrates an ascending slope. An antegrade pyelogram (**E**) shows no evidence of obstruction thereby confirming that the cause of the transplant dysfunction is cyclosporine nephrotoxicity.

marily suffering from another acute cause of graft dysfunction. Hence, imaging methods that can adequately differentiate acute rejection from other forms of acute graft dysfunction thereby obviating the need for renal biopsy have been extensively investigated. Acute rejection may occur at any time following transplantation, but most commonly such episodes occur between the 1st and 10th week after graft placement.

Acute rejection is suggested on radionuclide studies when there is deterioration of ^{99m}Tc-DTPA perfusion studies. This is best demonstrated by an analysis of perfusion curves acquired during the first 1 minute of the passage of the radiotracer through the iliac vessels into the kidney (Fig. 21.5). Rejection is characterized by prolongation of the interval between the peak of activity in the aorta and the peak of activity in the transplant itself

and by flattening of the ascending and descending slopes of the time-activity curve of the kidney when this curve is normalized to that of the aorta. In addition, there is a diminution in the kidney peak to plateau ratio. Characteristically in acute cellular rejection, there is relatively less impairment in a renogram curve performed with Hippuran. Such curves frequently show flattening of the excretory phase of the curve or may have a frankly ascending slope, but these abnormalities are proportionally less than the abnormalities present in the perfusion curve. Imaging studies may show patchy areas of perfusion. To establish the diagnosis of acute rejection, baseline radionuclide studies are frequently helpful and if this method is utilized to follow the status of the transplanted kidney, such baseline studies should be obtained either on the day of or the day following the initial surgery.

Other investigators have studied the use of ^{111}In platelets to detect acute transplant rejection. While this method offers a relatively high sensitivity in diagnosing rejection, it does not reliably differentiate rejection from cyclosporine nephrotoxicity, however, because of their high cost such studies are not widely performed.

Since the initial report of Maklad et al. in 1979, sonography has played a major role in the diagnosis of acute renal transplant rejection. Sonographic characteristics of rejection include an increased size of the transplanted kidney, increased size and decreased echogenicity of the renal pyramids, and a decrease in the echogenicity of the renal cortex (Fig. 21.6). The earliest sign appears to be an increase in the size of the medullary pyramids with the later appearance of cortical abnormalities. Hricak et al. have also reported that a change in the amplitude and distribution of renal sinus echoes is a sensitive indicator

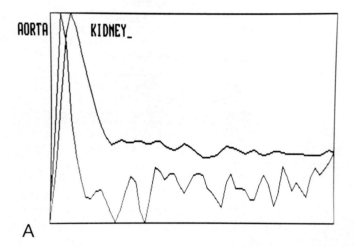

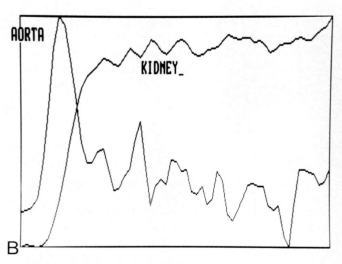

Figure 21.5. Acute rejection. Immediate posttransplant ^{99m}Tc-DTPA perfusion curve (**A**) is normal. Ten days later (**B**) a repeat study demonstrates diminution of the kidney peak to plateau ratio and flattening of the ascending and descending kidney curve in comparison to that of the aorta.

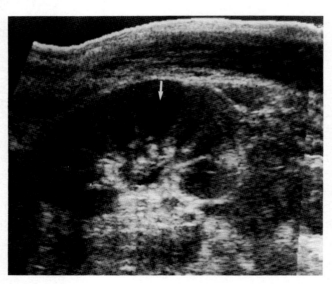

Figure 21.6. Acute rejection. A longitudinal ultrasound examination demonstrates an enlarged kidney with sonolucent pyramids (*arrow*) characteristic of acute rejection.

of transplant rejection. With advanced rejection, there is a decrease in the echogenicity of the renal sinus so that the renal sinus blends into the surrounding parenchyma. As with the radionuclide study, a baseline study is frequently helpful in establishing the diagnosis of acute rejection on sonography. The sonographic findings are believed to mirror the pathophysiology of acute rejection, with the decrease in echogenicity related to edema of the pyramids and ischemia of the cortex. Several reports suggest that these findings may, at the early stage, be focal in nature and therefore random needle biopsy of the transplanted kidney may not truly establish the correct diagnosis. For this reason, biopsy of the most abnormal regions under sonographic guidance has been advocated.

The sonographic diagnosis of acute rejection is largely subjective and interobserver and intraobserver variation may be present in as many as 80% of the cases, especially among relatively inexperienced sonographers. The accuracy of sonography in predicting renal transplant rejection has been variably reported. Singh and Cohen report a sensitivity of 70% and a specificity of 100%. Hoddick et al. report somewhat less encouraging results. In their study, which included 100 consecutive patients in whom sonographic guided biopsies of transplanted kidneys were performed, these investigators showed that the accuracy of a positive prediction of rejection was relatively high (83–90%), however, the accuracy of a negative prediction of rejection was uniformly low (17–30%) and they were unable to differentiate rejection from other causes of transplant dysfunction when sonographic findings of rejection were not present. Thus, when typical US findings of rejection are present, the specificity of US will be relatively high; when typical findings are not present, US cannot be utilized to exclude rejection. This is particularly true when the biopsy demonstrates a mild or predominantly interstitial type of rejection.

In an attempt to improve the objective assessment of sonography, the medullary pyramid index (MPI) may be utilized to quantitate the degree to which hypoechoic pyramids are present. Medullary index is calculated as follows:

$$MPI = \frac{\frac{1}{2}(\text{pyramid length} \times \text{pyramid width})}{\text{cortical thickness}}$$

There are little data, however, to show that the calculation of such an index improves the sensitivity of the sonographic diagnosis of acute rejection.

Recently, attempts to improve the sensitivity of US for the diagnosis of rejection have been made utilizing duplex Doppler examinations (Fig. 21.7) and color flow Doppler sonography. Rigsby et al., reported in a study of 24 patients who had received renal allografts, that increased pulsatility of the wave form by qualitative analysis indicated acute rejection. They reported a 60% sensitivity

and a 95% specificity for the diagnosis of rejection utilizing this method. In a subsequent report, the same authors calculated a pulsatility index (PI), which was defined as the ratio of the peak systolic frequency shift minus the minimal diastolic frequency shift divided by the mean frequency shift of a signal obtained from an interlobar artery. With a threshold PI of 1.5, the sensitivity of this technique for the diagnosis of acute rejection was reported as 75% with a specificity of 90%.

Rifkin et al. (1987) have advocated the use of the resistive index (RI) to evaluate patients with suspected rejection. They reported that the RI ([peak systolic frequency shift − lowest diastolic frequency shift]/peak systolic frequency shift) has a positive predictive value for rejection of 100% when a value greater than 0.90 was calculated. If the RI was less than 0.70, the negative predictive value for rejection was 94%. Allen et al., in a prospective study, demonstrated no significant difference between PI and RI and showed that scintigraphy more reliably differentiated rejection from ATN.

Buckley et al. have suggested that duplex sonography may be of particular value in patients with acute rejection in whom vascular changes on biopsy predominate; in their study patients with predominantly interstitial rejection and those with cyclosporine nephrotoxicity demonstrated normal duplex studies.

MRI was thought to hold great promise in differentiating acute rejection from other causes of renal transplant dysfunction. Hricak et al. reported that rejection could be diagnosed with accuracy on T1-weighted images because of a loss of the corticomedullary contrast and specifically that these findings were not present in patients in whom graft function was compromised by cyclosporine nephrotoxicity. Subsequent studies, however, have demonstrated that the loss of the corticomedullary contrast is a relatively nonspecific finding on MRI and this finding may be present in a wide variety of pathologic processes unrelated to allograft rejection. In a prospective study, Steinberg et al. reported that Doppler ultrasound was significantly superior to MRI in identifying rejection because of a higher sensitivity (95% versus 70%), specificity (95% versus 73%), and accuracy (95% versus 71%). The role of magnetic resonance spectroscopy, however, has yet to be defined.

Angiography in acute rejection shows an enlarged kidney with poor filling of the interlobar, arcuate, and cortical arteries. There is a prolonged arterial phase with poor washout. The nephrogram demonstrates patchy opacification and there is poor definition of the corticomedullary junction. Arteriovenous (AV) shunting may be present. The angiographic findings of acute rejection may not affect the entire kidney uniformly; they may be quite focal affecting only a relatively small portion of the kidney.

Experimental angiography in animal models of acute

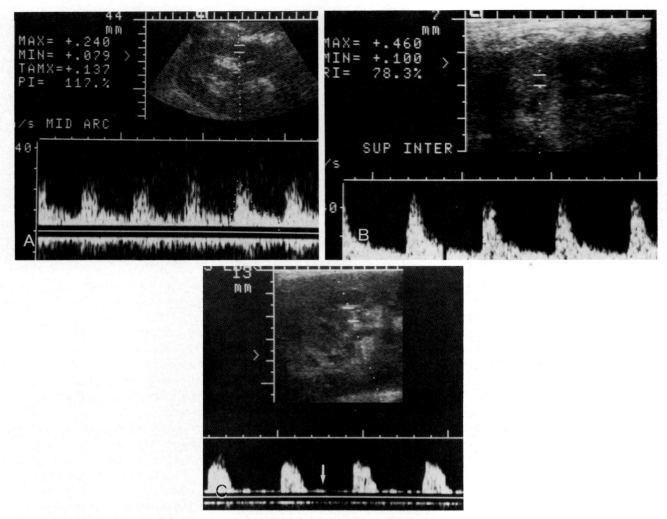

Figure 21.7.   Duplex Doppler ultrasonograms. **A**, Normal duplex study with a PI of 1.17. **B**, Mild rejection; RI = 0.78, PI = 1.7. **C**, Severe rejection with virtually complete absence of diastolic flow (*arrow*).

rejection shows that the vascular changes develop from the outer cortex inward and that medullary obliteration occurs after the cortical changes are apparent. Arteriovenous communications are a late manifestation of rejection and are demonstrated at the cortical, preglomerular, and postglomerular capillary levels.

Currently, angiography is rarely performed to evaluate the possibility of acute rejection. The angiographic findings indicating rejection, however, may be encountered when this procedure is performed to evaluate other suspected pathology.

Chronic Rejection

The term "chronic rejection" is used to signify a group of morphologic changes in the transplanted kidney that occur over a prolonged period of time. Prominent vascular changes including endothelial swelling, smooth muscle proliferation, and glomerular change are typically present. Segmental fibrosis and diffuse cellular infiltra-

tion may be found within the transplanted kidney. In contrast to acute rejection, the functional result of chronic rejection is a slow deterioration that progresses over months or years. In general, these changes are irreversible and lead to progressive azotemia and hypertension. On examination, the chronically rejected kidney is small with a decrease in cortical thickness.

In patients suffering from chronic rejection, angiography typically shows a small kidney. There is a reduction in the number of parenchymal vessels and there is diffuse narrowing of the vascular tree and multiple small irregular stenoses may be present. Frank areas of renal infarction may be demonstrated. In contrast to acute rejection, the arterial washout time is typically normal or only minimally prolonged. As in acute rejection, angiography is rarely performed to establish this diagnosis, but the findings of chronic rejection are frequently encountered when angiography is performed to evaluate renal vascular complications.

Infection

Thirty to 60% of patients receiving renal allografts are treated for urinary tract infection within the first 4 months following placement of the graft. One-fourth of these patients develop frank sepsis. The incidence and severity of the infection depends on the degree and duration of the immunosuppressive therapy such patients receive. Patients at risk for developing complications from urinary tract infection may be those with preexisting infection or those in whom urinary tract infection coexists with other forms of acute graft dysfunction. Diabetics, in particular, have a higher risk for the development of bacturia than other transplant patients, however, this does not appear to predispose such patients to an increased risk of sepsis.

The organisms found in transplant patients are the usual Gram-negative urinary pathogens found in nonimmunosuppressed patients. In addition, however, cytomegalovirus (CMV) and herpes simplex viral urinary tract infections are also found.

Four cases of emphysematous pyelonephritis in transplant patients have been reported in the radiologic literature. In these cases the diagnosis was established by CT (Fig. 21.8), US, or both. In one of the cases reported, percutaneous drainage utilizing CT guidance and parenteral antibiotics resulted in graft salvage.

As with other patients with urinary tract infection, patients following transplantation who present with recurrent episodes of pyelonephritis should be evaluated radiologically to detect the presence of vesicoureteral reflux (Fig. 21.9). If the reflux is significant and thought to be responsible for the infections, ureteroneocystostomy should be considered.

Renal Transplant Rupture

Renal transplant rupture is a dramatic complication of transplantation that usually occurs within the first 2

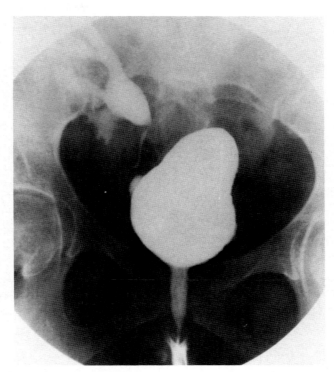

Figure 21.9. A voiding cystourethrogram shows reflux in to the transplanted kidney.

weeks following transplant placement. Transplant rupture occurs in 3–5% of renal allografts. The precise etiology of rupture of the transplant is not known, however, acute rejection, ATN, and vascular occlusion are thought to be predisposing causes. It has been speculated that transplant rupture occurs when the venous drainage of the kidney becomes compromised. This results in an increase in arterial pressure such that when the arterial pressure exceeds the renal capsular pressure, rupture can occur. This process may be enhanced by previous biopsies that reduce the amount of pressure the capsule is capable of withstanding. Clinically, patients experiencing transplant rupture have pain and swelling at the graft site, hematuria, and experience a fall in hematocrit. Signs of graft dysfunction are also present. Graft rupture usually occurs at the posterior and convex surface of the kidney and presents as a deep laceration in the renal parenchyma.

Sonography in such cases shows a hypoechoic mass (Fig. 21.10) within the renal parenchyma associated with a perinephric fluid collection. The hypoechoic mass represents the blood-filled laceration within the kidney.

Vascular Complications

Thrombosis

Thrombosis of the renal artery may occur in the immediate postoperative period as the result of kinking of the renal artery at the time of closure of the surgical

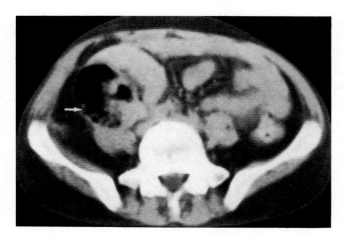

Figure 21.8. Emphysematous pyelonephritis. A CT scan demonstrates air (*arrow*) diffusely infiltrating the transplant kidney in the right iliac fossa.

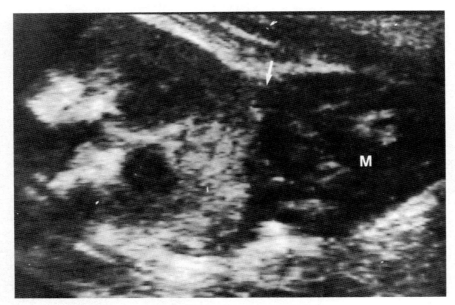

Figure 21.10. Transplant rupture. A longitudinal sonogram demonstrates a hypoechoic mass (M) in the inferior portion of the kidney at the site of the rupture (*arrow*).

incision or as a result of an intimal flap created during the vascular anastomosis. Such complications result in an absence of urinary output in the early posttransplant period. Radionuclide perfusion scans demonstrate no perfusion of the transplant; in the immediate postoperative period, this represents a surgical emergency and immediate reexploration of the kidney is usually performed. Renal artery thrombosis may also occur as the result of hyperacute rejection and is more common in kidneys containing more than one renal artery (Fig. 21.11).

Renal Artery Stenosis

Renal artery stenosis is reported to occur in 0.6–16% of patients following successful allograft placement. The real incidence of renal transplant artery stenosis, however, is difficult to estimate since asymptomatic cases may not be detected unless studied with angiography. Lacombe et al. in a prospective study evaluated 100 consecutive recipients and found a transplant renal artery stenosis in 23% of the patients. Such stenoses result in a decline in renal function, may cause hypertension, and eventually may lead to frank occlusion of the renal artery. A bruit may be present on physical examination.

The causes of transplant renal artery stenosis depend on the location at which the stenosis occurs. Preanastomotic stenoses may be related to host vessel arteriosclerosis, particularly in patients with diabetes or extensive vascular disease, or may be related to trauma to the vessels at the time of surgery. Anastomotic stenoses (Fig. 21.12) are said to be related to faulty suture technique, perfusion injury, or a local reaction to suture material. Postanastomotic stenoses may be related to either rejec-

tion, disturbed local hemodynamics, or extrinsic compression. Smooth tubular stenoses are more common following end-to-side anastomoses, whereas stenoses following end-to-end anastomosis may either be focal or tubular in nature. Kinking of the renal artery after placement of the graft within the surgical incision may also result in a long stenosis (Fig. 21.13).

Posttransplant renal artery stenosis requires angiography for accurate evaluation. Because 24–60% of patients who receive kidney transplants may have hypertension related to a variety of causes other than renal artery stenosis, a method by which transplant renal artery stenosis can be diagnosed noninvasively has widely been sought. At present, radionuclide studies appear to be too insensitive to reliably detect this complication. Taylor et al. reported that duplex Doppler US was able to suggest this diagnosis in four of seven patients who subsequently required angioplasty.

Intravenous DSA has been reported to be successful in screening posttransplant patients with hypertension for the presence of renal artery stenosis. Of the 10 patients studied by Flechner et al., renal artery stenosis was demonstrated to be present in two cases by the intravenous study and verified by standard catheter angiography.

Percutaneous transluminal angioplasty (PTA) has become the preferred method by which such stenoses are treated. Raynoud et al. performed technically successful angioplasty in 35 out of 43 renal transplant patients studied. After one month of follow-up, 74% of the patients were categorized as improved. PTA was technically successful on the first attempt in 91% of the patients with end-to-side anastomoses, but in only 75% of patients with

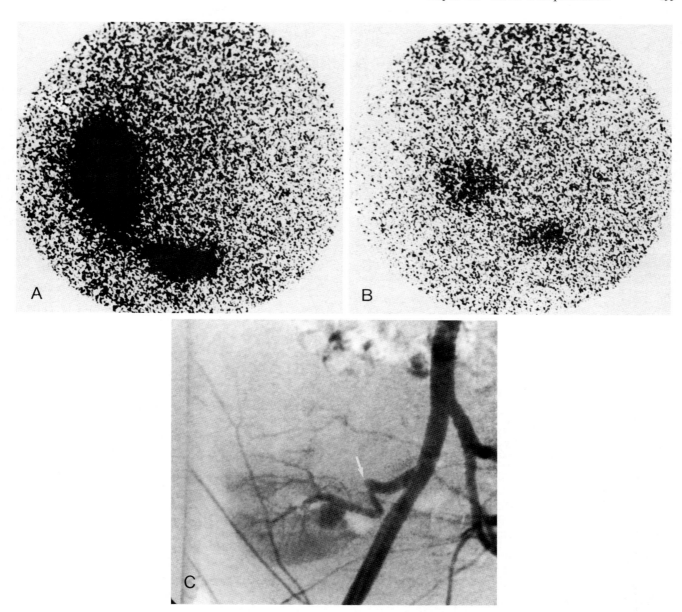

Figure 21.11. Renal artery thrombosis. **A,** Initial radionuclide scan shows excellent uptake and excretion of the labelled Hippuran. A study 2 weeks later demonstrates excretion in only a small inferior portion of the kidney (**B**). Emergency intraarterial digital arteriogram (**C**) shows thrombosis of the main renal artery (*arrow*) just distal to the site where a second polar vessel has been anastomosed.

end-to-end anastomoses. Spasm was a frequent complication of the angioplasty procedure and was treated with intraarterial nitroglycerin or papaverine. There were three complications reported in this group of patients including one dissection of the renal artery, one perforation of the artery by the guidewire, and one peripheral embolus. Sniderman et al. (1980b) reported one dissection in 12 transplant recipients undergoing PTA.

Renal Arteriovenous Fistula

The incidence of renal AV fistula that occur as a sequelae of biopsy in transplanted kidneys is difficult to estimate. These fistulas are most commonly small, asymp-tomatic, and close spontaneously. In 1–2% of patients, however, such fistulas persist and may be the cause of transplant dysfunction or significant AV shunting (Fig. 21.14). The incidence of these persistent symptomatic fistulas appears to be significantly higher in patients treated with cyclosporine when compared with a group of transplant patients treated with azathioprine. Such AV fistulas may be amenable to transarterial embolization with Gianturco coils (Fig. 21.15), Gelfoam, or detachable balloons. If this therapy is not successful, nephrectomy may be necessary due to a progressive reduction in renal function.

Uncommon vascular complications of transplantation

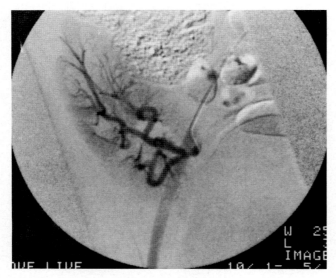

Figure 21.12.   Renal artery stenosis. An arteriogram shows a stenosis at the site of anastomosis of the renal artery and the internal iliac artery.

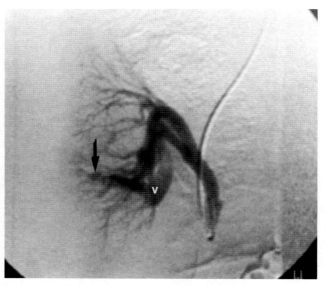

Figure 21.14.   Arteriovenous fistula. A selective transplant arteriogram shows an arteriovenous fistula (*arrow*) with early filling of the renal vein (v).

that have been reported include renal vein thrombosis thought to be related to extrinsic compression of the renal vein by a lymphocele, abscess, or urinoma; the formation of pseudoaneurysms (Fig. 21.16) that are usually mycotic in origin; and the development of perirenal hematomas secondary to technical problems with the vascular anastomosis that are not recognized at the time of surgery.

Vascular complications including AV fistula, pseudoaneurysm, and renal vein thrombosis require angiography for accurate delineation.

Urologic Complications

The incidence of urologic complications following renal transplantation has been variably reported to be between 0.9 and 30%. In most series, however, the incidence of these complications is between 10 and 13%.

Urinary Leakage

Urinary leakage or extravasation as a result of faulty surgical technique or unsuspected injury to the donor organ generally occurs within the first 3 months after transplantation and most commonly occurs 10–20 days following graft placement. Urinary leakage may occur as a result of leakage at the site of the ureterovesicle anastomosis outside of the bladder, may result from leakage from the bladder itself, secondary to inadequate closure of the vesicostomy, or may occur from a rent in the renal pelvis (Fig. 21.17). Despite the origin, such extravasation generally results in the formation of a urinoma.

Ureteral Necrosis

Necrosis or slough of the distal ureter is the most common urologic complication following transplantation and results in urinary extravasation (Fig. 21.18). This may occur in up to 4% of patients, usually before the sixth month following transplantation. The etiology of distal ureteral sloughing is thought to be related to ischemia of the distal ureter as the result of a compromise of the

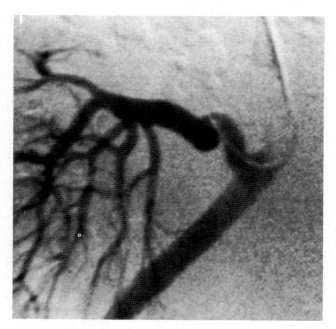

Figure 21.13.   A long tubular stenosis is present as a result of kinking of the artery during graft placement.

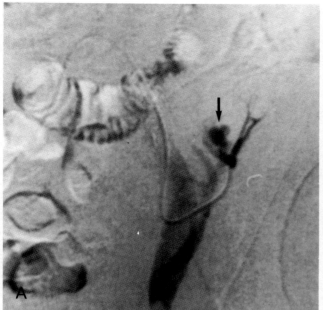

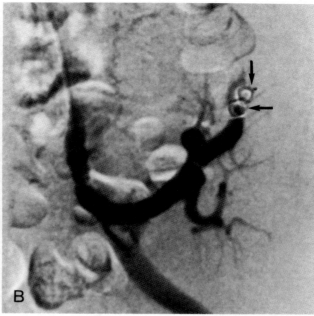

Figure 21.15. A subselective renal angiogram (**A**) shows a large arteriovenous fistula (*arrow*). After embolization with Gianturco coils (*arrows*), a repeat arteriogram (**B**) shows closure of the fistula.

blood supply of the ureter that occurs during the surgical dissection of the donor ureter prior to allograft placement, or from an overly constricted mucosal tunnel in the bladder. Ischemia of the ureter may also occur as a result of rejection. In either case, such necrosis results in the formation of a urinoma.

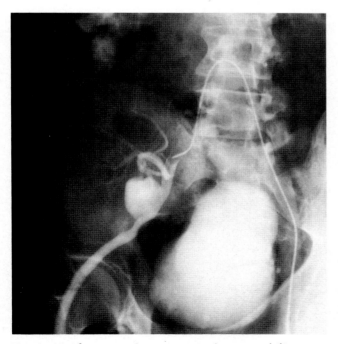

Figure 21.16. A pseudoaneurysm in the external iliac artery adjacent to the transplant anastomosis is present.

Ureteral Obstruction

Transient ureterovesicle obstruction in the early post-transplant period usually is related to postoperative edema at the ureteroneocystostomy. Rarely, acute obstruction from blood clots, calculi, fungus balls, or sloughed papilla may be the cause of ureteral obstruction. Ureteral obstruction as a late complication of transplantation usually occurs in the distal ureter. It may be the result of pressure on the ureter from a peritransplant fluid collection, however, more commonly it is the result of stricture formation of the ureter as a result of either vascular insufficiency or rejection.

Miscellaneous Urologic Complications

Ureterocutaneous fistulas occur when ureteral complications have not been promptly recognized. This complication is more common in donor kidneys that have multiple renal arteries and there has been inadvertent sacrifice of a polar vessel. This is a particularly devastating complication and the majority of patients eventually lose their graft.

Urinary calculi are reported to occur in approximately 1% of renal allografts. Underlying predisposing conditions for the formation of calculi are thought to be present in the majority of such cases. Additionally, undetected calculi in donor kidneys may occasionally be the source of such complications. If the calculus migrates into the ureter, the patient may experience pain and swelling of the graft that simulates acute rejection (Fig. 21.19). In such cases, there is also the sudden onset of

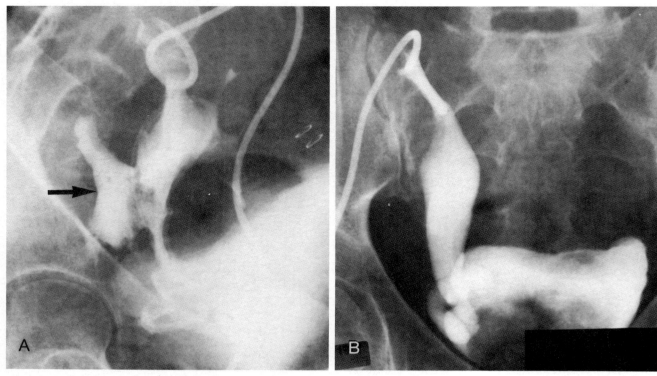

Figure 21.17. An oblique view from a nephrostogram (**A**) demonstrates extravasation from a tear of the renal pelvis. Fol-

lowing removal of the ureteral stent and several weeks of nephrostomy drainage, the leak has completely healed (**B**).

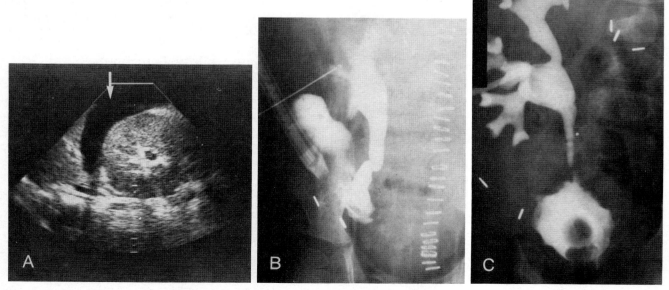

Figure 21.18. Ureteral necrosis. **A**, An ultrasound examination demonstrates fluid around the transplant kidney (*arrow*). **B**, Antegrade pyelogram shows extravasation from distal ureter

as a result of ureteral necrosis. **C**, Following percutaneous nephrostomy and stent placement, a nephrostogram shows complete healing.

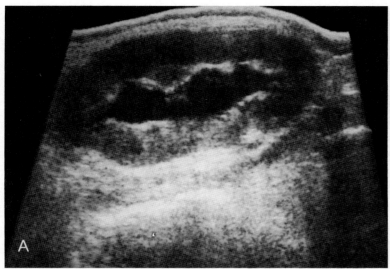

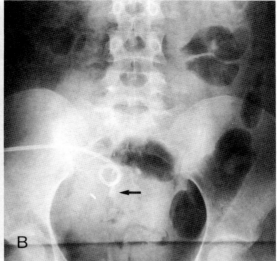

Figure 21.19. **A**, An ultrasound scan performed to evaluate the sudden onset of oliguria and pain in a transplant patient demonstrates hydronephrosis. **B**, A percutaneous nephrostomy was placed under ultrasound guidance. A follow-up radiograph shows that a stone (*arrow*) which has become lodged in the UPJ is the cause of the transplant dysfunction. Percutaneous nephrostolithotomy was subsequently performed.

oliguria or anuria depending on the degree of obstruction that is present. Bladder calculi originating on suture material that acts as a nidus for their formation are not uncommon.

A variety of radiologic investigations may be helpful in establishing the diagnosis of these urologic complications. Plain films may show the presence of a soft tissue mass as a result of urinary leakage and subsequent urinoma formation. Stones may also be visualized on such plain films, particularly if this diagnosis is suspected.

With the advent of newer imaging modalities, urography is rarely performed to elucidate the cause of transplant dysfunction. This is probably related to a reluctance to utilize contrast material in a patient with already compromised renal function, as well as the recognition that newer imaging studies may give information more directly (i.e., direct visualization of the fluid collection). Ureteral necrosis resulting in urinary extravasation (Fig. 21.20) may be diagnosed on urography if the patients level of renal function is sufficient to allow visualization.

Retrograde pyelography, while in theory well suited to demonstrate urologic complications of transplantation, is in practice difficult to perform because of difficulty in catheterizing ureteroneocystostomies, especially those made utilizing the Ledbetter-Politano technique. It should probably be attempted as a second-line procedure when other techniques to demonstrate the etiology of the dysfunction are not successful. Cystography is helpful in establishing the presence of urinary leak when the source of the leak is in the urinary bladder itself. The most common source of leakage, however, is related to necrosis of the distal ureter, and in such cases cystography does not demonstrate the source of extravasation.

Radionuclide examinations are commonly performed as an initial study to investigate the source of transplant dysfunction. In the early posttransplant period, radionuclide studies in patients with urinary extravasation using ^{131}I-Hippuran may demonstrate a photopenic area which represents the urinoma; this area will gradually accumulate activity if delayed images are obtained (Fig. 21.21).

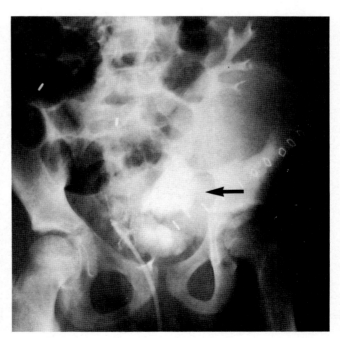

Figure 21.20. An excretory urogram demonstrating contrast extravasation (*arrow*) as a result of leakage from the ureteroneocystostomy site.

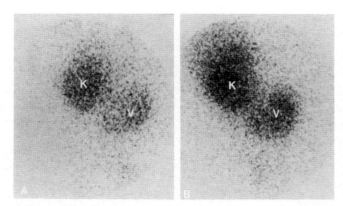

Figure 21.21. Initial (**A**) and delayed (**B**) images from ^{131}I-Hippuran radionuclide scan show increasing activity around the transplanted kidney (K) as the result of urinary extravasation. Activity is also present in the bladder (V).

Patients demonstrating ureteral obstruction may also be identified on radionuclide studies. The perfusion portion of the examination with DTPA shows relatively preserved perfusion while on the Hippuran examination there is relatively prompt uptake of the radiopharmaceutical by the transplant kidney. The excretory portion of the Hippuran study is prolonged and the renogram curve has an ascending slope (Fig. 21.22). These findings are similar to those accompanying ATN and cyclosporine nephrotoxicity, however, the time frame and clinical situation are frequently helpful in distinguishing among these possibilities.

Ultrasound studies are also extremely useful in establishing the diagnosis of urologic complications. Sonography shows the presence of hydronephrosis, renal calculi, and peritransplant fluid collections. A component of hydronephrosis is a frequent finding in patients experiencing ureteral sloughing and urinary extravasation.

Sonography may also be used to guide fine needle antegrade pyelography, with which many urologic complications may be diagnosed directly. Computed tomography may be used instead of US, but is most helpful when contrast enhanced studies are obtained (Fig. 21.23).

Fine needle antegrade pyelography (Fig. 21.24) in transplant recipients has been reported in several series to be extremely useful in the diagnosis of transplant ureteral obstruction and in detecting the presence of ureteral fistulas. Bennett et al. reported a series that included 79 antegrade pyelograms performed in a series of 686 transplant patients over a 5-year period. These investigators were able to diagnose ureteral obstruction in 40 patients, elucidate the cause of extravasation in 12 patients, and demonstrate the presence of a perirenal fluid collection in 10 patients. There were six procedure related complications including three cases of pelvicalyceal hemorrhage, however, the majority of these complications were related to subsequent interventional radiologic procedures that were performed.

Antegrade pyelography is also utilized to perform a Whitaker test (Chapter 14). In 28 of the 30 patients reported in Bennett's series in whom this procedure was performed, the result of the Whitaker test demonstrated that the hydronephrosis was not functionally significant, thereby, obviating the need for more invasive procedures.

Modern interventional uroradiologic procedures may now be utilized to treat or temporize most urologic complications. Percutaneous nephrostomy provides relief of obstruction. In addition, nephrostomy may be used as a diagnostic tool to establish the relative contribution of urinary tract obstruction to overall transplant dysfunction. Mild ureteral strictures may be successfully treated with percutaneous ureteral stent placement.

Bennett et al. demonstrated that in seven of nine

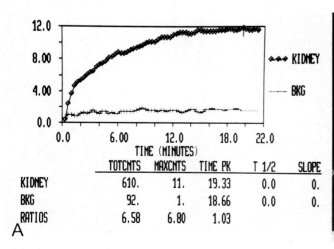

	TOTCNTS	MAXCNTS	TIME PK	T 1/2	SLOPE
KIDNEY	610.	11.	19.33	0.0	0.
BKG	92.	1.	18.66	0.0	0.
RATIOS	6.58	6.80	1.03		

Figure 21.22. Transplant obstruction. **A**, A renogram curve demonstrates an ascending slope compatible with obstruction.

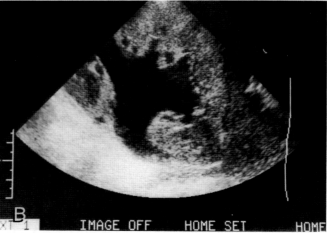

B, Ultrasound examination confirms that transplant hydronephrosis is present.

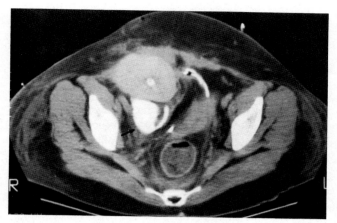

Figure 21.23. Computed tomography demonstrates a collection of extravasated contrast (*arrow*) behind the transplanted kidney.

more severe ureteral strictures treated by percutaneous balloon dilatation, this method of treatment was successful in relieving the obstruction with follow-up periods ranging from 8 to 45 months. The remaining two patients failed percutaneous dilatation and eventually required surgical procedures. Even when percutaneous dilatation of a ureteral stricture is not successful or is deemed inadvisable, percutaneous nephrostomy drainage allows the kidney to recover sufficient function so that definitive surgical therapy may be performed. Percutaneous extraction of renal and ureteral calculi through a percutaneous

nephrostomy tract in transplant patients has also been successfully accomplished.

Urinary leaks may be successfully managed with percutaneous diversion and internal stent placement (Fig. 21.24). In Bennett's series, in five of eight patients treated by this method the site of extravasation healed without further surgical intervention. The mean period of stent placement was 6 weeks. On theoretical grounds, it may be necessary to use a longer period of stenting than might otherwise be necessary in nontransplant patients since the majority of these patients are on chronic immunosuppression with prednisone and are therefore felt to have delayed wound healing. Concerns that the use of these percutaneous techniques may result in devastating infections in these immune compromised patients have not been substantiated.

Peritransplant Fluid Collection

Fluid collections around the transplanted kidney represent urinomas, hematomas, abscesses, or lymphoceles. Urinomas and hematomas have been discussed in Urologic Complications.

Lymphoceles are the most common peritransplant fluid collection, occurring in one to 15% of all transplant patients. They generally occur 4–6 weeks after transplantation and are frequently associated with a prior episode of rejection. The origin of the lymphocele is attributed to disruption and incomplete ligation of the recipients lymphatics at the time of allograft placement. As a result, fluid

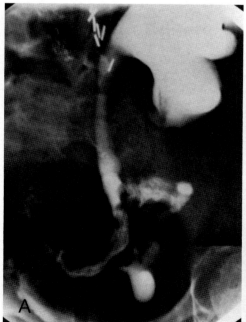
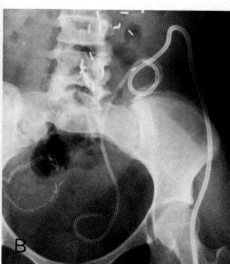
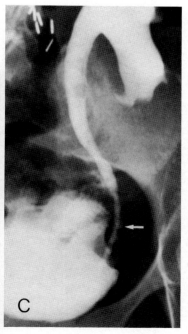

Figure 21.24. **A**, An antegrade pyelogram shows extravasation from the mid ureter. **B**, A percutaneous nephrostomy and double-J ureteral stent were placed for a period of 6 weeks. Follow-up nephrostogram (**C**) shows a small pseudodiverticulum in the distal ureter (*arrow*) but no further extravasation.

is allowed to accumulate around the transplanted kidney. Although controversial, some authorities believe that lymphoceles may also originate from disruption of the lymphatics of the donor kidney.

Lymphoceles may be largely asymptomatic, however, when large they may compress the collecting system of the kidney or the ureter and thereby cause a ureteral obstruction and impairment of function. In addition, a palpable mass may be present and there may be ipsilateral leg pain and edema.

Lymphoceles may be detected by a variety of imaging modalities (Fig. 21.25). On radionuclide examinations, lymphoceles are seen as a photopenic area between the transplanted kidney and the bladder that does not accumulate activity on delayed views, thereby distinguishing them from urinomas. Sonography demonstrates a sep-

tated fluid-filled mass that is otherwise indistinguishable from a urinoma. The fluid collection is usually demonstrated at the inferior margin of the transplant between the kidney and the urinary bladder. Rarely, a lymphocele may be present in the hilus of the kidney and may be confused with hydronephrosis.

On CT scans, lymphoceles are demonstrated as round or oval collections with sharp borders and attenuation values that range from 10 to 20 HU. Without the use of contrast enhancement, these collections may be difficult to distinguish from urinomas, however, if contrast material is utilized, lymphoceles are usually easily distinguishable because of the absence of contrast enhancement of these lesions. However, Nakstad et al. were able to differentiate lymphoceles from urinomas and hydronephrosis in 81% of the cases without the use of contrast material.

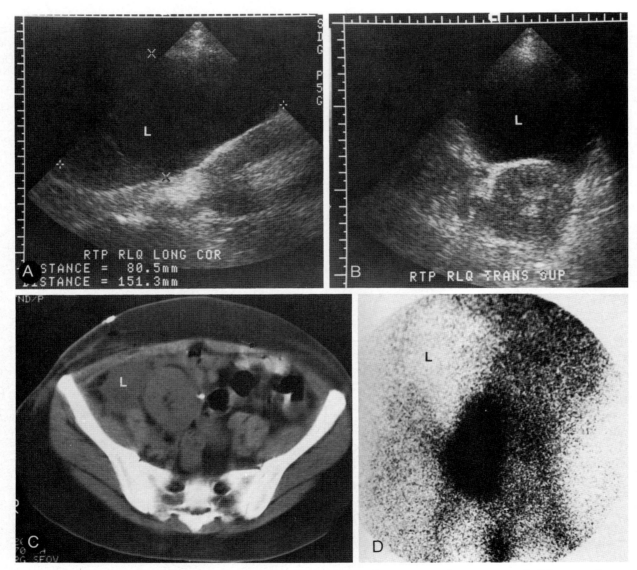

Figure 21.25.   Lymphocele (L). **A**, longitudinal ultrasonogram, **B**, transverse ultrasonogram, **C**, CT scan, and **D**, radionuclide scan.

The role of percutaneous drainage of lymphoceles is controversial. Either percutaneous aspiration or catheter drainage of a lymphocele was attempted in seven patients in the series of Bennett et al. In three of the patients the procedure was repeated on multiple occasions because of reaccumulation. In another small series, one of three lymphoceles aspirated reoccurred and required surgical drainage. Surgical therapy is considered by many to be the preferred method of treatment.

The incidence of peritransplant abscess is difficult to estimate from the reported series. Most peritransplant abscesses occur as a complication of pyelonephritis although abscess as a direct complication of surgery may occur as well. In addition, other peritransplant fluid collections such as urinomas, hematomas, or lymphoceles may become infected either due to manipulation or due to seeding from sepsis. Computed tomography and US are the most helpful imaging modalities in detecting the presence of a peritransplant abscess. In the clinical setting of fever in a transplant patient, the detection of a fluid collection around the kidney is presumptive evidence that the fluid is infected; needle aspiration is then performed for confirmation. Percutaneous drainage has been successfully reported in a variety of such cases including those associated with emphysematous pyelonephritis.

Long Term Complications of Renal Transplantation

There is an increased incidence of malignancy in patients treated with immunosuppressive drugs over a long period of time. Penn classified these patients into five groups of which three are pertinent to the renal transplant patient: (*a*) there is a 36% incidence of neoplasia in transplant recipients who receive organs from donors with an existing carcinoma; (*b*) the risk of a de novo malignancy at some time after transplantation is 6% or 100 times greater than that of the general population in the same age range; (*c*) there is a 53% incidence of recurrence for patients receiving a renal transplant because of a renal cell carcinoma if the interval between the treatment of the cancer and the transplantation is 1 year or less.

Of the organ recipients who developed a de novo malignancy, approximately 25% had lymphomas, 40% had tumors of the skin and lips, while the remainder developed a variety of solid tumors.

Frick et al. have reported the CT appearance of abdominal lymphoma which develops after renal transplantation. In this series, the incidence of abdominal lymphomas in the transplant population was 1.3%. They reported that posttransplant lymphomas differed from non-transplant related malignancies in that they frequently involve extranodal sites, especially in the central nervous system.

On CT, these posttransplant lymphomas presented as a bulky abdominal mass with inhomogeneous attenuation.

SUGGESTED READINGS

General References

Becker JA, Kutcher R: The renal transplant: rejection and acute tubular necrosis. *Semin Roentgenol* 13(4):352, 1978.

Caroline DF, Pollack HM, Banner MP, et al: Self-limiting extravasation in the unused urinary bladder. *Radiology* 155:311, 1985.

Halasz NA, Gambos EA, Ward DM, et al: Kidney transplantation in the cyclosporine era. *Arch Surg* 122:1001, 1987.

Hanto DW, Simmons RL: Renal transplantation: clinical considerations. *Radiol Clin North Am* 25(2):239, 1987.

Kahan BD, Flechner SM, Lorber MI, et al: Complications of cyclosporine-prednisone immunosuppression in 402 renal allograft recipients exclusively followed at a single center for from one to five years. *Transplantation* 43(2):197, 1987.

Maklad NF: Ultrasonic evaluation of renal transplants. *Semin Roentgenol* 2(1):88, 1981.

McEnery PT, Fine R, Sacher N, et al: Renal transplant immunity and immunosuppression. *Am J Kidney Dis* 7(4):312, 1986.

Monaco AP: Clinical kidney transplantation in 1984. *Transplant Proc* 17(1):5, 1985.

Stuck KJ, Jafri SZH, Adler DD, et al: Ultrasound evaluation of uncommon renal transplant complications. *Urol Radiol* 8:6, 1986.

Donor Evaluation

Flechner SM, Sandler CM, Houston GK, et al: 100 living-related kidney donor evaluations using digital subtraction angiography. *Transplantation* 40(6):675, 1985.

McElroy J, Novick AC, Streem SB, et al: A prospective analysis of the accuracy and cost-effectiveness of digital subtraction angiography for living related renal donor evaluation. *Transplantation* 42(1):23, 1986.

Infection

Balsara VJ, Raval B, Maklad NF: Emphysematous pyelonephritis in a renal transplant: sonographic and computed tomographic features. *J Ultrasound Med* 4:97, 1985.

Peterson P, Anderson RC: Infection in renal transplant recipients. Current approaches to diagnosis, therapy and prevention. *Am J Med* 81(Suppl 1A):2, 1986.

Potter JL, Sullivan BM, Flournoy JG, et al: Emphysema in the renal allograft. *Radiology* 155:51, 1985.

Radionuclide Studies

Fill H, Spielberger M, Leidlmair K, et al: Nephrography and radioactive Hippuran in transplanted kidneys: interpretation, limitations and usefulness. *Eur J Nucl Med* 11:171, 1985.

Kim EE, Pjura G, Lowry P, et al: Cyclosporin-A nephrotoxicity and acute cellular rejection in renal transplant recipients: correlation between radionuclide and histologic findings. *Radiology* 159:443, 1986.

Kirchner PT, Rosenthall L: Renal transplant evaluation. *Semin Nucl Med* 12(4):370, 1982.

Klintmalm GBG, Klingensmith WC, Iwatsuki S, et al: 99mTc DTPA and 131I Hippuran findings in liver transplant recipients treated with cyclosporin A. *Radiology* 142:199, 1982.

Marcos CS, Koyle MA, Darcourt J, et al: Evaluation of the utility of Indium 111 oxide platelet imaging in renal transplant patients on cyclosporine. *Clin Nucl Med* 11(12):834, 1986.

Tisdale PL, Collier BD, Kauffman HM, et al: Early diagnosis of acute postoperative renal transplant rejection by indium 111 labeled platelet scintigraphy. *J Nucl Med* 27:1266, 1986.

Thomsen HS, Munck O: Use of 99mTc radionuclides to show nephrotoxicity of cyclosporin A in transplanted kidneys. *Acta Radiol* 28:59, 1987.

Acute Rejection—Ultrasound Studies

Fried AM, Woodring JH, Loh FK, et al: The medullary pyramid index: an objective assessment of prominence in renal transplant rejection. *Radiology* 149:787, 1983.

Griffin JF, Short DC, Lawler W, et al: Diagnosis of disease in renal allografts: correlation between ultrasound and histology. *Clin Radiol* 37:59, 1986.

Heckemann R, Rehwald U, Jacubowski HD, et al: Sonographic criteria for renal allograft rejection. *Urol Radiol* 4:15, 1982.

Hoddick W, Filly RA, Backman U, et al: Renal allograft rejection: US evaluation. *Radiology* 161:469, 1986.

Hricak H, Romanski RN, Eyler WR: The renal sinus during allograft rejection: sonographic and histopathologic findings. *Radiology* 142:693, 1982.

Linkowski GD, Warvariv V, Filly RA, et al: Sonography in the diagnosis of acute renal allograft rejection and cyclosporine nephrotoxicity. *AJR* 148:291, 1987.

Maklad NF, Wright CH, Rosenthal SJ: Gray scale ultrasonic appearances of renal transplant rejection. *Radiology* 131:711, 1979.

Raiss GJ, Bree RL, Schwab RE, et al: Further observations in the ultrasound evaluation of renal allograft rejection. *J Ultrasound Med* 5:439, 1986.

Singh A, Cohen WN: Renal allograft rejection: sonography and scintigraphy. *AJR* 135:73, 1980.

Acute Rejection—Duplex Sonography

Allen KS, Jorkasky DK, Arger PH, et al: Renal allografts: prospective analysis of Doppler sonography. *Radiology* 169:371, 1988.

Buckley AR, Cooperberg PL, Reeve CE, et al: The distinction between acute renal transplant rejection and cyclosporine nephrotoxicity: value of duplex sonography. *AJR* 149:521, 1987.

Murphy AM, Robertson RJ, Dubbins PA: Duplex ultrasound in the assessment of renal transplant complications. *Clin Radiol* 38:229, 1987.

Needleman L, Kurtz AB: Doppler evaluation of the renal transplant. *J Clin Ultrasound* 15:661, 1987.

Rifkin MD, Needleman L, Pasto ME, et al: Evaluation of renal transplant rejection by duplex Doppler examination: value of resistive index. *AJR* 148:759, 1987.

Rifkin MD, Pasto ME, Goldberg BB: Duplex Doppler examination in renal disease: evaluation of vascular involvement. *Ultrasound Med Biol* 11(2):341, 1985.

Rigsby CM, Burns PN, Weltin GG, et al: Doppler signal quantitation in renal allografts: comparison in normal and rejection transplants, with pathologic correlation. *Radiology* 162:39, 1987.

Rigsby CM, Taylor KJW, Weltin G, et al: Renal allografts in acute rejection: evaluation using duplex sonography. *Radiology* 158:375, 1986.

Rejection—Angiographic Studies

Clark RL, Mandel SR, Webster WR: Microvascular changes in canine renal allograft rejection: a correlative microangiographic and histologic study. *Invest Radiol* 12:62, 1977.

Foley WD, Bookstein JJ, Tweist M, et al: Arteriography of renal transplants. *Radiology* 116:271, 1975.

Kaude JV, Hawkins IF Jr: Angiography of renal transplant. *Radiol Clin North Am* 14:295, 1976.

Magnetic Resonance Imaging

Baumgartner RB, Nelson RC, Ball TI, et al: MR imaging of renal transplants. *AJR* 147:949, 1986.

Geisinger MA, Risius B, Jordan ML, et al: Magnetic resonance imaging of renal transplants. *AJR* 143:1229, 1984.

Halasz NA: Differential diagnosis of renal transplant rejection: is MR imaging the answer? *AJR* 147:954, 1986.

Hricak H, Terrier F, Demas BE: Renal allografts: evaluation by MR imaging. *Radiology* 159:435, 1986.

Klehr HU, Spannbrucker N, Molitor D, et al: Magnetic resonance imaging in renal transplants. *Transplant Proc* 19(5):3716, 1987.

Steinberg HV, Nelson RC, Murphy FB, et al: Renal allograft rejection: evaluation by Doppler US and MR imaging. *Radiology* 163:337, 1987.

Yap HK, Dietrich RB, Kangarloo H, et al: Acute renal allograft rejection. *Transplantation* 43(2):249, 1987.

Transplant Rupture

Ostrovsky PD, Carr L, Goodman JC, et al: Ultrasound findings in renal transplant rupture. *J Clin Ultrasound* 13:132, 1985.

Rahatzad M, Henderson SC, Borch GS: Ultrasound appearance of spontaneous rupture of renal transplant. *J Urol* 126:535, 1981.

Susan LP, Braun WE, Banowsky LH, et al: Ruptured human renal allograft. *Urology* 11:53, 1978.

Computed Tomography

Ehrman KO, Kopecky KK, Wass JL, et al: Parapelvic lymph cyst in a renal allograft mimicking hydronephrosis: CT diagnosis. *J Comput Assist Tomogr* 11(4):714, 1987.

Letourneau JG, Day DL, Feinberg SB: Ultrasound and computed tomographic evaluation of renal transplantation. *Radiol Clin North Am* 25(2):267, 1987.

Nakstad P, Kolmannskog A, Kolbenstvedt A, et al: Computed tomography in surgical complications following renal transplantation. *J Comput Assist Tomogr* 6(2):286, 1982.

Vascular Complications

Flechner SM, Sandler CM, Childs T, et al: Screening for transplant renal artery stenosis in hypertensive recipients using digital subtraction angiography. *J Urol* 130:440, 1983.

Hohnke C, Abendroth D, Schleibner S, et al: Vascular complications in 1200 kidney transplantations. *Transplant Proc* 19(5):3691, 1987.

Lancombe M: Arterial stenosis complicating renal allotransplantation in man: a study of 38 cases. *Ann Surg* 134:400, 1977.

Raval B, Balsara V, Kim EE: Computed tomography detection of transplant renal artery pseudoaneurysm. *CT: J Computed Tomogr* 9(2):149, 1985.

Raynaud A, Bedrossian J, Remy P, et al: Percutaneous transluminal angioplasty of renal transplant arterial stensosis. *AJR* 146:853, 1986.

Sniderman KW, Sos TA, Sprayregen S, et al: Percutaneous transluminal angioplasty in renal transplant arterial stenosis for relief of hypertension. *Radiology* 135:23, 1980a.

Sniderman KW, Sprayregen S, Sos TA, et al: Percutaneous transluminal dilation in renal transplant arterial stenosis. *Transplantation* 30(6):440, 1980b.

Taylor KJW, Morse SS, Rigsby CM, et al: Vascular complications in renal allografts: detection with duplex Doppler US. *Radiology* 162:31, 1987.

Urologic Complications

Becker JA, Kutcher R: Urologic complications of renal transplantation. *Semin Roentgenol* 13(4):341, 1978.

Bennett LN, Voegeli DR, Crummy AB, et al: Urologic complications following renal transplantation: role of interventional radiologic procedures. *Radiology* 160:531, 1986.

Bushnell DL, Wilson DG, Lieberman LM: Scintigraphic assessment of perivesical urinary extravasation following renal transplantation. *Clin Nucl Med* 9(2):92, 1984.

Cohen RH, Saeed M, Schwab SJ, et al: Povidone-iodine sclerosis of pelvic lymphoceles: a prospective study. *Urol Radiol* 10:203, 1988.

Curry NS, Cochran S, Barbaric ZL, et al: Interventional radiologic procedures in the renal transplant. *Radiology* 152:647, 1984.

Glanz S, Gordon DH, Butt K, et al: Percutaneous transrenal balloon dilatation of the ureter. *Radiology* 149:101, 1983.

Glanz S, Rotter MR, Gordon DH, et al: Interventional radiologic procedures in the management of the renal transplant patient. *Urol Radiol* 7:97, 1985.

Loughlin KR, Tilney NL, Richie JP: Urologic complications in 718 renal transplant patients. *Surgery* 95:297, 1984.

Schmeller NT, Schuller J, Hofstetter A, et al: Fine needle antegrade pyelography of transplanted kidneys. *Urol Radiol* 7:19, 1985.

Streem SB, Novick AC, Steinmuller DR, et al: Percutaneous techniques for the management of urological renal transplant complications. *J Urol* 135:456, 1986.

Van Gansbeke D, Zalcman M, Matos C, et al: Lithiasic complications of renal transplantation: the donor graft lithiasis concept. *Urol Radiol* 7:157, 1985.

vanSonnenberg E, Wittich GR, Casola G, et al: Lymphoceles: imaging characteristics and percutaneous management. *Radiology* 161:593, 1986.

Voegeli DR, Crummy AB, McDermott JC, et al: Percutaneous management of the urological complications of renal transplantation. *Radiographics* 6(6):1007, 1986.

Long Term Complications of Renal Transplantation

Frick MP, Salomonowitz E, Hanto DW, et al: CT of abdominal lymphoma after renal transplantation. *AJR* 142:97, 1984.

Penn I: Malignancies associated with immunosuppressive or cytotoxic therapy. *Surgery* 83(5):492, 1978.

CHAPTER 22

INTERVENTIONAL URORADIOLOGY

PERCUTANEOUS NEPHROSTOMY

Percutaneous nephrostomy (PCN) is the single most valuable interventional technique in uroradiology. It re-lieves obstruction of the urinary tract and provides access to the collecting system for a variety of diagnostic and therapeutic procedures.

Indications

A PCN is indicated in a large variety of clinical situations (Table 22.1). Each patient must be considered individually, and some may have both indications and contraindications to the procedure. The decision whether or not to undertake a PCN must depend on other available options.

Obstruction

The most common indication for PCN is relief of obstruction, but there are several subcategories. Infection in an obstructed collecting system requires urgent decompression. If the patient is toxic, PCN may be an emergency procedure.

Acute obstruction often causes ureteral colic as the ureter attempts to overcome the obstruction with active peristalsis. Analgesics are usually employed to control pain until the obstruction can be relieved. Occasionally, decompression with a PCN may be elected until the obstruction can be relieved.

Chronic obstruction results in dilation of the collecting system, tubular damage, parenchymal loss, and deterioration of renal function. PCN may be used to prevent renal damage if the cause of obstruction cannot be adequately treated (Fig. 22.1). If there is bilateral obstruction, impaired renal function may result in electrolyte abnormalities (Fig. 22.2).

Most urinary tract infections respond to appropriate antibiotics. If there is obstruction, however, even sensitive bacteria will not be eradicated. Drainage of the closed infection can be readily performed with a PCN in most patients.

A nephrostomy performed for an elective indication should be delayed until the urinary tract infection is erad-

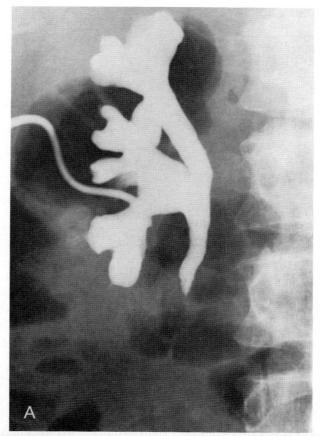

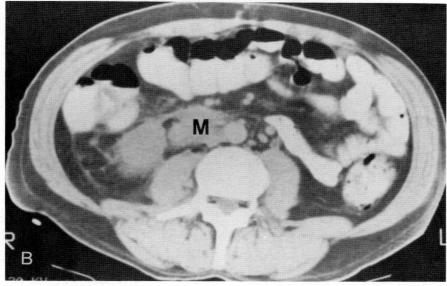

Figure 22.1. Percutaneous nephrostomy. **A**, Antegrade pyelogram after PCN demonstrates proximal ureteral obstruc-tion. **B**, Computed tomography demonstrates a tumor mass (M) causing the ureteral obstruction.

Table 22.1.
Percutaneous Nephrostomy Indications

Relief of obstruction
    Preserve renal function
    Treatment of infection
    Relieve pain
Urinary diversion
    Heal leak or fistula
Diagnostic study
    Antegrade pyelogram
    Whitaker test
    Biopsy or brushing for cytology
Removal of solid material
    Stone
    Foreign body removal
Access for ureteral intervention
    Stricture dilation
    Stenting
    Ureteral occlusion
Infusion of chemolytic agents
Access for nephroscopy

icated. However, obstruction must be relieved before the infection can be cleared. Thus, a PCN must be performed as an urgent procedure despite the contraindications.

Urinary Diversion

Traumatic extravasation from the urinary tract usually heals spontaneously. If there is continued urine flow through the leak, however, healing will be delayed and a chronic fistula may develop. Even those cases that heal spontaneously may have a large urinoma that is fed by extravasated urine until the perforation seals. These patients are usually helped by a diverting nephrostomy.

When a nephrostomy catheter is placed in the renal pelvis, urine takes the path of least resistance and flow out the catheter. The amount of urine flowing out the site of extravasation is markedly reduced, promoting healing (Fig. 22.3).

In patients who are incontinent, a variety of methods, including catheter drainage of the bladder, may be used to prevent continued urine leak and soiling of the patient. Occasionally a nephrostomy may be needed to divert the urine before it reaches the bladder.

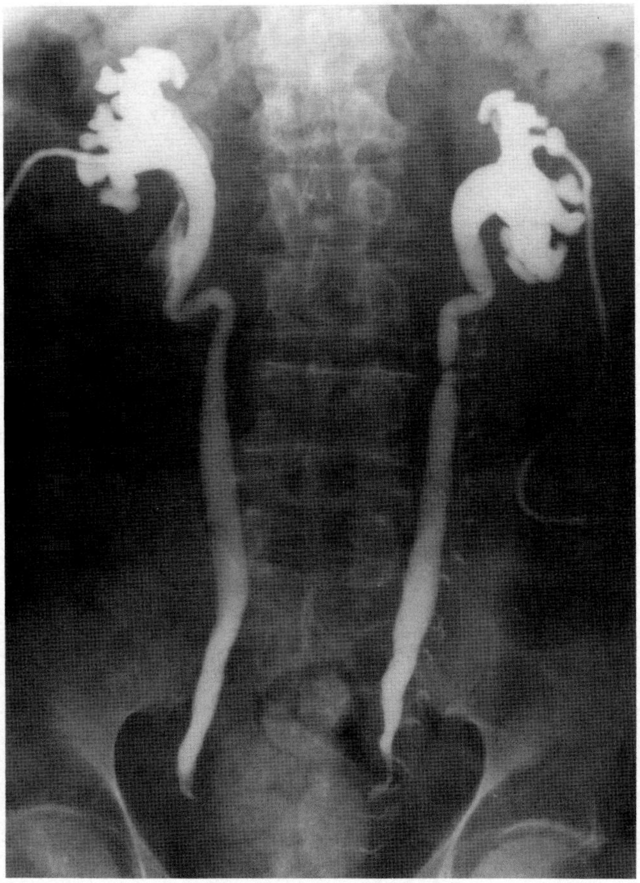

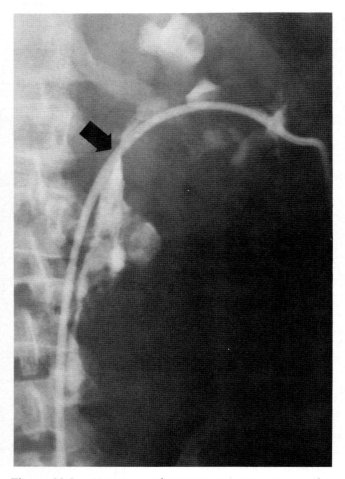

Figure 22.2.   Bilateral PCN. Obstruction of both distal ureters by prostate cancer necessitated bilateral nephrostomies.

Figure 22.3.   Diverting nephrostomy. Traumatic injury to the ureter has resulted in persistent leak (*arrow*) with urinoma formation. PCN with urinary diversion and ureteral stenting.

Diagnostic Studies

The collecting system is better imaged with direct contrast injection than with excretory urography. Retrograde pyelography requires cystoscopy and cannulation of the distal ureter. Even with this method, the intrarenal collecting system may not be optimally imaged, especially if there is a ureteral lesion causing some degree of obstruction.

Antegrade pyelography allows direct opacification of the intrarenal collecting system (Fig. 22.3). It may be necessary to use this method to image the proximal ureter if there is a high degree of obstruction.

A PCN also provides access to the collecting system for brushing or aspiration biopsy of lesions within the collecting system. Samples for cytologic evaluation may be obtained directly.

It is not uncommon to see dilatation of the collecting system, but not know whether or not obstruction exists. This occurs more commonly in children, especially those patients who have had previous surgical procedures which further confuses the evaluation. Antegrade pyelography with direct instillation of contrast material allows evaluation of urine flow through the collecting system and does not rely upon contrast material excreted by the kidney. This technique is often helpful as many of these patients have impaired renal function so that opacification of the dilated collecting system is poor.

Urodynamic techniques take this one step further by measuring the pressure gradient between the intrarenal collecting system and the bladder (Chapter 14).

Removal of Stones or Foreign Bodies

The PCN is the first step in extracting solid material from the collecting system. The most common use is nephrostolithotomy, discussed in Chapter 10. However, other materials such as broken catheters or ureteral stents may also be removed (Fig. 22.4). Simple guide wire snares are used most frequently, as they require the least dilation of the nephrostomy track, however, any number of other instruments including grasping forceps may be used for this purpose.

Access for Ureteral Intervention

A PCN is also used to gain access to the ureter for interventional techniques. Stricture dilation and ureteral stenting are discussed later in this chapter and in Chapter 14. Rarely there may be a desire to occlude the ureter. Temporary occlusion is readily accomplished with a balloon catheter. However, the pressure of the balloon against the ureteral mucosa may create sufficient ischemia to induce necrosis or stricture formation. Deposition of embolic materials, such as cyanoacrylate and vascular coils, has also been used to accomplish ureteral occlusion.

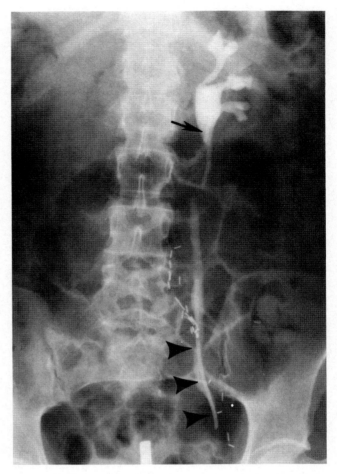

Figure 22.4. Broken ureteral stent. A double-J ureteral stent catheter has broken into three pieces. A PCN was used for access to remove the portions from the renal pelvis (*arrow*) and distal ureter (*arrowheads*).

Infusion of Chemolytic Agents

Chemical stone dissolution is discussed in Chapter 10. Two catheters are often required, one for infusion and a second for drainage. They should be placed on either side of the stone to obtain maximal bathing of the calculus.

Other therapeutic agents can also be instilled via a PCN. This technique allows a high concentration of the drug in the collecting system with a minimal systemic level.

Access for Nephroscopy

In the past 2 years there has been a dramatic increase in endourologic procedures. Most of these require access to the collecting system via a PCN. Earlier instruments were rigid and a straight track was needed. Furthermore, the position of the nephrostomy limited access to only one portion of the collecting system. Flexible nephroscopes alleviate this problem to a large degree, but still may not provide access to the entire collecting system.

Thus, the exact position of the PCN contributes significantly to the success or failure of the procedure.

Anatomy

The kidneys are retroperitoneal organs surrounded by perinephric fat and enclosed by Gerota's fascia. Their axis parallels the psoas muscle so that the upper pole is medial and slightly more posterior than the lower pole. During normal development the kidney ascends and rotates medially about its vertical axis such that the renal hilum is directed anteromedially at an angle of approximately 30° from horizontal.

The pleura extends down to the 12th vertebral body, posteriorly, then extends laterally crossing the 12th, 11th, and 10th ribs as they angle caudally. Although there is great normal variation, approximately half of the right kidney and one-third of the left kidney lie above this posterior reflection of the pleural surface.

The liver is anterolateral to the upper pole of the right kidney. In occasional patients, however, a portion of the right lobe of the liver may extend posterolateral to the upper pole of the kidney.

The position of the spleen is more variable. It classically lies superolateral to the kidney but is often adjacent to the lateral margin and may frequently be posterolateral to the upper pole.

The colon may also lie along the proposed route of the nephrostomy (Fig. 22.5). The descending colon lies in the anterior pararenal space and its position depends upon the position of the lateroconal fascia. In approximately 10% of patients the descending colon lies behind a horizontal line at the posterior edge of the left kidney. In 1% of patients the descending colon actually extends

behind the left kidney. Thus, in 1% of patients the descending colon would be punctured if the standard nephrostomy approach is used. Occasionally, the ascending colon is seen posterolateral to the right kidney, medial to the liver.

The calyces are generally arranged in two rows, anterior and posterior. At either pole, fusion results in compound calyces. In the interpolar region anterior calyces are often seen "end on" during urography while posterior calyces are seen extending laterally. This appearance reflects the classic description by Brodel. However, there is significant normal variation. In fact, Hodson described the typical kidney as having a mirror image position with the posterior calyces seen enface and the anterior calyces extending more laterally. The significant normal variation in this anatomy requires that the urogram include anteroposterior and both oblique views that can be carefully examined before the nephrostomy route is chosen.

The main renal artery and vein lie anterior to the renal pelvis. There is, however, a posterior branch of the renal artery which courses behind the renal pelvis to supply the dorsal segments. The segmental arteries divide into interlobar and the arcuate arteries which enter the renal parenchyma, usually at the corticomedullary junction. The closer to the calyx, the smaller the artery has become. Thus, a puncture into the calyx traverses a much smaller artery than a needle passing into an infundibulum.

Technique

A percutaneous nephrostomy is performed by visualizing the target, identifying the tract for the PCN, and placing the catheter. The procedure may be guided with fluoroscopy, ultrasound, or even CT. Fluoroscopy is the most convenient method of guidance and is used for the vast majority of these procedures. Visualization of the collecting system requires its opacification by contrast material. This may be accomplished either by renal excretion after intravenous injection or blind percutaneous puncture of renal pelvis.

Ultrasound may be used in conjunction with fluoroscopy to eliminate the need for contrast material to opacify the collecting system. This is most conveniently done by moving an ultrasound unit to the fluoroscopy table. Ultrasound can not only identify the targeted collecting system but also assure that adjacent organs do not lie along the proposed nephrostomy tract.

Many variations on the basic PCN technique may be used depending upon the clinical setting and specific patient anatomy. The two basic procedures are the trocar technique and the needle–guidewire–catheter exchange system described by Seldinger for arterial catheterization.

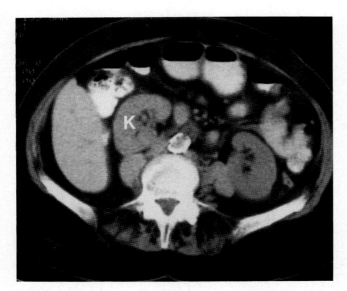

Figure 22.5. Anterior position of right kidney (K) places liver and colon along proposed percutaneous nephrostomy tract.

The trocar technique consists of passing a draining catheter and trocar needle together into the collecting system. The trocar is removed and the catheter is secured in position. Because this involves an initial puncture with a large needle, it is used primarily for large, superficial targets.

This trocar method can also be adapted to a two-puncture technique. An initial puncture with a small (22- or 23-gauge) needle is made through which contrast media can be injected to optimally opacify the collecting system. The trocar can then be placed more confidently in the desired location.

As experience with interventional techniques increases, however, most radiologists prefer variations on the Seldinger technique. With this method a smaller needle, usually 20- to 22-gauge, is used for the initial puncture. Thus, if needle placement is undesirable, it can be withdrawn and repositioned after having created only a small perforation.

If the collecting system is not well seen due to poor renal function, a direct puncture of the renal pelvis with a 22-gauge needle may be performed. Contrast can then be introduced to opacify the collecting system (Fig. 22.6). This technique is also used when there is no dilation of the intrarenal collecting system. A 0.018-inch guidewire is passed through the 22-gauge needle. After removal of the needle, a 3 French multiside-hole catheter is passed over the guidewire into the renal pelvis. Injection of contrast material not only opacifies but also dilates the collecting system.

The percutaneous nephrostomy may be performed in the prone, prone-oblique, or supine-oblique positions. The prone position is the most stable for the patient, but requires an angled needle approach. This is facilitated if C- or U-arm fluoroscopy is available. The prone-oblique position elevates the ipsilateral side 30–45° so that a vertical puncture can be made. Thus, patient positioning compensates for a fixed fluoroscope. The supine-oblique position consists of elevation of the ipsilateral side and a horizontal needle entry. It is used for very sick or immobile patients.

The collecting system should be punctured through the kidney. Direct access to the renal pelvis has a higher incidence of vascular complications. The needle should pass through the least vascular plane of the kidney (Brodel's line). A needle traversing this route into a calyx avoids all but the smallest intrarenal arteries. This long route through the renal parenchyma increases catheter purchase and minimizes urine leakage or catheter dislodgement. This posterolateral track results in catheter exit near the posterior axillary line which allows the patient to lie supine without kinking the catheter or causing undue discomfort.

Results

The results of PCN procedures are excellent. In 1978, Stables et al. reported a technical success rate greater than 90% and major complications of only 4%. With increased experience and improvements in equipment and

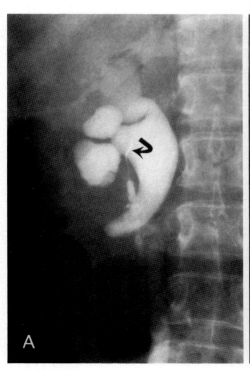
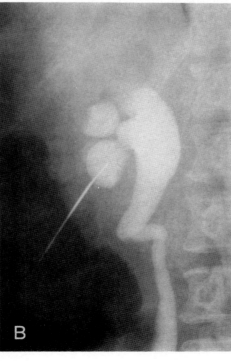

Figure 22.6. PCN technique. **A,** A 3 French dilator (*arrow*) has been passed over a 0.018-inch guide wire and is used to opacify the collecting system. **B,** With good opacification, the desired calyx can be punctured.

technique even better results can be expected. A successful PCN placement should be accomplished in almost every obstructed system if there is dilation of the collecting system. Failure is more likely in the rare case of nondilated obstruction, or in patients with urinary leaks or fistulas which keep the collecting system decompressed.

Similar excellent success rates can be achieved in infants and children by modifying the equipment and paying close attention to the special needs of these very young patients. Stanley et al. were successful in each of 28 PCNs performed in children ranging in age from 1 day to 18 years, while Ball et al. reported a 98% success rate in 61 interventional uroradiologic procedures.

Complications

The most common complications of PCN are related to bleeding, urine extravasation (Fig. 22.7), and infection. The kidney is a highly vascular organ and puncture of at least small intrarenal arteries cannot be avoided (Fig. 22.8). However, the PCN catheter usually provides sufficient tamponade to prevent significant blood loss. Retro-

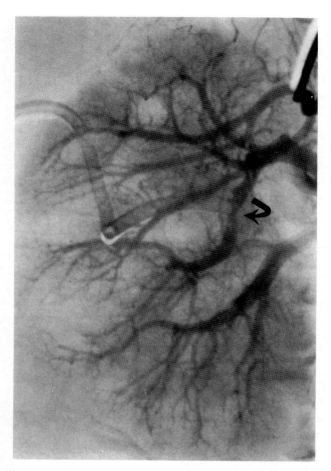

Figure 22.8. Arterial injury. Persistent hematuria after PCN prompted this selective renal arteriogram. Note the arterial damage (*arrow*) adjacent to the PCN catheter.

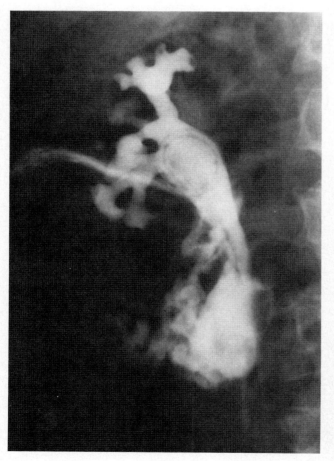

Figure 22.7. Extravasation. Inadvertent puncture of the renal pelvis has resulted in contrast extravasation. This condition usually heals within 2 days with nephrostomy drainage.

peritoneal hemorrhage will be an even greater problem in patients with clotting deficiencies. However, these patients may not be surgical candidates and PCN is still appropriate if the collecting system is dilated and no technical difficulties are anticipated in catheter placement.

In addition to hematoma formation (Fig. 22.9), an AV fistula or a pseudoaneurysm may be created. Either of these may result in delayed bleeding or bleeding when the PCN catheter is removed. Arteriography with selective renal artery injection is indicated in these patients to better define the source of bleeding. In many patients selective occlusion of a branch renal artery can be performed and surgery avoided.

Infection is the other common complication of PCN. It is more likely to be a problem in patients with preexisting pyonephrosis which is exacerbated by the procedure. Catheter manipulation or injection of contrast into an infected closed space may force bacteria into the circulation and cause septicemia or septic shock. Thus, a urinary tract infection is a contraindication to PCN placement.

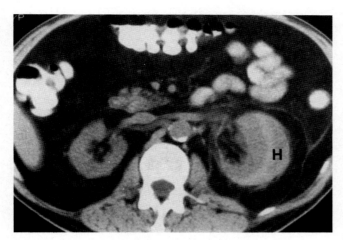

Figure 22.9. Subcapsular hematoma. A left subcapsular hematoma (H) is seen on this unenhanced CT scan.

However, infection of an obstructed collecting system is often a medical emergency requiring percutaneous relief. In these patients antibiotics are often administered before beginning the procedure. If the sensitivity of the infecting organism is unknown, a broad-spectrum antibiotic should be used. The PCN should be placed with as little manipulation as possible, and only small amounts of contrast, if any, should be used to confirm catheter position. Larger contrast injections for diagnostic purposes (antegrade pyelogram) should be delayed at least 1 day until the infection is under control.

An indwelling nephrostomy catheter will become colonized with bacteria. However, as long as there is adequate drainage of the collecting system, either through the ureter or the PCN, infection will not be a problem.

Recently, Cronan et al. studied a series of patients with indwelling percutaneous nephrostomy catheters and urinary tract infections to see how often bacteremia occurred during catheter manipulation and whether or not antibiotics affected the incidence of bacteremia. Asymptomatic bacteremia was documented in 11 of 104 (11%) nephrostomy tube exchanges, but there was no difference in incidence between the group receiving prophylactic antibiotics and those patients which did not have antibiotic coverage.

Failure to respond to percutaneous drainage may indicate a perinephric abscess. The most common etiology of a retroperitoneal abscess is a urinary tract infection, and the development of a perinephric abscess in a patient undergoing PCN should occur only in patients with preexisting pyonephrosis. Perinephric abscesses require ultrasound or CT for detection, and are usually amenable to percutaneous catheter drainage.

Occasionally adjacent organs are traversed during nephrostomy placement. This is more likely to occur if a specific portion of the collecting system must be entered such as for percutaneous nephrostolithotomy or in patients with variations of normal anatomy.

Pneumothorax is more likely to occur if the upper-pole collecting system must be entered. In many patients an entry site above the 11th or 12th rib is selected and the pleural space is traversed. An expiratory chest film should be obtained to look for pneumothorax when a high puncture is used. Most small pneumothoraces resolve spontaneously and only observation is required. Large or symptomatic pneumothoraces can be treated by the radiologist with a small chest tube.

Variations of normal anatomy may result in liver, spleen or colon lying in the path of the nephrostomy tract. In many patients the position of the kidneys or the identification of bowel gas may suggest this interposition. An ultrasound or CT examination may be very helpful in confirming the position of the interposed organ and identifying a path through which the nephrostomy can be safely placed (Fig. 22.5).

URETERAL INTERVENTION

With the nephrostomy catheter providing access to the collecting system, interventional procedures can be performed in the ureter. This direct antegrade approach avoids problems associated with traversing the urethra, bladder, and ureterovesicle junction. Ureteral stents may be placed to bypass obstruction, to heal a ureteral leak, or to prevent stricture formation. In patients in whom a stricture has already occurred, angioplasty balloon catheters may be used to dilate the stricture. Stone removal has been discussed in Chapter 10, but other solid materials such as broken ureteral catheters may often be removed easier through this antegrade approach than with retrograde catheterization of the ureter.

Stenting

Once access to the renal pelvis has been gained, catheterization of the ureter is seldom difficult. A variety of torque control catheters can be used to direct the guide wire down the ureter.

If the ureter is obstructed, especially by an extrinsic mass, the guidewire and catheter can usually be passed beyond the obstruction into the bladder. If the obstruction cannot be passed, decompression of the collecting system decreases the caliber of the dilated ureter and diminishes the edema at the site of obstruction. A second attempt at crossing the obstruction after decompression is often successful.

If there is a leak from the ureter, care must be taken not to pass the guidewire or catheter through the perforation into the retroperitoneum. This is likely to enlarge the hole and may contaminate the retroperitoneal space. Careful manipulation of the catheter and wire, and the use of contrast to identify the ureteral tear will aid in accessing the distal ureter. If the catheter cannot be passed beyond the perforation into the distal ureter, decompression with a PCN, and diversion of urine flow may allow healing of the tear so that the ureter may be negotiated at a later date.

The initial ureteral stent is often a long percutaneous catheter that extends through the intrarenal collecting system, down the ureter, and into the bladder. Holes are punched in the catheter to allow urine flow into the catheter at the renal pelvis. This requires measurement of the patient's internal anatomy. This can be simply done using a long angiographic guidewire. The tip of the guidewire is placed in the middle of the bladder using fluoroscopic guidance. The guidewire is then crimped where it exits the skin. The guidewire is then withdrawn until the tip is in the renal pelvis (a catheter is left in the bladder so that access is not lost), and a second crimp is made at the skin. The distance between these two crimps is the distance between the renal pelvis and the bladder. This measuring technique can be used to determine the length of an indwelling ureteral stent or to determine the position of holes for drainage of urine in the renal pelvis.

For initial ureteral stenting, polyurethane angiographic pigtail catheters are most commonly employed. If long-term catheterization is needed, a longer silicone copolymer catheter that is softer and less likely to obstruct may be used. However, these soft catheters are more difficult to place and overdilation of the nephrostomy tract may be required.

If long-term catheterization is anticipated, an internal stent may be chosen. The length of the ureteral stent is measured using the guidewire technique described above. Once the ureteral stent has been placed, an external nephrostomy catheter is no longer required (Fig. 22.10). However, the PCN is often left in place for 1–2 days to preserve access should problems arise.

After the PCN has been removed there is no easy access to the collecting system. Stent patency can be confirmed by demonstrating intrarenal reflux during cystography. Removal of the ureteral stent catheter requires cystoscopy. If necessary, however, a PCN can be placed and the proximal end of the stent snared and withdrawn through the PCN tract.

Fistula Management

Ureteral fistulas are often the result of surgery or penetrating trauma (Fig. 22.11). These fistulas have the best prognosis, as there is adequate blood supply and the ureter is otherwise healthy. Other causes are due to abnormalities of the ureteral tissue such as invasion by neoplasm, inflammatory changes, and radiation injury (Chapter 14).

Care must be taken in crossing the site of the fistula so that the hole is not enlarged or the urinoma contaminated. A straight guide wire with a long floppy tip introduced through a torque control catheter under careful fluoroscopic guidance is usually successful. Diversion of urine via a nephrostomy or ureteral stent is often successful in closing the fistula. The indwelling stent is also used to prevent stricture formation.

Figure 22.10. Ureteral stent. **A**, Moderate hydronephrosis of the right kidney is seen on an excretory urogram. **B**, After placement of a double-J ureteral stent catheter, the collecting system returns toward normal.

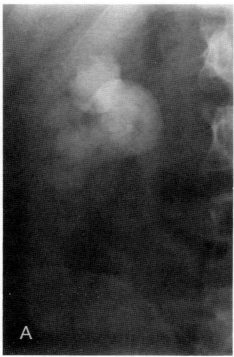
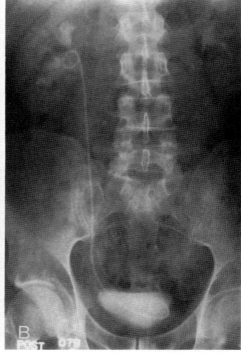

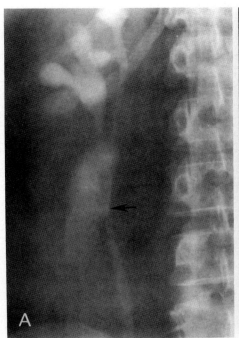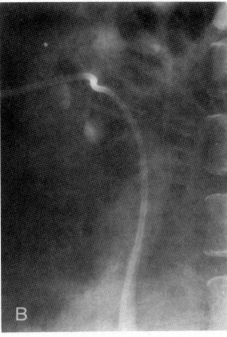

Figure 22.11. Penetrating trauma. (**A**) resulting in persistent urine leak (*arrow*) and urinoma formation. (**B**) Percutaneous nephrostomy and ureteral stenting were performed to divert the urine and to prevent stricture formation.

Stricture Dilation

There are many etiologies of ureteral strictures including both benign and malignant causes (Chapter 14). Benign etiologies include trauma, inflammation, radiation therapy, and retroperitoneal fibrosis. Among the more common causes are a response to ureteral stones, attempts at their removal, or various surgical manipulations of the ureter.

Malignant strictures include both primary tumors of the renal pelvis, ureter, or bladder and secondary involvement of the ureter via direct or hematogenous invasion.

The ureteral stricture may be negotiated with a variety of catheter and guidewire combinations. However, a straight-tipped wire passed through a torque control catheter with a slight bend at the tip, such as a visceral cobra catheter, is often successful. Once the guidewire has negotiated the stricture, the catheter will usually follow. In resistant cases decompression of the collecting system and resolution of edema may help.

Another manipulation in particularly difficult cases involves capturing the distal end of the guidewire in the bladder and pulling it out through the urethra. Once both ends of the wire are controlled, the catheter will cross almost any stricture.

Dilation of the ureteral stricture is accomplished with balloon angioplasty catheters. This is performed under fluoroscopic guidance to confirm the location of the balloon and the success of the dilation. A "waist" is seen as the balloon is dilated. As the stricture is stretched, the waist disappears.

Many ureteral strictures require more than one dilation. Ureteral strictures are dilated for 30 seconds to several minutes at this time. The procedure may be repeated again 1 or 2 days after the initial dilation. The technical success of the dilation can be judged by disappearance of the "waist." However, the stricture often reappears on subsequent procedures and multiple dilations over several days are often required for a more durable result.

Ureteral stenting after stricture dilation appears to be an important adjunct of this procedure, but it is not clear how large a stent is required or how long it should be left in place. We have arbitrarily elected to maintain ureteral stenting for 3 months after dilation. After this time, the catheter is removed but a wire left across the stricture. An antegrade nephrostogram is performed to assess the success of the dilation. If narrowing recurs, the dilation can be repeated, otherwise, the catheter can be removed.

The results of ureteral stricture dilation depend on the etiology of the stricture. The best results are obtained from benign strictures with good blood supply (Fig. 22.12). Ischemic strictures, such as those found at ureteroilial anastomoses, strictures with dense fibrosis, and those due to underlying malignancy are not likely to respond to percutaneous dilation techniques.

Banner et al. reported successful dilation in 13 (48%) of 27 benign postoperative ureteral stricture. Lang and Glorioso reported a similar 50% success rate in percutaneous dilation of 127 benign ureteral strictures. The most successful subgroup were those patients with fresh strictures and no evidence of vascular compromise. A successful outcome was achieved in over 90% of these pa-

Figure 22.12. Ureteral dilation. **A**, A stricture at the ureteropelvic junction was felt to be due to stone disase. **B**, A urogram after stricture dilation demonstrates an excellent result.

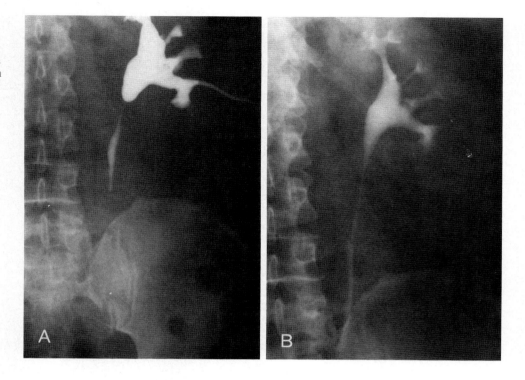

tients. However, success was gained in less than 20% of patients with evidence of devitalization.

Complications of ureteral stricture dilation are rare. The most common untoward event is perforation of the ureter. However, these usually heal without sequelae. Because serious complications are so unlikely, percutaneous stricture dilation is often undertaken as the initial therapeutic maneuver. If this technique fails, surgery is not compromised.

PERCUTANEOUS BIOPSY

Percutaneous biopsy has become a common radiologic procedure. Using a variety of imaging modalities, cutting needles provide tissue for histologic evaluation. Aspirating needles provide material for cytopathology and may be used to diagnose the primary tumor, but they are more commonly used to confirm the presence of malignant tissue, especially metastases when the primary tumor has been diagnosed previously.

Needle Selection

Needles ranging from 23 to 14 gauge are frequently used for radiologically guided percutaneous aspiration biopsy. In general, the smaller needles offer greater safety than the larger needles. However, smaller needles less consistently obtain an adequate sample for diagnosis. The specific needle choice should be individualized for each patient, biopsy target and clinical setting. Furthermore, the experience of both the radiologist and the pathologist as well as the guiding modality must also be considered.

Fine 22- or 23-gauge needles achieved popularity in the early experience of radiologically guided percutaneous biopsy. They were used for fluoroscopically guided lung biopsies and then applied to abdominal lesions where CT or ultrasound were used as the guiding modality. Using 22-gauge needles, Wittenberg et al. reported an overall accuracy of 85% in percutaneous biopsy of 150 patients with suspected abdominal tumors.

However, these thin needles are frequently difficult to direct into a small, deep lesion. The 22- and 23-gauge needles take the path of least resistance and often "bow" out of the line of direction during insertion. Thus, greater skill may be required to direct these needles into the target or more passes may have to be made. This can be expected to decrease patient comfort and increase the complication rate.

Medium-size needles, 18–20 gauge, provide larger samples than the 22- or 23-gauge needles. Andriole et al. reported the average weight of the liver biopsy specimen using a variety of needles (Table 22.2). They demonstrated a progressive increase in sample weights as larger needles were used. They also demonstrated that for any given needle size, the more acute angle of the bevel (usually 30°), provided more tissue than needles with a flat 90° bevel.

These medium-size needles are easier to direct into the target which enables the biopsy procedure to be performed more quickly. The larger diameter of the needle

Table 22.2
Size of Biopsy Specimen

Needle	Sample Weight (mg)
22 gauge	4.0
20 gauge	7.6
19 gauge	12.5
18 gauge	16.2
16 gauge	37.3

From Andriole JG, Haaga JR, Adams RB, et al: Biopsy needle characteristics assessed in the laboratory. *Radiology* 148:659–662, 1983.

makes it more apparent under fluoroscopy or ultrasound guidance. When CT is used, these needles are easier to keep within the axial scan plane and this requires fewer images to track the course of the needle. Recently 18- and 20-gauge Percu-cut (E-Z-EM, Westbury, NY) needles have been developed to obtain samples adequate for histology consistently. They consist of a tooth biopsy needle and a spear-tipped stylet.

Cutting needles are often employed when the diagnosis of the primary tumor has not yet been made. The target mass should be large enough that the entire specimen can be obtained from the suspected tumor. Adjacent structures, especially arteries, must be avoided. The most commonly used cutting needles are those with a "slot" or cutting gap into which the sample falls before it is cut off by a sheath. Cutting needles used for percutaneous biopsy are usually 18–14 gauge.

To improve the consistency of biopsy samples, a spring-loaded biopsy gun was developed by Lindgren. A model marketed by Bard (Biopty gun) achieved popularity for ultrasound-directed prostate biopsies. Although designed for use in prostate biopsies, it has been applied to a variety of organs.

Parker et al. recently reported their results using a biopsy gun for 182 percutaneous biopsies from a variety of anatomic sites. They obtained high-quality histopathologic specimens in 177 (97%) of their biopsies. "Crush" artifact and obscuring blood were eliminated and patient discomfort was decreased.

The biopsy gun is designed for an 18-gauge slotted cutting needle. The spring-loaded gun is cocked and the hub of the needle is placed into the gun. The covering panel of the gun is closed and the needle tip advanced into the patient. When released, the spring of the gun moves the needle 2.3 cm further into the patient and then advances the sheath which cuts off the core specimen. Thus, the needle tip must be positioned in front of the target to be sampled. A 1 × 17 mm core of tissue is consistently obtained. The speed of the needle movement seems to lessen patient discomfort.

The biopsy gun is ideal for ultrasound-guided biopsies, however, it can be readily applied to procedures guided by fluoroscopy. The density of the metal device makes CT-directed biopsies more difficult. However, the needle can be passed into the patient and poised in front of the lesion. The gun can then be attached to the needle hub, although some slight adjustment of the needle is usually required.

Adrenal Biopsy

Indications

Adrenal biopsy is indicated when there is the need for more certainty about the nature of an adrenal mass. The combination of the morphologic characteristics of the mass determined by imaging modalities and the clinical setting allow a presumptive diagnosis in many cases. However, situations may arise which require a more definitive diagnosis.

Because the adrenal glands are a frequent site of metastatic disease, they are included in the staging and disease monitoring evaluation for many tumors. An adrenal mass in the presence of other metastatic disease is most likely another metastatic deposit. There is seldom need to provide confirmation as systemic therapy is already required, and other followable disease is present. However, if there is no other evidence of metastases, it may be critically important to know if it is a benign adrenal mass or an adrenal metastasis.

A newly discovered adrenal mass in a patient without an underlying primary tumor also presents a diagnostic problem. Hyperfunctioning adrenal masses, especially pheochromocytoma, should be sought for by serum or urine hormone measurements. However, this does not absolutely exclude a nonfunctioning pheochromocytoma which may be stimulated to secretion by the biopsy. If there is no underlying tumor, an adrenal metastasis is unlikely but could arise from an occult carcinoma. Other morphologic characteristics gained from CT, ultrasound, MRI, or radionuclide examinations may indicate the nature of the mass. However, if a diagnosis cannot be made with a high degree of confidence, percutaneous biopsy may be needed.

The adrenal glands may be involved in a variety of systemic infections which result in unilateral or bilateral adrenal masses. Percutaneous aspiration may be performed to acquire material for diagnostic staining and culture. Biopsy may also be performed to confirm that the adrenal mass is another manifestation of the systemic process.

Technique

Because the adrenal glands are small structures located near the center of the body, percutaneous biopsies are usually directed by CT. However, large lesions, especially those involving the right gland, may be approached with ultrasound guidance.

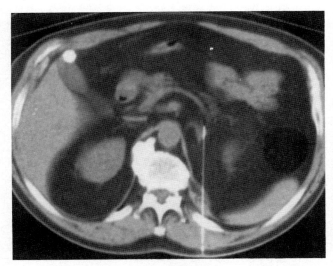

Figure 22.13. Adrenal biopsy. A direct posterior approach was used to biopsy this left adrenal mass. Cytology demonstrated metastatic melanoma.

If possible, a posterior approach should be used. Often a direct path is available which traverses only the posterior muscles and the perinephric fat (Fig. 22.13). Care must be taken, however, to avoid the pleura if possible. This posterior approach results in less respiratory motion than the anterior or transhepatic approaches and should facilitate needle placement.

If lung or pleura lie in the proposed needle path to the adrenal mass, an angled posterior approach may be taken. This requires triangulation to determine the direction of the needle toward the mass (Fig. 22.14). The skin is punctured below the pleura and the needle directed upward into the mass.

On the right side a transhepatic path may be chosen (Fig. 22.15). Although the liver is a vascular structure, bleeding complications are unlikely if the patient has a normal coagulation profile. Transgression of the spleen for adrenal biopsy is not recommended.

Results

Many studies quote low accuracies for percutaneous biopsies of the adrenal glands, but in these studies excretory urograms and ultrasound were often used as guidance modalities. The accuracy of CT-guided sampling of adrenal masses ranges from 90 to 94%. Bernardino reported a series of 58 CT-guided percutaneous adrenal gland biopsies in 53 patients. A correct tissue diagnosis was obtained from the initial biopsy in 83% of patients on lesions ranging from 1.5 to 9 cm in size. Some of the initial insufficient tissue biopsies underwent a second biopsy for an overall diagnostic accuracy of 90.6% when first and second biopsies were combined. In many departments, an immediate preliminary cytopathology report regarding the adequacy of aspirated tissue can be obtained allowing prompt rebiopsy if the initial sample is inadequate.

Complications

Complications of adrenal gland biopsy include pneumothorax (Fig. 22.16) and hemorrhage. If an effort is made to avoid the pleura with angled or transhepatic approaches, the risk of pneumothorax can be greatly reduced.

In Bernardino's series of 58 biopsies, hemorrhage occurred in six patients (12%). Five patients had a fall in hematocrit of three to six points and two required transfusions. There are two reports of hemorrhage leading to death. One was after biopsy of a pheochromocytoma with

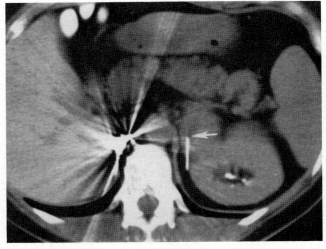

Figure 22.14. Adrenal biopsy. Lung and pleura prevent a direct posterior approach. Triangulation was used to avoid the lung and direct the needle tip (*arrow*) into the left adrenal mass. Note artifact arising from surgical clips from right nephrectomy.

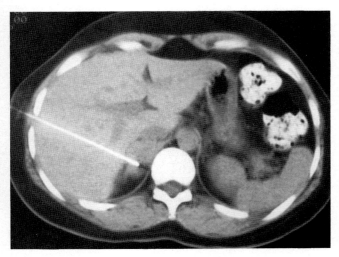

Figure 22.15. Adrenal biopsy. A transhepatic approach may be chosen for right adrenal masses.

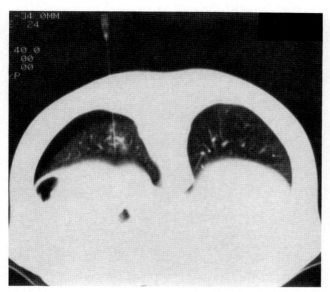

Figure 22.16. Pneumothorax. Small pneumothoraces can easily be detected after CT-directed biopsies. The needle can be seen through the lung during this adrenal biopsy.

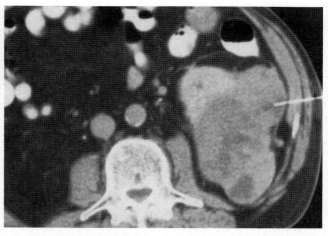

Figure 22.17. Renal biopsy. A large inhomogeneous renal mass is suspicious for adenocarcinoma. This was confirmed by percutaneous biopsy.

hemorrhage and subsequent hypertensive crisis; the other occurred after biopsy of an angiosarcoma.

Renal Biopsy

Indications

Percutaneous renal biopsies may be performed in a variety of clinical settings. A solid renal mass or complicated cystic mass considered suspicious for renal adenocarcinoma is amenable to percutaneous renal biopsy. If the tumor is resectable or can be completely removed via nephrectomy, the surgical procedure is often elected. A biopsy that is positive for malignancy would lead to nephrectomy. A negative biopsy does not exclude renal carcinoma with sufficient confidence to exclude malignancy, so surgery is still needed.

Thus, percutaneous biopsy is seldom performed in this clinical setting unless the patient is a very poor surgical risk.

In patients in whom there is evidence of metastatic disease and nephrectomy would not be performed, a percutaneous biopsy of the renal mass may be used to diagnose the renal malignancy (Figs. 22.17 and 22.18). These patients might then be treated with chemotherapy or receive palliative therapy only.

Metastases to the kidneys are not often seen on imaging studies. However, they are being detected with increasing frequency due to more sensitive examinations, especially CT, and the more aggressive management of oncologic patients.

Patients with an underlying malignancy and a solitary renal mass may have either a second primary tumor (renal adenocarcinoma) or a metastasis to the kidney. Earlier CT literature indicated that although renal metastases were more common than primary renal adenocarcinoma, the masses that were detected radiographically were more likely to be new primary renal adenocarcinomas. This was due to the fact that most metastases to the kidney were small, occurred late in the course of the disease, and were usually found at autopsy. However, more recent work suggests that the sensitivity of CT has improved to the point that a new renal mass is more likely to represent metastatic disease than renal adenocarcinoma. This may also reflect the more frequent use of imaging modalities, such as CT, late in the course of the patient's disease.

Percutaneous renal biopsy is also frequently performed to diagnose a variety of other renal diseases. However, there are many entities that affect the kidney globally and do not require direction of the needle into a mass lesion by an imaging modality. In many institutions ultrasound is used to localize the kidneys and increase the success rate of what would otherwise be a blind biopsy.

Results

The accuracy of a renal biopsy depends on the quality of the sample obtained and the skill of the pathologist looking at the cytologic or histologic preparation. The results also reflect the type of lesion aspirated. Solid tumors, either primary renal adenocarcinomas or metastases, result in a relatively high accuracy. Sarcomas are more difficult to identify on cytologic preparation and histologic preparations are often needed. Inflammatory masses must be interpreted with caution as they may reflect tissue response to either a benign or a malignant stimulus.

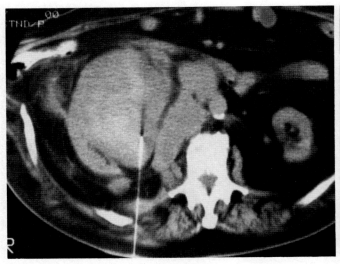

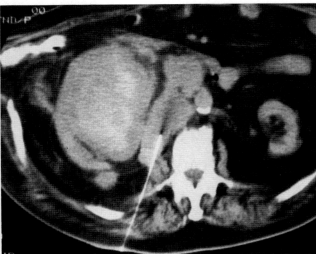

Figure 22.18. Renal biopsy. A renal mass with lymphadeno-pathy was seen on an unenhanced CT scan. Percutaneous bi-opsy was used to (**A**) prove the primary renal malignancy and (**B**) confirm regional lymph node involvement.

Accuracy can be increased by performing several passes rather than relying on a single specimen. Nadel et al. reported an 87% sensitivity in their series of 51 renal biopsies, which increased to 97% after a second biopsy.

Complications

The most common complication of renal biopsy is hemorrhage (Fig. 22.19). If all patients were examined with CT after renal biopsy, it is likely that almost all would have at least a small perirenal hematoma. These subcapsular or perinephric bleeds are seldom clinically significant. Occasionally, however, sufficient blood may be lost to require transfusion. Patients in renal failure or with other clotting deficiencies are more likely to have a significant hemorrhage.

Vascular complications including pseudoaneurysm formation or development of an arteriovenous fistula may also occur. They may be treated with selective arterial catheterization and occlusion. If the specific feeding artery cannot be cannulated, surgery may be elected. These are more common when large cutting needles are used.

Tumor seeding of the needle tract is rare, but has been reported after biopsy of many different tumors. The incidence has decreased further with the use of smaller needles but has been reported after biopsy with a 22-gauge needle.

Retroperitoneal Biopsy

Indications

Indications for percutaneous biopsy of the retroperitoneum are the presence of a mass or adenopathy in a patient with a suspected neoplasm or infection. The most common clinical settings in which retroperitoneal biopsy is needed include:

- Staging a known malignancy
- Diagnosing a primary retroperitoneal tumor
- Distinguishing benign from malignant retroperitoneal lymphadenopathy

Although ultrasound and fluoroscopic guidance have been used, these modalities do not visualize the retroperitoneal abnormalities, adjacent organs, or vessels as well as CT. Needle placement can be guided so precisely

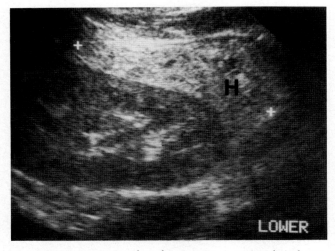

Figure 22.19. Perinephric hematoma. A perinephric hematoma (H) is seen after this ultrasound-directed renal biopsy.

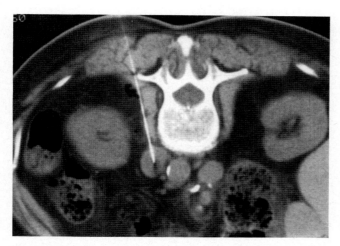

Figure 22.20. Retroperitoneal biopsy. Computed tomography is used to direct a 20-gauge needle into this enlarged paraaortic lymph node.

with CT that even paraaortic and paracaval masses can be safely sampled (Fig. 22.20).

Technique

Retroperitoneal biopsies are generally performed from a posterior approach with the patient lying prone. However, the position and approach must be adjusted depending on location of the mass and its relationship to adjacent organs. Masses between the inferior vena cava and aorta (aortocaval) are usually approached anteriorly.

The size and type of needle depends on the type and location of the lesion to be biopsied. If the mass is in a critical anatomic area, a smaller needle (20–22 gauge) is more appropriate. More tissue will be needed for lymphomas or sarcomas and a larger cutting needle should be used when these tumors are suspected.

For possible metastatic disease from a known primary tumor, an 18- to 22-gauge aspiration needle can be used to obtain a cytologic sample. Whenever possible, and especially for undiagnosed or unknown tumors, a 14- to 18-gauge cutting needle should be used. This is most important if lymphoma is possible since cytologic specimens alone are not adequate for confident diagnosis or subclassification of lymphomas. If adequate tissue is obtained from a cutting needle biopsy, a diagnosis of lymphoma can be confidently made, Hodgkin's lymphoma differentiated from non-Hodgkin's lymphoma, and subclassification of the non-Hodgkin's lymphomas performed. Subclassification of Hodgkin's disease that is based on evaluation of nodal architecture is not possible on percutaneous biopsy specimens, however.

Results

The accuracy of retroperitoneal biopsy varies with the modality used, the size of the needle, and tissue type. When fluoroscopy is used to biopsy tissue later found to be lymphoma, the accuracy is only 40%, but it rises to 94% when CT guidance and 14-gauge cutting needles are used.

Ferrucci reported biopsy of 22 retroperitoneal masses with 22- and 23-gauge aspiration needles, only half of which were with CT guidance. Sixteen malignancies were identified for a success rate of 78%. Of the 11 biopsies with CT guidance, however, 10 were positive for an accuracy rate of 91% even with the small needles. Zornoza noted a success rate of 76% in 25 biopsies of retroperitoneal nodes or masses with five false-negatives. However, only 20- to 22-gauge aspiration needles were used and the guidance modality was not CT.

When CT is used for guidance in the retroperitoneum, accuracies have ranged from 82 to 96%.

Complications

Serious complications from percutaneous biopsy of the retroperitoneum are rare. The major potential complication is hemorrhage. In a combined series of 128 retroperitoneal biopsies there were no complications and no patients required surgery or blood transfusions.

ABSCESS DRAINAGE

Retroperitoneal abscesses are particularly well suited to percutaneous drainage. They can usually be approached posteriorly such that peritoneum, bowel, and other organs are not traversed. In most patients percutaneous drainage results in cure and surgery can be avoided.

Indications

An *abscess* is an abnormal fluid collection that has become infected. To be successfully treated with percutaneous drainage, a retroperitoneal abscess must be well defined and sufficiently liquid that it can drain out a catheter (Fig. 22.21). The wall of the abscess collapses around the draining catheter and residual bacteria are cleared by the patient's white cells and normal immune response in conjunction with an appropriate systemic antibiotic.

A diffuse infection is not amenable to percutaneous drainage and must be treated medically (Fig. 22.22). Most acute infections respond to antibiotic therapy. Chronic or recurrent infections should undergo radiographic evaluation to look for a morphologic abnormality that is pre-

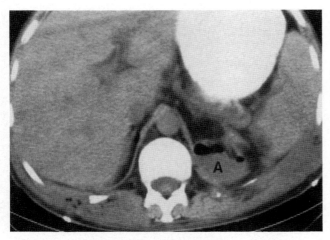

Figure 22.21. Postoperative abscess. An abnormal fluid collection with gas (A) is seen in the left renal bed after nephrectomy.

venting successful medical treatment. Multiple abscesses or diffuse infection that does not respond to antibiotics may be better treated with surgery.

Not all abscesses are appropriate for percutaneous therapy. If the pus and debris are too thick, they may not flow out through the draining catheter. This most commonly occurs when a hematoma becomes infected. Clotted blood will not drain until the hematoma liquifies.

In a rare patient there may not be a good access route. These patients may be better treated with surgery where organs may be displaced rather than traversed by the draining catheter. However, this occurrance is very unlikely in the retroperitoneum where abscesses can be approached posteriorly.

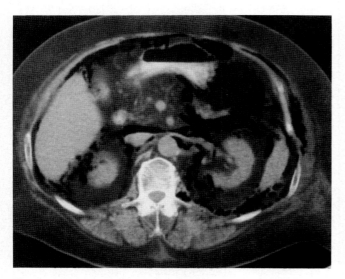

Figure 22.22. Retroperitoneal gas. Gas is seen in retroperitoneum, mesentary and along the chest wall. However, it is not well defined nor does it contain significant fluid and is not amenable to percutaneous drainage.

Occasionally there may be medical contraindications to percutaneous abscess drainage. The most common contraindication to abscess drainage is a bleeding diathesis. Although each case must be individualized, the patient's coagulopathy can often be improved with platelets or fresh frozen plasma so that safe percutaneous drainage can be performed. Furthermore, the surgical option is usually more hazardous in these patients.

Abscesses are usually detected by an enhanced CT examination. Abundant oral contrast is needed to opacify the bowel so that a fluid-filled loop is not confused with an abscess. The drainage route can be determined from the CT delineation of the abscess and adjacent organs.

Ultrasound may also be used to detect or drain a retroperitoneal abscess (Fig. 22.23). It is most often useful in directed examinations where the clinical setting points to a specific location. Ultrasound is also valuable in examining children as ionizing radiation is avoided.

The CT and ultrasound features are not specific for abscess. An abnormal fluid collection may not be infected. Thus, an uninfected hematoma, urinoma (Fig. 22.24), or lymphocyst may have an appearance identical to an abscess. Percutaneous aspiration is indicated to clarify further the nature of these collections.

Technique

In a patient with signs and symptoms of a retroperitoneal abscess, an abnormal fluid collection must be presumed to be an abscess. Percutaneous aspiration is indicated. This should be done with a large needle (18 gauge) which will allow aspiration of the pus. If purulent fluid is found, the track can be dilated using sequential fascial dilators passed over a guidewire. The draining catheter is then placed and the abscess cavity evacuated.

If the fluid collection is not an abscess, the aspirated fluid is usually diagnostic. The most likely etiologies include a urinoma, lymphocyst, hematoma, or seroma.

The route of the aspirating needle determines the track of the draining catheter. Thus, a direct route that transgresses as few anatomic planes as possible is desirable. Pus may track along the catheter and infection of intervening spaces such as the pleura should be avoided.

A posterolateral entrance is usually best for retroperitoneal abscesses. This allows the patient to lie supine without kinking the drainage catheter or causing discomfort.

There are numerous catheters available for abscess drainage. They range from small pigtail or self-retaining catheters to large sump catheters. The choice is a matter of personal preference, but Gobien et al. found that 88% of abdominal abscesses can be successfully drained with a 8 French catheter. A self-retaining catheter helps to prevent inadvertent dislodgement.

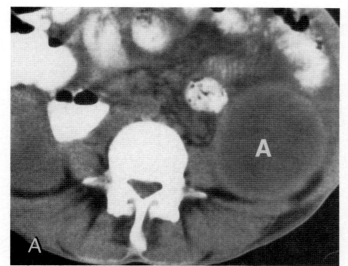

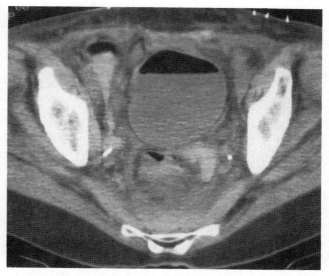

Figure 22.24.   Urinoma. A well-defined fluid collection with gas and a thick wall is indistinguishable from an abscess.

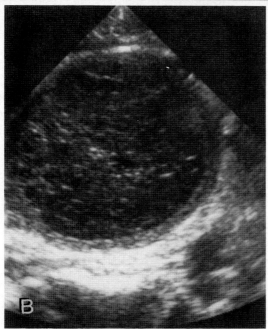

Figure 22.23.   Retroperitoneal abscess. **A**, An abnormal fluid collection (A) is seen on CT. **B**, Ultrasound demonstrates increased through transmission confirming its fluid nature. The multiple internal echoes reflect pus and debris.

Most patients respond to percutaneous abscess drainage within the first 24 to 48 hours. They feel better, defervesce, and the leukocytosis begins to subside. The amount of drainage from the catheter should be monitored daily. If the patient has responded medically the drainage catheter can be removed when output reaches about 5 ml/day. If the patient has not responded, a repeat CT scan should be performed to see if there are other cavities or loculations that are not being drained adequately.

Results

Most patients with a renal, perirenal, pararenal, or retroperitoneal abscess can be cured with percutaneous drainage. Lang reported success in curing 31 of 33 (94%) patients with such abscesses. Patients who are not cured may still benefit from the procedure. The abscess cavity is usually decreased in size and culture of the fluid allows the most effective antibiotics to be selected. Thus, percutaneous drainage may serve as a temporizing procedure to improve the patient's condition and make subsequent surgery less complicated.

The complications of percutaneous abscess drainage include bleeding, spread of infection into a previously uninfected space, and exacerbating bacteremia or sepsis during manipulation. Bleeding is seldom a problem unless the renal parenchyma or hilar vessels have been traversed during puncture. Hilar vessels are easily identified and can usually be avoided when CT is used as the guiding modality. The drainage catheter should provide sufficient tamponade for any vessels punctured within the kidney.

Because infected material may track along the drainage catheter, uninfected spaces should be avoided, if possible. The only major complication reported by Lang was a pyopneumothorax from a catheter that violated the pleural space.

During catheter manipulation, evacuation of the abscess cavity, and subsequent lavage, bacteria may enter the blood stream and create an acute bacteremia or even gram-negative sepsis. This occurred in four patients in Lang's series. During the initial placement of the drainage catheter, care should be taken to minimize manipulations. Pus should be evacuated, but lavage should be withheld for at least 24 hours. During subsequent lavage, the goal is to wash out the cavity gently and prevent adhesions and loculations. Too vigorous a fluid injection will distend the abscess cavity and force bacteria into the bloodstream.

PERCUTANEOUS SUPRAPUBIC CYSTOSTOMY

Percutaneous suprapubic cystostomy is indicated for temporary bladder diversion in patients in whom it is not possible to place a Foley catheter (i.e., acute urethral injury, stricture disease), patients who need continuing temporary bladder diversion but for whom prolonged Foley catheter drainage may be hazardous, and in those who need long-term bladder drainage but are not candidates for other methods of bladder diversion (i.e., patients whose neurologic status precludes the use of clean intermittent self-catheterization).

Blind suprapubic cystostomy has been the method used by urologists for many years. With this technique the lower abdomen is percussed to be certain that the bladder is distended. The skin and soft tissues in the midline 2–3 cm above the symphysis pubis are infiltrated with local anesthetic. An 18- to 20-gauge spinal needle is then inserted straight down until urine is successfully aspirated. A small skin incision is then made adjacent to the spinal needle and a 12 or 14 French mushroom-tipped catheter on a trocar (e.g., Stamey suprapubic catheter, Cook Urological, Spencer, IN) is then advanced parallel to the spinal needle. When urine is aspirated, the catheter is pushed off the trocar. Continued urine drainage confirms its location in the bladder. The catheter is then sutured to the anterior abdominal wall to secure it in place.

Fluoroscopically guided percutaneous suprapubic cystostomy should be used in patients whose pelvic anatomy is distorted, those with a small bladder capacity and by those who feel more comfortable with a guided technique. The bladder is generally filled with dilute contrast material via a Foley catheter, or if this is not possible, via excreted contrast material after intravenous injection. A puncture site is chosen as close to the midline as possible just above the base of the bladder using fluoroscopic guidance. After infiltration with local anesthetic, either a trocar catheter technique or a needle–guidewire technique may be chosen. The Stamey catheter may be utilized, but has a major disadvantage in that it is not radiopaque. If the needle–guidewire technique is selected, the track is dilated to an appropriate size so that a drainage catheter may be placed in the bladder. A locking loop catheter of 10–12 French provides excellent drainage and has the advantage of not requiring skin sutures. If a large-bore catheter is desired, the track can be dilated with an 8- to 10-mm balloon catheter and a 24–26 French peel-away sheath placed. A short-tipped Foley catheter or

a Malecot-tipped catheter can then be placed into the bladder through the sheath to provide long term drainage.

Once the track has formed, catheter replacement on an outpatient basis can be accomplished without the use of fluoroscopy. The needle–guidewire technique may also be used to gain antegrade access to the urethra for urethral stricture dilatation.

URETHROPLASTY

Benign Prostatic Hypertrophy

Dilation of the prostatic urethra is performed to relieve symptoms of bladder outlet obstruction. After preliminary animal and cadaver studies, the technique has been applied to humans with good initial results.

Indications

Balloon dilation of the prostatic urethra may be undertaken in patients in whom a surgical transurethral resection of the prostate (TURP) would otherwise be performed. If early good results and lack of complications are confirmed by further experience, the indications may be relaxed to include only mildly symptomatic patients.

Technique

Retrograde transurethral balloon dilation of the prostatic urethra is performed under fluoroscopic guidance and may be done as an outpatient procedure.

A catheter specifically designed for this technique with a 25 mm dilation balloon is used. After mild sedation and topical anesthesia, the urethroplasty balloon catheter is introduced over a guidewire. The location of the external sphincter must be precisely defined. A retrograde urethrogram is performed for this purpose and the external sphincter is marked with a needle or clamp. The position of the balloon is carefully monitored to avoid damage to the external sphincter. The balloon is then inflated for approximately 10 minutes to dilate the prostatic urethra.

The mechanism of urethroplasty is not completely understood. In humans, the prostatic capsule is quite strong, and it is likely that exhaustion of the elasticity of this capsule is necessary. Tearing or splitting of the prostatic lobes may also contribute to a successful urethral dilatation.

Results

The initial results of transurethral balloon dilation of the prostatic urethra have been excellent. Patients have noted a decrease in frequency of micturation and an improvement in urinary stream.

Castaneda et al. reported successful dilation in four of five patients with benign prostatic hypertrophy. The single failure was in a patient with predominant middle lobe hypertrophy. In these patients, urethral dilation may merely displace the middle lobe which falls back to compress the urethra when the catheter is withdrawn.

Patients experience transient dysuria and hematuria. However, incontinence is avoided if the external sphincter is not damaged.

The reported experience with balloon urethroplasty is still small, however, the results are encouraging. If patients with predominant median lobe hypertrophy are excluded, successful dilatation with clinical improvement can be expected. Because urethroplasty can be performed safely on an outpatient basis, it may be appropriate to use as the first-line therapy for symptomatic patients. If symptoms recur, the procedure may be repeated or surgical resection offered. Further work is needed to confirm the subjective improvement reported in these early studies as objective urodynamic parameters have not yet documented significant changes after balloon urethroplasty.

Urethral Strictures

Most urethral strictures are the result of either trauma or inflammation. Congenital urethral strictures are rare.

Traditionally urethral strictures have been treated with bougies, filiforms, or sounds. The strictures often recurred and repeated dilations were required. Furthermore, the shearing force created by dilation with a fixed, rigid instrument often denuded the mucosa and subjected the urethra to further injury from bleeding, infection or the creation of false passages.

Angioplasty balloon catheters have been adapted for use in the ureter and may also be applied to the urethra. The guidewire that is used to cross even tight strictures usually also allows placement of the balloon dilation catheter. If the stricture cannot be passed in a retrograde manner, suprapubic catheterization with an antegrade approach may succeed. Because radial force is created by the dilating balloon, the strictures can be "overdilated" with little risk to the urethra.

It is too early to determine how often or how quickly these strictures recur after balloon dilation. However, early reports are encouraging. Furthermore, redilation with balloon catheters under fluoroscopic guidance should be less traumatic to the urethra than traditional dilation methods.

SUGGESTED READINGS

Percutaneous Nephrostomy

Dunnick NR, Illescas FF, Mitchell S, et al: Interventional uroradiology. *Invest Radiol* 24:831, 1989.

Hopper KD, Yakes WF: The posterior intercostal approach for percutaneous renal procedures: risk of puncturing the lung, spleen, and liver as determined by CT. *AJR* 154:115, 1990.

Kay KW, Reinke DB: Detailed caliceal anatomy for endourology. *J Urol* 132:1085, 1984.

Matalon TAS, Silver B: US guidance of interventional procedures. *Radiology* 174:43, 1990.

Pfister RC: Percutaneous nephrostomy. In Lang EK (ed): *Percutaneous and Interventional Urology and Radiology*. Berlin, Springer Verlag, 1986, pp. 1–28.

Sherman JL, Hopper KD, Greene AJ, et al: The retrorenal colon on computed tomography: a normal variant. *J Comput Assist Tomogr* 9(2):339, 1985.

Seldinger, SI: Catheter replacement of needle in percutaneous arteriography: new technique. *Acta Radiol* (STOCKH) 39:368, 1953.

Silverman SG, Mueller P, Pfister RC: Hemostatic evaluation before abdominal interventions: an overview and proposal. *AJR* 154:233, 1990.

Spies JB, Rosen RJ, Liebowitz AS: Antibiotic prophylaxis in vascular and interventional radiology: a rational approach. *Radiology* 166:381, 1988.

Stables DP, Ginsberg NJ, Johnson ML: Percutaneous nephrostomy: a series and review of the literature. *AJR* 130:75, 1978.

Stanley P, Bear JW, Reid BS: Percutaneous nephrostomy in infants and children. *AJR* 141:473, 1983.

Winfield WC, Kirchner SG, Brun ME, et al: Percutaneous nephrostomy in neonates, infants and children. *Radiology* 151:617, 1984.

Ureteral Intervention

Banner MP, Pollack HM, Ring EJ, et al: Catheter dilatation of benign ureteral strictures. *Radiology* 147:427, 1983.

Ball WS Jr, Towbin R, Strife JL, Spencer R: Interventional genitourinary radiology in children: a review of 61 procedures. *AJR* 147:791, 1986.

Beckmann CF, Roth RA, Bihrle W III: Dilation of benign ureteral strictures. *Radiology* 172:437, 1989.

Johnson CD, Oke EJ, Dunnick NR, et al: Percutaneous balloon dilatation of ureteral strictures. *AJR* 148:181, 1987.

Lang EK, Glorioso LW III: Antegrade transluminal dilatation of benign ureteral strictures: long-term results. *AJR* 150:131, 1988.

Maillet PJ, Pelle-Francoz D, Leriche A, et al: Fistulas of the upper urinary tract: percutaneous management. *J Urol* 138:1382, 1987.

Mitty HA, Train JS, Dan SJ: Antegrade ureteral stenting in the management of fistulas, strictures and calculi. *Radiology* 149:433, 1983.

Papanicolaou N, Pfister RC, Yoder IC: Interventional uroradiology: percutaneous occlusion of ureteral leaks and fistulae using nondetachable balloons. *Urol Radiol* 7:28, 1985.

Percutaneous Biopsy

Andriole JG, Haaga JR, Adams RB, et al: Biopsy needle characteristics assessed in the laboratory. *Radiology* 148:659, 1984.

Bernardino ME, Walther MM, Phillips VM, et al: CT-guided adrenal biopsy: accuracy, safety and indications. *AJR* 144:67, 1985.

Bret PM, Fond A, Casola G, et al: Abdominal lesions: a prospective study of clinical efficacy of percutaneous fine-needle biopsy. *Radiology* 159:345, 1986.

Casola G, Nicolet V, vanSonnenberg E, et al: Unsuspected pheochromocytoma: risk of blood-pressure alterations during percutaneous adrenal biopsy. *Radiology* 159:733, 1986.

Casola G, vanSonnenberg E, Keightley A, et al: Pneumothorax: radiologic treatment with small catheters. *Radiology* 166:89, 1988.

Charboneau JW, Reading CC, Welch TJ: CT and sonographically guided needle biopsy: current techniques and new innovations. *AJR* 154:1, 1990.

Ferrucci J, Wittenberg J, Mueller P, et al: Diagnosis of abdominal malignancy by radiologic fine-needle aspiration biopsy. *AJR* 134:323, 1980.

Haaga JR, LiPuma JP, Bryan PJ, et al: Clinical comparison of small- and large-caliber cutting needles for biopsy. *Radiology* 146:665, 1983.

Jeffrey RB: Coaxial technique for CT-guided biopsy of deep retroperitoneal lymph node. *Gastrointest Radiol* 13:271, 1988.

Kaufman RA: Technical aspects of abdominal CT in infants and children. *AJR* 153:549, 1989.

Koenker RM, Mueller PR, vanSonnenberg E: Interventional radiology of the adrenal glands. *Semin Roentgenol* 22(4):314, 1988.

Matalon TS, Silver B: US guidance of interventional procedures. *Radiology* 174:43, 1990.

Mostbeck GH, Wittich GR, Derfler K, et al: Optimal needle size for renal biopsy: in vitro and in vivo evaluation. *Radiology* 173:819, 1989.

Nadel L, Baumgartner BR, Bernardino ME: Percutaneous renal biopsies: accuracy, safety and indications. *Urol Radiol* 8:67, 1986.

Parker SH, Hooper KD, Yakes WF, et al: Image-directed percutaneous biopsies with a biopsy gun. *Radiology* 171:663, 1989.

Welch TJ, Sheedy PF, Johnson CD, et al: CT-guided biopsy: prospective analysis of 1,000 procedures. *Radiology* 171:493, 1989.

Whitney W, Dunnick NR: Biopsy techniques in uroradiology. *Radiol Report* 2:302, 1990.

Wittenberg J, Mueller PR, Ferrucci JT Jr, et al: Percutaneous core biopsy of abdominal tumor using 22 gauge needle: further observations. *AJR* 139:75, 1982.

Yankaskas BC, Staab EV, Craven MB, et al: Delayed complications from fine-needle biopsies of solid masses of the abdomen. *Invest Radiol* 21(4):325, 1986.

Zornoza J, Wallace S, Goldstein HM, et al: Transperitoneal percutaneous retroperitoneal lymph node aspiration biopsy. *Radiology* 122:111, 1977.

Abscess Drainage

Butch RJ, Mueller PR, Ferrucci JT Jr, et al: Drainage of pelvic abscesses through the greater sciatic foramen. *Radiology* 158:487, 1986.

Cronan JJ, Amis ES Jr, Dorfman GS: Percutaneous drainage of renal abscesses. *AJR* 142:351, 1984.

Cronan JJ, Horn DL, Marcello A, et al: Antibiotics and nephrostomy tube care: preliminary observations. *Radiology* 172:1043, 1989.

Deyoe LA, Cronan JJ, Lambiase RE, Dorfman GS: Percutaneous drainage of renal and perirenal abscesses: results in 30 patients. *AJR* 155:81, 1990.

Glass CA, Cohn I Jr: Drainage of intra-abdominal abscesses: a comparison of surgical and computerized tomography guided catheter drainage. *Am J Surg* 147:315, 1984.

Gobien RP, Stanley JH, Schabel SI, et al: The effect of drainage tube size on adequacy of percutaneous abscess drainage. *Cardiovasc Intervent Radiol* 8:100, 1985.

Lang EK: Renal, perirenal and pararenal abscesses: percutaneous drainage. *Radiology* 174:109, 1990.

Mueller PR, White EM, Glass-Royal M, et al: Infected abdominal tumors: percutaneous catheter drainage. *Radiology* 173:627, 1989.

vanSonnenberg E, Wing VW, Casola G, et al: Temporizing effect of percutaneous drainage of complicated abscesses in critically ill patients. *AJR* 142:821, 1984.

Yoder IC, Pfister RC, Lindors KK, et al: Pyonephrosis: imaging and intervention. *AJR* 141:735, 1983.

Gordon RL, Banner MP, Pollack HM: Selected endourologic techniques. *Radiol Clin North Am* 24:633, 1986.

Urethroplasty

Castaneda F, Hulbert JC, Letourneau JG, et al: Perineal abscess after prostatic urethroplasty with balloon catheter: report of a case. *Radiology* 174:49, 1990.

Castaneda F, Isorna S, Hulbert JC, et al: The importance of separation of prostatic lobes in relief of prostatic obstruction by balloon catheter urethroplasty: studies in dogs and humans. *AJR* 153:1301, 1989.

Castaneda F, Reddy P, Wasserman N, et al: Benign prostatic hypertrophy: retrograde transurethral dilation of the prostatic urethra in humans. *Radiology* 163:649, 1987.

Goldenberg SL, Perez-Marrero RA, Lee LM, Emerson L: Endoscopic balloon dilation of the prostate: early experience. *J Urol* 144:83, 1990.

Mohammed SH, Wirima J: Balloon catheter dilatation of urethral strictures. *AJR* 150:327, 1988.

Quinn SF, Dyer R, Smathers R, et al: Balloon dilatation of the prostatic urethra. *Radiology* 157:57, 1985.

Percutaneous Suprapubic Cystostomy

Papanicolaou N, Pfister RC, Nocks BN: Percutaneous, large-bore, suprapubic cystostomy: technique and results. *AJR* 152:303, 1989.

INDEX

Page numbers in *italics* denote figures; those followed by "t" denote tables.